CLINICAL PSYCHOMOTOR SKILLS

Ninth edition

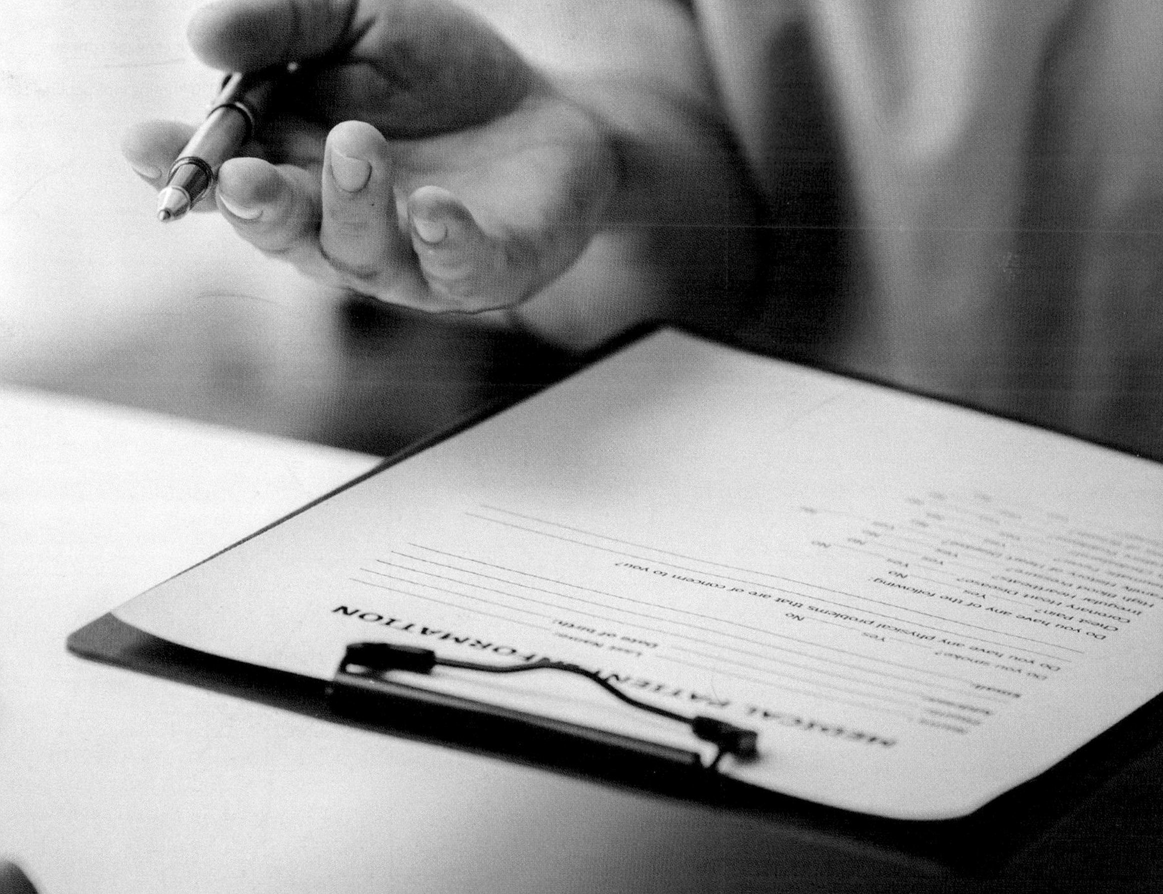

HEALTH + NURSING SERIES

JOANNE TOLLEFSON • ELSPETH HILLMAN

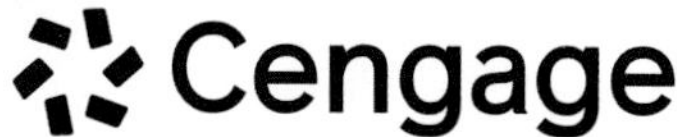

Clinical Psychomotor Skills: Assessment Tools for Nurses
9th Edition
Joanne Tollefson
Elspeth Hillman

Senior Product manager: Michelle Aarons
Content developer: Caitlin Bush/Mickayla Borthwick
Associate Content project manager: Ananya Sarkar
Text designer: Cengage Creative Studio
Cover designer: Cengage Creative Studio
Project designer: Nikita Bansal
Editor: Anne Mulvaney
Proofreader: Sylvia Marson
Permissions/Photo researcher: Lumina Datamatics
Cover: Daenin/stock.adobe.com
Typeset by KGL

Any URLs contained in this publication were checked for currency during the production process. Note, however, that the publisher cannot vouch for the ongoing currency of URLs.

Eighth edition published in 2022

For product information and technology assistance,
in Australia call **1300 790 853;**
in New Zealand call **0800 449 725**

For permission to use material from this text or product, please email
aust.permissions@cengage.com

National Library of Australia Cataloguing-in-Publication Data
ISBN: 9780170477413
A catalogue record for this book is available from the National Library of Australia

Cengage Learning Australia
Level 7, 80 Dorcas Street
South Melbourne, Victoria Australia 3205

For learning solutions, visit **cengage.com.au**

Printed in China by 1010 Printing International Limited.
1 2 3 4 5 6 7 27 26 25 24 23

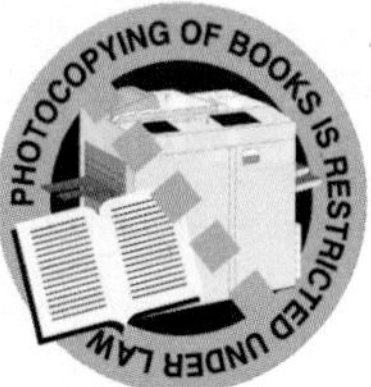

CONTENTS

Guide to the text v
Guide to the online resources ix
New to this edition x
About the authors xi
Acknowledgements xi

PART 1

INTRODUCTION 1

1 Psychomotor skills 2
2 Clinical thinking 6
3 Person-centred practice 10
4 Professional communication 13

PART 2

ASEPTIC NON TOUCH TECHNIQUE 17

5 Hand hygiene 18
6 Personal protective equipment 24
7 Aseptic Non Touch Technique 31
8 Aseptic/clinical hand hygiene 37
9 Surgical gowning and gloving 42

PART 3

ASSESSMENT 47

10 Temperature, pulse and respiration measurement 48
11 Blood pressure measurement 56
12 Pulse oximetry – measuring oxygen saturation 62
13 Pain assessment 67
14 Blood glucose measurement 72
15 Physical assessment 78
16 Mental status assessment 85
17 Focused cardiovascular health history and physical assessment 90
18 12-lead electrocardiogram 96
19 Focused respiratory health history and physical assessment 101
20 Focused neurological health history and physical assessment 109
21 Neurovascular observations 116
22 Focused gastrointestinal health history and abdominal physical assessment 121
23 Height, weight and waist circumference measurements 126
24 Focused musculoskeletal health history and physical assessment and range of motion exercises 132

PART 4

PROFESSIONAL COMMUNICATION 146

25 Clinical handover 147
26 Documentation 152
27 Healthcare teaching 157

PART 5

ASSISTING WITH FLUID AND NUTRITIONAL STATUS 165

28 Assisting with meals 166
29 Nasogastric tube insertion 171
30 Administering enteral nutrition 177
31 Intravenous therapy – assisting with establishment 185
32 Intravenous therapy – management 192

PART 6

ASSISTING WITH ELIMINATION 201

33 Assisting with elimination needs 202
34 Administering an enema 209
35 Suprapubic catheter care – catheter irrigation 215
36 Urinary catheterisation 221

PART 7

MEDICATION ADMINISTRATION 231

37 Oral medication 232
38 Enteral medication 241
39 Topical medication 247
40 Optic medication 254
41 Otic medication 260
42 Vaginal medication 265
43 Rectal medication 271
44 Inhaled medication 278
45 Parenteral medication 285
46 Intravenous medication administration – volume-controlled infusion set 295
47 Intravenous medication administration – intravenous container 301
48 Intravenous medication administration – bolus 306

PART 8

PAIN MANAGEMENT 319

49 Non-pharmacological pain management intervention – dry heat and cold therapy 320
50 Patient-controlled analgesia and other syringe-driven medication 324
51 Subcutaneous infusions 333

PART 9
PERIOPERATIVE CARE 340
52 Preoperative care 341
53 Post-anaesthesia care and handover 349
54 Postoperative care 357

PART 10
ASSISTING WITH PERSONAL HYGIENE, SKIN INTEGRITY AND MOBILISING 368
55 Bed bath or assisted shower 369
56 Oral care, hair care, nail care and shaving 375
57 Assisting a person to reposition 381
58 Assisting a person to mobilise 387
59 Pressure area care – preventing pressure injuries 392

PART 11
RESPIRATORY SKILLS 402
60 Oxygen therapy via nasal cannula or various masks 403
61 Oropharyngeal and nasopharyngeal suctioning 411
62 Artificial airway suctioning 417
63 Tracheostomy care 426
64 Chest drainage system assessment and management 435

PART 12
TRANSFUSION AND BLOOD PRODUCTS 441
65 Blood transfusion 442
66 Venipuncture 449

PART 13
WOUND MANAGEMENT 457
67 Dry dressing technique 458
68 Complex wounds: drain care and suture, staple or clip removal 464
69 Complex wounds: wound irrigation 471
70 Complex wounds: filling a wound; Negative Pressure Wound Therapy 477

PART 14 (ALL ONLINE)
ADVANCED SKILLS
71 Caring for a person with a central venous access device
72 Assisting with stoma care
73 Seclusion management
74 Electroconvulsive therapy care
75 Non-pharmacological pain management interventions – therapeutic massage
76 Non-pharmacological pain management interventions – conventional transcutaneous electrical nerve stimulation
77 Infant – daily care
78 Caring for a person who is unconscious
79 Continuous bladder irrigation
80 Continuous abdominal peritoneal dialysis

Appendix A: NMBA *Registered Nurse Standards for Practice* 2016 487
Appendix B: NMBA decision-making framework summary 495
Index 496

Guide to the text

As you read this text you will find a number of features in every chapter to enhance your study of clinical skills and help you understand how the theory is applied in the real world.

PART OPENING FEATURES

Refer to the **Chapter list** for an outline of the chapters in each part.

PART 2

ASEPTIC NON TOUCH TECHNIQUE

5 HAND HYGIENE
6 PERSONAL PROTECTIVE EQUIPMENT
7 ASEPTIC NON TOUCH TECHNIQUE
8 ASEPTIC/CLINICAL HAND HYGIENE
9 SURGICAL GOWNING AND GLOVING

Note: These notes are summaries of the most important points in the assessments/procedures and are not exhaustive on the subject. References of the materials used to compile the information have been supplied. The student is expected to have learnt the material surrounding each skill as presented in the references. No single reference is complete on each subject.

CHAPTER OPENING FEATURES

Indications sections identify the clinical reasons to perform the skill outlined in the chapter.

CHAPTER 6

PERSONAL PROTECTIVE EQUIPMENT

INDICATIONS

Personal protective equipment (PPE) is anything used or worn to minimise health or safety risks, including face masks, goggles, gloves and aprons. PPE is worn to prevent microorganism transmission (e.g. SARS-CoV-2) from a reservoir to a susceptible host, such as from healthcare workers to recipients of care or family and friends, and vice versa. PPE also prevents spray or splash injuries from chemicals and hazardous medications. PPE is an integral component of standard and transmission-based precautions in healthcare facilities. Preventable healthcare-associated infections (HCAIs) increase a person's pain; may result in lifelong disabilities or death; extend length of stays, reducing available bed access; and increase health systems' economic burden (Australian Commission on Safety and Quality in Health Care [ACSQHC], 2021; Magtoto, 2023; National Health and Medical Research Council [NHMRC], 2019). Preventing and controlling HCAIs is Standard 3 of the *National Safety and Quality Health Service Standards,* aiming to stop people from acquiring preventable HCAIs and to effectively manage these infections using evidence-based strategies (ACSQHC, 2021).

Using PPE singly or in combination interrupts transmission of contaminated material, contamination of sterile materials (e.g. when preparing medications, intravenous fluids) and exposure of mucous membranes, eyes, broken skin, or clothing to another person's bodily secretions, blood, excretions or hazardous substances. You need a sound understanding of the modes of microorganism transmission for effective infection prevention and control measures. Additionally, you need to be aware of the occupational requirements for safe handling of hazardous medications and chemicals. Your decision to use PPE should be based on an assessment of risks associated with the person and the care activity you are undertaking, or the potential for contamination from microorganisms or hazardous chemicals.

FEATURES WITHIN CHAPTERS

Gather equipment tables list and explain each item of equipment you will need to perform the clinical skill.

GATHER EQUIPMENT

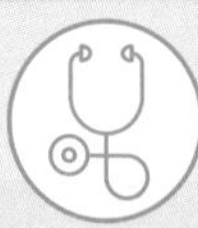

The equipment required depends on the procedure and the facility's procedural guidelines. Planning the procedure and having all equipment ready for use beforehand are part of an effective time-management strategy and reduce the amount of time that the critical aseptic field will be exposed to the air. A critical aseptic field left unattended is considered to be contaminated.

EQUIPMENT	EXPLANATION
A trolley	• Collect and clean with the facility's recommended solution to establish a clean (not sterile) work surface • Removing much of the microbial load from the trolley surfaces helps to prevent cross-contamination
Dressing equipment	• Gather dressing equipment while the trolley dries, to save time and eliminate microorganism transfer via moisture • Place the dressing pack on the top shelf and all other unopened plastic-, paper- and cloth-wrapped items and required personal protective equipment on the trolley's bottom shelf, leaving the top surface as clean as possible for the aseptic procedure (Peters, 2017)
A plastic bag	• Attach a plastic bag large enough to collect used materials to the side of the trolley closest to the person, which avoids contaminated material being brought over the critical aseptic field • Open the mouth of the bag wide enough so that material can easily be dropped into the bag, preventing contamination of forceps or gloves

NEW **The person living with severe obesity** boxes highlight where there is a specific focus on the patient with severe obesity.

THE PERSON LIVING WITH SEVERE OBESITY

NEW

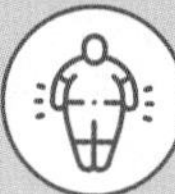

It is difficult to obtain an accurate BP reading on someone who is severely obese (see **Clinical Skills 15 and 23** for brief discussions of people living with severe obesity). The circumference of their upper arms often precludes the use of even the largest cuffs, and even large cuffs cannot accommodate the cone shape of the limb (Eley et al., 2019). The thick layer of tissue between the cuff/stethoscope and the artery muffle the pulse and make registering a BP difficult (Eley et al., 2019). As well, severely obese people usually have hypertension (due to increased circulating blood volume needed to oxygenate the excess tissue, plus increase in some hormones and possible kidney damage). You will need to obtain a sufficiently large conical-shaped cuff (a bariatric cuff – usually from central supply) and a Doppler to hear the pulse, or use an automated BP machine with a bariatric cuff, which is preferable.

NEW **Elder care** boxes highlight where there is a specific focus on the elderly.

ELDER CARE

NEW

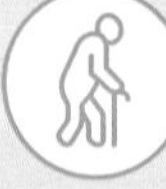

Knowing the baseline BP of elderly people is important in assessing their current BP. Their normal systolic readings may be high due to reduced compliance of the arteries and a 'normal' reading might then indicate shock (Mattu et al., 2016).

Arterial stiffness is associated with a widening pulse pressure (systolic BP minus diastolic BP). This, in turn, is associated with increased frailty, decreased functioning (Chuang et al., 2022) and increased sarcopenia (Rong et al., 2020). Sarcopenia is a decline in skeletal muscle mass and strength. Target systolic BP for those over 65 years is less than 130 mmHg with no recommendations made for a target diastolic BP (Flack & Adekola, 2020).

Hypertension is associated with ageing, with 79 per cent of those over 80 years old affected. Hypertension is asymptomatic, but has devastating effects on the cardiovascular, renal and neurological systems over time (Siedlinski et al., 2023).

Hypotension has also been linked to increased mortality in the elderly (Yamaguchi et al., 2023). Postural (also called orthostatic) hypotension is a significant contributor to falls in the elderly (Jones et al., 2023). Kubota et al. (2022) demonstrated the effectiveness of drinking cold/carbonated water in raising the BP in someone with postural hypotension in addition to repositioning.

If...Then boxes present a common challenge you may face when performing a clinical skill and examining how this can be overcome.

> If the person has poor perfusion or a low-quality signal message is displayed, the oximeter probe needs to be moved to another site to obtain the best signal and most accurate reading (Pretto et al., 2014).

Chapter linkages refer you back to important foundational skills and highlight the connection between similar tasks, procedures and skills.

Aseptic/clinical hand hygiene
Wash hands thoroughly using the facility's antimicrobial soap for one minute using the technique outlined for routine/social hand hygiene in **Clinical Skill 5**. A reduction of transient and resident flora is effectively accomplished with an antiseptic liquid soap preparation (ACSQHC, 2021). Rinse carefully.

Do not touch taps with clean hands. Avoid contaminating your hand by using paper towels to turn taps off if elbow or foot controls are unavailable.

ICONS

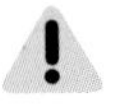
Safety

Safety icons indicate when you should be aware of a particular safety issue when performing a clinical skill.

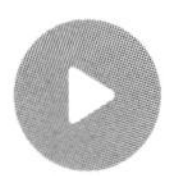
Video

Video icons direct you online where you can find a suite of videos that take you through each skill, step-by-step.

LOOK
LISTEN
FEEL
SMELL

Look, Listen, Feel, Smell icons are a call to action for you to reflect and apply the skill knowledge you have learned.

END-OF-CHAPTER FEATURES

At the end of each chapter you'll find a **clinical skills assessment table** for you to review, practise and record your growing competency for each clinical skill.

- The key **performance criteria** for an entire skill are listed, not just a task or procedure, and the relevant **NMBA National Competency Standards** are included.
- There is space for students and clinical facilitators to record your performance and progress using the **five-point scale** – Dependent (1), Marginal (2), Assisted (3), Supervised (4), Independent (5).
- **Signature section** for students and clinical facilitators to record assessment.

CLINICAL SKILLS ASSESSMENT

Personal protective equipment

Demonstrates the ability to assess and select appropriate personal protective equipment (PPE) for risks associated with the procedure or care activity and utilises PPE to prevent transmission of microorganisms transmitted by contact, droplet or airborne modes, or to prevent injury from hazardous medications or chemicals. Incorporates the *National Safety and Quality Health Service Standards*: 2 Partnering with Consumers, 3 Preventing and Controlling Healthcare-Associated Infection, 5 Comprehensive Care, 6 Communicating for Safety, and 8 Recognising and Responding to Acute Deterioration (ACSQHC, 2021).

Performance criteria	1	2	3	4	5
(Numbers indicate NMBA *Registered Nurse Standards for Practice*)	(Dependent)	(Marginal)	(Assisted)	(Supervised)	(Independent)
1. Identifies the indication (1.1, 1.4, 3.5)	☐	☐	☐	☐	☐
2. Evidence of therapeutic interaction with the person, carers or visitors (1.2, 2.1, 2.2, 2.9, 6.1)	☐	☐	☐	☐	☐
3. Demonstrates clinical reasoning abilities, such as risk assessment and obtaining PPE prior to performing hand hygiene (1.1, 1.4)	☐	☐	☐	☐	☐
4. Identifies and gathers appropriate PPE (1.1, 1.2, 1.4): ■ plastic apron ■ gowns ■ long-sleeved gown (full body gown) ■ sterile gown ■ goggles and safety glasses ■ surgical masks ■ face shield ■ P2 respirator (N95) ■ non-sterile gloves ■ sterile gloves ■ synthetic gloves, e.g. nitrile or polyvinyl chloride (PVC) ■ sharps container	☐	☐	☐	☐	☐
5. Performs hand hygiene (1.1, 6.1)	☐	☐	☐	☐	☐
6. Safely and effectively puts on, uses and removes PPE (6.1)	☐	☐	☐	☐	☐
7. Cleans, replaces and disposes of equipment appropriately (1.1, 3.6, 6.1)	☐	☐	☐	☐	☐
8. Demonstrates the ability to link theory to practice (1.1, 3.3, 3.4, 3.5)	☐	☐	☐	☐	☐

Student:

Clinical facilitator: Date:

Guide to the online resources

FOR THE INSTRUCTOR

Cengage Learning is pleased to provide you with a selection of resources that will help you prepare your lectures and assessments when you choose this textbook for your course. Log in or request an account to access instructor resources at au.cengage.com/instructor/account for Australia or nz.cengage.com/instructor/account for New Zealand.

INSTRUCTOR'S MANUAL

The Instructor's Manual includes:

- Simple task-oriented questions to test student preparedness
- Higher level critical thinking questions for further discussion

CASE STUDIES

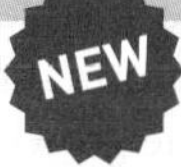

NEW case studies which demonstrate how clinical psychomotor skills are applied in a specific scenario.

CLINICAL SKILLS VIDEOS

These videos provide relevant and engaging visual teaching demonstrations allowing instructors to illustrate in class the clinical skills covered in the new 9th edition of Clinical Psychomotor Skills. These visual resources are available to instructors prescribing the text.

COGNERO® TEST BANK

A **bank of questions** has been developed in conjunction with the text for creating quizzes, tests and exams for your students. Create multiple test versions in an instant and deliver tests from your LMS, your classroom, or wherever you want using **Cognero**. Cognero test generator is a flexible online system that allows you to import, edit, and manipulate content from the text's test bank or elsewhere, including your own favourite test questions.

CLINICAL SKILLS ASSESSMENT TABLES

Add the 5-point and 3-point clinical skills assessment tables into your course management system, use them in student handouts, or copy them into your lecture presentations.

ARTWORK FROM THE TEXT

Add the digital files of graphs, tables, pictures and flow charts into your course management system, use them in student handouts, or copy them into your lecture presentations.

FOR THE STUDENT

ONLINE STUDY TOOLS

Resources on the Student Website are included with this text. This collection of bonus online tools includes clinical skills assessment tables and online advanced skills chapters.

Access the resources at https://au.cengage.com/

NEW TO THIS EDITION

The Nursing and Midwifery Board of Australia's *Registered Nurse Standards for Practice* (2016) are again used in this edition to underpin skills development and to reflect the progression of thinking within the nursing profession. Assessment incorporates the National Safety and Quality Health Service Standards as applicable to each skill. Many of the skills have been restructured to make content clearer and easier to navigate.

People who are severely obese are becoming an ever-growing part of nursing practice, and to acknowledge their requirements, more brief discussions of 'People living with severe obesity' have been added to relevant skills. The wording around the information about obesity has been altered to reflect the growing concerns about respectful and sensitive discussion of this topic.

Many of the skills have additional information on 'Elder care', where information or precautions specific to older people are highlighted.

The boxed feature 'If … then', which highlights to students common challenges, scenarios or clinical questions that might arise throughout their practice, and then provides practical solutions for how to deal with these challenges, has again been used and expanded where necessary.

To assist students to develop a structured holistic assessment approach, many of the assessments (where applicable) are presented in the LOOK, LISTEN, SMELL and FEEL format, with specific parameters listed under these headings.

As always, nursing and associated literature was consulted to ensure that the information is as current as possible. Available evidence-based information has been included in this edition. The information that forms the theory underlying the skills in this book comes from a number of sources. Nursing fundamentals texts were used as a base, and searches of various databases found recent, research-based material to make the information as current as possible. This edition includes evidence-based material published between 2020 and the time this book went to print. The databases searched were CINAHL, Medline, Cochrane Library, Joanna Briggs Institute and ProQuest 5000 as well as Google Scholar. Government, medical and health-related websites were accessed for recent evidence-based information as well. This edition has incorporated information from Joanna Briggs Institute (2021–24) evidence-based summaries and clinician information.

Adjustments to some of the skills were made using the recommendations of clinicians and clinical facilitators, students and preceptors, who have kindly critiqued the skills and sent their comments to us. Professionals who reviewed content for specific skills are acknowledged.

ABOUT THE AUTHORS

Joanne Tollefson (RN, BGS, MSc, PhD) was Senior Lecturer in the School of Nursing Sciences at James Cook University. She is a registered nurse with many years of clinical experience in several countries and extensive experience in nursing education at both the hospital and tertiary levels. Her research interests include competency-based education and clinical assessment, development of reflective practitioners for a changing work environment, chronic pain and arbovirus disease in the tropics. She is a two-time recipient of the National Awards for Outstanding Contributions to Student Learning (Carrick Award, 2007 and Australian Teaching and Learning Council Award, 2008). Since retirement, she has maintained an interest in nursing through researching, writing and editing nursing textbooks.

Elspeth Hillman (RN, BN, MN) is a lecturer and Academic Lead: Professional Practice in nursing at James Cook University, with an interest in nursing education research. She has extensive experience in several Australian states in a range of clinical situations from rural to critical care nursing. Her experience includes facilitation of both undergraduate nursing students in various clinical facilities, and of postgraduate nursing students in high-dependency units.

ACKNOWLEDGEMENTS

The publisher would like to thank the following reviewers for their incisive and helpful comments:

- Kelli Wain, Victoria University
- Karen Missen, Federation University
- Elyse Coffey, Deakin University
- Martina Costello, Edith Cowan University
- Bianca Viljoen, University of Southern Queensland
- Tamara Page, University of Adelaide
- Jan Alderman, University of Adelaide
- Carol Crevacore, Edith Cowan University
- Danny Sidwell, University of Tasmania – Hobart
- Meg Pollock, Deakin University

PART 1

INTRODUCTION

1 PSYCHOMOTOR SKILLS

2 CLINICAL THINKING

3 PERSON-CENTRED PRACTICE

4 PROFESSIONAL COMMUNICATION

Note: These notes are summaries of the most important points in the assessments/procedures and are not exhaustive on the subject. References of the materials used to compile the information have been supplied. The student is expected to have learnt the material surrounding each skill as presented in the references. No single reference is complete on each subject.

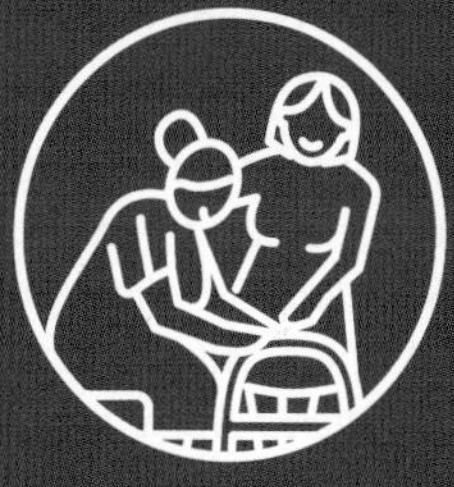

CHAPTER 1

PSYCHOMOTOR SKILLS

Fundamental nursing care is at the core of the nursing profession and thus critical to the practice of nursing (Mudd et al., 2020). Caring for a person's basic needs (nutrition, hydration, elimination, hygiene, mobility, safety and medication management) are each addressed in this text, as well as assessment skills and many of the more technically advanced skills you will need as you progress through your course.

Psychomotor skills are those that require an integration of motor dexterity, related knowledge, values, and in the case of nursing, orientation towards and inclusion of the person in care. Psychomotor skills require practice to master and are developed over time, initially with a concentrated effort on coordinating movement and reflexes along with incorporating appropriate interpersonal skills. As you develop skills in nursing, you will be expected to meet the standards of care that have been set by the Nursing and Midwifery Board of Australia (NMBA) – the chief nursing body in Australia. These standards are the basis for the nursing course you are undertaking, which meets the Australian Nursing and Midwifery Accreditation Competencies (ANMAC, 2019) that deal with such nursing education criteria as course content, amount and type of clinical placement, English proficiency and student progression.

NURSING STANDARDS

In 1990, the nursing bodies in Australia developed the Australian Nursing and Midwifery Council (ANMC) *National Competency Standards for the Registered Nurse* as the minimum requirements for registration as a nurse. The concept of competency was later updated and defined as:

> The combination of skills, knowledge, attitudes, values and abilities that underpin effective and/or superior performance in a profession/occupational area.
>
> ANMC (2006), p. 8

Since then, these competencies have been further revised and updated. The ANMC's *National Competency Standards for the Registered Nurse* (2006) were adopted by the NMBA, and in 2016 were replaced by the *Registered Nurse Standards for Practice* (NMBA, 2016), which remains the current standard. (This document is available in the Appendix of this book.) These standards are instrumental in determining the model for tertiary nursing.

The *Registered Nurse Standards for Practice* outlines an entry-level standard across a global range of nursing activities to uphold, including critical thinking and analysis, legal accountability, an individual's rights, excellent communication skills, patient safety and trust. Two of the outcomes of utilising these standards include professional pride and the transferability of skills. However, because much of the work done by nurses is interpersonal, competency is very difficult to determine and measure. The complexity in assessing skill competency is addressed in the NMBA's *Framework for Assessing National Competency Standards* (2015).

Clinical Psychomotor Skills outlines the practical aspects necessary for the skill assessment of entry-level registered nurses (RNs). The text is structured to enable theoretical knowledge to be applied experientially. This assists you to effectively master the practical applications of the theory you are learning. The tools in this book minimise the difficulties in assessing your clinical skills and are already used extensively throughout Australian nursing schools.

PSYCHOMOTOR SKILLS ASSESSMENT

The actual 'motor skill' is only one aspect of the overall competency of an individual nurse. Other aspects include specialised knowledge, cognitive skills, technical skills, interpersonal skills and personal traits, which are demonstrated when you perform psychomotor skills. The observer or expert nurse assessor will reassess overall performance as new 'cues' are added to the observation dataset. From this, over time, an idea about your abilities can be derived.

According to the NMBA (2016), assessment is conducted using five principles:

- *Accountability* – the assessor is accountable to the public and the nursing profession to validly and reliably assess you in a practice setting.
- *Performance-based assessment* – the assessment is undertaken in the context of a range of

interactions between you and the person receiving care to enable global assessment of your knowledge, skills, values and attitudes.

- *Evidence-based assessment* – you will be observed, interviewed and asked to reflect on your performance, your documentation is examined, tests are given (e.g. medication calculations, questions about anatomy and physiology), others are consulted for their views (peers, supervisors and individuals receiving care), and this information is analysed using the assessor's professional judgement to form a conclusion about your competence.
- *Validity and reliability* – a knowledgeable, skilled nurse assessor gathers evidence from a variety of sources and, using reflection and judgement, determines if the assessment meets the intended outcome (validity) and if the assessment process is consistent and accurate (reliability).
- *Participation and collaboration* – the assessment process is based on participation and collaboration between you and your nurse assessor, involving high levels of communication, reflection on the process by both of you and reinterpretation of the evidence.

As a beginning practitioner, you will benefit from guidelines and direction, and having complex interactions simplified into recognisable and achievable steps will enhance your learning, reduce stress and allow you to better concentrate on the complexities of the situation.

Initially, skills are learnt in the safety of the laboratory through demonstrations and discussions with the laboratory leader, who is a skilled current nursing practitioner. The skills and the linked theory are read, digested, conceptualised and discussed before you attempt a new skill in the clinical environment. The equipment is handled and explored to gain dexterity and confidence. These processes increase confidence and foster clinical reasoning and judgement. Stimulating clinical reasoning from the beginning of academic education increases performance of skills (Carvalho, Oliveira-Kumakura & Morais, 2017). Critical thinking, clinical judgement, decision making and problem solving (among others) are essential for professional excellence and accurate clinical decision making (Giuffrida et al., 2023). Lifelong learning and systematic use of evidence-based practice education are other factors that positively affect clinical decision making (Vaajoki et al., 2023).

USING THIS ASSESSMENT TOOL

This book has been developed to guide you when learning a new skill. When you are on professional experience placements, the book will need to be used in conjunction with the facility's relevant procedural guidelines. Clinical reasoning skills are enhanced by providing evidence-based explanations.

The information provided here is generic and must be adapted to and integrated within the specific clinical context. The facility type (e.g. acute care, aged care), geographical location, staff availability, shift, time of day, day of the week and season will influence how the procedural information is used. Individual differences between people, including age and developmental stage, culture, gender, wellness level, stress levels and their ability to communicate, will alter the procedure as well.

This book contains many of the major psychomotor skills taught throughout the entire undergraduate nursing program and is intended to be used both on professional experience placement and theory-building encounters throughout the entire three years of study. Upon completion, you will have a record of the clinical skills assessed and the results achieved during undergraduate nursing education.

You can use this book in skills laboratories or during demonstrations and discussions by the laboratory leader. We have minimised the use of diagrams and photographs (the 'visuals' specific to a skill [e.g. charts, documentation] and the requisite equipment [e.g. oxygen equipment, intravenous (IV) cannulae], all of which will be presented and discussed in your laboratory) and lengthy explanations so the book can be easily carried into and used in clinical, laboratory and assessment situations. Your facilitator or preceptor can also use it as either a formative or a summative assessment tool to provide a structured assessment and assist in facilitating objective, comprehensive and constructive feedback on your performance. They can assess the various aspects of your clinical skills performance as exemplars of your ability to demonstrate domain criteria of the NMBA *Registered Nurse Standards for Practice* (2016). It thus fits well with the Australian Nursing Standards Assessment Tool (ANSAT, 2017), which is used in many Australian universities (Ossenberg, Henderson & Mitchell, 2020).

Each chapter is called a 'Clinical Skill', and these are cross-referenced in bold throughout the text where relevant; for example, 'see **Clinical Skill 53**' is directing you to Chapter 53. Each Clinical Skill has two or three pages that provide the required underpinning theoretical components. The information presented is not exhaustive in relation to the subject, but it does provide you and the assessor with a mutual basic understanding of each procedure. Foundational nursing texts and medical surgical texts must be used to support and supplement the material in the theoretical links to practice.

Many skills are not available in the clinical settings that you will attend (e.g. intravenous medication administration is not usually undertaken in a community setting). Take advantage of the skills available for practice and assessment (physical assessment skills, communication skills, interviewing), and do not worry that you are 'missing out' on some skills. They will be available in another context or setting. Skills need practice to master (Sterling-Fox et al., 2020). Do not fool yourself that taking a blood pressure or assessing a limb a few times is sufficient. To become proficient, a skill set needs a great deal of repetition, with attention to the nuances between individuals and using the skills of professional communication, observation and clinical reasoning concurrently. You must practise individual skills until they become ingrained and automatic to perform, and then further learning and practice are needed in the clinical setting to make you truly proficient in the skill.

The Clinical Skills encompass entire skills, not just individual tasks or procedures. Nursing students with limited exposure to clinical situations must still demonstrate a level of competence to demonstrate safe practice. The balance and integration of the skills and knowledge you acquire determine your ability, not within just one skill, but in your overall readiness for nursing. You are assessed on your ability to interact with the person you are caring for, to solve problems and to effectively manage the time and resources at your disposal. You are also assessed on your ability to complete the procedure efficiently and safely, to ensure the person is clean and comfortable, to document their care and to dispose of waste afterwards.

The evidence-based information that forms the theory underlying the skills in this book comes from a number of sources. However, some fundamental nursing-care skills in this book still do not have a great deal of solid evidence or research-based foundations. You are expected to read widely, attend professional experience workshops, and discuss issues with the laboratory leader, clinical educator or RN, in order to broaden your knowledge prior to implementing a skill in the clinical setting.

PERFORMANCE CRITERIA

In the Clinical Skills Assessment table at the end of each Clinical Skill, each criterion is linked to one or more of the NMBA *Registered Nurse Standards for Practice* (2016). Standards' reference numbers are listed beside each criterion to facilitate linking your performance with the relevant NMBA Standards criteria. The facilitator can gather many cues in relation to the specific Standards criteria before giving you a formal judgement of your performance and verbal or written assessment feedback of your progress for the relevant NMBA Standard.

Even though the performance criteria have been broken into arbitrary sections, the entire skill should be seamless. You should not be assessed on your first attempt to complete a procedure; practice improves performance and fosters your confidence.

The five-point Bondy rating scale is used in this edition. This scale considers three areas: professional standards, competence and independence. There are five 'levels' of performance, as follows:

- *Independent* – you can complete the procedure or skill safely, accurately and efficiently, without any cues from the clinical facilitator. You can discuss the theory as it relates to the person's clinical situation. You use appropriate vocabulary and excellent communication and show appropriate affect. You use your time well and are confident in your actions. The clinical facilitator would feel confident that you are able to perform this procedure, or one similar, independently.
- *Supervised* – you can complete the procedure, safely and accurately; however, you may require direction, prompting or more time to complete the skill. You focus on the person in your care and your affect is appropriate. You can discuss the theory behind the procedure in a general way. Conversely, you may be able to complete the psychomotor skill but not discuss the rationale behind what you are doing. The clinical facilitator would not feel confident enough to allow you to complete this or a similar procedure without some supervision.
- *Assisted* – you can accomplish the procedure safely and accurately; however, you may have difficulties with time management, with focusing on the person rather than yourself or the skill, with your affect, with anxiety or with communication, or your knowledge base may be lacking and you cannot provide a rationale for your actions. Your clinical facilitator may have to provide directive cues as well as supportive cues to help you through the procedure and would need to supervise this or a similar procedure in the future.
- *Marginal* – you cannot complete the procedure accurately, safely or without directive assistance from the assessor, and you have difficulty in linking theory to the practice. You may be anxious and lack confidence, you take too much time to finish and cannot focus on the person in care due to focusing on the procedure or on yourself. The clinical facilitator would not allow you to complete this or a similar procedure without supervision.
- *Dependent* – you are unable to complete the procedure and your performance is unsafe and inaccurate. You are uncoordinated, lack knowledge of the theory, do not focus on the person and require so much direction and assistance that the assessor is essentially performing the procedure (Bondy, 1983).

NOTE TO THE CLINICAL EDUCATOR OR FACILITATOR

Foster, Evans and Alexander (2023) emphasise the importance of mentoring and supporting colleagues – especially younger ones ('generativity' or passing one's knowledge and experience on to the next generation) – to build confident and more effective professional nurses. Moon and Chang (2023) agree on the crucial role clinical educators play in developing knowledge, values, skills and professional attributes. These authors also assert that clinical educators, in their mentoring role for professional socialisation, are instrumental in helping prevent the attrition of new graduates.

Several recent studies have demonstrated the importance of the clinical educator/facilitator's role in fostering the learning of nursing students, using strategies such as:

- role modelling
- creating a safe environment
- clinical supervision
- providing experiential learning opportunities
- setting realistic expectations
- goal setting
- providing feedback and stimulating learning (Calaguas, 2023; Karani et al., 2014; Ossenberg et al., 2023).

Using these teaching strategies will assist the student to develop the core professional characteristics of the RN: care, compassion, courage, communication, competence, collegiality, commitment, empathy, respect, confidentiality, reflection, integrity, honesty, morality and ethical conduct (Artim et al., 2020; Baillie, 2017; Cruess et al., 2011; Foster et al., 2023; Moon & Chang, 2023). These professional characteristics are enhanced by focusing on the social, cultural and ethical dimensions of the nurse–person interaction, as well as the knowledge and motor skills of competent care that are easier to teach and assess.

Please refer to the *ANSAT Resource Manual* (2018) for information and helpful hints about assessing students and providing feedback. As a gatekeeper to our profession, you will need both confidence and courage to honestly assess each student fairly. You will also probably need the support of your colleagues and of the university if/when it comes to failing a student for unsafe care. We hope you will use your skills to help students to become grounded in a nursing culture of excellence.

CHAPTER 2

CLINICAL THINKING

Critical thinking is a process. It is a purposeful act that uses careful, deliberate thought, creativity, intuition, reflective thinking, fair and open mindedness, logic, analysis and evaluation to arrive at a decision or an understanding that is cognisant of the social, political, economic and environmental implications (Giacomazzi, Fontana & Camilli Trujillo, 2022). Critical thinking fosters the ability to analyse, evaluate and reconstruct information in order to make a decision and act on it (Haghparast, Nasaruddin & Abdullah, 2013, cited in Mahanal et al., 2019). In nursing, critical thinking forms the basis for clinical decision making. Berg, Philipp and Taff (2021) state that 'critical thinking exposes assumptions, biases, and beliefs that influence clinical reasoning'. Professional and theoretical knowledge, as well as technical skills, self-confidence and self-efficacy, are prerequisites to clinical decision making (Wijbenga, Bovend'Eerdt & Driessen, 2019).

Clinical reasoning, the basis of clinical decision making, is a subset of critical thinking that focuses on the care of a person within the healthcare system. Using the critical thinking processes, clinical reasoning takes into consideration:

- medical and nursing knowledge about the person's diagnosis (e.g. anatomy and physiology, pharmacology, communications, clinical psychomotor skills)
- the legal, ethical and other professional standards
- safety
- evidence-based knowledge
- your knowledge of the person and their clinical situation
- your clinical experience to determine, prevent and manage care situations (i.e. to problem-solve).

Sound clinical reasoning takes time to develop. As well as theoretical knowledge from your nursing courses and clinical knowledge from your clinical experiences, practice and reflection on your clinical experience are needed. Clinical reasoning underlies safety and good outcomes for people in your care and the preservation of professional nursing standards (Alfaro-LeFevre, 2017).

Clinical judgement is an essential component of competent nursing practice and an extension of critical thinking, and is a complex process. It takes clinical reasoning (i.e. the 'cues', such as data, signs and symptoms, 'normal' and 'abnormal' findings that you identified with the person), your own nursing knowledge, best evidence, learned theories and knowledge from other disciplines, and applies pattern recognition and intuition to determine if there is a nursing problem/something wrong with the person. Lastly, the available alternatives to solve the problem are sorted through (using flexibility and prioritisation [Tsang et al., 2023]) and the best solution is determined. Arriving at decisions with the person about their care using clinical reasoning and clinical judgement is known as *clinical decision making*. Its application is bound to real life. It is contextual (Shirazi & Heidari, 2019; Tsang et al., 2023), and thus depends on the person in your care and their individual situation.

Your clinical facilitators or registered nurses (RNs) with whom you are working may assist you to develop your clinical reasoning and judgement. For instance, they may ask you to analyse a care episode or case study (see the example clinical scenario on pages 7–8) or to talk through your reasoning and decision making following an interaction with someone in your care. Timely feedback in a respectful environment plays an essential part in assisting you to develop and reinforce clinical decision making (Huang et al., 2023; Koharchik et al., 2015). It is also a skill that many RNs find provides deep satisfaction throughout their career.

According to Levett-Jones et al. (2010), the eight steps in clinical reasoning (as shown in **FIGURE 2.1**) are:

1. *Looking* – noticing signs, being aware of the person and looking for change during any interaction, and scanning the person at each encounter.
2. *Collecting* – purposeful observation and assessment, data collection, review handover, charts, history, results of investigations, recall related information (e.g. anatomy and physiology, pharmacology, therapeutics, culture) and context of care.
3. *Processing* – cognition, including new relationships, cue clusters, what is relevant, not relevant, normal versus abnormal, nursing knowledge of past situations you have seen, deciding on significance of

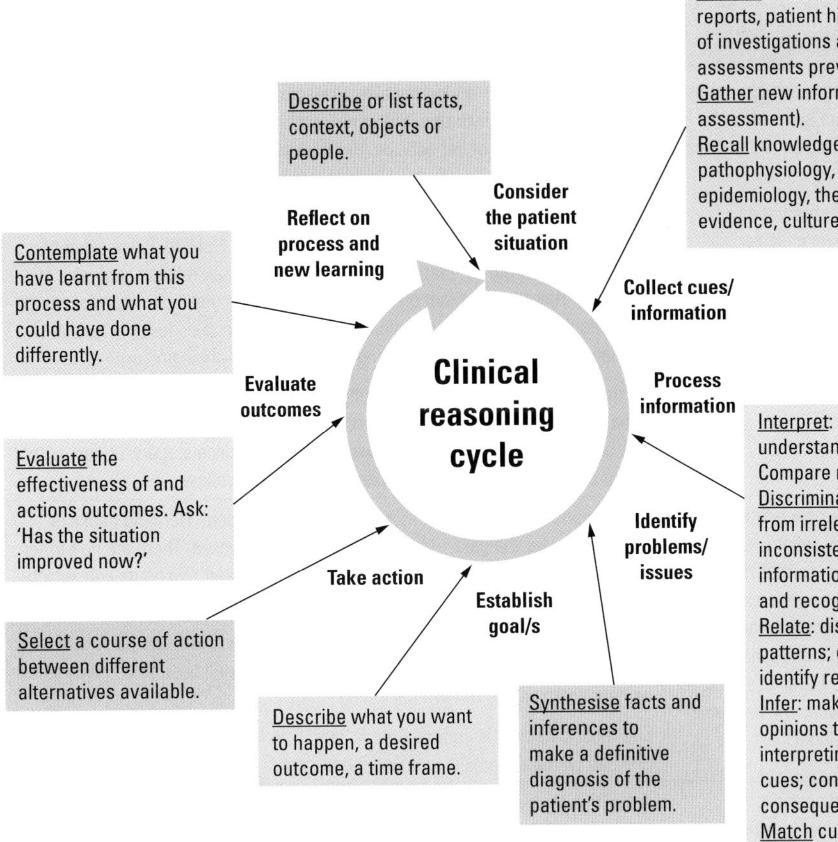

FIGURE 2.1 The clinical reasoning process with descriptors

SOURCE: REPRINTED FROM THE 'FIVE RIGHTS' OF CLINICAL REASONING: AN EDUCATIONAL MODEL TO ENHANCE NURSING STUDENTS' ABILITY TO IDENTIFY AND MANAGE CLINICALLY 'AT RISK' PATIENTS, LEVETT-JONES, T., HOFFMAN, K., DEMPSEY, J., JEONG, S., NOBLE, D., NORTON, C., ROCHE, J., & HICKEY, N., *NURSE EDUCATION TODAY*.

data in this person's situation and questioning what will happen if nothing is done.

4. *Deciding* – review and analysis, generating ideas and using theoretical and experiential knowledge to define the problem.
5. *Planning* – determining with the person which course of action is most appropriate to achieve the best clinical outcomes for the person, stating a time frame and feeling confident that you have made the best choice.
6. *Acting* – carrying out the chosen course of action.
7. *Evaluating* – determining if the action was the best choice to improve the situation and why or why not.
8. *Reflecting* – thinking back, including questioning what could have been done differently and asking yourself probing questions about the entire process in order to learn from it; both in a clinical and a personal sense.

Ideally, all nurses, from novices to experts, use these steps. Expert nurses may not seem to use the steps, but they do – just very quickly and using their experience to inform the processes. These steps can occur out of sequence, overlap or blur into each other; however, all are essential in nursing care. A ninth critical step, which precedes all the others, is anticipation. Know the person you are caring for, their diagnosis and their problems, and anticipate what could go wrong. Your anticipation results in vigilance for signs of probable difficulties and helps you to recognise subtle indications early.

TABLE 2.1 Analysis of example scenario using the clinical reasoning process

CLINICAL REASONING ACTION	DESCRIPTION	CLINICAL EXAMPLE
Looking	Noticing signs and symptoms, being aware and looking for change during any interaction	2345h. Mrs Gardiner is alert (awakes to voice), her colour is good (pink), and her skin is dry and well hydrated. She is moving well in bed and she has drunk most of the litre of water at her bedside. Her IV is infusing at 125 mL/hour. There is about 200 mL left to be infused. Her blanket is bunched up on the side of her bed
Collecting	Purposeful observation and assessment, data collection, review handover, charts, history, results of investigations, recall related information	She returned from theatre seven hours ago. Her vital signs are stable at: TPR: 36.9 °C, 84/14; BP: 145/90 (on admission it was 154/88). Pulse oximetry 96 per cent on room air; states minimal pain (had a slow release analgesic at 2200 hrs). Right leg and foot elevated. Toes are warm, nails pink, can feel touch and wriggle toes, dressing remains intact, unable to access foot pulses due to bandaging. Moonboot on. IV infusing well and IV site clean and dry
		On the surgical chart, she had 2 L of fluid in theatre, and has only the current litre remaining of the order. She fasted from 0600 hrs. She is eating and drinking well. She has been up to the toilet with assistance twice since surgery, urinary output is approximately 350 mL/void – urine clear and pale yellow
Processing	Cognition – new relationships, cue clusters, what is relevant, not relevant, normal vs not normal, nursing knowledge of past situations you have seen, deciding on significance of data in Mrs Gardiner's clinical situation, what will happen if nothing is done?	Mrs Gardiner is recovering from surgery without incident. Her fluid intake is good (3.8 L over the past 18 hours) and she has no nausea. There are no further IV orders after the current litre. She had analgesia about two hours ago, which is effective The IV line and pump are waking her up. If left in, the IV line and pump will keep her awake periodically throughout the night and she will need to be awakened in an hour and a half to remove the IV line She reports being hot. Temperature is 36.9 °C. Ambient temperature is 24 °C. She had warmed blankets on following theatre
Deciding	Review and analysis, generating ideas, using theoretical and experiential knowledge to define the problem	If the IV is removed, there is no direct access to veins if a need for rapid administration of medications or fluid is needed (following surgery, this is not a good choice) The hospital protocol allows the IV cannula to be left in situ and capped for the night. Lowering the air conditioning may increase her comfort
Planning	Determining with Mrs Gardiner which course of action is appropriate to get the best outcome for her, stating a time frame, feeling confident that it is the best choice	In this instance, capping the cannula now permits Mrs Gardiner to sleep through until the next observation period at 0400 hrs, taking advantage of the peak analgesic period, although she will miss out on about 200 mL of fluid. Since her intake for the day is more than adequate, this is a reasonable choice. Set the air conditioning at 22 °C
Acting	Carrying out the chosen course of action	Cap the cannula and take away the line and volumetric pump. Provide Mrs Gardiner with a fresh litre of water and ask her to drink some now. Change the setting on the air conditioner
Evaluating	Determining if the action was the best choice to improve the situation and why or why not	Determine if Mrs Gardiner is sleeping during each round throughout the night. Check if she still has a blanket on At 0600 hrs, when you come to take the observations, ask Mrs Gardiner how she slept and assess her pain levels
Reflecting	Thinking back asking yourself what you could have done differently, and asking yourself probing questions about the entire process in order to learn from it – both in a clinical sense and a personal sense	I needed to look up the hospital protocol for leaving an IV cannula capped. This is a common occurrence and one I could have anticipated. I will have to be more alert to common protocols in the future. I had read about the surgery, and studied her chart before I went to her room (anticipation), so I felt confident about what observations to make I checked with the RN about my clinical reasoning and she agreed with my thinking and what I decided I felt proud that I made the right clinical decisions

The following is a clinical scenario and analysis (see TABLE 2.1) to illustrate the practical use of the eight steps in clinical reasoning.

You are working a night shift and it is 2345 hours. You have been asked to do the postoperative observations for Mrs Gardiner, who returned from orthopaedic surgery (right foot) at 1700 hours. She is dozing when you enter her room but wakens when you call her name. Her vital signs have been within acceptable limits, she states that her pain is minimal (3/10), she is drinking and eating without experiencing any nausea, and she has been up to the toilet and voided a good amount of urine twice since surgery. Mrs Gardiner has D5S infusing into her left cephalic vein (forearm). She states that the intravenous (IV) line keeps pulling and waking her up and the lights and beeping of the pump are annoying, and asks you to remove it. She also feels hot and has tossed the blanket off.

As you progress through your studies, you will encounter increasingly complex clinical situations; therefore, developing clinical reasoning skills is an essential part of becoming an RN. It demands a deeper and more sophisticated understanding of the knowledge underpinning practice and of the person in your care. The basis for developing effective clinical reasoning is a sound core of the essential knowledge of the profession. Your clinical observation skills need to be nurtured and honed. Beginning nurses often have difficulties differentiating between a situation that needs immediate attention and one that does not, and also in processing large amounts of complex clinical data when under time pressure. In the beginning, deciding on a course of action, then asking more experienced RNs for their input and critique is a good strategy to develop your clinical decision-making skills. There are also frameworks that look at physiological cues in acutely ill people (early warning systems) to assist you in determining if the person's condition is stable or deteriorating.

Situational awareness is a process nurses use to avert poor outcomes in people with unstable conditions and that may deteriorate quickly. This type of clinical reasoning begins with knowing the person, their diagnosis, what is likely to go wrong and what could go wrong. From here you notice their environment and apply:

- *vigilance* – look for indications of problems; for example, altered vital signs, reduced urine output, poor colour, sweaty skin, saturated dressing, empty IV bag
- *perception* – notice the differences in the person from the last time you saw them or from the handover you received; for example, increased pain, confusion, less alert, restlessness.

You can then use clinical reasoning to identify important elements, decide what cues to look for, and from these cues predict what might happen. At this point, you intervene if you can (e.g. apply oxygen, give pain relief as ordered) or communicate your findings and prediction to a senior colleague who can address them (e.g. contact the medical team, initiate a unit protocol for electrocardiograms).

Competent professional nursing care is never a superficial or habitual activity. Nursing practice requires a fully engaged mind using critical, reflective thinking and the sound reasoning of an intelligent mind developed and dedicated to safe, effective care. Nurses using well-developed clinical reasoning skills positively impact on an individual's recovery and wellbeing. Nurses who do not think critically become part of the problem (Shirazi & Heidari, 2019). Nurses with poorly developed clinical reasoning skills may be unable to determine when an individual is beginning to deteriorate or to recognise the onset of a complication (Tsang et al., 2023). They may also be unable to diagnose a problem or start appropriate treatment for the problem or complication. They are not as effective in providing safe care as they could be.

CHAPTER 3

PERSON-CENTRED PRACTICE

Person-centred practice is a way of thinking about and doing things in a healthcare setting that reflects the person as an individual with unique life stories, preferences, values and needs. It places the individual at the centre of the care being offered. Person-centred practice is defined by the Nursing and Midwifery Board of Australia (NMBA) *Registered Nurse Standards for Practice* (2016, p. 6) as a 'collaborative and respectful partnership built on mutual trust and understanding through good communication' and has been adopted for the NMBA's *Codes of Conduct for Nurses and Midwives* (NMBA, 2018b). Person-centred care that incorporates good communication, holism, trust, sharing of knowledge and decision making, a tailored approach and reciprocal respect is important for effective treatment of most illnesses. Registered nurses (RNs) base person-centred care on the recognition and use of the individual's resources, needs and preferences (Ski et al., 2023). Person-centred care also recognises that each individual is part of a social system, is in various relationships and has both a past and future that impact on their behaviour and decisions (Tieu et al., 2022). We try to humanise health care by valuing people as individuals, using their strengths and capabilities to facilitate active participation in their own care. Knowing the person's values and beliefs enables RNs to make decisions with the individual and be responsive to meet the individual's needs. Nurses need to see an individual as expert about their own life, choices, health and care. We need to 'do with the person', not 'do to the person'.

The components of person-centred practice (adapted from Health Innovation Network [2017]; Phelan et al. [2020]; and Rathert et al. [2015]) are:

- knowing the person as an individual
- being responsive
- providing care that is meaningful, coordinated and integrated
- respecting the individual's values, preferences and needs and putting them at the centre of care
- fostering trusting caregiving relationships, with good communication, information sharing and education
- emphasising freedom of choice with access to appropriate care when it is needed (shared decision making)
- promoting physical and emotional comfort
- involving the person's family and friends, as appropriate
- ensuring continuity of care between and within healthcare services.

Part of person-centred care is cultural safety. Culturally safe and respectful practice means you must be aware of your own culture, values, attitudes, biases and beliefs. This enables you to respect the culture of others while understanding that only they can determine what is safe and respectful; acknowledge the cultural, social, behavioural and economic influences on health of people and communities; adopt practices that respect diversity (e.g. gender, disability, race, ethnicity, religious belief, sexuality, age) to avoid bias, discrimination and racism; and support an inclusive environment for the safety and security of the individual and their family. This includes your colleagues as well as the people in your care (adapted from the NMBA's *Code of Conduct for Registered Nurses* [NMBA, 2018a]).

A person's emotional and spiritual wellbeing is also part of person-centred care. Spiritual care can be religious or non-religious and reflects values, relationships, purpose and what is of intrinsic meaning to the individual (Ebenau, 2023). Kegl et al. (2023) add the caring relationships within the healthcare team as contributing to effective person-centred care.

On the healthcare system side, we need to consider the person's whole experience and promote continuity and coordination ensuring that the physical, cultural and psychosocial environment of health services supports person-centred care. Healthcare professionals must be supportive, good communicators and strive to put people at the centre of their own care. The term 'person-centred' is as applicable to our interactions with our colleagues as to the people for whom we care.

Even though 'patient-centred care' is often used to mean the same as 'person-centred practice', the latter avoids the terms 'patient', 'consumer' or 'client' as politically and economically created terms that ignore the individuality of each person. Anyone who comes into contact with the healthcare system is vulnerable because they seek help beyond their own knowledge and ability to self-care. The word 'patient' places an individual in a position of increased vulnerability and powerlessness as the healthcare system, including nurses, becomes the provider of and gateway to care. The use of the word 'patient' depersonalises an interaction and places the focus on the nursing needs and medical diagnosis that take priority over personal needs of the care receiver. 'Client' and 'consumer' are economically constructed terms that evoke the notion that the person receiving care is a paying customer who must get what they want to have a satisfactory outcome. The terms 'person' and 'people' are used in the NMBA *Registered Nurse Standards for Practice* (2016, p. 6) to refer to 'individuals who have entered into a therapeutic and/or professional relationship with a registered nurse' and include families, carers, community groups, colleagues and students as well as those requiring direct nursing care who come within the scope and context of practice of the registered nurse.

Healthcare workers have a greater understanding of the disease processes, interventions and treatments. Individuals know their own values, needs, preferences, goals and experiences. Shared decision making is dependent on the carer and the individual exchanging this knowledge. Relationship-centred care means the individual is treated, rather than the disease, fostering feelings of respect, trust and support, and enabling the person to take part in decisions about their care. Chu et al. (2022) found that having a sympathetic presence and engagement with the individual were especially important for interacting with people who have dementia.

Please do not use diagnostic 'labels' (e.g. the diabetic in 204, or the laparotomy in 616) for identifying people. Use their names, and if clarification is required, something like 'Mrs Jones, the woman with diabetes'. Using diagnostic labels demoralises and dehumanises the individual, and may actually change the care given to the person as we are treating the disease, not the person.

HOW DOES PERSON-CENTRED PRACTICE BENEFIT THE PERSON?

Person-centred practice:

- is informed by evidence
- incorporates the individual's needs, capabilities and goals
- is a collaboration between the person and the nurse
- includes family involvement
- takes into account the context
- is cost-effective.

Nursing interventions based on person-centred practice help individuals get the care they need when they need it, help them to be more independent and active in their own health care, improve the quality of available healthcare services, reduce some health and social services pressures (Moyle et al., 2015), and provide dignity, compassion and respect (Hunter-Jones et al., 2023). Person-centred care improves the quality of care for individuals as well as job satisfaction for nurses (Kim, Kim & Lee, 2022). Wolf, Vella and Fors (2019) assessed person-centred care versus standard care in adults and found an improvement in the information gained by the person and their family (especially in those with lower educational attainment), more involvement in care decisions, significantly better individual–physician communication and improved documentation. Person-centred care can improve the individual's experience of care and their satisfaction with it. It can help people to lead healthier lifestyles; for example, by supporting them to make healthier life choices, such as exercising and eating healthily. It involves people in their care decisions so that the services and support provided are what they need at the time, and it can impact on their health outcomes (e.g. education and support tailored to the individual assist in reducing blood pressure, stabilising blood glucose levels).

Person-centred practice benefits the healthcare system by reducing the frequency of the use of services, which may then reduce the overall cost of care. It also benefits nurses by improving the confidence nurses have in themselves and in the care they provide. Person-centred care enhances the satisfaction nurses feel in their caregiving.

There are barriers to providing person-centred care. These include the nurse's task orientation, risk minimisation (e.g. limiting necessary mobilisation to reduce falls in those deemed to be high-risk) and time limitations (Tobiano et al., 2016). Damant et al. (2023) found barriers to using person-centred care included staff levels and skills, attitudes and availability, as well as the quality of care leadership. Boggatz (2020) added that economic constraints, low qualification of caregivers and a hierarchical organisation of work also negatively impacted on the effectiveness of person-centred care. Kong, Kim and Kim (2021) cited insufficient resources, lack of education, negative mindset and poor relationships in aged care facilities. These authors emphasised that success in implementing person-centred practice hinges on excellent communication skills.

Personal bias is another barrier to providing person-centred care (think of the severely obese individual or someone who is addicted to illicit substances). Nurses need to be aware of these barriers to enable themselves to improve their person-centred practice. Nurses are committed to caring equally for all. Often, the health needs of lesbian, gay, bisexual, transgender, intersex and queer (LGBTIQ+) people are ignored because of our own bias, our own lack of knowledge and the challenges of initiating difficult conversations with colleagues and with LGBTIQ+ people about their health needs (McEwing et al., 2022). These difficulties need to be recognised and addressed if excellent person-centred care is to be achieved.

Use your interpersonal skills to establish a warm relationship with the person. Smile when you see them, ask about their life, truly listen to them, answer questions as honestly as you can and respond with warmth and genuine interest to build a person-centred relationship. Never forget that they are 'there' (e.g. when two healthcare professionals are performing a procedure, often the person is 'talked over' as if they are invisible), that they may be anxious and stressed and in pain. People who seek or need health care are often at a low point in their lives, with fear, sadness, despair and grief as predominant emotions and pain, fatigue and immobility as predominant physical effects. Your humanity and compassion, shown by interest in them and acting with gentleness and kindness, will go a long way to easing some of these emotional and physical burdens. Simple empathetic listening is a powerful tool in alleviating suffering and gaining trust. Empathy (experiencing another's emotions while being aware that they are not your own emotions), humaneness, concern and the desire for another's wellbeing contribute to compassion (Cura & Atay, 2022).

Trauma-informed care

In addition to person-centred care, trauma-informed care is an increasingly recognised approach to care. It acknowledges that many people have endured some sort of trauma (physical, emotional or psychological [e.g. post-traumatic stress disorder, judgemental health care, marginalisation]) that results in stress. This stress is caused by the negative impacts of trauma and occurs when individuals are uncertain about how to ensure their own social, physical or mental wellbeing. Stress impacts a person's ability to cope, to learn and to understand what is told to them, and can be exacerbated by the experience of hospitalisation. Trauma-informed care should be implemented for each person in our care (Brown et al., 2022). Trauma-informed care is closely associated with person-centred care, but further emphasises the importance of safety (physical and emotional); trustworthiness and transparency; empowerment, voice, choice; use of peer support; and cultural, historical and gender responsiveness (Fleishman, Kamsky & Sundborg, 2019). The aim of trauma-informed care is to build a working relationship with the person, empower them to make their own choices and reduce any trauma-triggering situations. Implementing trauma-informed care involves such easily accomplished acts as introducing yourself and your role at every encounter with the person (they may not remember your name or your position, for example); using non-threatening body positioning, such as sitting at the bedside during an interview; providing information about what is going to happen to them (e.g. dressing change schedules, medication rounds); asking for permission to touch them; and ensuring their privacy, including by privately asking if they want their family members to leave during a procedure or interview. In addition, trauma-informed care requires transparency and consistency of information to decrease confusion. Use plain language and ask the person to 'teach back' (see **Clinical Skill 27**) to determine their understanding and ability to implement their own care.

CHAPTER 4

PROFESSIONAL COMMUNICATION

Professional communication (or therapeutic communication/interaction) is a specific type of verbal and non-verbal communication used by health professionals to help the people for whom they are caring. It is different from social communication. The Nursing and Midwifery Board of Australia (NMBA) *Codes of Conduct for Nurses and Midwives* (NMBA, 2018b) has adopted the term 'professional communication' (p. 4) in preference to therapeutic communication. Use of professional communication reduces the apprehension, anxiety and fear of people in care to increase relaxation, and assists them to provide information to participate in their care and thus influences the outcome of the health-based interaction. You can use specific communication techniques to gain information about the person's unique life story, preferences, values and needs, circumstances, health problem and state of mind. Professional communication is foundational to the practice of mental health nursing (Hercelinskyj & Alexander, 2020, p. 80). Communication is one of the explicit assessment items of the Australian Nursing Standards Assessment Tool (ANSAT, 2017). Using professional communication can provide support and information to assist a person to deal with and understand their situation and emotional reactions to it. This improves the comfort and safety of the person, their trust in nurses and the healthcare system, and ultimately their health and wellbeing.

Part of gaining a person's trust is using the appropriate pronoun when talking to or about someone. It is courteous and denotes respect and understanding of their gender identity. Assuming the person's pronoun preference can be offensive, harmful and oppressive (Zambon, 2021). Most people's gender (a spectrum of the social construct of values, roles, behaviour and identity of the person) will align with their sex (reproductive anatomy at birth, physical characteristics, gene expression and hormones). However, some of the people you care for will have a different gender identity (e.g. non-binary or transgender) and use a pronoun (he/him, she/her or they/their) that differs from how they may appear to you. It is respectful to ask about preferred pronouns when meeting someone, and using those pronouns when interacting with or discussing the person. If you make a mistake in pronoun use, simply apologise to the person and move on with the conversation. Also, avoid gender-laden words (e.g. lovely, handsome) when talking to someone whose gender identity is diverse. These actions help create an inclusive environment.

Professional communication is generally taught as part of a required subject in nursing courses, so this discussion is a brief introduction to this topic. Some specific communication techniques can be found in TABLE 4.1.

TABLE 4.1 Techniques for professional communication

TECHNIQUE NAME	EXPLANATION	EXAMPLE
Active listening	A potent communication device foundational to professional communication. It involves being attentive to the person – being 'with' the person, calmly and actively	Maintain appropriate eye contact; face the person at their level, if possible, and lean towards them; also use accessible language (no jargon)
Give recognition	Acknowledge the person as an individual without any value judgements	Call the person by title or name, using their preferred pronoun; note any changes, such as they have applied make-up, shaved or changed into their own clothes
Use open questions	Open questions require an explanation and therefore elicit more information. Ask only one question at a time and explore that topic thoroughly before moving on to another In contrast, closed questions require only a brief answer (e.g. yes or no) and are used if the situation warrants (e.g. if the person is in severe pain or respiratory distress)	Examples of open questions include: 'Tell me how you are feeling' and 'What makes your pain worse?' Examples of closed questions include: 'Do you feel nauseated?' and 'What is the level of your pain on a scale from zero to ten?'
Share observations	Talk with the person about what you have seen or heard, then remain silent to allow the person to respond	'You haven't been out of bed much today'

TABLE 4.1 (Continued)

TECHNIQUE NAME	EXPLANATION	EXAMPLE
Use empathy	Demonstrate an understanding of another person's feelings and then wait for a response	'It must be very frustrating to have to stay in bed all day'
Acceptance	Accept what the person says without judgement to acknowledge them	This could just be a nod, a smile or saying 'Mmm'
Touch	Touch the person appropriately to offer comfort	Gentle touch, usually on their hand, arm or shoulder
Use humour	Humour used appropriately promotes friendliness, sharing and relaxation. Use with care	This is situational. What may be humorous to one person may be insulting or derogatory to another
Provide factual information	Information helps the individual to make decisions, feel safe, secure and to reduce anxiety	'Your surgery is scheduled for 11 this morning' 'Your IV can come out when this litre is completed'
Clarify	Ensure an accurate understanding of what you have heard (usually by restating)	'I'm not sure I understood what you meant when you said that you feel "down" just now'
Explore	Learn more about a situation (usually used if the person remains on a superficial level) using broad, then focused questions to delve into an experience or situation	'Tell me more about …', then ask further specific questions about the situation
Focus on a single idea	Explore a symptom or idea in greater depth	'You have pain in that ankle? Can you tell me your level of pain on a scale of zero to ten?' 'Can you point to where it hurts most?' 'What makes it feel worse? Better?' 'Can you move the joint?'
Paraphrase	Use different words to sum up the person's message. Paraphrases are usually shorter and use different but similar words. Usually tentative – wait for the person to give you feedback in their response	The person tells you: 'My foot is aching and the arch feels like it has broken glass in it. I don't want to get up and walk or do the exercises' You could paraphrase with: 'You are reluctant to exercise your foot because it is so painful?'
Summarise	Sum up the person's information so they know you understand the key parts of the interaction	'Since you had the ibuprofen an hour ago, you have been able to take part in the physiotherapy for your foot and partial weight bear without much pain'
Self-disclosure	Telling someone about your own experiences, using honesty and genuineness to demonstrate empathy and focus the person on a difficult situation. This is only used infrequently and if the situation is both true and relevant, and the nurse feels comfortable disclosing the information about themselves to this person	When looking after a person who is grieving – for example, 'I had a still birth between two normal pregnancies a few years ago and I felt totally alone and bereft at the time despite a really supportive family. I went to see a grief counsellor, and it really did help. Do you think it would help you to see a counsellor?'
Plan for action	Helping the person to formulate a way to deal with a stressful situation and prevent anxiety from escalating	Ask the person: 'The next time the doctor comes in, how are you going to express your concerns to her?' Perhaps suggest rehearsing or keeping a list of questions

Setting boundaries for a professional relationship, and understanding how to terminate the relationship, are also important techniques for you to learn early. There are many more professional communication techniques that you will learn and use throughout your nursing career.

Throughout this text, we suggest you use these communication techniques to:

- understand who the person is, so you can incorporate their preferences within their care
- elicit information essential to their health and care
- establish the person's understanding of a procedure, medication or outcome
- determine their readiness to learn a technique or undergo a procedure, so you can incorporate the appropriate health teaching
- provide information, explanations and the reason for a procedure
- elicit any concerns the person has about a procedure or medication, to be able to address these and increase safety and comfort
- make the person aware of the steps and sensations of a procedure, to gain their cooperation, reducing apprehension and anxiety and promoting relaxation during a procedure
- gain a person's trust and confidence
- provide support.

We hope you find this book helpful in your clinical skills development so that you can provide excellent nursing care.

Joanne Tollefson, RN, BGS, MSc, PhD
Elspeth Hillman, RN, BN, MN

REFERENCES

Alfaro-LeFevre, R. (2017). *Critical thinking, clinical reasoning and clinical judgement: A practical approach* (6th ed.). Philadelphia, PA: Elsevier.

Artim, D. E., Smallidge, D., Boyd, L. D., August, J. N. & Vineyard, J. (2020). Attributes of effective clinical teachers in dental hygiene education. *Journal of Dental Education, 84*, 308–15. https://doi.org/10.21815/JDE.019.188

Australian Nursing and Midwifery Accreditation Council (2019). *Australian Nursing and Midwifery Accreditation Standards.* Canberra: ANMAC. https://www.anmac.org.au/search/publication

Australian Nursing and Midwifery Council (ANMC) (2006). *National Competency Standards for the Registered Nurse* (4th ed.). Dickson, ACT: Australian Nursing and Midwifery Council.

Australian Nursing Standards Assessment Tool (ANSAT) (2017). *Australian Nursing Standards Assessment Tool (ANSAT).* http://www.ansat.com.au/home/tools

Australian Nursing Standards Assessment Tool (ANSAT) (2018). *Resource Manual.* https://drive.google.com/file/d/1R4VF7057GOoxnmRvOzasu-PgePwcqYsR/view

Baillie, L. (2017). An exploration of the 6Cs as a set of values for nursing practice. *British Journal of Nursing, 26*(10). https://doi.org/10.12968/bjon.2017.26.10.558

Berg, C., Philipp, R. & Taff, S. (2021). Scoping review of critical thinking literature in healthcare education. *Occupational Therapy In Health Care, 37*(1), 18–39. https://doi.org/10.1080/07380577.2021.1879411

Boggatz, T. (2020). Person-centred care and quality of life. In T. Boggatz (ed.), *Quality of life and person-centred care for older people.* Cham, Switzerland: Springer, p. 449. https://doi.org/10.1007/978-3-030-29990-3_7

Bondy, K. N. (1983). Criterion referenced definitions for rating scales in clinical evaluation. *Journal of Nursing Education, 22*(9), 376–82.

Brown, T., Ashworth, H., Bass, M., Rittenberg, E., Levy-Carrick, N., Grossman, S., Lewis-O'Connor, A. & Stoklosa, H. (2022). Trauma-informed care interventions in emergency medicine: A systematic review. *Western Journal of Emergency Medicine, 23*(3), 334–44. https://doi.org/10.5811/westjem.2022.1.53674

Calaguas, N. (2023). Mentoring novice nurse educators: Goals, principles, models, and key practices. *Journal of Professional Nursing*, 44, 8–11. https://www.sciencedirect.com/science/article/pii/S8755722322001624

Carvalho, E., Oliveira-Kumakura, A. & Morais, S. (2017). Clinical reasoning in nursing: Teaching strategies and assessment tools. *Revista Brasiliera Enfermagen* [Internet], *70*(3), 662–8. https://doi.org/10.1590/0034-7167-2016-0509

Chu, C. H., Quan, A. M. L., Gandhi, F. & McGilton, K. S. (2022). Perspectives of substitute decision-makers and staff about person-centred physical activity in long-term care. *Health Expectations, 25*, 2155–65. https://doi.org/10.1111/hex.13381

Cruess, R. L., Cruess, S. R., Snell, L., Ginsburg, S., Kearney, R., Ruhe, V., Ducharme, S. & Sternszus, R. (2011). *Teaching, learning and assessing professionalism at the post-graduate level.* Members of the Future of Medical Education in Canada Consortium (Post-Graduate). Montreal, Canada.

Cura, S. & Atay, S. (2022). Correlation between mindfulness, empathy and compassion levels of nursing students: A cross-sectional study. *Archives of Psychiatric Nursing, 42*, 92–6. https://doi.org/10.1016/j.apnu.2022.12.017

Damant, J., Ettelt, S., Perkins, M., Williams, L., Wittenberg, R. & Mays, N. (2023). Facilitators of, and barriers to, personalisation in care homes in England: Evidence from Care Quality Commission inspection reports. *Policy Press*, 7(1). https://doi.org/10.1332/239788221X16426133095792

Ebenau, A. F. (2023). Exploring the spiritual dimension and life values of people with severe illness: Towards an inclusive and person-centered approach to care. Dissertation, Radboud University. https://repository.ubn.ru.nl/handle/2066/286390

Fleishman, J., Kamsky, H. & Sundborg, S. (2019). Trauma-informed nursing practice. *Online Journal of Issues in Nursing, 24*(2). https://www.medscape.com/viewarticle/922155_4

Foster, K., Evans, A. & Alexander, L. (2023). Grace under pressure: Mental health nurses' stories of resilience in practice. *International Journal of Mental Health Nursing, 00*,1–9. https://doi.org/10.1111/inm.13130

Giacomazzi, M., Fontana, M. & Camilli Trujillo, C. (2022). Contextualization of critical thinking in sub-Saharan Africa: A systematic integrative review. *Thinking Skills and Creativity, 43*, 100978. https://www.sciencedirect.com/science/article/pii/S1871187121001930

Giuffrida, S., Silano, V., Ramacciati, N., Prandi, C., Baldon, A. & Bianchi, M. (2023). Teaching strategies of clinical reasoning in advanced nursing clinical practice: A scoping review. *Nurse Education in Practice, 67*, 103548. https://www.sciencedirect.com/science/article/pii/S1471595323000100

Health Innovation Network (2017). *What is person-centred care and why is it important?* https://healthinnovationnetwork.com/system/ckeditor_assets/attachments/41/what_is_person-centred_care_and_why_is_it_important.pdf

Hercelinskyj, G. & Alexander, L. (2020). *Mental health nursing: Applying theory to practice.* South Melbourne, VIC: Cengage Learning.

Huang, H., Huang, C., Lin, K., Yu, C. & Cheng, S. (2023). Development and psychometric testing of the clinical reasoning scale among nursing students enrolled in three types of programs in Taiwan. *Journal of Nursing Research, 31*(2), e263. https://doi.org/10.1097/jnr.0000000000000547

Hunter-Jones, P., Sudbury-Riley, L., Al-Abdin, A. & Spence, C. (2023). The contribution of hospitality services to person-centred care: A study of the palliative care service ecosystem. *International Journal of Hospitality Management.* https://doi.org/10.1016/j.ijhm.2022.103424

Karani, R., Fromme, H., Cayea, D., Muller, D., Schwartz, A. & Harris, I. (2014). How medical students learn from residents in the workplace: A qualitative study. *Academic Medicine, 89*(3), 490–6.

Kegl, B., Fekonja, Z., Kmetec, S., McCormack, B. & Mlinar Reljič, N. (2023). 8 elements of person-centred care of older people in primary healthcare: A systematic literature review with thematic analysis. In K. Čuček Trifkovič, M. Lorber, N. Mlinar Reljič & G. Štiglic (eds), *Innovative nursing care: Education and research.* Berlin, Boston: De Gruyter, pp. 103–24. https://doi.org/10.1515/9783110786088-008

Kim, J. M., Kim, N. G. & Lee, E. N. (2022). Emergency room nurses' experiences in person-centred care. *Nursing Reports, 12*(3), 472–81. https://doi.org/10.3390/nursrep12030045

Koharchik, L., Caputi, L., Robb, M. & Culleiton, A. (2015). Fostering clinical reasoning in nursing students. *American Journal of Nursing, 15*(1), 58–61. https://doi.org/10.1097/01.NAJ.0000459638.68657.9b

Kong, E.-H., Kim, H. & Kim, H. (2022). Nursing home staff's perceptions of barriers and needs in implementing person-centred care for people living with dementia: A qualitative study.

Journal of Clinical Nursing, 31, 1896–906. https://doi.org/10.1111/jocn.15729
Levett-Jones, T., Hoffman, K., Dempsey, J., Jeong, S., Noble, D., Norton, C., Roche, J. & Hickey N. (2010). The 'five rights' of clinical reasoning: An educational model to enhance nursing students' ability to identify and manage clinically 'at risk' patients. *Nurse Education Today, 30*(6), 515–20.
Mahanal, S., Zubaidah, S., Sumiati, I., Sari, T. & Ismirawati, N. (2019). RICOSRE: A learning model to develop critical thinking skills for students with different academic abilities. *International Journal of Instruction, 12*(2). https://files.eric.ed.gov/fulltext/EJ1211048.pdf
McEwing, E., Black, T., Zolobczuk, J. & Dursun, U. (2022). Moving beyond the LGBTQIA+ acronym: Toward patient-centered care. *Rehabilitation Nursing, 47*(5), 162–7. https://doi.org/10.1097/RNJ.0000000000000378
Moon, S. & Chang, S. J. (2023). Professional socialization of hospital nurses: A scale development and validation study. *BMC Nursing, 22*, 2. https://doi.org/10.1186/s12912-022-01169-6
Moyle, W., Rickard, C., Chambers, S. K. & Chaboyer, W. (2015). Partnering with patients model of nursing interventions: A first step to a practice theory. *Healthcare, 3*(2), 252–62. https://doi.org/10.3390/healthcare3020252
Mudd, A., Feo, R., Conroy, T. & Kitson, A. (2020). Where and how does fundamental care fit within seminal nursing theories: A narrative review and synthesis of key nursing concepts. *Journal of Clinical Nursing, 29*, 3652–66. https://doi.org/10.1111/jocn.15420
Nursing and Midwifery Board of Australia (NMBA) (2015). *Framework for assessing national competency standards.* Canberra: Nursing and Midwifery Board of Australia.
Nursing and Midwifery Board of Australia (NMBA) (2016). *Registered nurse standards for practice.* Dickson, ACT: Nursing and Midwifery Board of Australia.
Nursing and Midwifery Board of Australia (NMBA) (2018a). *Code of conduct for registered nurses.* Dickson, ACT: Nursing and Midwifery Board of Australia.
Nursing and Midwifery Board of Australia (NMBA) (2018b). *Codes of conduct for nurses and midwives.* Dickson, ACT: Nursing and Midwifery Board of Australia.
Ossenberg, C., Henderson, A. & Mitchell, M. (2020). Adoption of new practice standards in nursing: Revalidation of a tool to measure performance using the Australian registered nurse standards for practice. *Collegian, 27*(4), 352–60.
Ossenberg, C., Mitchell, M., Burmeister, E. & Henderson, A. (2023). Measuring changes in nursing students' workplace performance following feedback encounters: A quasi-experimental study. *Nurse Education Today, 121*, 105683. https://www.sciencedirect.com/science/article/pii/S0260691722004208
Phelan, A., McCormack, B., Dewing, J., Brown, D., Cardiff, S., Cook, N., Dickson, C., Kmetec, S., Lorber, M., Magowan, R., McCance, T., Skovdahl, K., Štiglic, G. & van Lieshout, F. (2020). Review of developments in person-centred healthcare. *International Practice Development Journal.* https://doi.org/10.19043/ipdj.10Suppl2.003
Rathert, C., Williams, E. S., McCaughey, D. & Ishqaidef, G. (2015). Patient perceptions of patient-centred care: Empirical test of a theoretical model. *Health Expectations, 18*, 199–209. https://doi.org/10.1111/hex.12020
Shirazi, F. & Heidari, S. (2019). The relationship between critical thinking skills and learning styles and academic achievement of nursing students. *Journal of Nursing Research, 27*(4), e38. https://doi.org/10.1097/jnr.0000000000000307
Ski, C., Cartledge, S., Foldager, D., Thompson, D., Fredericks, S., Ekman, I. & Hendriks, J. (2023). Integrated care in cardiovascular disease: A statement of the Association of Cardiovascular Nursing and Allied Professions of the European Society of Cardiology, *European Journal of Cardiovascular Nursing*, zvad009. https://doi.org/10.1093/eurjcn/zvad009
Sterling-Fox, C., Smith, J., Gariando, O. & Charles, P. (2020). Nursing skills video selfies: An innovative teaching and learning strategy for undergraduate nursing students to master psychomotor skills. *SAGE Open Nursing, 6*, 1–6. https://doi.org/10.1177/2377960820934090
Tieu, M., Mudd, A., Conroy, T., Pinero de Plaza, A. & Kitson, A. (2022). The trouble with personhood and person-centred care. *Nursing Philosophy, 23*, e12381. https://doi.org/10.1111/nup.12381
Tobiano, G., Marshall, A., Bucknall, T. & Chaboyer, W. (2016). Activities patients and nurses undertake to promote patient participation. *Journal of Nursing Scholarship, 48*(4), 362–70.
Tsang, M., Martin, L., Blissett, S., Gauthier, S., Ahmed, Z., Muhammed, D. & Sibbald, M. (2023). What do clinicians mean by 'good clinical judgment': A qualitative study. *International Medical Education, 2*(1), 1–10. https://doi.org/10.3390/ime2010001
Vaajoki, A., Kvist, T., Kulmala, M. & Tervo-Heikkinen, T. (2023). Systematic education has a positive impact on nurses' evidence-based practice: Intervention study results. *Nurse Education Today, 120*, 105597. https://www.sciencedirect.com/science/article/pii/S0260691722003331
Wijbenga, M., Bovend'Eerdt, T. & Driessen, E. (2019). Physiotherapy students' experiences with clinical reasoning during clinical placements: A qualitative study. *Health Professions Education, 5*(2), 126–35. https://doi.org/10.1016/j.hpe.2018.05.003
Wolf, A., Vella, R. & Fors, A. (2019). The impact of person-centred care on patients' care experiences in relation to educational level after acute coronary syndrome: Secondary outcome analysis of a randomised controlled trial. *European Journal of Cardiovascular Nursing, 18* i(4), 299–308. https://doi.org/10.1177/1474515118821242
Zambon, V. (2021). What to know about gender pronouns. *Medical News Today.* https://www.medicalnewstoday.com/articles/gender-pronouns#definition

PART 2

ASEPTIC NON TOUCH TECHNIQUE

5 HAND HYGIENE

6 PERSONAL PROTECTIVE EQUIPMENT

7 ASEPTIC NON TOUCH TECHNIQUE

8 ASEPTIC/CLINICAL HAND HYGIENE

9 SURGICAL GOWNING AND GLOVING

Note: These notes are summaries of the most important points in the assessments/procedures and are not exhaustive on the subject. References of the materials used to compile the information have been supplied. The student is expected to have learnt the material surrounding each skill as presented in the references. No single reference is complete on each subject.

CHAPTER 5

HAND HYGIENE

INDICATIONS

Contaminated hands of healthcare workers are a primary source of healthcare-associated infections (HCAIs). Hand hygiene is defined as 'the reduction of harmful infectious agents by the application of alcohol-based hand rubs (ABHR) without the addition of water, or by hand washing with plain or medicated/antimicrobial soap and water' (Porritt, 2022). There are three types of hand hygiene techniques:

- routine/social
- aseptic/clinical
- surgical (Australian Commission on Safety and Quality in Health Care [ACSQHC], 2019).

There are two groups of microorganisms found on skin:

- *resident microorganisms*, which rarely cause infection unless introduced into body tissue by trauma or in conjunction with foreign bodies, such as intravenous catheters
- *transient microorganisms*, which include pathogens carried on healthcare workers' hands and are responsible for most HCAIs resulting from cross-infection. Transient organisms are easily removed by effective hand cleansing technique (ACSQHC, 2019).

The National Health and Medical Research Council (NHMRC, 2019, p. 24) emphasises a person-centred approach to hand hygiene and that people have the right to question healthcare workers about their hand hygiene performance. Hand hygiene is the single most important strategy to reduce HCAIs and applies to everyone – staff, recipients of care and their visitors (ACSQHC, 2019; NHMRC, 2019).

See **FIGURE 5.1** for the National Hand Hygiene Initiative five moments for hand hygiene.

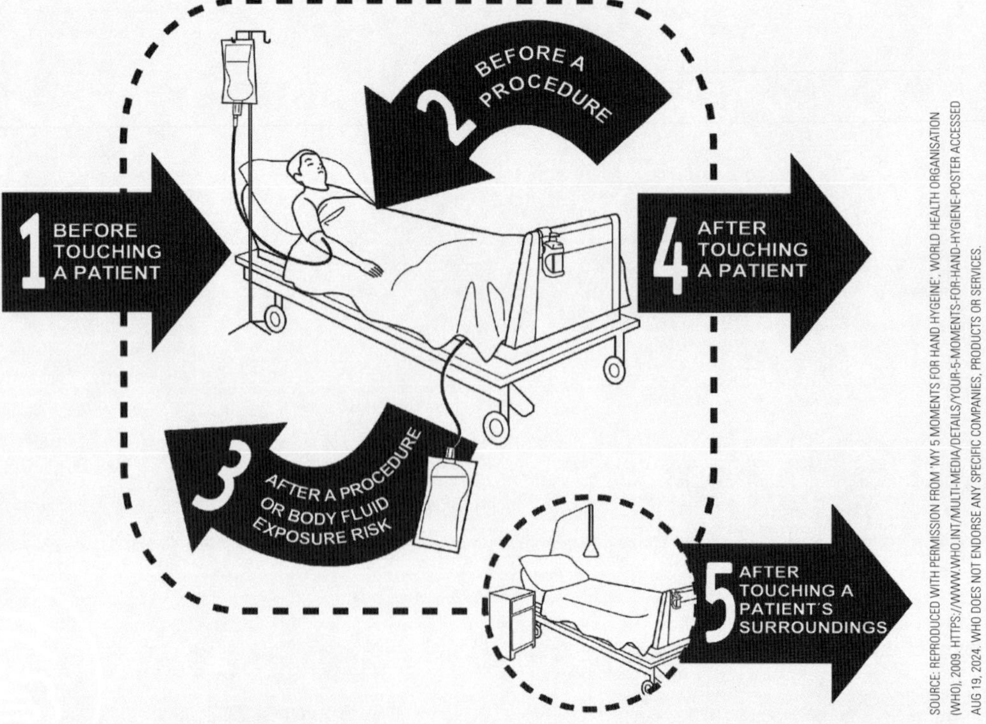

FIGURE 5.1 Five moments for hand hygiene

1 BEFORE TOUCHING A PATIENT	**When:** Clean your hands before touching a patient and their immediate surroundings. **Why :** To protect the patient against acquiring harmful germs from the hands of the HCW.
2 BEFORE A PROCEDURE	**When:** Clean your hands immediately before a procedure. **Why :** To protect the patient from harmful germs (including their own) from entering their body during a procedure.
3 AFTER A PROCEDURE OR BODY FLUID EXPOSURE RISK	**When:** Clean your hands immediately after a procedure or body fluid exposure risk. **Why :** To protect the HCW and the healthcare surroundings from harmful patient germs.
4 AFTER TOUCHING A PATIENT	**When:** Clean your hands after touching a patient and their immediate surroundings. **Why :** To protect the HCW and the healthcare surroundings from harmful patient germs.
5 AFTER TOUCHING A PATIENT'S SURROUNDINGS	**When:** Clean your hands after touching any objects in a patient's surroundings when the patient has not been touched. **Why :** To protect the HCW and the healthcare surroundings from harmful patient germs.

FIGURE 5.1 (Continued)

Washing hands with liquid soaps has minimal effect on antimicrobial activity and is suitable for routine/social hand washing (ACSQHC, 2019; NHMRC, 2019). ABHR is the gold standard of care for all Standard Aseptic Non-Touch Technique (ANTT) procedures in healthcare settings, whereas hand washing is reserved for situations when hands are visibly dirty or contaminated with protein-based material, soiled with blood or other body fluids, or exposed to potential spore-forming organisms or non-enveloped viruses, or after using the bathroom (ACSQHC, 2019; Porritt, 2022). (See **Clinical Skill 7** for ANTT and surgical procedures.)

HAND PREPARATION

Limit the amount of jewellery (e.g. rings, bracelets and wrist watches) worn to work. Be aware of the healthcare facility's hand hygiene, jewellery and dress code policy. Many health facilities have a 'bare below the elbows' policy as jewellery harbours microorganisms in its nooks and crannies and between the jewellery and the skin. Limiting jewellery provides better soap or ABHR solution access and friction to underlying skin. A plain wedding band may be worn but must be moved about on the finger during hand hygiene, enabling the solution and friction to be applied to the metal and the underlying skin to dislodge dirt and microorganisms. Simple bands should be removed in high-risk settings (NHMRC, 2019).

The National Hand Hygiene Initiative does not recommend acrylic nails for those working in clinical areas. Long or artificial nails and nails with chipped or old nail polish harbour four times more microorganisms than unpolished or freshly polished nails (ACSQHC, 2019). Therefore, your nails should be clipped short and nail polish removed.

Inspecting your hands for any lesions allows you to select an appropriate hand hygiene method and dictates further precautions; for example, covering lesions with an occlusive/waterproof dressing.

If personal protective equipment is required, apply this prior to commencing hand hygiene to avoid contaminating clean hands by touching your hair or clothing.

GATHER EQUIPMENT

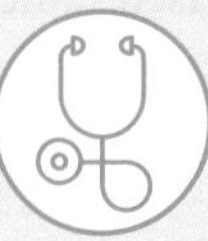

The following equipment is required to wash hands:

EQUIPMENT	EXPLANATION
Warm running water	• Less damaging to your skin than hot water, which opens pores, removes protective oils and causes irritation
Wash area	• The sink should be a convenient height and large enough to minimise splashing, because damp clothing encourages the multiplication and transmission of microorganisms, and wet floors increase the risk of slipping
Soap or an antimicrobial solution	• Used to cleanse your hands. The choice is dictated by the person's condition • Effective hand washing with plain soap removes dirt, soil, various organic substances and loosely adherent transient microorganisms, rendering your hands socially clean and suitable for social contact and most non-invasive clinical care activities (ACSQHC, 2019; Porritt, 2022) • Aseptic/clinical hand hygiene is required for any care activity involving direct or indirect contact with a mucous membrane, non-intact skin or an invasive procedure (ACSQHC, 2019; NHMRC, 2019)
A convenient dispenser (preferably non-hand-operated)	• Increases hand hygiene compliance
Disposable paper towels	• Preferred for drying hands because they prevent the transfer of microorganisms • Ensure you do not contaminate the remaining paper towels, which can lead to cross-infection (Porritt, 2022)

HAND WASHING

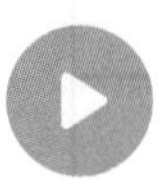
Video

Prepare your hands

Ensure your arms are bare below the elbows, fingernails are short, clean, and free from false nails and nail polish. Cuts and abrasions must be covered with waterproof dressings.

Turn on the water flow

Using the available mechanism (hand, elbow, knee, foot or sensor control), establish a flow of warm water to rinse dirt and microorganisms from your skin and flush these into the sink.

Thoroughly wet hands and apply soap

When wetting hands, do not touch the inside or outside of the sink, which is contaminated; touching it transfers microorganisms onto your hands. As you wash your hands, take care not to contaminate the taps, sink or soap dispenser nozzle with dirt or organic material washed off your hands (Dougherty, Lister & West-Oram, 2015). Wet hands to above the wrists; keeping hands lower than elbows prevents water from flowing onto your arms and later contaminating your clean hands. Apply enough liquid soap or an antimicrobial cleanser to cover all surfaces of your hands; generally, this is 5 mL or the effective amount recommended by the manufacturer – less does not effectively remove microbes, and more than that wastes resources. If only bar soap is available, lather and rinse the bar to remove microbes before starting to wash your hands, and do not put the bar down until there is sufficient lather for the duration of the wash. Lather hands to above the wrists.

Clean under the fingernails

Under the nails is a highly soiled area with high concentrations of transient microbes. Clean debris from under your nails by using the nails of the opposite hand. Cleaning this area under flowing water is most effective for removing debris.

Wash hands with soap or antiseptic solution

Effective hand washing technique takes 40 to 60 seconds and involves three stages: preparation, washing and rinsing, and drying (ACSQHC, 2019). Friction, caused by vigorously rubbing one hand with the other, is effective in dislodging dirt and transient microorganisms. Dirt and microorganisms lodge in skin creases, so pay particular attention to your palms, backs of hands, knuckles, and webs of fingers. Lather and scrub up over wrists and onto your lower forearms to remove dirt and microorganisms from this area. Wrists and forearms are considered less contaminated than hands; scrubbing these after your hands prevents microorganism transmission to a less contaminated area. Wash your hands for 15 to 30 seconds following the sequence in FIGURE 5.2.

Rinse hands

Rinse your forearms, hands and fingers, in this order (Porritt, 2022), under running water to wash transient microorganisms and dirt from the least contaminated area, over a more contaminated area and off into the sink. Rinse well to prevent residual soap from irritating your skin (see FIGURE 5.2).

Note: this sequence differs from aseptic/clinical and surgical scrub requirements for ANTT and surgical procedures.

Dry hands

Using paper towels, pat your fingers, hands and forearms to dry your skin well (see FIGURE 5.2). Damp hands are a source of microbial growth and transmission, and contribute to chapping and hand lesions developing.

Turn off taps

To turn off hand-manipulated taps, use dry paper towels, taking care not to contaminate hands on the sink or taps (see FIGURE 5.2). Carefully discard paper towels so that your hands are not contaminated.

Turn off other types of taps with a foot, knee or elbow as appropriate.

ALCOHOL-BASED HAND RUB

Hand hygiene using a waterless alcohol-based hand rub (ABHR) is more effective against most bacteria and many viruses than using liquid or antimicrobial soap. However, if your hands are visibly soiled they must be washed with soap and water (ACSQHC, 2019; NHMRC, 2019; Porritt, 2022). ABHR is not effective against *Clostridium difficile* and non-enveloped viruses such as norovirus, will not remove dirt and some organic material, and is not effective in some outbreak situations (ACSQHC, 2019; Porritt, 2022).

Although ABHR is more expensive than soap or antiseptic hand-washing solutions, it has been demonstrated to save time, increase compliance and reduce infections (Porritt, 2022). Alcohol-based hand rubs should be routinely used for hand hygiene, in combination with washing with soap/antiseptic agents and water (Porritt, 2022).

Apply the solution to dry, visibly clean hands and rub vigorously over all hand and finger surfaces for 20 to 30 seconds, until your hands are thoroughly dry. Pay attention to palms, back of the hands, finger webs, knuckles and wrists as you would while hand washing. Apply ABHR to hands following the sequence in FIGURE 5.3.

MAINTAINING HAND HEALTH

Part of hand hygiene is maintaining healthy and intact skin. Moisturising your hands contributes to healthy skin (Johal, 2022) by restoring moisture and oils removed by repeated use of soap or ABHR solutions. Applying emollients compatible with the facility's ABHR or antiseptic soap ensures no reduction in their effectiveness. You should apply moisturiser a minimum of three times per shift to reduce chapping and drying. Applying the lotion prior to tea and meal breaks and when going off-duty is a good routine.

Remember that many people in healthcare facilities are bed-bound and unable to perform hand hygiene. Offering ABHR or soap with a water basin and a towel to people unable to independently attend to hand hygiene before meals, visiting hours, or before settling for the night or after they use a bed pan/urinal allows the person to maintain their hand hygiene and reduces their infection risk.

Duration of the entire procedure: 40–60 seconds

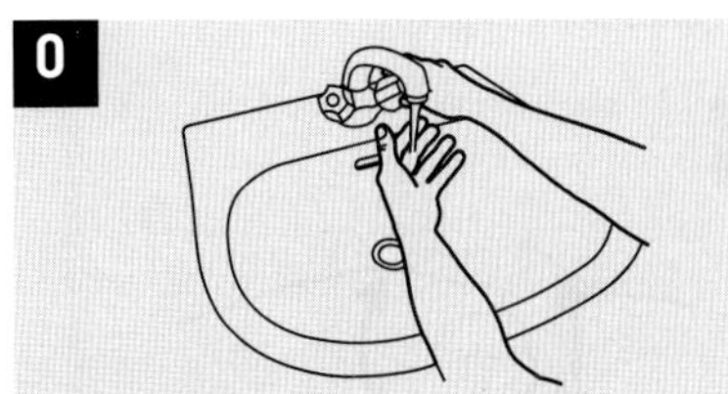

Wet hands with water

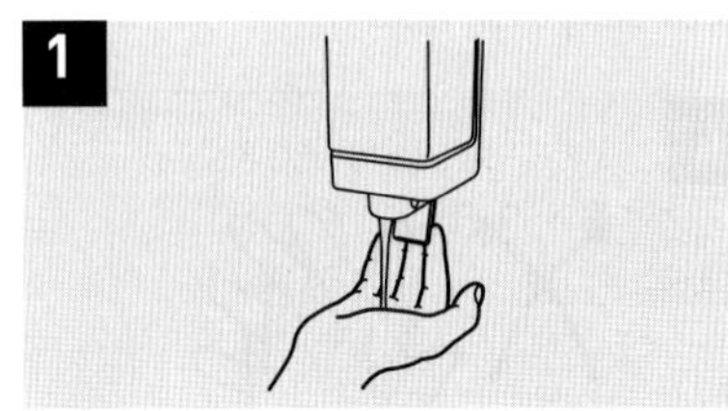

Apply enough soap to cover all hand surfaces

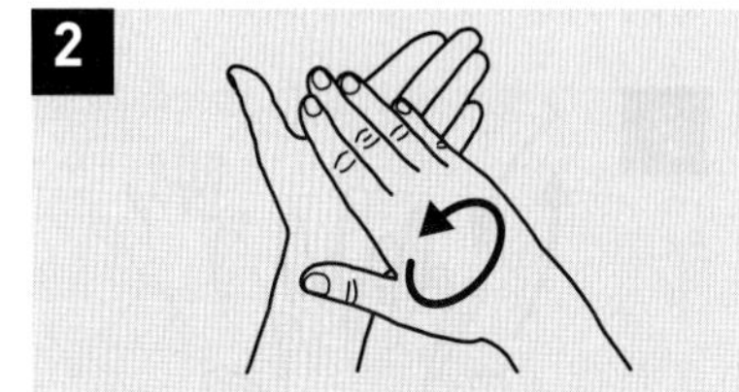

Rub hands palm to palm

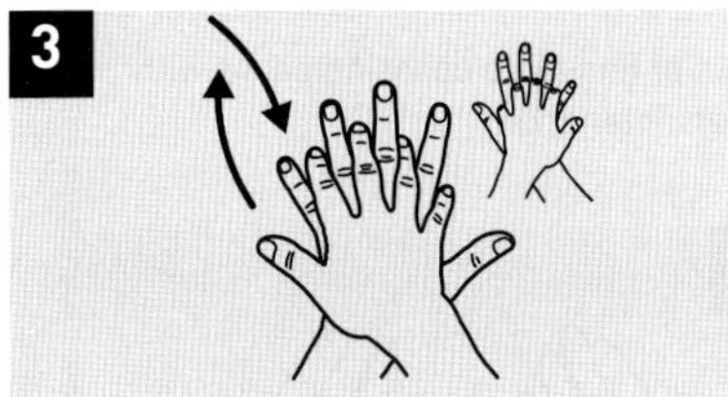

Right palm over left dorsum with interlaced fingers and vice versa

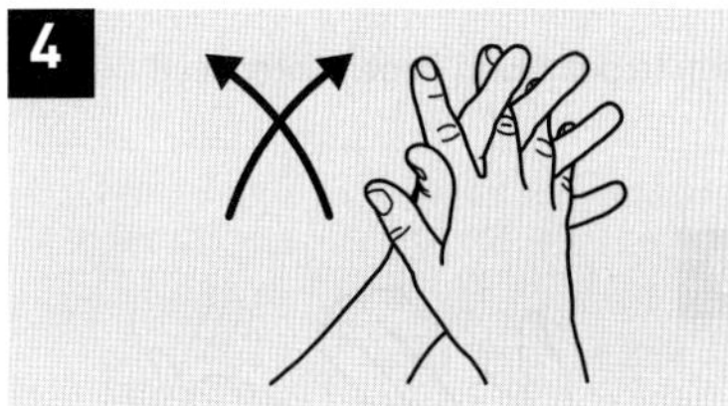

Palm to palm with fingers interlaced

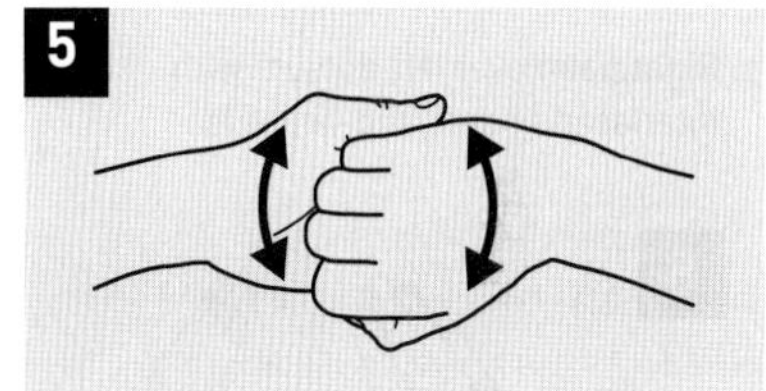

Backs of fingers to opposing palms with fingers interlocked

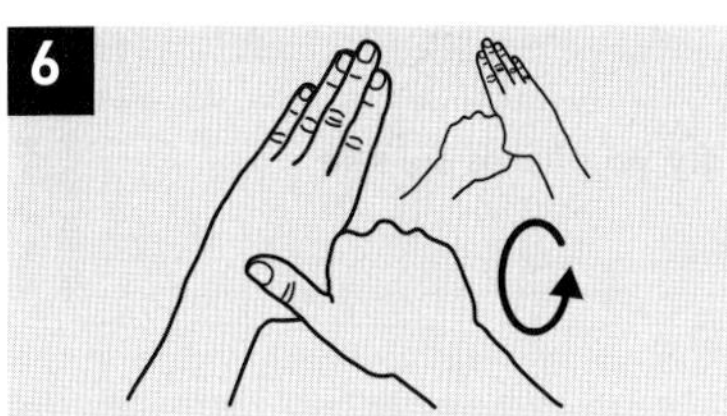

Rotational rubbing of left thumb clasped in right palm and vice versa

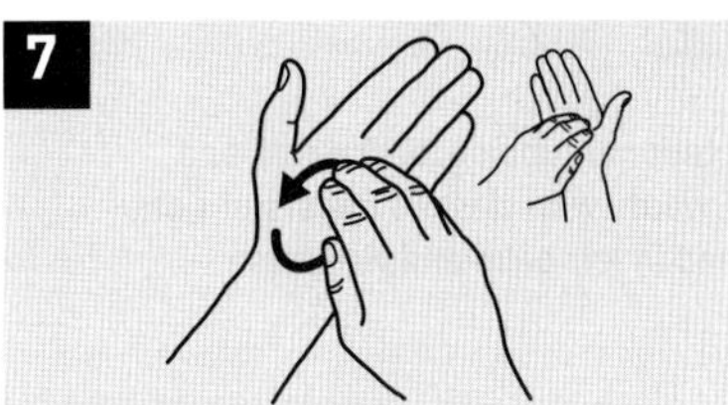

Rotational rubbing, backwards and forwards with clasped fingers of right hand in left palm and vice versa

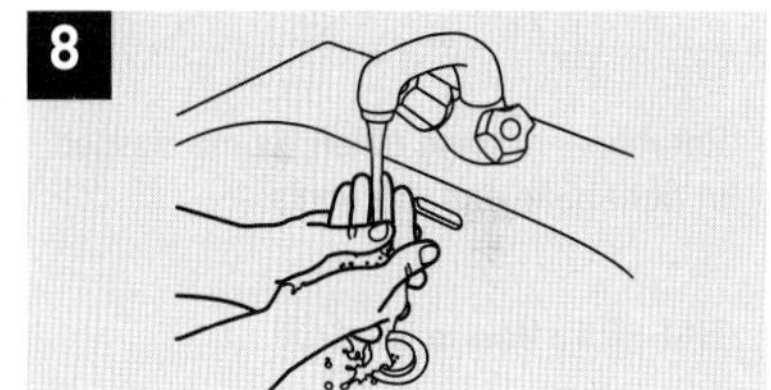

Rinse hands with water

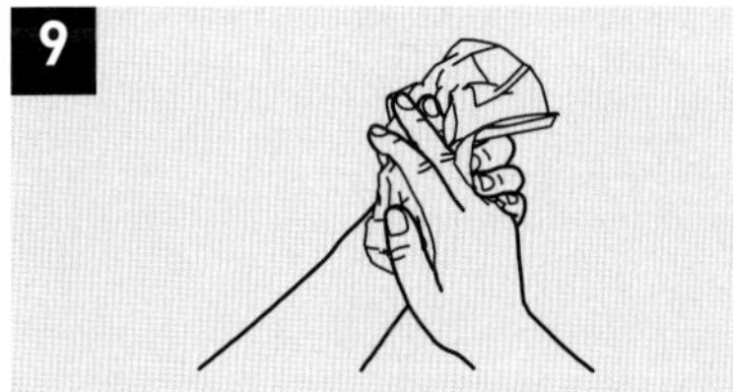

Dry hands thoroughly with a single use towel

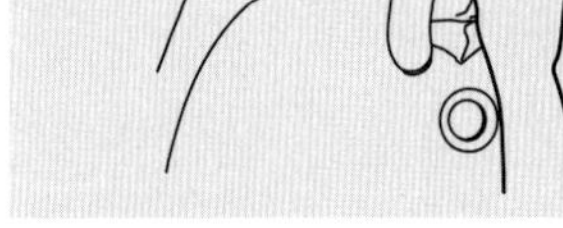

Use towel to turn off tap

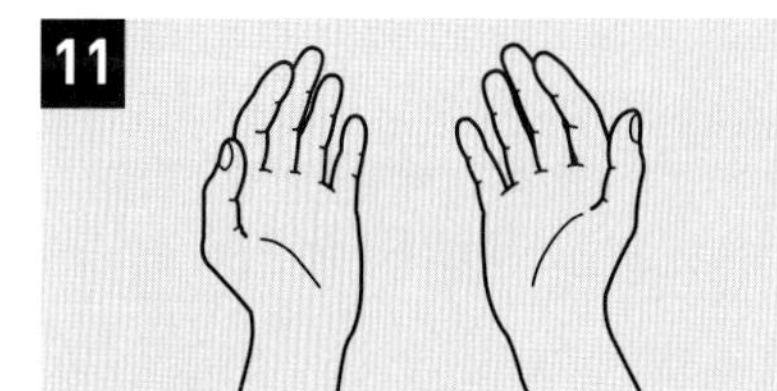

Your hands are now safe

FIGURE 5.2 How to hand wash

Duration of the entire procedure: 20–30 seconds

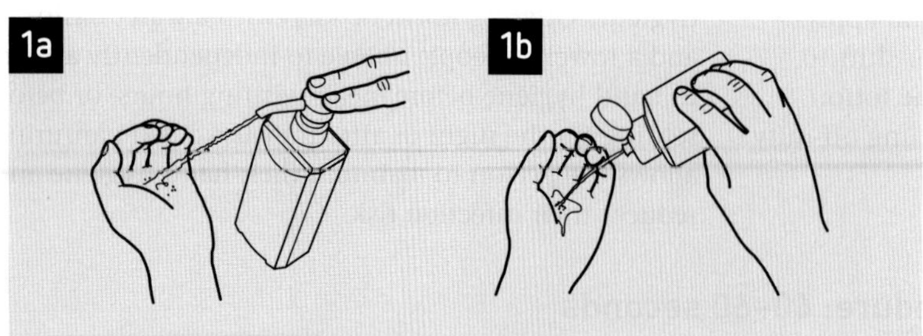

Apply a palmful of the product in a cupped hand, covering all surfaces

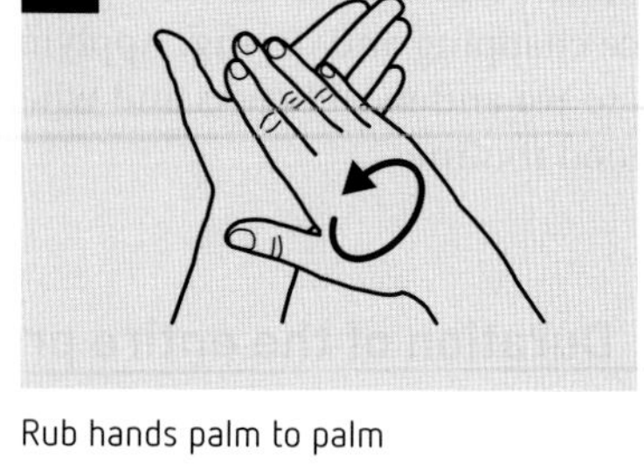

Rub hands palm to palm

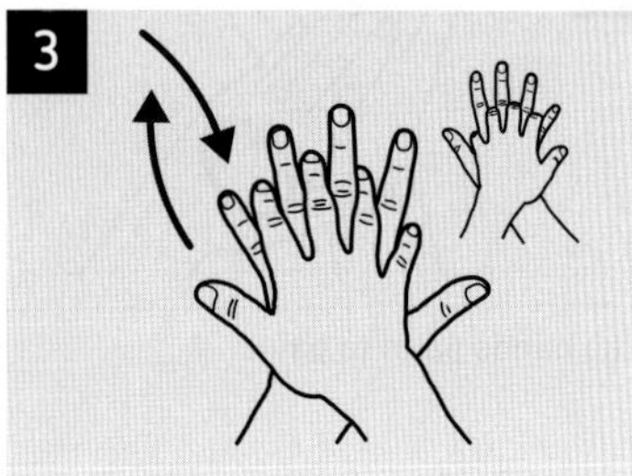

Right palm over left dorsum with interlaced fingers and vice versa

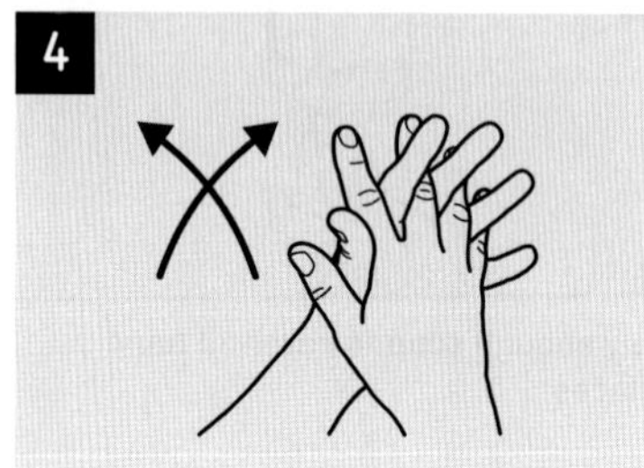

Palm to palm with fingers interlaced

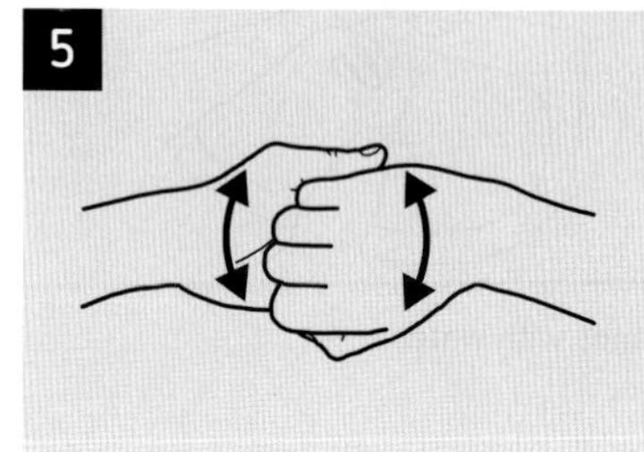

Backs of fingers to opposing palms with fingers interlocked

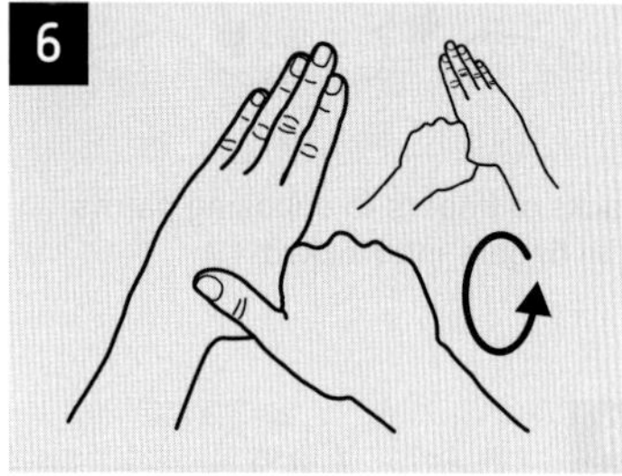

Rotational rubbing of left thumb clasped in right palm and vice versa

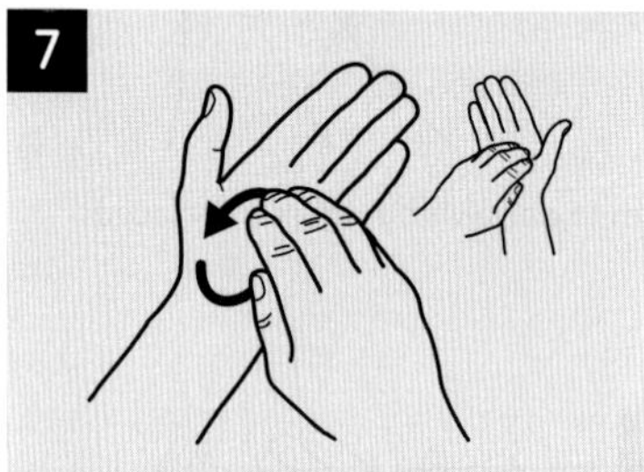

Rotational rubbing, backwards and forwards with clasped fingers of right hand in left palm and vice versa

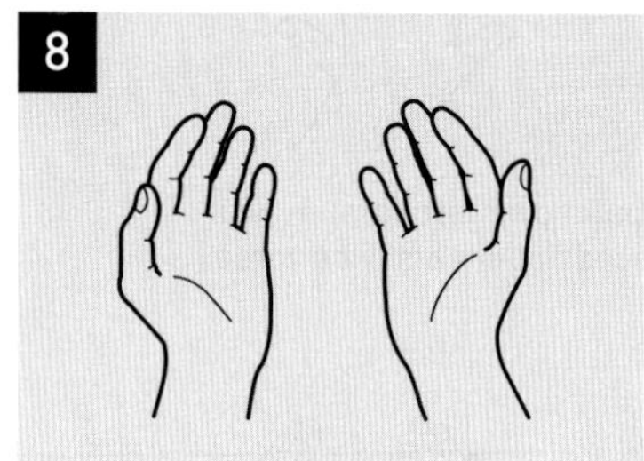

Once dry, your hands are safe

FIGURE 5.3 How to hand rub

SOURCE: REPRODUCED FROM 'HOW TO HANDRUB?', WORLD HEALTH ORGANIZATION, COPYRIGHT 2009, HTTP://WWW.WHO.INT/GPSC/5MAY/HOW_TO_HANDRUB_POSTER.PDF?UA=1, ACCESSED 25/05/21.

CLINICAL SKILLS ASSESSMENT

Hand hygiene

Demonstrates the ability to effectively reduce infection risk by performing social hand wash or hand rub. Incorporates the *National Safety and Quality Health Service Standards*: 2 Partnering with Consumers, 3 Preventing and Controlling Healthcare-Associated Infection, 5 Comprehensive Care, 6 Communicating for Safety, and 8 Recognising and Responding to Acute Deterioration (ACSQHC, 2021).

Performance criteria	1	2	3	4	5
(Numbers indicate NMBA *Registered Nurse Standards for Practice*)	(Dependent)	(Marginal)	(Assisted)	(Supervised)	(Independent)
1. Identifies the indication (1.1, 1.4, 3.5)	☐	☐	☐	☐	☐
2. Identifies National Hand Hygiene Initiative five moments for hand hygiene (1.1, 6.2)	☐	☐	☐	☐	☐
3. Undertakes hand preparation (1.1, 6.2), e.g. bare below the elbows, skin intact, no rashes, cuts or abrasions; no acrylic/artificial nails; natural nails are clean and manicured	☐	☐	☐	☐	☐
4. Gathers equipment (1.1, 6.2): ■ warm running water ■ soap or an antimicrobial solution ■ a convenient dispenser (preferably non-hand-operated) ■ disposable paper towels	☐	☐	☐	☐	☐
5a. Turns on and adjusts water flow (1.1, 6.2)	☐	☐	☐	☐	☐
5b. Wets hands, applies enough appropriate liquid to cover all hand surfaces (1.1, 6.2)	☐	☐	☐	☐	☐
5c. Cleans under fingernails (1.1, 6.2)	☐	☐	☐	☐	☐
5d. Thoroughly washes hands by rubbing hands together vigorously, distributing solution over palms, back of hands, between fingers and wrists as per sequence in **FIGURE 5.2** (1.1, 6.2)	☐	☐	☐	☐	☐
5e. Rinses hands thoroughly under running water, allowing water to drip from fingertips (1.1, 6.2)	☐	☐	☐	☐	☐
5f. Dries fingers, hands and forearms (1.1, 6.2)	☐	☐	☐	☐	☐
5g. Turns off the water without contaminating hands (1.1, 6.2)	☐	☐	☐	☐	☐
ABHR application 6a. Applies appropriate amount of solution into cupped hands ensuring all hand surfaces covered (1.1, 6.2)	☐	☐	☐	☐	☐
6b. Rolls hands distributing solution over palms, back of hands, between fingers, and wrists (1.1, 6.2). Follows sequence in **FIGURE 5.3**	☐	☐	☐	☐	☐
7. Rubs hands together until all surfaces are dry (1.1, 6.1)	☐	☐	☐	☐	☐
8. Demonstrates ability to incorporate theory into clinical practice (1.1, 1.2, 6.2)	☐	☐	☐	☐	☐

Student:

Clinical facilitator: Date:

CHAPTER 6

PERSONAL PROTECTIVE EQUIPMENT

INDICATIONS

Personal protective equipment (PPE) is anything used or worn to minimise health or safety risks, including face masks, goggles, gloves and aprons. PPE is worn to prevent microorganism transmission (e.g. SARS-CoV-2) from a reservoir to a susceptible host, such as from healthcare workers to recipients of care or family and friends, and vice versa. PPE also prevents spray or splash injuries from chemicals and hazardous medications. PPE is an integral component of standard and transmission-based precautions in healthcare facilities. Preventable healthcare-associated infections (HCAIs) increase a person's pain; may result in lifelong disabilities or death; extend length of stays, reducing available bed access; and increase health systems' economic burden (Australian Commission on Safety and Quality in Health Care [ACSQHC], 2021; Magtoto, 2023; National Health and Medical Research Council [NHMRC], 2019). Preventing and controlling HCAIs is Standard 3 of the *National Safety and Quality Health Service Standards*, aiming to stop people from acquiring preventable HCAIs and to effectively manage these infections using evidence-based strategies (ACSQHC, 2021).

Using PPE singly or in combination interrupts transmission of contaminated material, contamination of sterile materials (e.g. when preparing medications, intravenous fluids) and exposure of mucous membranes, eyes, broken skin, or clothing to another person's bodily secretions, blood, excretions or hazardous substances. You need a sound understanding of the modes of microorganism transmission for effective infection prevention and control measures. Additionally, you need to be aware of the occupational requirements for safe handling of hazardous medications and chemicals. Your decision to use PPE should be based on an assessment of risks associated with the person and the care activity you are undertaking, or the potential for contamination from microorganisms or hazardous chemicals.

EVIDENCE OF THERAPEUTIC INTERACTION

Incorporating a person-centred approach to practice and enabling people to actively participate in their care process is more than just explaining treatment risks. It requires considering and incorporating the person's needs at every level (McCormack & McCance, 2016). Before putting on PPE, explain to the person that these are routine aspects of infection prevention and control strategies used for everyone's safety (NHMRC, 2019). Wearing PPE could indicate to the person that they are 'dirty' and are being treated differently to others. People should be familiarised with the facility's infection prevention and control strategies and informed of their specific requirements. The person and visitors should be encouraged to minimise infection risks by following hand and respiratory hygiene practices, and be provided with necessary information and instructions to be able to adhere to these. People must be informed of their right to ask healthcare professionals if hand hygiene was performed and whether PPE should be used.

GATHER EQUIPMENT

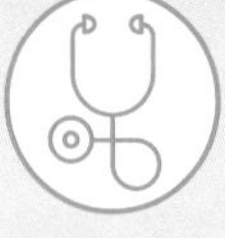

Gather the equipment before you initiate the care activity. PPE used as part of standard precautions includes aprons, gowns, gloves, surgical masks, protective eyewear and face shields (NHMRC, 2019). PPE selection is based on risk assessment of:

- transmission of infectious microorganisms
- contamination of your clothing or skin or that of other people by blood, body substances, secretions or excretions
- the facility's policies and current health and safety legislation (NHMRC, 2019, p. 46).

Gowns and aprons

Gowns or aprons are recommended PPE for procedures or care activities when close contact with the person, materials or equipment leads to contamination of your skin, uniform or other clothing with infectious agents or hazardous medications or chemicals (NHMRC, 2019). The apron or gown type required depends on the risk, the anticipated contact with infectious material and the potential for blood, body substances or hazardous materials to penetrate through to your clothes or skin. Appropriate gowns or aprons need to be worn for a single procedure or care episode and removed where the care episode took place. The following table provides a summary of apron and gown types, characteristics and considerations for appropriate selection.

EQUIPMENT	EXPLANATION
Plastic apron	• Single-use • Plastic • Impervious to liquids • Disposable • Protects your uniform from contamination by droplets or sprayed substances • Worn when there is a low risk that clothing or your arms will be exposed to blood or body substances (generally environmental) during low-risk procedures • Worn during contact precautions when contact with the person or their environment is likely
Gowns	• Single-use • Disposable • Worn to protect your skin and clothing from blood, body substances (except sweat), secretions or excretions during procedures or care activities associated with splashing or sprays of blood or body substances • Worn when there is close contact with the person, when equipment or materials may contaminate your skin or uniform, or to protect the person from the microbes you carry

Long-sleeved gown (full body gown)	• Single-use
	• Fluid-resistant
	• Long-sleeved, closed-fronted and elastic/knit-closed cuffs (under which gloves are tucked); worn:
	  • during procedures or care activities during which there will be contact between your skin and a person's broken skin
	  • during extensive skin-to-skin contact (e.g. repositioning a person with extensive burns)
	  • during contact with or splashing from uncontained blood or body substances (vomiting, uncontrolled diarrhoea)
	  • when there is a risk of exposure to large amounts of body substances during an operative procedure
	  • when handling cytotoxic agents

Sterile gown	• Sterile prepackaged gowns • Worn for procedures requiring aseptic fields

SOURCES: S. MARIN (2020). *APRONS, GOWNS, FACE MASKS AND EYE PROTECTION.* ADELAIDE, SA: JOANNA BRIGGS INSTITUTE; NHMRC (2019). *AUSTRALIAN GUIDELINES FOR THE PREVENTION AND CONTROL OF INFECTION IN HEALTHCARE.* COMMONWEALTH OF AUSTRALIA.

Face and eye protection

Face and eye protection includes goggles or safety glasses (with side protection), surgical masks or full-face shields. These are required when there is a risk of airborne, droplet or spray contamination of your mucous membranes (eyes, nose and mouth) or non-intact skin surfaces, which are entry portals for microorganisms. Face and eye protection is required to prevent splashes, spray or dust from cytotoxic medications or hazardous chemicals (Marin, 2020). The ties, earpieces and headbands securing face and eye protection are considered 'clean'. These are safe to touch with bare hands (NHMRC, 2019).

Masks are worn once and discarded promptly when damp or soiled, or when the procedure is completed. Do not leave your mask dangling around your neck.

The following table provides a summary of face and eye protection.

EQUIPMENT	CHARACTERISTICS	REQUIRED FOR
Goggles and safety glasses	• Rigid plastic • Usually reusable	• Procedures involving the respiratory tract or those generating splashes and sprays (NHMRC, 2019)
Surgical masks	• Loose-fitting items protecting your mouth and nose • Pleated face • Two to three polypropylene layers • Filtration via mechanical impaction • Fluid-resistant • Ties at crown and bottom of head	• Procedures requiring surgical ANTT to protect the person from exposure to infectious microorganisms carried in your nose or mouth • Routine care of people requiring droplet precautions (NHMRC, 2019)
Face shields	• Extend from the chin to the crown • Provide better protection of your face and eyes from splashes and sprays than wrap-around style, as the sides reduce splashes around the shield's edges (NHMRC, 2019)	• Procedures generating splashes or sprays of large blood droplets, body substances, secretions, excretions, or hazardous medications or chemicals

EQUIPMENT	CHARACTERISTICS	REQUIRED FOR
P2 respirators (N95)	• Raised dome or duckbill • Four to five layers (polypropylene outer, charged polypropylene centre) • Sturdier than and fit better than surgical masks (NHMRC, 2019) • Offering greater protection against airborne and droplet infection as well as from contact from splashes and sprays • Filtration via mechanical impaction and electrostatic capture • Ties at crown and bottom of head, pliable metal nose bridge • Fit testing and fit checking required	• Routine care of people requiring airborne precautions • Bronchoscopy or other high-risk procedures in a person of unknown infectious status • Procedures involving particle aerosolisation containing specific pathogens

SOURCE: ADAPTED FROM NHMRC (2019). *AUSTRALIAN GUIDELINES FOR THE PREVENTION AND CONTROL OF INFECTION IN HEALTHCARE*. COMMONWEALTH OF AUSTRALIA.

The following table provides a summary of face and eye protection usage requirements.

PROCEDURE OR CARE ACTIVITIES	CLINICAL EXAMPLES	REQUIRED FACE AND EYE PROTECTION
Routine care	• Assessing vital signs • Physical assessment	• Not required unless caring for a person on droplet precautions (surgical mask) or airborne precautions (P2 respirator)
Procedures generating splashes or sprays	• Emptying wound or urinary drainage bag, bed pans or urinals • Administering intravenous cytotoxic medications	• Surgical mask • Protective eyewear/full-length face shield
Procedures involving respiratory tract and mouth	• Intubation • Nasopharyngeal suctioning	• Protective eyewear • Surgical mask or, if required, P2 respirator

SOURCE: NHMRC (2019). *AUSTRALIAN GUIDELINES FOR THE PREVENTION AND CONTROL OF INFECTION IN HEALTHCARE*. COMMONWEALTH OF AUSTRALIA

Gloves

Glove use plays a key role in reducing microorganism transmission between the person and you, and vice versa. Gloves also assist in preventing your skin from being exposed to chemicals and hazardous medications (Marin, 2020). As with all PPE, which gloves are used is determined by risk assessment of the procedure or care activity, contamination type, whether an aseptic or clean technique is required, and if you or the person has a latex allergy (Marin, 2020). Gloves should also be fit for purpose and avoid interference with your dexterity, and not cause friction, excessive sweating, or finger and hand muscle fatigue (NHMRC, 2019).

Non-sterile gloves should remain in their original box until needed to maintain their integrity (Marin, 2020). Keeping gloves in your pocket contaminates the gloves from your hands or pocket debris. Put gloves on immediately before undertaking a procedure and remove them immediately after completing it. Discard gloves into a contaminated waste bin. Gloves are changed after each care episode and between individuals. Ensure you perform effective hand hygiene before putting on gloves and immediately after you remove your gloves (ACSQHC, 2019). Remember: wearing gloves is no substitute for effective hand hygiene (ACSQHC, 2019; NHMRC, 2019).

The following table provides a summary of glove types and clinical examples of their use.

EQUIPMENT	REQUIRED FOR	CLINICAL EXAMPLES
Non-sterile gloves	• Potential exposure to blood, body substances, secretions or excretions • Contact with non-intact skin or mucous membranes	• Emptying urinary drainage bags • Nasogastric aspiration • Vaginal examinations • Management of minor cuts or abrasions
Sterile gloves	• Potential exposure to blood, body substances, secretions or excretions • Contact with susceptible sites or clinical devices requiring that sterile conditions be maintained	• Surgical Aseptic Non Touch Technique complex dressings • Dressing changes for central venous line insertion sites • Clinical care of acute surgical wounds and drainage sites
Synthetic gloves, e.g. nitrile or polyvinyl chloride (PVC)	• Procedures involving a high risk of exposure to blood-borne viruses or where high barrier protection is required	• Preparing or administering cytotoxic medications

SOURCES: ACSQHC (2019). *NATIONAL HAND HYGIENE INITIATIVE MANUAL*; NHMRC (2019). *AUSTRALIAN GUIDELINES FOR THE PREVENTION AND CONTROL OF INFECTION IN HEALTHCARE*. COMMONWEALTH OF AUSTRALIA; WHITEHORN (2020). *CYTOTOXIC AGENTS: SAFE HANDLING AND ADMINISTRATION* [EVIDENCE SUMMARY]. ADELAIDE, SA: JOANNA BRIGGS INSTITUTE.

Sharps containers

Sharps containers are important in reducing risks from sharp devices. There are a number of devices available designed to eliminate sharps injuries (e.g. needleless and retractable safety devices); however, many procedures require sharp instruments. When sharps are used, handling must be minimised – instruments rather than fingers are used to grasp sharps when possible; use of neutral zones such as basins for scalpel transfer; disposable needles should not be bent, broken or recapped after use. The person using a disposable sharp instrument is responsible for its safe management and immediate disposal after use (NHMRC, 2019). All used disposable sharps (e.g. blades, needles, catheter stylets and glass vials) must be placed into clearly labelled, puncture-proof, leakproof and untippable point-of-use containers to minimise sharps injury or contamination (Valdez, 2022).

PUT ON AND REMOVE PERSONAL PROTECTIVE EQUIPMENT

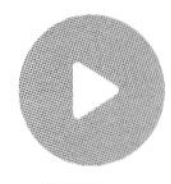
Video

To minimise the risk of transmitting microorganisms, the NHMRC (2019, pp. 123–4) recommends the following sequence for safely and effectively putting on PPE (see TABLE 6.1) and removing PPE (see TABLE 6.2).

Hand hygiene

Hand hygiene must be performed before putting on PPE and after removing PPE (ACSQHC, 2019; NHMRC, 2019). Perform appropriate hand hygiene (see **Clinical Skill 5**). Put on PPE before contact with the person, and generally before entering the person's room (NHMRC, 2019).

Put on personal protective equipment (donning)

Remove all personal items (e.g. watches, pens). PPE is donned prior to entering at the PPE station or outside the person's room, or in the anteroom (if airborne precautions in use).

TABLE 6.1 Putting on PPE

Aprons • Place over your head and fasten the ties behind your back **Gowns** • Pick up and hold out by the neckline in front of you and allow to unfold (without being contaminated by body or substances) • Slide your arms and hands into the sleeves • Fully cover your body from neck to knees, arms to end of wrists, and wrap around the back • Fasten at the back of your neck and waist	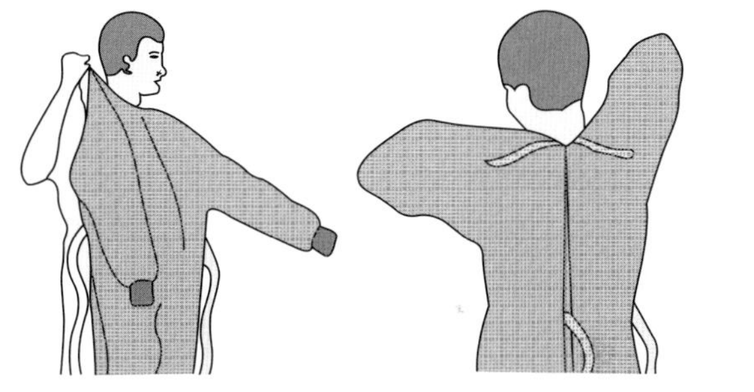
Masks or face shields Don the correct mask **Droplet:** Surgical mask for people with suspected or confirmed pneumonia, and clinically well • Hold upper ties, and place over your nose and mouth. Upper ties are tied at the back of your head or strung over your ears and tied under your chin • Lower ties are tied at the nape of your neck or the top of your head to secure a firm fit over your face. Smooth aluminium strip over your nose • If you wear glasses, fit your mask under your glasses to reduce clouding from exhalation **Airborne:** N95/P2 mask (fit check required) for clinically ill people with suspected or confirmed pneumonia and/or requiring aerosol-generating procedures **Fitting an N95/P2 respirator** N95/P2 are available in different designs – please review the specific fitting guidelines • Position respirator over mouth and nose • Position tapes above and below ears at back of head • Using the adjustors, fit snugly at bridge of nose and under chin	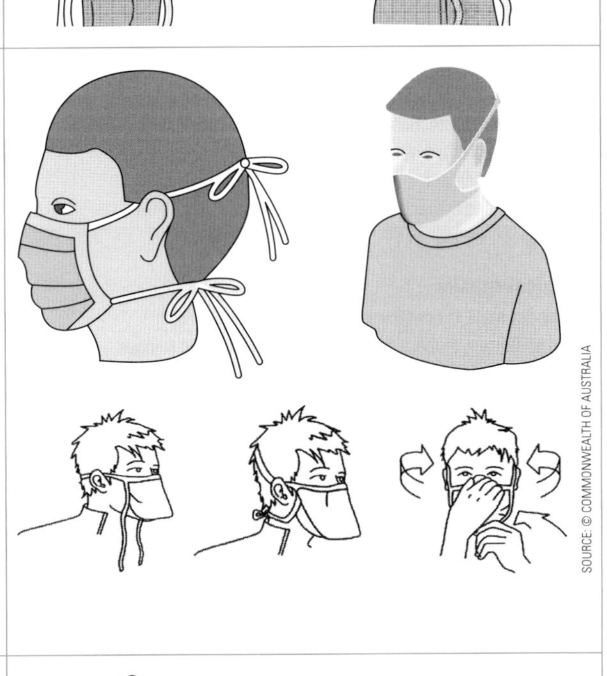
Protective eyewear (goggles or safety glasses, face shields) • Place over your eyes and face, and adjust to fit your face (and over glasses) comfortably	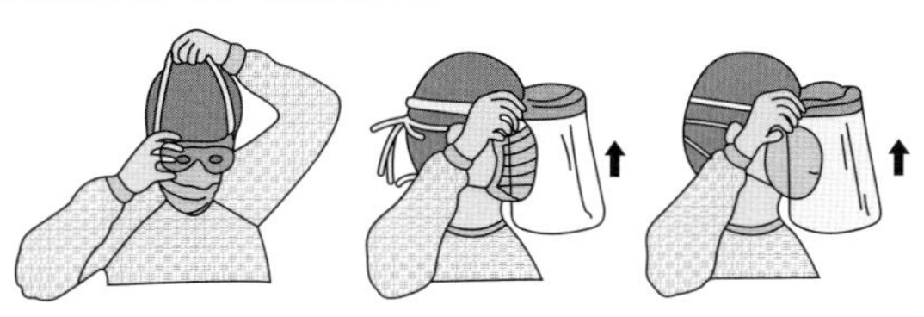

TABLE 6.1 (Continued)

Gloves (clean) • If wearing a gown, pull the gloves up over the cuffs • If no gown, extend gloves to protect your wrists (see **Clinical Skill 9** for putting on sterile gloves)	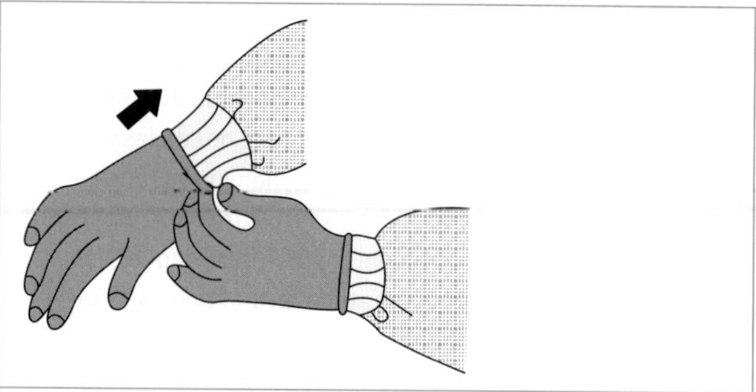

SOURCES: ACSQHC (2019). *NATIONAL HAND HYGIENE INITIATIVE MANUAL*; NHMRC (2019). *AUSTRALIAN GUIDELINES FOR THE PREVENTION AND CONTROL OF INFECTION IN HEALTHCARE*. COMMONWEALTH OF AUSTRALIA.

TABLE 6.2 Removing PPE

Step 1 **Gloves** • Outside of gloves is contaminated • Grasp outside of glove with opposite gloved hand; peel glove off this hand • Keep removed glove in gloved hand • Slide fingers of your ungloved hand under the wrist of remaining glove; peel it off over your first glove • Discard glove bundle into contaminated waste bin • Perform hand hygiene by washing hands or using ABHR	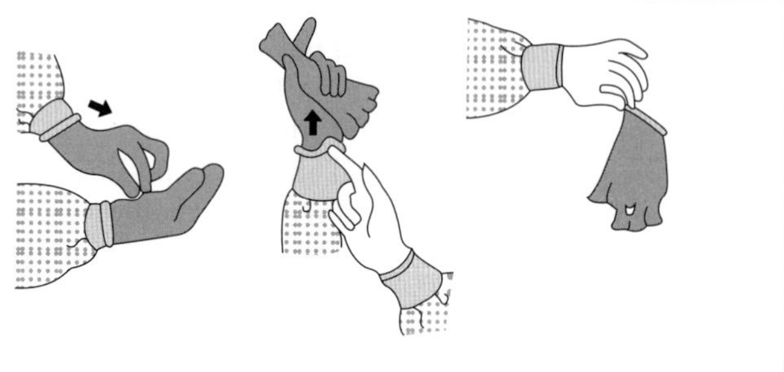
Step 2 **Apron or gown** • Apron front or gown front and sleeves are contaminated • Unfasten ties • Pull gown away from your neck and shoulders, only touching the inside of apron or gown • Turn apron or gown inside out • Fold or roll into bundle • Discard apron or single-use gown into contaminated waste bin • Place cloth gowns into appropriate linen skip • Alternatively, gloves and gown can be removed as one step • Perform hand hygiene by washing hands or using ABHR	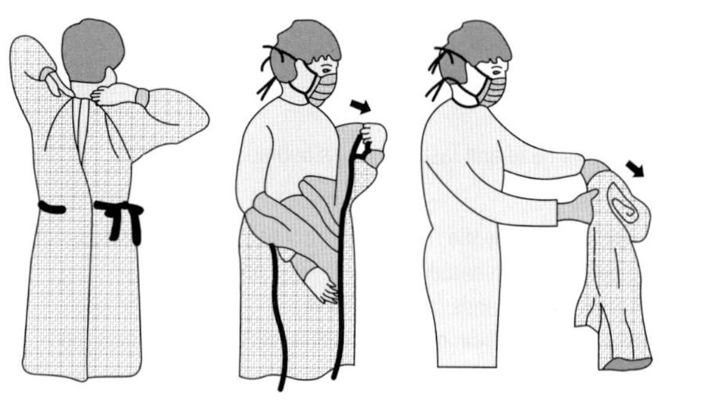
Step 3 **Protective eyewear or face shield** • Outside of eye protection or face shield is contaminated • Remove eye protection by touching only headband or earpieces • Discard single-use items into the contaminated waste bin • Place reusable items into cleansing container • Perform hand hygiene by washing hands or using ABHR	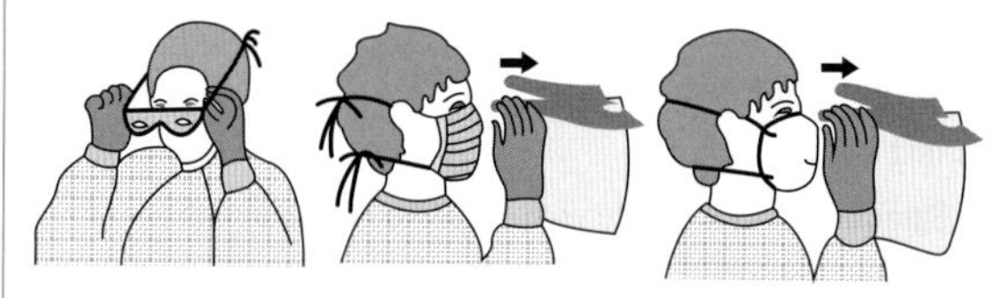
Step 4 **Surgical masks** • Front of mask is contaminated – do not touch • Grasp bottom of mask, then top ties or elastic and remove • Discard mask into contaminated waste bin **P2 respirator** • Perform hand hygiene • Step outside room or into anteroom before removing • With clean hands, grasp tapes at the back of head and remove by only handling the tapes • Discard mask into appropriate closed container • Perform hand hygiene by washing hands or using ABHR • If exiting an anteroom, hand hygiene must be attended to after exiting	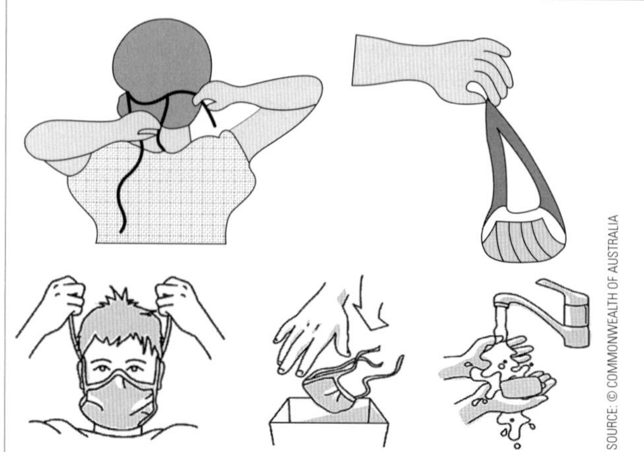 SOURCE: © COMMONWEALTH OF AUSTRALIA

SOURCES: ACSQHC (2019). *NATIONAL HAND HYGIENE INITIATIVE MANUAL*; NHMRC (2019). AUSTRALIAN GUIDELINES FOR THE PREVENTION AND CONTROL OF INFECTION IN HEALTHCARE. COMMONWEALTH OF AUSTRALIA.

If door handles or curtains are touched when entering a room, gloves are to be removed, hand hygiene performed, and new gloves donned.

During a care episode, ensure gloves are removed, hand hygiene performed, and new gloves donned as per the five moments for hand hygiene principles.

If you are contaminated during care procedures, PPE must be changed as per the donning and doffing sequence.

Remove personal protective equipment (doffing)

PPE is designed to be used once and must be removed when a specific procedure or care activity is completed. This prevents other sites, people or the environment being contaminated.

PPE is removed at a designated doffing area or anteroom if airborne precautions are in use.

CLEAN, REPLACE AND DISPOSE OF EQUIPMENT

Dispose of single-use safety equipment in the contaminated-waste receptacle in the dirty utility room. Non-disposable items such as goggles or face shields will require cleaning according to the manufacturer's instructions and the facility's policy. The front of face shields and goggles is considered contaminated and should not be touched with bare hands. Generally, cleansing with a mild detergent and warm water, and drying well prior to replacing the equipment is sufficient. If there is gross contamination or contaminating material is infectious, disinfection using an instrument-grade disinfectant is required (NHMRC, 2019, p. 51). Hand hygiene is performed as the final infection prevention and control measure when cleaning is completed.

CLINICAL SKILLS ASSESSMENT

Personal protective equipment

Demonstrates the ability to assess and select appropriate personal protective equipment (PPE) for risks associated with the procedure or care activity and utilises PPE to prevent transmission of microorganisms transmitted by contact, droplet or airborne modes, or to prevent injury from hazardous medications or chemicals. Incorporates the *National Safety and Quality Health Service Standards*: 2 Partnering with Consumers, 3 Preventing and Controlling Healthcare-Associated Infection, 5 Comprehensive Care, 6 Communicating for Safety, and 8 Recognising and Responding to Acute Deterioration (ACSQHC, 2021).

Performance criteria	1	2	3	4	5
(Numbers indicate NMBA *Registered Nurse Standards for Practice*)	(Dependent)	(Marginal)	(Assisted)	(Supervised)	(Independent)
1. Identifies the indication (1.1, 1.4, 3.5)	☐	☐	☐	☐	☐
2. Evidence of therapeutic interaction with the person, carers or visitors (1.2, 2.1, 2.2, 2.9, 6.1)	☐	☐	☐	☐	☐
3. Demonstrates clinical reasoning abilities, such as risk assessment and obtaining PPE prior to performing hand hygiene (1.1, 1.4)	☐	☐	☐	☐	☐
4. Identifies and gathers appropriate PPE (1.1, 1.2, 1.4): ■ plastic apron ■ gowns ■ long-sleeved gown (full body gown) ■ sterile gown ■ goggles and safety glasses ■ surgical masks ■ face shield ■ P2 respirator (N95) ■ non-sterile gloves ■ sterile gloves ■ synthetic gloves, e.g. nitrile or polyvinyl chloride (PVC) ■ sharps container	☐	☐	☐	☐	☐
5. Performs hand hygiene (1.1, 6.1)	☐	☐	☐	☐	☐
6. Safely and effectively puts on, uses and removes PPE (6.1)	☐	☐	☐	☐	☐
7. Cleans, replaces and disposes of equipment appropriately (1.1, 3.6, 6.1)	☐	☐	☐	☐	☐
8. Demonstrates the ability to link theory to practice (1.1, 3.3, 3.4, 3.5)	☐	☐	☐	☐	☐

Student:

Clinical facilitator: Date:

CHAPTER 7

ASEPTIC NON TOUCH TECHNIQUE

INDICATIONS

Surgical Aseptic Non Touch Technique (ANTT) or Standard ANTT is used when preparing for and undertaking any invasive procedure penetrating the body's natural defence of intact skin and mucous membrane. ANTT principles incorporate the following:

- sterile objects remain sterile only when touched by another sterile object
- only sterile objects may be placed in an aseptic field
- sterile objects or aseptic fields become contaminated by prolonged exposure to air
- sterile objects or aseptic fields should be kept in view
- a sterile surface coming in contact with a wet contaminated surface becomes contaminated by capillary action
- fluid flows in the direction of gravity or by capillary action
- the edges of an aseptic field are considered contaminated
- skin cannot be made sterile; however, washing reduces the number of microorganisms on it
- sterile gloves are used to further prevent transfer of microorganisms
- conversation should be minimised to reduce the spread of droplets
- sterile objects opened for one person can only be used for that person
- unused sterile supplies are discarded or resterilised if these are to be used for another person (Australian College of Operating Room Nurses [ACORN], 2023; Marin & Valdez, 2023).

These principles are similar to and compatible with standard and transmission-based precautions recommended by the National Health and Medical Research Council (NHMRC) (2019). Conscientiousness, alertness and honesty are essential qualities in maintaining asepsis. Unless these principles and guidelines are strictly followed, safety is compromised and infection may occur. You must assess people for whom you are caring for risks associated with the procedure and use the appropriate ANTT and protective barriers (Marin & Valdez, 2023; NHMRC, 2019; Rowley & Clare, 2019).

The following is a general guideline for Surgical ANTT (e.g. dressing change or catheterisation) conducted in a non-operating theatre environment.

BACKGROUND TO ASEPTIC NON TOUCH TECHNIQUE

Aseptic Non Touch Technique (ANTT®) is a specific type of aseptic technique with a unique theory and practice framework (Rowley & Clare, 2019). ANTT protects individuals during invasive clinical procedures by utilising infection-prevention measures to minimise the introduction of sufficient quantities of microorganisms to cause an infection by hands into susceptible sites, surfaces or equipment (Marin & Valdez, 2023; NHMRC, 2019). Preventing and controlling healthcare-associated infections (HCAIs) is Standard 3 of the *National Safety and Quality Health Service Standards*, aiming to stop people from acquiring preventable HCAIs and to effectively manage these infections using evidence-based strategies (Australian Commission on Safety and Quality in Health Care [ACSQHC], 2021).

ANTT is the recommended standardised aseptic technique adopted within Australian healthcare facilities (NHMRC, 2019). It uses a concept called key-part and key-site protection to achieve asepsis by identifying and then protecting procedure key-parts and key-sites from contamination. This is achieved by:

1. appropriate and effective hand hygiene
2. maintaining Non Touch Technique (NTT)
3. using new sterilised equipment
4. disinfecting existing key-parts to a standard rendering these aseptic before use (NHMRC, 2019).

Although based on the same principles, in practice the type of ANTT is determined according to risk assessment of the procedure (Marin & Valdez, 2023; NHMRC, 2019; Rowley & Clare, 2019).

Aseptic fields provide the vital controlled aseptic working space that is necessary to maintain asepsis during clinical procedures. In ANTT, the types of aseptic fields utilised depend on whether Standard or

Surgical ANTT is being used. Larger, sterile drape-type aseptic fields are termed *critical aseptic fields* and are used in surgical ANTT when key-parts and/or key-sites (usually due to their size or number) cannot be easily protected with individual covers or caps, or be handled at all times by NTT. These include insertion of peripherally inserted central cannula (PICC) lines, complex wound care and in operating theatres. This approach demands more sterilised equipment, sterile gloves, and other barriers, such as gowns (Marin & Valdez, 2023; Rowley & Clare, 2019). *Critical micro aseptic fields* involve covering or protecting key-parts with syringe caps, sheaths, covers or packaging. The cap and covers inside are sterile, providing optimal aseptic fields for key-parts. Used along with NTT, these provide an aseptic field for key-parts and contribute to a *general aseptic field*, promoting asepsis.

The core infection-control components of ANTT are summarised below:

- *Key-part and key-site identification and protection* – determine the key-part (e.g. the equipment part, dressing or cleansing material) that comes into contact with the susceptible key-site (the person's vulnerable site, such as incisions or open wounds). Key-part protection means that only these areas come into contact with other key-parts or the key-site. A vital aspect of maintaining asepsis is the use of NTT on the key-part. For example, where the key-site is an incision, it is only touched by an aseptically clean key-part: sterilised gauze squares dampened with sterile normal saline using sterilised forceps.
- *Non Touch Technique (NTT)* – not touching key-parts directly by using sterile instruments, dressings or solutions.
- *Hand hygiene* – an essential ANTT component (see **Clinical Skills 5 and 8**).
- *Sterile gloves* – used if it is necessary to directly touch any key-parts or key-sites. If not, *non-sterile gloves* are usually used. Your risk assessment determines whether you can perform the procedure and maintain asepsis without touching either the key-part or the key-site and contaminating it. Complex procedures are usually more difficult, and inexperience often dictates the need for sterile gloves rather than non-sterile gloves, or the use of additional barrier precautions. Rowley et al. (2010) originated two types of ANTT as follows:

1. *Standard ANTT* procedures generally require less than 20 minutes and are technically simple clinical procedures involving relatively few and small key-sites and key-parts (see FIGURE 7.1). These require a main general aseptic field and non-sterile gloves, using critical micro aseptic fields and NTT to protect key-parts and key-sites. Examples include intravenous (IV) therapy, simple wound dressing and, for experienced health professionals, urinary catheterisation or IV cannulation. Less-experienced healthcare workers, however, may require a critical aseptic field (NHMRC, 2019).
2. *Surgical ANTT* procedures are technically complex, require more than 20 minutes to complete, and involve large open key-sites, or large or numerous key-parts. Surgical ANTT procedures require critical aseptic fields, sterile gloves and full-barrier precautions (see FIGURE 7.1). Surgical ANTT procedures continue to utilise critical micro aseptic fields and NTT when practical to do so (NHMRC, 2019). Examples include complex dressings, insertion of central venous catheters (CVC) and surgery.

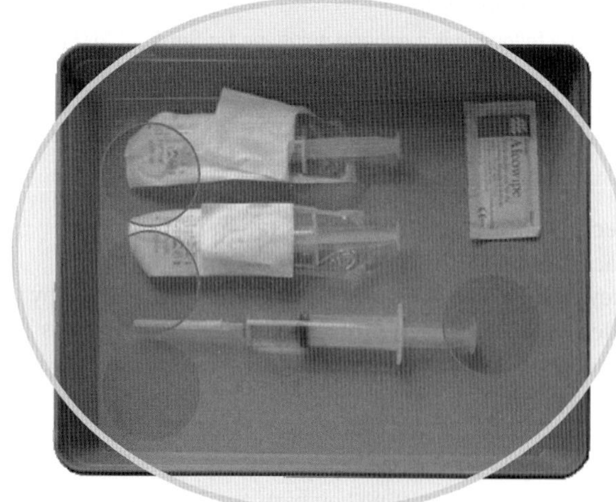

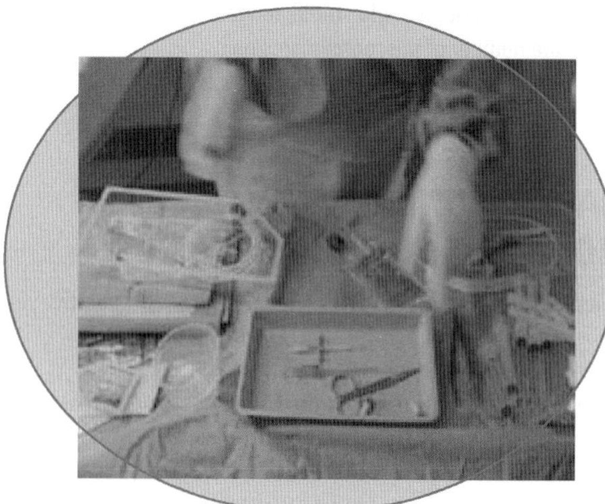

SOURCE: © ASEPTIC NON TOUCH TECHNIQUE (ANTT)

FIGURE 7.1 Use of Standard and Surgical ANTT

EVIDENCE OF THERAPEUTIC INTERACTION

Introduce yourself and advise the person of your designation. Confirm the person's identity. Inform the person about the procedure and obtain their verbal consent to proceed. Clarify their immediate concerns regarding the procedure. Discuss with the person the most comfortable position for them during the procedure and their expectations of the procedure. Including the person in their care incorporates Standard 2 (Partnering with Consumers), Standard 5 (Comprehensive Care) and Standard 6 (Communicating for Safety) of the *National Safety and Quality Health Service Standards* (ACSQHC, 2021). By explaining how the person can assist you, you enable them to actively participate in their care and reduce the risk they will touch or contaminate sterile items, and will also reduce the need to talk during the procedure.

DEMONSTRATE CLINICAL REASONING

Environment control

Before conducting an aseptic procedure, you need to ensure that there are no avoidable risk factors, such as bed making or people using commodes (NHMRC, 2019).

Position the person

Consider the person's position in relation to the duration of the procedure, and the location of the treatment site. Positioning the person comfortably reduces or eliminates movement during the procedure, reduces their discomfort and avoids unnecessary contamination of items. Ensure that you administer the required analgesia approximately 30 minutes before the procedure. Anticipate toileting requirements and attend to these before you position the person or set up the critical aseptic field. Maintain privacy to enhance the person's comfort and dignity.

PERFORM ASEPTIC NON TOUCH TECHNIQUE

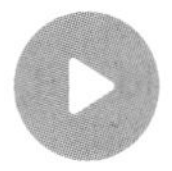
Video

Hand hygiene

This should be performed using an alcohol-based rub or another surgical hand wash prior to performing ANTT as your hands will have been contaminated by touching the packaging while adding sterile items to the critical aseptic field (Marin & Valdez, 2023). Depending on the facility's policy or your risk assessment, you may need sterile gloves and other personal protective equipment (Rowley & Clare, 2019) (see **Clinical Skills 6 and 9**).

Confirm the sterility of the packages and solution

Inspect items to confirm that they remain sterile. The colour-change sterility indicator should indicate that the package is sterile, the item should be within its use-by date and the packaging must be dry and intact, with no water damage or stains, and bottles must be unopened. Tears and punctures create a pathway for microorganisms to access the interior of the packaging. Stains, dampness and water damage indicate that the wrapping has been wet, allowing microorganisms to enter the package by capillary action. A broken seal on a bottle indicates that the contents have been exposed to the air and have possibly been contaminated.

GATHER EQUIPMENT

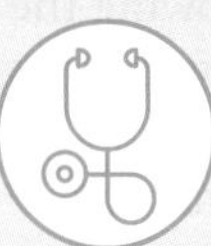

The equipment required depends on the procedure and the facility's procedural guidelines. Planning the procedure and having all equipment ready for use beforehand are part of an effective time-management strategy and reduce the amount of time that the critical aseptic field will be exposed to the air. A critical aseptic field left unattended is considered to be contaminated.

EQUIPMENT	EXPLANATION
A trolley	• Collect and clean with the facility's recommended solution to establish a clean (not sterile) work surface • Removing much of the microbial load from the trolley surfaces helps to prevent cross-contamination
Dressing equipment	• Gather dressing equipment while the trolley dries, to save time and eliminate microorganism transfer via moisture • Place the dressing pack on the top shelf and all other unopened plastic-, paper- and cloth-wrapped items and required personal protective equipment on the trolley's bottom shelf, leaving the top surface as clean as possible for the aseptic procedure (Peters, 2017)
A plastic bag	• Attach a plastic bag large enough to collect used materials to the side of the trolley closest to the person, which avoids contaminated material being brought over the critical aseptic field • Open the mouth of the bag wide enough so that material can easily be dropped into the bag, preventing contamination of forceps or gloves

Perform hand hygiene. Take the trolley and all items required for the procedure to the person's bedside.

Prepare the critical aseptic field

Initially, remove the outer plastic wrap (in pre-packaged supplies) and drop the inner, sterile, still-wrapped tray package (e.g. dressing or catheter tray) on the trolley's top surface. With the initial folded flap facing you, touch only the wrapper's outside surface to maintain the sterility of the inner surface. Using your thumb and forefinger, grasp the flap and fold out, away from you, which eliminates reaching over the exposed sterile contents and contaminating these.

To avoid reaching over sterile content, carefully using your right hand for the right-side flap and your left hand for the left-side flap, fold out the sides. Finally, the last flap is folded towards you to form a critical aseptic field. Adjustments of the critical aseptic field's position are made from underneath the outside surface of the wrapper. The main critical aseptic field for sterile items (dressing tray, catheter tray, dressings) is formed 5 cm inside the border edges.

Add sterile supplies

Stand back from the established critical aseptic field while opening all packages to avoid contaminants from the outside of the packaging material falling onto the field. Ensure that only sterile items come into contact with your critical aseptic field.

Open sterile packages

Grasp the opposite edges of the two sides of the wrapper and carefully peel them down to fully expose the item (gauze squares, instruments, IV catheters). Without reaching across the critical aseptic field or touching non-sterile wrappings on the critical aseptic field, drop the item from the wrapper onto the critical aseptic field, avoiding the 5 cm border edges. Dropping sterile items from about 15 cm avoids packaging material or your hand touching the critical aseptic field. Alternatively, after you open the package and fold back the packaging sides, hold the package in one hand. Carefully pick up the top forceps by the handle with your other hand, using the forceps to position the sterile item within your critical aseptic field. Remember that the forceps tips and body remain sterile; this section is placed within the critical aseptic field, ensuring the forceps handle section you touched is within the 5 cm non-sterile edge of your critical aseptic field.

Unwrap hospital-wrapped items

Hold the item in your non-dominant hand and open the top flap away from you. Remove the sterilisation tape and, using your dominant hand, open the flap away from you, folding the corners well back from the item. Take care not to touch the wrapper's contents as you carefully and fully expose the item by folding the side and front flaps away from the contents. Grasp the wrapper's loose corner material and secure it at your wrist with your dominant hand (to keep the unsterile wrapping material from inadvertently contaminating the critical aseptic field) before carefully dropping the item onto the critical aseptic field.

Open the solution bottles

Generally, there is a container within the basic dressing pack available for solutions. Read the label three times – before you place the bottle on the trolley, before you pour the solution into the container, and before you replace it on the trolley's bottom shelf – to ensure that the correct solution is used. Break the bottle's seal and remove the cap. Either keep the cap in one hand or place the cap on a clean surface, inside up. Check the label and then cover it with your palm to prevent inadvertent splashes or dribbles obscuring the writing. Hold the bottle approximately 5 cm directly above the container to prevent accidentally touching the critical aseptic field and pour slowly to prevent splashes contaminating the field by facilitating microorganism movement through the drape. Some facilities consider previously opened bottles to remain sterile for 24 to 48 hours, after which the contents must be discarded. If this is the case, recap the bottle immediately without touching the inside of the lid to maintain sterility. Write a time and date clearly on the label and initial it. To reuse, cleanse the bottle's lip by pouring a small amount of the contents into a sink or plastic bin prior to pouring the solution into the sterile container on the critical aseptic field.

Manipulate sterile items

Rearrange sterile items on the critical aseptic field with the sterile forceps included in the commercial dressing tray. These are a different colour and are the most easily accessible of the forceps. As some sterile trays do not include extra forceps, add one with the other sterile supplies. After all additional items have been placed on the critical aseptic field, carefully pick up the forceps, touching nothing else. Following the principles of asepsis, use the forceps to conveniently manipulate the items on the field. If the forceps are used for anything wet, keep the tip lower than your wrist to prevent liquid from running down the forceps by gravity and then back to the tips, making the forceps unsterile. When the items are organised to your satisfaction, discard the forceps either into the disposal bag (if plastic) or on the bottom shelf of the trolley (if metal). If you are wearing sterile gloves, you can manipulate the items on the field directly with your fingers.

Perform the required procedure using Aseptic Non Touch Technique

Perform the required procedure using Surgical ANTT. Following the procedure, ensure the person is comfortable. Any articles or possessions moved during the procedure should be replaced within the person's reach.

CLEAN, REPLACE AND DISPOSE OF EQUIPMENT

Contaminated disposables should be wrapped in the disposable wrapper and placed in the plastic bag. This material is then placed in the clinical waste bin in the dirty utility room.

Clean the trolley with the recommended solution. If the trolley is grossly contaminated or contaminated with infectious material, disinfect it using an instrument-grade disinfectant (NHMRC, 2019). Return the cleaned trolley to the unit's service area. Put reusable solutions in front of unopened solutions to ensure that these are used, to avoid waste.

Clean and place non-disposable items in the appropriate container in the dirty utility room to be returned to the central sterile services department (CSSD) for resterilisation. Place non-disposable linens in the appropriate linen skip for return to the laundry. Perform hand hygiene as the final infection prevention and control measure once the cleaning has been completed.

DOCUMENTATION

ANTT is a process used to perform procedures and generally does not require documentation. There are some procedures that require documentation, for which it should be noted that ANTT was performed during that procedure.

CLINICAL SKILLS ASSESSMENT

Aseptic Non Touch Technique

Demonstrates the ability to effectively and safely establish and maintain a critical aseptic field incorporating Aseptic Non Touch Technique (ANTT) principles. Incorporates the *National Safety and Quality Health Service Standards*: 2 Partnering with Consumers, 3 Preventing and Controlling Healthcare-Associated Infection, 5 Comprehensive Care, 6 Communicating for Safety, and 8 Recognising and Responding to Acute Deterioration (ACSQHC, 2021).

Performance criteria	1	2	3	4	5
(Numbers indicate NMBA *Registered Nurse Standards for Practice*)	(Dependent)	(Marginal)	(Assisted)	(Supervised)	(Independent)
1. Identifies indication (1.1, 3.3, 3.4)	☐	☐	☐	☐	☐
2. Evidence of therapeutic interaction with person, e.g. informs person about procedure, obtains verbal consent and gives explanation (1.4, 1.5, 2.1, 2.2, 3.2)	☐	☐	☐	☐	☐
3. Demonstrates clinical reasoning abilities, e.g. performs risk assessment to identify appropriate ANTT, positions the person (1.1, 1.2, 1.3, 4.1, 4.2, 6.1)	☐	☐	☐	☐	☐
4. Gathers equipment (1.1, 5.5, 6.1) ■ cleaned trolley ■ dressing equipment ■ plastic bag	☐	☐	☐	☐	☐
5. Performs hand hygiene (1.1, 3.4, 6.1)	☐	☐	☐	☐	☐
6. Confirms the sterility of all items (1.1, 6.1)	☐	☐	☐	☐	☐
7. Opens the tray/package (1.1, 6.1)	☐	☐	☐	☐	☐
8. Adds necessary sterile supplies without contaminating critical aseptic field or items (1.1, 6.1)	☐	☐	☐	☐	☐
9. Manipulates sterile items without contaminating critical aseptic field or items or self (1.1, 6.1)	☐	☐	☐	☐	☐
10. Performs required procedure incorporating Surgical ANTT principles (1.1, 6.1)	☐	☐	☐	☐	☐
11. Cleans, replaces and disposes of equipment appropriately (1.1, 3.6, 6.1)	☐	☐	☐	☐	☐
12. Ensures person's comfort and safety following procedure (1.1, 6.1)	☐	☐	☐	☐	☐
13. Demonstrates the ability to link theory to practice (1.1, 3.3, 3.4, 3.5)	☐	☐	☐	☐	☐

Student:

Clinical facilitator: Date:

CHAPTER 8

ASEPTIC/CLINICAL HAND HYGIENE

INDICATIONS

Aseptic/clinical hand hygiene is done to remove as many transient microorganisms as possible from your arms and hands, and to limit the growth of resident microorganisms by leaving an antimicrobial residue on your skin (Australian Commission on Safety and Quality in Health Care [ACSQHC], 2019; National Health and Medical Research Council [NHMRC], 2019). Clinical hand hygiene is undertaken prior to any care activity involving direct or indirect contact with a person's mucous membrane, non-intact skin or an invasive medical device, to limit microorganism transmission (NHMRC, 2019).

Surgical hand wash or scrubbing is undertaken to remove transient microorganisms from hands before undertaking invasive procedures, and also aims to inhibit further microorganisms growth for several hours (ACSQHC, 2019; Marin & Mbinji, 2022). Surgical hand washes are done before procedures in operating theatres or birthing suites, and before complex procedures. The Australian College of Operating Room Nurses (ACORN) *Standards for Safe and Quality Care in the Perioperative Environment (SSQCPE) for Individuals* (2023) advocate a five-minute scrub time for your first scrub of the day and a three-minute scrub time for subsequent scrubs.

The following is a guide, as each facility has procedural guidelines for clinical hand hygiene and surgical hand washing. Review the facility procedural guidelines to determine the scrub time required.

Preventing and controlling healthcare-associated infections is Standard 3 of the *National Safety and Quality Health Service Standards*, aiming to stop people from acquiring preventable healthcare-associated infections (HCAIs) and to effectively manage these infections using evidence-based strategies (ACSQHC, 2021).

DEMONSTRATE CLINICAL REASONING

Hand hygiene effectiveness is improved when your skin is intact; your nails are natural, short and unvarnished; your hands and forearms are free from jewellery; and your sleeves are above the elbows (ACORN, 2023; ACSQHC, 2021; NHMRC, 2019; World Health Organization [WHO], 2009). Adjust clothing to expose your upper arms, which prevents your clothing from getting wet or interfering with effective hand hygiene. Tucking in any loose clothing at your waist reduces the risk of inadvertently contaminating your hands. Securely tying back your hair ensures it does not become loose and contaminate your critical field (ACORN, 2023).

> ? If you have cuts or abrasions, these need to be covered with appropriate dressings.

Before commencing your surgical hand wash, prepare your gown pack and gloves so these can be donned immediately. Place them appropriately close to the scrub sink. Use Aseptic Non Touch Technique (ANTT) to open both packs to expose the towel and the gown in the pack. Use this towel to dry your hands. If required, put on appropriate personal protective equipment and your scrub cap. Ensure that all your hair is covered, because hair is a source of microbial contamination.

PERFORM ASEPTIC/CLINICAL HAND HYGIENE

Aseptic/clinical hand hygiene

Wash hands thoroughly using the facility's antimicrobial soap for one minute using the technique outlined for routine/social hand hygiene in **Clinical Skill 5**. A reduction of transient and resident flora is effectively accomplished with an antiseptic liquid soap preparation (ACSQHC, 2021). Rinse carefully.

Do not touch taps with clean hands. Avoid contaminating your hand by using paper towels to turn taps off if elbow or foot controls are unavailable.

GATHER EQUIPMENT

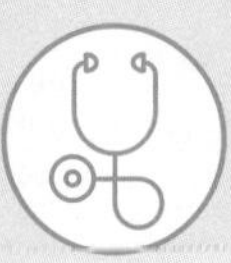

Gather items and take them to a scrub sink with running hand-hot water. Once you have commenced your clinical hand hygiene or surgical hand wash, touching unsterile items causes contamination, so you will need to begin the procedure again.

EQUIPMENT	EXPLANATION
Antimicrobial wash solution	• Surgical scrubbing with chlorhexidine gluconate is the most effective aqueous scrub • The WHO (2009) emphasises important differences between routine or social hand hygiene and surgical hand preparation, which must reduce the resident flora, eliminate transient microorganisms and also inhibit bacteria growth under gloved hands
Sterile scrub sponge and nail cleaner	• Supplied in a sealed pack, which should be opened using ANTT and left in an easy-to-reach space • Some sponges are impregnated with an antimicrobial solution or Betadine solution, others have no antimicrobial properties • Some are a combination of sponge and brush for nails while others are just sponges
Sterile hand towel	• Generally situated on top of the gown in the gown pack • Use a sterile towel pack if gown packs are unavailable. Use ANTT to expose the towel, which allows it to be picked up without contaminating your hands or the gown

Using clean paper towels, pat your hands dry. A study by Suen et al. (2019) examining the hygienic efficacy of different hand-drying methods found that paper towels dry hands efficiently, remove bacteria effectively and cause less cross-contamination associated with jet air dryer use. The study recommended hand drying in hospital and other high-risk environments should be performed using paper towels.

If hands are not visibly soiled, perform hand hygiene using application of alcohol-based hand rub (ABHR).

> If your hands are visibly soiled or contaminated with organic material, then perform hand hygiene with soap and water as outlined in **Clinical Skill 5**.

Into cupped hands, apply the manufacturer's recommended quantity of ABHR hand hygiene solution. Use the technique outlined in **Clinical Skill 5** to perform routine/social ABHR hand hygiene.

Surgical hand wash

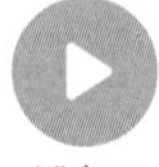

Video

The ACORN Standards (2023) recommend the following:

- A five-minute surgical hand wash is undertaken as the first scrub of the day. It incorporates cleaning fingernails.
- Subsequent scrubs of three minutes (without cleaning fingernails) are performed between cases.
- Hands are kept higher than elbows at all times to allow water to run from clean to dirty (hands to elbows). Note the difference between social and clinical hand hygiene.
- Nailbrush bristles are only used to clean fingernails.
- Arms are washed in a circular motion, from hands to elbows without returning to hands.
- The antimicrobial soap used for the first scrub of the day should continue to be used for subsequent scrubs.

Adjust the water temperature

Turn taps on and leave on throughout the clinical hand hygiene or surgical hand wash so that you do not touch them. Scrub sink taps usually have knee, foot or sensor controls. The WHO (2009) notes that although there are issues of skin tolerance and comfort, water temperature does not appear to be a critical factor in removing microbes during hand washing. Johal (2022) suggested water temperature between 21.1 and 26.7 °C assists with reducing skin irritation.

Run the water at a flow rate that prevents splashing. Direct water flow away from the plug hole, as it is likely to be contaminated with microorganisms, which could be transferred to you or the environment if splashing occurs (Lister, Hofland & Grafton, 2020).

The first five-minute scrub

First step (one minute)

Open the sponge pack

Check the pack for holes to ensure sterility (gently squeeze it – it should resist). Carefully peel the edges back to expose the sponge. The fully open sponge pack with an orange stick or similar is placed at a convenient location (usually at the back of the sink) so that you can access it when needed without touching the packaging or the sink. Wet your forearms (fingertips to elbows), apply antimicrobial scrub solution and clean under your fingernails with the orange stick.

Start timing

Keep your hands higher than your elbows at all times to avoid contaminating them with bacteria-laden soap and water. Wet your hands from fingertips to wrists to elbows and apply sufficient antimicrobial soap to ensure your skin is adequately covered to 2.5 cm above your elbow.

Apply 5 mL of antimicrobial solution, following the manufacturer's instructions, without touching the container with your hands. Most containers at scrub sinks use elbow, knee or foot triggers to access the solution. Some facilities use single-use disposable brush-sponges impregnated with antimicrobial soap.

With your hands under gently running water, remove the debris from under your fingernails with the nail cleaner. Rinse the nail cleaner between nails so contaminated material is not transferred from one nail to another. The antimicrobial soap remains in contact with your skin while you clean your fingernails.

Safely discard nail cleaner.

Starting at your fingertips, rinse your hands by passing your hands in one direction through the water. Avoid moving your hand back and forth through the water.

Second step (two minutes)

Apply antimicrobial soap to the sponge-brush bristles and continue cleaning your fingernails.

Apply antimicrobial soap to the sponge and wash all surfaces of your hands and forearms, working from your nail beds and between your fingers before washing up to your elbows using circular hand motions. All surfaces must be washed – visualise each finger, hand and arm as having four sides. Wash each finger and thumb, the webs (front and back) between your fingers, lateral surfaces, the back and the palm of each hand. Be vigilant about washing palm creases, knuckles and wrists.

Apply more antimicrobial soap if necessary.

> ?
> If your hand touches anything during your surgical scrub, your scrub must be lengthened by one minute for the contaminated area.

On completion, safely dispose of the sponge-brush. Rinse your hands and forearms by passing them through the water in one direction only, from fingertips to elbow. Do not move the arm back and forth through the water. During the scrub procedure, take care not to splash water onto your clothes.

Third step (two minutes)

Wash your hands and forearms again using the same principles and procedures as in the second step; however, this time you stop at your mid-forearm. Rinse your hands and forearms.

Next, wash your hands again using the same principles and procedures.

Finally, rinse your hands and forearms thoroughly. Remember to keep your fingertips higher than your elbows when rinsing to remove the loosened bacteria and sediment. When all lather traces are rinsed off, turn the taps off with the foot/elbow control.

Remain at the scrub sink until your hands are free from excess water, being careful to avoid splashes, contamination or injury on wet surfaces.

Subsequent scrubs of the day (three minutes)

First step (two minutes)

Preliminary step: rinse your hands and arms, and wash with sufficient antimicrobial soap to 2.5 cm above the elbows (20 seconds). This ensures adequate skin coverage and contact time during the next step.

Without rinsing, apply additional antimicrobial soap and wash all surfaces of your hands and forearms, working from the nail beds and between fingers before proceeding to wash the forearms to the level of the elbows using circular motions. Apply more antimicrobial soap if necessary. On completion, rinse your hands and forearms well.

Second step (one minute)

Wash your hands and forearms again using the same principles and procedures above; however, this time stop at your mid-forearms.

On completion, rinse your hands and forearms. Finally, rinse your hands and forearms thoroughly as described in the third step of the five-minute surgical hand wash.

Approach the gown trolley and carefully grasp the sterile towel to avoid contamination of the sterile field by contact with drips from your hands, which are clean, not sterile.

Step back from the sterile field with your hands outstretched and allow the towel to unfold.

Use half of the towel to dry one hand and arm from fingertips. Pat dry or wipe the opposite fingers and hand, moving down your forearm in a circular motion to your elbow without returning to your hand. This method avoids moving contaminants from the less-clean areas to the cleaner areas. Once this half of the towel comes in contact with the skin above your elbow, you are unable to use it any more.

Holding the towel with the still-wet hand, pick up the dry end with the dry hand and dry the remaining hand. Be sure to dry thoroughly. Moist skin is subject to chapping and breakdown. Also, it is difficult to put on gloves with damp skin.

Drop the towel into an appropriate container. Be careful to avoid being contaminated when discarding the towel.

Scrub using an alcohol-based hand rub solution procedure

The following guidelines are for a five-minute standardised scrubbing procedure undertaken prior to your first scrubbing procedure of the day using an ABHR solution. Use the ABHR solution in conjunction with the manufacturer's instructions. ACORN (2020) and WHO (2009) recommend a minimum of three applications or steps, to be used for three to five minutes.

Before commencing your scrub using ABHR, inspect your hands and arms to ensure there is no physical evidence of soiling.

Rinse and thoroughly dry hands prior to commencing the rub procedure. You must perform a social hand wash prior to subsequent scrubbing procedures using ABHR solution and rinse and dry hands. Always ensure you have sufficient ABHR to keep hands and forearms wet throughout the procedure.

First step

Use your right elbow to operate the dispenser. Dispense approximately 5 mL (three doses) of ABHR solution into the palm of your left hand.

Dip your right-hand fingertips into the ABHR solution to decontaminate under your nails. Smear the ABHR onto your right forearm up to the elbow. Ensure the whole skin area is covered by using circular movements around the forearm until the hand rub has completely evaporated. Repeat the procedure for your left arm.

Using your left elbow dispense approximately 5 mL (three doses) of ABHR into your right palm. Dip your left-hand fingertips into the ABHR solution to decontaminate under the nails. Smear the ABHR onto your left forearm up to the elbow. Ensure the whole skin area is covered by using circular movements around the forearm until the hand rub has completely evaporated.

Second step

Cover the whole surface of your hands up to the wrist with ABHR, rubbing palm against palm with a rotating movement until the hand rub has completely evaporated.

Third step

Rub the backs of your hands, including the wrists, moving back and forth. Rub palm against palm back and forth with fingers interlinked. Rub the back of your fingers in the palm of your other hand with a sideways back and forth movement and rub your thumbs by rotating the thumb in your clasped palm.

Allow your hands and forearms to dry thoroughly prior to putting on your sterile surgical clothing and gloves.

Continue with gowning and gloving

Keep your dry, clean hands in front of you above your waist and below your shoulders to prevent accidental contamination (see **Clinical Skill 9**).

Safety

General hand hygiene must be performed immediately after you remove your surgical gloves and before any further activities are undertaken. Gloves are not a substitute for good hand hygiene.

CLINICAL SKILLS ASSESSMENT

Aseptic/clinical hand hygiene

Demonstrates the ability to effectively and safely perform aseptic/clinical hand hygiene or surgical hand wash. Incorporates the *National Safety and Quality Health Service Standards*: 2 Partnering with Consumers, 3 Preventing and Controlling Healthcare-Associated Infection, 5 Comprehensive Care, 6 Communicating for Safety, and 8 Recognising and Responding to Acute Deterioration (ACSQHC, 2021).

Performance criteria	1	2	3	4	5
(Numbers indicate NMBA *Registered Nurse Standards for Practice*)	**(Dependent)**	**(Marginal)**	**(Assisted)**	**(Supervised)**	**(Independent)**
1. Identifies indication: is able to identify when to use aseptic/clinical hand hygiene or surgical hand wash and can differentiate between when (1.1, 1.4, 6.2)	☐	☐	☐	☐	☐
2. Demonstrates clinical reasoning abilities; e.g. skin is intact; nails are natural, short and unvarnished; hands and forearms are jewellery-free; sleeves are above the elbows; prepares gown pack and gloves before scrubbing; adjusts clothing to expose upper arms; ties back hair (as appropriate); dons appropriate personal protective equipment before scrubbing (1.1, 1.4, 6.2).	☐	☐	☐	☐	☐
3. Adheres to Hand Hygiene Australia's five moments for hand hygiene (1.1, 3.4, 6.1)	☐	☐	☐	☐	☐
4. Gathers equipment to the sink with running hand-hot water (1.1, 4.1, 6.2): ■ antimicrobial wash solution ■ sterile scrub brush/sponge and nail cleaner ■ sterile hand towel	☐	☐	☐	☐	☐
5. Adjusts water temperature and opens sponge-brush pack (1.1, 6.2)	☐	☐	☐	☐	☐
6. Wets hands and applies antiseptic scrub solution (1.1, 6.2)	☐	☐	☐	☐	☐
7. Washes hands and cleans beneath fingernails (1.1, 6.2) – five-minute surgical hand wash	☐	☐	☐	☐	☐
8. Rinses hands (1.1, 6.2)	☐	☐	☐	☐	☐
9. Applies antiseptic solution and washes hands and forearms (1.1, 6.2)	☐	☐	☐	☐	☐
10. Dries hands and arms (1.1, 6.2)	☐	☐	☐	☐	☐
11. Continues with gowning and gloving (1.1, 6.2)	☐	☐	☐	☐	☐
12. Demonstrates the ability to link theory to practice (1.1, 3.2, 3.3, 3.5, 6.2)	☐	☐	☐	☐	☐

Student:

Clinical facilitator: Date:

CHAPTER 9

SURGICAL GOWNING AND GLOVING

INDICATIONS

Surgical site infections (SSIs) are serious postoperative complications associated with increased length of hospital stays and increased costs for the healthcare facility (Australian Commission on Safety and Quality in Health Care [ACSQHC], 2019; National Health and Medical Research Council [NHMRC], 2019). Protective barriers such as sterile gowns and gloves assist in minimising people's SSI risks, disease transmission and health professionals' exposure to blood and other body fluids contamination (NHMRC, 2019). Maintaining a Surgical Aseptic Non Touch Technique (ANTT) when donning and wearing sterile gowns and gloves reduces the risk of wound contamination and SSI (Johal, 2022).

Intraoperative team members have a higher incidence of percutaneous injuries compared with other healthcare workers, increasing their risk of exposure to blood-borne pathogens and acquiring blood-borne illnesses (NHMRC, 2019; Sai Sivapuram, 2020). Double gloving (using two layers of surgical gloves) or the use of indicator gloves (coloured latex gloves worn underneath sterile gloves) or glove liners are recommended, as these significantly reduce perforation risks to the inner gloves and do not affect surgical performance (NHMRC, 2019; Pamaiahgari, 2023).

GATHER EQUIPMENT

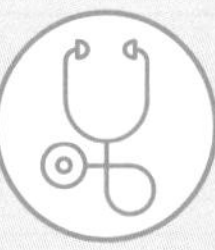

Equipment used for surgical gowning and gloving includes the following:

EQUIPMENT	EXPLANATION
A gown pack	• Contains a gown of appropriate size and a sterile towel, and is brought to an appropriate area near the scrub sink prior to starting the surgical scrub • The outer wrapping is opened to produce a sterile field • The sterile towel should be on top of the gown and readily accessible
Sterile gloves (two pairs)	• Ensure that the gloves are the appropriate size: the underneath glove should be half a size larger than the top gloves, which are your usual size • Open and place gloves in the inner wrapping on the sterile field using ANTT • Make sure gloves are placed so that the towel and the gown are accessible, as you will need to put on your gown before your gloves • Follow the facility's guidelines regarding sterile gloving policy

Sterile gloves (for open gloving, when a gown is not required) are removed from the outer packaging and placed in their sterile wrapper on a clean surface (e.g. the over-bed table) that has been wiped with an antiseptic solution and thoroughly dried. The surface must be at or above waist height to comply with the principles of asepsis.

Latex-free surgical gloves have been developed due to increasing latex hypersensitivity. Bayuo (2022) recommends healthcare workers use low-protein, non-powdered natural latex gloves to reduce latex sensitivities. Inform the staff in the clinical area if you have a latex sensitivity.

PROCEED WITH GOWNING AND GLOVING

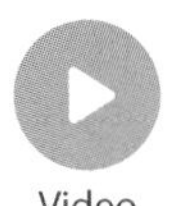
Video

Surgical scrub

A surgical scrub is carried out for the length of time required by the agency or the procedure (see **Clinical Skill 8**). Before commencing the scrub, apply your cap, mask, eyewear and footwear (as required by the facility's guidelines). Ensure that you keep your surgical attire dry (Johal, 2022). Your hands must be thoroughly dried prior to gowning and gloving to prevent maceration and chapping of your hands and dampening of the gown (Johal, 2022). Dry hands are also essential for ease of gloving.

Gowning

Gowns are folded inside out. To put on your gown, hold it at the neckline's seam with your thumbs and forefingers, and with your remaining fingers grasp the bulk of the gown and step back from the trolley or table.

Extend your arms to shoulder height. Continue holding your gown with your thumbs and forefingers, then release your remaining fingers and allow the gown to unfold to its full length without touching anything.

Place one hand inside the gown's shoulder. Repeat with your other hand and work both hands down the inside of the gown's arms. Do not touch any part of the outside of the gown, or the entire gown becomes unsterile. Make sure your hands remain inside the cuffs and encased in the sleeves. Use the sleeves as mittens.

A co-worker will be required to assist you. They will touch only the inside of the gown. They will adjust the neckline of your gown so that your uniform is entirely covered front and back. *The neck ties will be tied by your co-worker*. The waist ties remain tied in front of your waist until you have donned your gloves.

Closed gloving method

Closed gloving method is recommended for those involved in surgical procedures (Sai Sivapuram, 2020). The closed gloving process is described below.

Open the sterile wrapper containing the gloves

Follow the instructions printed on the inner sterile wrapping of the glove package. Remember to keep your hands encased within the cuffs of the sterile gown. Pinch the outside edges of the packaging to open fully. When the directions are followed the inner wrapping forms the sterile field. Ensure all folds remain open since any that close will contaminate your gloves.

Position a glove on your non-dominant hand

Pick up the appropriate glove with the sleeve-enclosed dominant hand and place it cuff to cuff along the palmar aspect of your non-dominant arm. The glove's palm should face downwards, fingers towards your elbow with the thumb of the glove overtopping your thumb. With your non-dominant hand still inside the sleeves of the sterile gown, grasp the cuff lying on top of the glove.

Pull on the first sterile glove

Grasp the upper, inner edge of the cuff with your sleeve-encased dominant hand and pull it over the top of your non-dominant hand. The glove cuff should encase your entire hand and gown cuff. With your dominant hand holding the gown's cuff, carefully advance your non-dominant hand into the glove. Do not be concerned if the glove is not properly fitted, you can adjust it once your second sterile glove is on your dominant hand.

To position the glove on your dominant hand

Pick up the remaining glove with your gloved non-dominant hand. Place the fingers in between the cuff and the glove to ensure that your gloved hand remains sterile. Take care to keep your gloved hand thumb well away from any area that can contaminate it. Place the glove palm down and cuff to cuff, with that glove's fingers extended towards your elbow along the palmar aspect of your dominant arm.

Pull on your second sterile glove

Proceed in a similar manner to the first sterile glove; however, this time you can use your gloved hand to carefully adjust the cuff of your second sterile glove. Again, carefully advance the hand into the glove. Adjust both gloves so that they fit comfortably and do not impair your circulation. Adjust both gloves' cuffs so that they extend comfortably and well above the gown's cuffs.

> ? If your ungloved fingers extend beyond your gown's cuff, this constitutes glove contamination. Your gown and gloves will need to be discarded and new gown and gloves donned.

Open gloving method

For the open gloving method, touch only the cuff of your glove with the ungloved hand, and then only glove to glove for the other hand (Sai Sivapuram, 2020). The open gloving method is described below.

Open the inner wrapper

Proceed according to the directions printed on the package. Make sure the folds are pulled firmly to keep them open and avoid contamination. The gloves should be positioned palms up, with thumbs to the outside and cuffs at the bottom.

Using your non-dominant hand, pick the glove for your dominant hand out of the wrapper

Touch only the inside of the cuff (i.e. the folded-over edge). Keep both hands above your waist level as you lift it above the wrapper, away from your body. Keep the thumb of your dominant hand folded against your palm and slide your fingers inside the glove, taking care not to contaminate its outer surface. Do not be concerned about the glove's fit at this point. Even if all of the fingers are not in position, you can adjust both gloves more easily later.

Slip the fingers of your gloved dominant hand under the cuff of the remaining glove

Keep your thumb extended and away from any exposed skin. Keep your wrist straight so there is no chance that the fingers of the second glove can contact exposed skin. Lift the glove away from the wrapper and slip your non-dominant hand's fingers into the glove.

Adjust both gloves

Make sure to touch only the sterile, outer surfaces of both gloves on the finger or palmar surfaces, as the cuffs are considered contaminated if there is no gown.

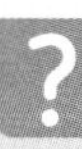

If you contaminate your gloves at any stage during this procedure, your gown and gloves must be discarded and new ones donned.

Tie the sterile gown's waist ties

Ask for assistance from your co-worker, who is 'scrubbed' and wearing sterile gloves to help with your waist ties. Carefully untie the waist ties in the front of the sterile gown, ensuring that the tie's entire length remains in your control. To do this, gather the ties into the palms of your hands before you untie the knot. Keep the front tie held in your left hand. Hand the furthest tip of the tie attached to the back of the gown to your co-worker. Take care not to contaminate your glove.

Carefully turn three-quarters of a circle, making sure no sterile areas are contaminated. Grasp the tie held by your co-worker no further than halfway along its length. Your co-worker will drop the distal end of the tie (or disengage it from the attached sterile card or haemostat). Tie the two ties together, making sure that you do not contaminate your hands on the distal portion of the tie.

Some facilities prefer that a sterile haemostat is used to hand off the tie. Some gowns have a sterile card attached to each tie; follow the facility's guidelines regarding how these gowns are tied.

Define surgically aseptic areas

Once you have been gowned and gloved, the front of the gown is considered sterile from your nipple line to the level of the sterile field and from your fingertips to your elbows (Overall, 2022). Any non-visible area is considered contaminated. All sterile procedures are performed without extraneous movement, as excessive movement increases contamination risks and creates air currents, which could transmit microorganisms to the person or to the sterile field (Overall, 2022).

Remove gown and gloves

When the procedure is finished, your gown is removed by pulling it over your gloved hands and discarding it in the appropriate waste container. Gloves should be removed without contamination to your hands, and discarded appropriately (Johal, 2022).

CLINICAL SKILLS ASSESSMENT

Surgical gowning and gloving

Demonstrates the ability to effectively and safely prepare for a surgical procedure. Incorporates the *National Safety and Quality Health Service Standards*: 2 Partnering with Consumers, 3 Preventing and Controlling Healthcare-Associated Infection, 5 Comprehensive Care, 6 Communicating for Safety, and 8 Recognising and Responding to Acute Deterioration (ACSQHC, 2021).

Performance criteria	1	2	3	4	5
(Numbers indicate NMBA *Registered Nurse Standards for Practice*)	**(Dependent)**	**(Marginal)**	**(Assisted)**	**(Supervised)**	**(Independent)**
1. Identifies indication (1.1, 1.4, 6.2)	☐	☐	☐	☐	☐
2. Gathers equipment (1.1, 6.2): ■ gown pack containing a gown of appropriate size and a sterile towel ■ two pairs of sterile gloves of appropriate size	☐	☐	☐	☐	☐
3. Washes and dries hands (surgical scrub) (1.2)	☐	☐	☐	☐	☐
4. Picks up the gown (1.2)	☐	☐	☐	☐	☐
5. Places hand inside the gown shoulder, works the arms down (1.2)	☐	☐	☐	☐	☐
6. Has a co-worker tie the neck ties (1.2)	☐	☐	☐	☐	☐
7. Opens the sterile wrapper containing the gloves (1.2)	☐	☐	☐	☐	☐
8. Positions the glove on the non-dominant hand (1.2)	☐	☐	☐	☐	☐
9. Pulls on the first sterile glove (1.2)	☐	☐	☐	☐	☐
10. Positions the glove on the dominant hand (1.2)	☐	☐	☐	☐	☐
11. Pulls on the second sterile glove (1.2)	☐	☐	☐	☐	☐
12. Ties the waist ties of the sterile gown (1.2)	☐	☐	☐	☐	☐
13. Defines the sterile areas (1.2, 6.2)	☐	☐	☐	☐	☐
14. Removes and disposes of the gown and the gloves appropriately (6.2)	☐	☐	☐	☐	☐
15. Demonstrates the ability to link theory to practice (1.1, 3.2, 3.3, 3.5, 6.2)	☐	☐	☐	☐	☐

Student:

Clinical facilitator: Date:

REFERENCES

Australian College of Operating Room Nurses (ACORN) (2023). *Standards for safe and quality care in the perioperative environment (SSQCPE) for individuals.* Lyndoch, SA: ACORN.

Australian Commission on Safety and Quality in Health Care (ACSQHC) (2019). *National hand hygiene initiative manual.* ACSQHC. https://www.safetyandquality.gov.au/sites/default/files/2020-09/nhhi_user_manual_-_sep_2020.pdf

Australian Commission on Safety and Quality in Health Care (ACSQHC) (2021). *National safety and quality health service standards* (3rd ed.). Sydney, NSW: ACSQHC.

Bayuo, J. (2022). *Latex allergy in health care workers: Management.* [Evidence summary]. Adelaide, SA: Joanna Briggs Institute.

Dougherty, L., Lister, S. & West-Oram, A. (eds) (2015). *The Royal Marsden manual of clinical nursing procedures* (9th ed.). Oxford, UK: Wiley-Blackwell.

Johal, J. (2022). *Surgical site infection: Surgical scrubbing, gowning and gloving.* [Evidence summary]. Adelaide, SA: Joanna Briggs Institute.

Lister, S., Hofland, J. & Grafton, H. (eds) (2020). *The Royal Marsden manual of clinical nursing procedures* (10th ed.). Oxford, UK: Wiley-Blackwell.

Magtoto, E. (2023). *Surgical site infection prevention: Dressings.* [Evidence summary]. Adelaide, SA: Joanna Briggs Institute.

Marin, S. (2020). *Aprons, gowns, face masks and eye protection.* Adelaide, SA: Joanna Briggs Institute.

Marin, T. & Mbinji, M. (2022). *Minor surgical procedures: Non-sterile and sterile gloves.* [Evidence summary]. Adelaide, SA: Joanna Briggs Institute.

Marin, T. & Valdez, F. C. (2023). *Aseptic techniques: Standard Aseptic Non-Touch Technique.* [Evidence summary]. Adelaide, SA: Joanna Briggs Institute.

McCormack, B. & McCance, T. (2016). *Person-centred practice in nursing and health care: Theory and practice* (2nd ed.). Oxford, UK: Wiley-Blackwell.

National Health and Medical Research Council (NHMRC) (2019). *Australian guidelines for the prevention and control of infection in healthcare.* Commonwealth of Australia. http://www.nhmrc.gov.au

Overall, B. (2022). *Surgical site infection: Effectiveness of a sterile field.* [Evidence summary]. Adelaide, SA: Joanna Briggs Institute.

Pamaiahgari, P. (2023). *Surgical settings (infection): Double-gloving with indicator gloves.* [Evidence summary]. Adelaide, SA: Joanna Briggs Institute.

Peters, M. (2017). *Asepsis: Clinician information* [Evidence summary]. Adelaide, SA: Joanna Briggs Institute.

Porritt, K. (2022). *Hand hygiene: Indications and general principles in primary, community and acute healthcare settings* [Evidence summary]. Adelaide, SA: Joanna Briggs Institute.

Rowley S. & Clare S. (2019). Right asepsis with ANTT® for infection prevention. In N. Moureau (ed.), *Vessel health and preservation: The right approach for vascular access.* Cham, Switzerland: Springer. https://doi.org/10.1007/978-3-030-03149-7_11

Rowley, S., Clare, S., Macqueen, S., & Molyneux, R. (2010). ANTT v2: An updated practice framework for aseptic technique. *British Journal of Nursing, 19*(5), S5–S11. https://doi.org/10.12968/bjon.2010.19.Sup1.47079

Sai Sivapuram, M. (2020). *Surgical site infection: Surgical hand scrubs and gloving.* Adelaide, SA: Joanna Briggs Institute.

Suen, L. K. P., Lung, V. Y. T., Boost, M. V., Au-Yueng, C. H. & Siu, G. K. (2019). Microbiological evaluation of different hand drying methods for removing bacteria from washed hands. *Scientific Reports, 9,* 13754. https://doi.org/10.1038/s41598-019-50239-4

Valdez, F. C. (2022). *Sharp and needle stick injuries.* [Evidence summary]. Adelaide, SA: Joanna Briggs Institute.

Whitehorn, A. (2020). *Cytotoxic agents: Safe handling and administration* [Evidence summary]. Adelaide, SA: Joanna Briggs Institute.

World Health Organization (WHO) (2009). *WHO guidelines on hand hygiene in health care: A summary. First global patient safety challenge – clean care is safer care.* Geneva, Switzerland: World Health Organization. http://whqlibdoc.who.int/hq/2009/WHO_IER_PSP_2009.07_eng.pdf

PART 3

ASSESSMENT

10 TEMPERATURE, PULSE AND RESPIRATION MEASUREMENT

11 BLOOD PRESSURE MEASUREMENT

12 PULSE OXIMETRY – MEASURING OXYGEN SATURATION

13 PAIN ASSESSMENT

14 BLOOD GLUCOSE MEASUREMENT

15 PHYSICAL ASSESSMENT

16 MENTAL STATUS ASSESSMENT

17 FOCUSED CARDIOVASCULAR HEALTH HISTORY AND PHYSICAL ASSESSMENT

18 12-LEAD ELECTROCARDIOGRAM

19 FOCUSED RESPIRATORY HEALTH HISTORY AND PHYSICAL ASSESSMENT

20 FOCUSED NEUROLOGICAL HEALTH HISTORY AND PHYSICAL ASSESSMENT

21 NEUROVASCULAR OBSERVATIONS

22 FOCUSED GASTROINTESTINAL HEALTH HISTORY AND ABDOMINAL PHYSICAL ASSESSMENT

23 HEIGHT, WEIGHT AND WAIST CIRCUMFERENCE MEASUREMENTS

24 FOCUSED MUSCULOSKELETAL HEALTH HISTORY AND PHYSICAL ASSESSMENT AND RANGE OF MOTION EXERCISES

Note: These notes are summaries of the most important points in the assessments/procedures and are not exhaustive on the subject. References of the materials used to compile the information have been supplied. The student is expected to have learnt the material surrounding each skill as presented in the references. No single reference is complete on each subject.

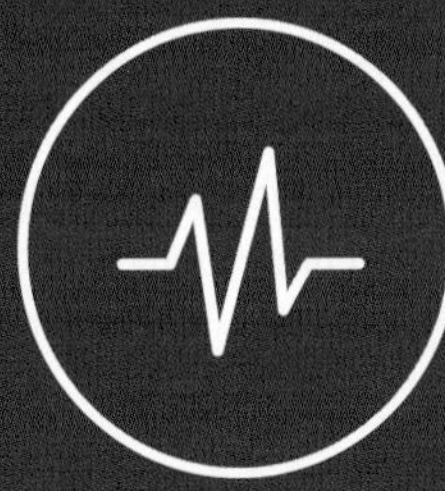

CHAPTER 10

TEMPERATURE, PULSE AND RESPIRATION MEASUREMENT

INDICATIONS

Temperature measurement

Indications for assessing temperature include:

- establishing a baseline for subsequent comparison
- identifying the core temperature reading
- evaluating responses to specific therapies, such as antipyretic medication
- identifying core temperature of anyone at risk for temperature alterations (e.g. infection, hypo- or hyperthermia, exposure to invasive procedures).

Infants do not conserve heat well because of immature thermoregulation, their greater body surface-area-to-mass ratio and decreased subcutaneous fat. Elderly people have poor responses to environmental temperature extremes resulting from slowed blood circulation, structural and functional changes in the skin, and overall decrease in ability to thermoregulate (Deering, 2023; Wang et al., 2022). Body temperature in the elderly is often 1 °C lower than in a younger person. Van Steen et al. (2019) found elderly women to be more affected by heat-wave conditions than elderly men. Men generally have a slightly lower body temperature than women, who often perceive greater thermal discomfort at the same absolute temperature (Greenfield et al., 2023).

Core body temperature is 36.7 (+/– 0.43) °C (Werner & Gunga, 2020, p. 477). Normal oral body temperature ranges between 36 and 38 °C although rigorous exercise, emotional upsets or cold morning temperatures can alter this to between 35.0 and 39.5 °C. Rectal temperatures register 0.4 to 0.5 °C higher than oral temperatures (Estes et al., 2020) and most closely reflect the core temperature. Therefore, consistency in the method of obtaining body temperature readings is important.

A body temperature registering above these values (i.e. 38 °C) is called fever or hyperthermia and a body temperature below 36 °C is called hypothermia (Dudhe et al., 2023; Marchand & Gin, 2022). An elevated temperature may indicate infection, systemic inflammatory responses or thermoregulatory function disorders, and is ultimately fundamental to the diagnosis and treatment of a person. Accurate monitoring enables triggering of an early warning system to initiate appropriate treatment.

Pulse measurement

Indications for assessing the pulse include:

- determining whether the pulse rate, rhythm and volume are within normal limits for the person
- establishing a baseline for subsequent comparison
- monitoring the person's health status
- comparing the qualities of peripheral pulses bilaterally
- monitoring anyone at risk for alterations in their pulse.

Pulse rate is a measure of the frequency of the heart's pumping action. With each beat a volume of blood is ejected from the heart into the aorta (stroke volume), causing a pressure wave against the arteries that is felt in the peripheries. Normal pulse rates for adults range from 60 to 100 beats per minute. The pulse rhythm is regular, with equal intervals between each beat. The pulse volume is the same with each beat. It can be felt with a moderate amount of pressure of the fingers and can be obliterated with greater pressure (Estes et al., 2020). Peripheral pulses (temporal, carotid, apical, brachial, radial, femoral, popliteal, posterior tibial and dorsalis pedis) are easily felt where arteries lie close to the surface. Alteration in pulse rate along with respiratory rate is often the first sign of deterioration in a person's condition.

Respiratory measurement

Indications for assessing respiration include:

- determining whether the respiratory rate, rhythm, quality and depth are within normal limits for the person
- establishing a baseline for subsequent comparison
- monitoring the person's health status
- assessing respirations prior to and following medication administration (e.g. anaesthesia, morphine, Ventolin)
- monitoring those at risk for alterations in their respiratory status (e.g. asthma, croup).

Normal respiratory rates for adults range from 12 to 20 breaths per minute (Depta et al., 2023). In the elderly, the respiratory rate is higher, ranging from 10 to 18 in those in their 60s to 13 to 21 in those in their 90s (Takayama, Nagamine & Kotani, 2019). Respiratory volume varies from short, shallow breaths (e.g. severe anxiety) to deep, noisy, gasping breaths (e.g. following heavy work, exercise).

Sighing breaths can be part of the normal respiratory effort because they open alveoli that quiet breaths do not. Understanding respiratory physiology is crucial to making use of the respiratory assessment. Xie et al. (2022) demonstrated that the respiratory rate is one of the most significant physiological indicators of severity of illness.

The respiratory rate helps predict clinical deterioration (Takayama, Yoshioka & Nagamine, 2023). Clinical deterioration is often preceded by changes in the vital signs that are detectable up to 48 hours before an adverse event (e.g. rapid deterioration, respiratory or cardiac arrest, death) and can alert caregivers to begin treatment and increase vigilance to prevent the event (Cornish et al., 2019). During clinical deterioration, the respiratory rate and heart rate rise in compensation before any other clinical signs (Olshansky, Ricci & Fedorowski, 2022). The respiratory rate is the vital sign most closely related to the outcome (changes predict deterioration) (Brekke et al., 2019).

Nurses usually initiate vital signs (temperature, pulse and respiration [TPR], blood pressure, pulse oximetry, level of consciousness, pain assessment) monitoring and/or follow a prescribed facility policy. TPR should be monitored any time you feel that the health status of the person warrants assessment.

Be aware of trends in TPR. As part of a person's vital signs, the pulse and respiratory readings are significantly associated with deterioration. These parameters should be carefully considered (using an early warning scoring [EWS] system is most efficient) when assessing a person in hospital (Holland & Kellet, 2023).

EVIDENCE OF THERAPEUTIC INTERACTION

Explanation helps to allay the person's anxiety and gains their cooperation. It reduces apprehension, which alters vital signs. The person needs to understand that the thermometer must remain in place for the entire time to obtain an accurate reading. However, because respiratory rates and patterns change when people are aware that you are counting their breaths, do not tell the person when you are assessing their respirations. Obtain consent (either verbal or tacit) before proceeding.

DEMONSTRATE CLINICAL REASONING

Prepare the environment. Ensure that the ambient temperature is comfortable without draughts and/ or provide a blanket for warmth. Sufficient light and quiet are needed so you can examine the person. Privacy is preferable (i.e. close the room door, draw the curtains and speak quietly) so you can concentrate on the sensation in your fingers when assessing the pulse or when listening to quiet respirations. You may need to ask family and friends to wait outside. Familiarise yourself with the forms used by the facility prior to obtaining the TPR. Most Australian hospitals use the Adult Deterioration Detection System (ADDS).

GATHER EQUIPMENT

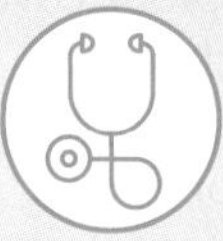

Gathering equipment is an organisational step that helps to create a positive environment for a successful interaction. It ensures that you have all needed material, boosts the person's confidence and trust in you, and increases your self-confidence. While gathering the equipment, you can mentally rehearse the procedure. Ensure you know how each piece of the equipment works. Equipment may include the following items:

EQUIPMENT	EXPLANATION
Oral thermometers	Oral readings are generally 0.5 °C lower than rectal readings (i.e. normal = 36.57 °C with a range of 36 to 38 °C) Oral readings are an accurate non-invasive method. However, oral thermometers can understate the temperature, so observation skills are mandatory (Reece & Hughes, 2022) *Electronic thermometers (most common and most accurate)* • Electronic machine with a digital readout • Consists of a thermistor rod probe that measures temperature accurately and quickly, a battery-operated electronic pack, and disposable probe covers • Can be used in the mouth, axilla (blue probe) or rectum (separate red probes for these) *Digital analogue thermometers* • Covered with a plastic disposable sheath • Record temperatures from 32 to 42 °C
Tympanic thermometer	Tympanic thermometers are the most accurate non-invasive measurement of temperature (Halford & Foran, 2022). Normal tympanic temperature is 36.64 °C with a range of 36 to 38 °C • Is a minimally invasive way to measure temperature. The covered (disposable) probe is inserted into the person's ear canal • Has a sensor at the end of the probe that records the infrared radiation emitted by the warmth of the tympanic membrane and surrounding tissues. The radiation is converted into a digital temperature reading • The temperature reading from the tympanic membrane consistent with core temperature because its blood supply is shared with the hypothalamus where the body temperature is regulated • These temperature readings are comparable with oral temperatures; however, the thermometer requires calibration to maintain accuracy (Halford & Foran, 2022)

EQUIPMENT	EXPLANATION
Temporal artery thermometer	• This non-invasive measure uses the infrared emissions from the temporal artery to produce an average reading over six seconds. The operator slides the probe across the forehead or behind the ear to obtain the reading • Fitzwater et al. (2019) found this thermometer is comparable in accuracy to the oral thermometer in normothermic adults, as did Man et al. (2023) with tympanic thermometers
Rectal thermometer	• Rectal temperatures are slightly higher (up to 0.5 °C) than normal oral readings with a normal of 37.04 °C and a range of 36.7 to 38 °C, but are considered to be closest to the core temperature (Hernandez & Upadhye, 2017) • Rectal probes for electronic thermometers are red and use disposable probes • Used when a person cannot cooperate with oral assessment, or has facial/mouth injuries when other, less invasive thermometers are not available or when greater temperature accuracy is required • Not used with people who have coagulation disorders, diseases or surgery of the rectum, severe haemorrhoids or diarrhoea, or who are immune suppressed
Sheath or probe covers	As required for the type of thermometer being used
Watch with a second hand	To calculate the pulse and respirations per minute
Clean gloves	To prevent contamination of hands with body fluid if taking a rectal temperature
Alcowipes	To disinfect the probe unit after rectal use

TAKE TEMPERATURE, PULSE AND RESPIRATION MEASUREMENT

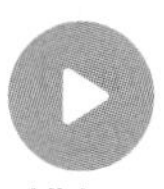

Hand hygiene

Hand hygiene (see **Clinical Skill 5**) removes microorganisms from your hands. It is the most effective preventative measure for cross-contamination, reducing incidences of nosocomial (i.e. hospital- or treatment-acquired) infection.

Temperature measurement

Select the thermometer according to the person's needs and what is available on the unit. Since values fluctuate between types of thermometers, ensure you consistently use the same type of device (Díaz-González et al., 2023). If you are unfamiliar with the type of thermometer provided, read the instructions and practise using it before taking it to the bedside.

Prepare the thermometer

Digital and electronic thermometers

Snap the disposable probe cover into place snugly. Various units have different configurations. You must become familiar with the one used in the facility where you are located.

Tympanic thermometer

Remove the thermometer from the base unit and ensure the lens is clean, shiny, dry, undamaged and free of debris. To clean the lens, use a lint-free swab, tissue or gauze. Refer to the manufacturer's guidelines if additional cleaning is required. Attach a probe cover to protect the tip of the probe. For the machine to function, it is necessary to firmly press the tip of the thermometer probe in the centre of the probe cover until the backing frame of the cover clicks into the base of the probe.

Rectal thermometers

The oral electronic machine is used and the probe attachment unit is changed from a blue to a red unit. The probe is sheathed in a plastic probe cover (as above) prior to lubrication with a water-soluble lubricant.

ELDER CARE

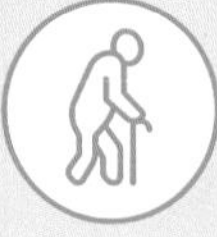

Older adults (age ≥60) register a lower temperature than younger adults by 0.23 °C in normal ambient temperatures (Geneva & Javaid, 2021). The thermoregulatory mechanisms of the ageing body decline over the years, reducing its ability to adapt to extremes in temperature (Cho et al., 2022). The physiological changes causing this decline include decreased basal metabolic rate, decreased cardiac output, delayed vasoconstriction and dilation, decreased and constricted skin blood flow, reduced ability to sweat and altered body fat distribution (increased central adiposity) (Younes et al., 2023). This means the older person is unable to adapt quickly to extremes of heat and their temperature will rise, sometimes to damaging levels. Extremes in environmental temperature (especially heat) increase the risks of morbidity and mortality in the elderly.

THE PEOPLE LIVING WITH SEVERE OBESITY

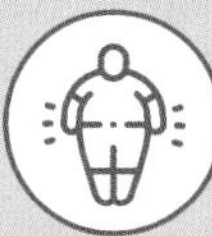

For people living with severe obesity, oral or tympanic temperature readings are preferable because of the following possible issues:

- increased perspiration affects the accuracy of temporal artery readings
- excess subcutaneous fat makes axillary temperatures difficult to accomplish and inaccurate
- decreased ability for the person to move to a side-lying position, and excess tissue in the buttocks make rectal readings difficult (an extra nurse would be required to hold the buttocks apart and allow visualisation of the anus).

See **Clinical Skills 15 and 23** for a brief explanation of some of the issues faced by people living with severe obesity.

Assess the person

Visually assess the person as you prepare to take their temperature. Observation is your most important tool when caring for people.

LOOK for flushing, sweating, shivering, pallor and dry mucous membranes.

LISTEN to reports of feeling hot or cold.

FEEL the skin for dampness, dryness and tactile warmth.

These observations take only a second but can alert you to alterations in the person's condition that require immediate intervention.

Ask the person if they have recently ingested hot or cold food or fluid, because this can affect the accuracy of oral temperature assessment. Recent exertion or smoking can alter oral temperatures, pulse and respirations. Also, if the person has received oxygen via mask, this can lower oral temperatures.

Oral temperature readings are *not* done on anyone who is confused, unconscious, has an active convulsive disorder, is younger than six years of age, has trauma or infection in the oral cavity, has had recent oral surgery or is a mouth breather (i.e. cannot breathe through their nose). People with these criteria may injure themselves, or the accuracy of the reading may be suspect. Temporal artery, tympanic or axillary temperature is taken for these people. Rectal temperatures are preferred when accuracy to core body temperature is important (e.g. hyper- or hypothermia) (Hernandez & Upadhye, 2017); however, it is invasive and distressing to most people.

The use of glass and axillary thermometers is no longer considered best practice because of inaccuracy and possible transmission of infection (especially since the beginning of 2020) – disposable oral, tympanic and temporal artery thermometer readings have demonstrated accuracy (Blake et al., 2019). Non-contact infrared thermometers (as used for mass screening during the SARS outbreak and COVID-19 pandemic) measure surface temperature of the skin by measuring electromagnetic wave emissions, which strengthen with an increase in body temperature. These thermometers have been demonstrated to be accurate, quick and easy to use and permit a non-contact reading in some clinical situations (e.g. febrile screening [van Zundert et al., 2022]). Exercise, metabolism and external environmental heat sources can affect skin temperature and the accessible body areas (neck, forehead and wrist), as surface areas are easily altered by external temperatures and skin cooling. This results in a lower temperature than from an oral reading. Lin et al. (2023) demonstrated the equivalent (to the oral value of 37.3 °C) temperature values for fever are 37.10 °C for the neck, 36.90 °C for the forehead and 36.80 °C for the wrists. In clinical situations where temperature accuracy triggers an EWS, these values must be taken into consideration. Other authors found tympanic and oral thermometers were consistently sensitive and accurate (Sharif Nia et al., 2022; Van Zundert et al., 2022).

Breda et al. (2023) have developed a smartphone application for use in the community that employs the touchscreen to capture heat transfer from the body. The 'Feverphone' demonstrated accuracy, sensitivity and specificity in their clinical study.

Take the temperature

Tympanic temperature

Ask or assist the person to turn their head to one side and inspect their ear. If necessary, remove a hearing aid and wait about 10 minutes. Do not use a tympanic thermometer in an ear that is inflamed, infected or draining; has an adjacent lesion; in which an incision is present or that the person has been lying on (Martin et al., 2022). Incorrect technique in the use of tympanic thermometers is a primary cause of inaccurate readings – probe placement is crucial to accuracy. The same ear is used in subsequent readings due to slight differences in left and right ears (Mah et al., 2021). Temperatures range from 34.5 °C at the opening of the ear canal to 36.4 °C on the canal wall and 37.3 °C at the tympanic membrane (Duncan et al., 2008). A firm seal within the ear canal is essential (Martin et al., 2022).

Before inserting the probe, use your non-dominant hand to gently pull the pinna upwards and backwards for an adult and downwards and backwards for a child. This ensures the probe is registering the temperature at the tympanic membrane rather than that of the skin, the external ear canal or wax. Insert the probe by centring and gently advancing it into the ear canal to make a firm seal that prevents air from entering and causing a false low measurement (Martin et al., 2022). Press and release the scan button to commence, then remove the probe tip from the person's ear as soon as the thermometer display reads 'done', which is usually indicated with a beep.

The measurement is generally completed within two seconds. Press the 'release/eject' button to discard the probe cover into the contaminated waste bin (the covers are for single-use only). Read and record the temperature displayed, then wipe the thermometer clean before replacing it into the base unit.

Oral temperature

Insert the distal end of the probe of the digital or electronic thermometer into the person's mouth. It should be under the tongue, on either side of the frenulum (the posterior sublingual fossa) and not in the area in front of the tongue (Mah et al., 2021). There may be a difference in temperature of up to 1.7 °C between these areas (Dougherty, Lister & West-Oram, 2015). The area on either side of the frenulum is close to the body's core temperature because the superficial arterioles, derived from the external carotid artery, are close to the surface. Ask the person to close their lips around the thermometer to prevent cooling by the ambient temperature. Instruct them not to clamp their teeth on the thermometer to avoid any breakage and subsequent possible injury. An electronic or digital thermometer takes between 20 and 90 seconds to register the temperature, and the unit will generally register completion by beeping.

After the temperature has registered, remove the probe cover of the electronic or digital thermometer and discard into the contaminated waste bin without contaminating your hands. The temperature will be displayed as a digital read-out on the unit.

Axillary temperature

This reading, although safe and non-invasive, is less desirable than other sites because it is difficult to achieve an accurate and reliable reading. The axilla is not close to major vessels (the axillary artery is deep), there are varying fat masses, and skin surface temperatures vary more with the ambient temperature (Marui et al., 2017). This method is used when an oral thermometer is unsuitable or the person cannot tolerate it. Do not compare axillary temperatures with other methods (i.e. compare with baseline axillary temperature).

To take an axillary temperature, assist the person to a comfortable position and expose the axilla area. Ensure the axilla area is dry, because presence of moisture may result in a false low reading. Place the thermometer in the centre of the axilla, as high up in the axilla as possible and with full skin contact. Ask the person to hold their arm firmly against their side or across their chest. A digital or electronic thermometer takes between one and two minutes to register an axillary temperature. Use the same axilla consistently (variation between the axillae is 0.1 and 0.9 °C) (Vardasca et al., 2019).

Temporal artery temperature

Place the probe on the forehead, press and hold down the activate button and slowly slide the probe across the forehead from centre to hairline. Make sure there is no hair under the probe and do not go down the side of the face. When the clicks stop (after about two to three seconds), the thermometer has registered the highest temperature, which will be displayed.

> ?
> If the person is diaphoretic, the temporal artery thermometer will not register an accurate temperature. In this instance, take the reading behind the ear to just below the mastoid bone and behind the earlobe.

Rectal temperature

Position the person in the left lateral or Sims' position to enable access to the anus. Wear non-sterile gloves, sheathe the probe in a plastic cover, and lubricate the sheathed probe for about 5 cm of its length. Expose the anus by lifting the upper buttock and ask the person to take slow deep breaths. Gently insert the thermometer for 3.5 cm. Never force the thermometer. If resistance is felt, stop inserting the thermometer, ask the person to breathe deeply, and very carefully and gently resume insertion. If there is still resistance, withdraw the thermometer. If no resistance is felt, leave the thermometer in the rectum until the device registers the maximum temperature and signals with a beep. Withdraw the thermometer. Remove and discard the plastic probe-cover, replace the red rectal probe attachment with the blue oral probe attachment. Wipe the red probe attachment with alcowipes. Return the thermometer to the charging unit.

Pulse measurement

Pulse assessment requires quiet and concentration to assist you to count the beats accurately.

Assess the person

For pulse rate readings, assess the person for age, medications and exposure to environmental heat or cold, smoking status, general fitness and exercise within the past 20 minutes. Women generally have a higher heart rate than men. Caffeine, pain, anxiety, exercise, elevated temperature and low blood pressure elevate the heart rate. Remember to observe the person:

LOOK	Are they pale, flushed, cyanotic; do they look comfortable; can you see carotid or temporal pulses?
LISTEN	Are they complaining of palpitations or a thumping heart?
FEEL	Is their skin warm or cool, dry, or moist and clammy?

Manual assessment of pulse is best practice. Electronic recording of pulse provides information on the rate; manual assessment provides information on rate, rhythm and amplitude. It also fosters a more trusting relationship.

ELDER CARE

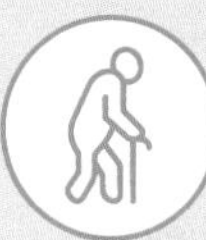

Deconditioning and diminished autonomic function due to ageing increase the resting heart rate (Sapra, Malik & Bhandari, 2023). Warm ambient temperatures tend to decrease the heart rate in older people (Tochihara et al., 2021). Dehydration, comorbidities and polypharmacy (common in older people) will also affect the heart rate. Heart rate in elders is often more irregular.

THE PERSON LIVING WITH SEVERE OBESITY

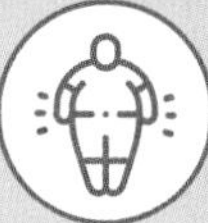

For people living with severe obesity (see **Clinical Skills 15 and 23** for a brief explanation of the problems encountered by people living with severe obesity), assessing the peripheral pulses manually may be impossible because of the thickness of tissues between your finger pad and the arterial wall. You may need to use a Doppler pulse assessment machine, which turns the waveform of the pulse into an audible sound. You will need to practise this and know the location of the pulse you are trying to assess to be successful.

Take the pulse

The radial pulse is normally used unless it cannot be exposed (because of a cast, for instance) or if there is a particular reason for assessing another peripheral pulse point (e.g. assessing pedal circulation). Pulse points that can be palpated easily are the temporal, carotid, brachial, radial, femoral, popliteal (rarely used), dorsalis pedis and posterior tibialis. Radial pulses are the most commonly used. Position the person so the pulse point is available for assessment – with the forearm resting across the chest (so respirations can be counted without the person's awareness), across the thigh or beside the body with the palm downwards.

Resting pulse is usually taken with the person supine to ensure consistency. Using two or three middle fingertips (not the thumb because your own pulse is discernible), locate the pulse. The radial pulse is on the thumb side of the wrist along the radial bone. Lightly hold your fingers over the pulse so that it is discernible but not occluded. Using the second hand on the watch, count the beat for one minute on an initial assessment, for a child or if the pulse is irregular to ensure accuracy. If the pulse is regular, the person is an adult and the assessment is not the first one, counting for 30 seconds and multiplying by two is acceptable. The heart rate of children under two is assessed by listening to the apical heart rate.

Assess the rhythm of the pulse by noting the pattern between beats. When there is a gross pulse irregularity, use a stethoscope to assess the apical heart rate (see **Clinical Skill 17**) and count the beats for 60 seconds.

Assess the amplitude of the pulse on a 0 to 3 scale, where:

- 0 is absent
- 1 is weak or thready (easily occluded with light touch)
- 2 is normal (i.e. the pulse can be occluded with moderate force)
- 3 is full or bounding (the pulse is difficult to occlude with moderate force).

Assess the person for other physical signs (e.g. pallor, cool peripheries) and, if appropriate, ask about symptoms of altered cardiac output (e.g. confusion) or altered regularity (e.g. palpitations).

To take an apical-radial pulse, ask another nurse to take the radial pulse at the same time as you auscultate the apical rate (at the 5th intercostal space, left midclavicular line). Signal to the other nurse when you start counting the heart rate and when the minute is up. A pulse deficit results from the ejection of a volume of blood that is too small to initiate a peripheral pulse wave (DeLaune et al., 2024, p. 590). The difference between the two rates should be documented.

Respiration measurement

If the person is aware that you are counting their respirations, their rate will change, so try to incorporate respiration measurement with pulse assessment.

Assess the person

For respiratory readings, assess the person for age, smoking status, medications and exposure to environmental heat or cold, anxiety, general fitness and exercise within the past 20 minutes. A resting respiratory assessment needs to be conducted a minimum of 20 minutes after exercise. The person's position is also pertinent in some cases (e.g. some respiratory diseases make breathing difficult if the person is lying down). These factors increase or decrease the rate and depth of respiration.

Remember to observe the person:

LOOK Are they breathing easily, is their colour good, are they resting comfortably and are they using accessory muscles to breathe?

LISTEN Do they have laboured breathing; can they talk in sentences?

FEEL Is their skin warm and dry or cool and clammy; is their chest rising/falling evenly?

PART 3

THE PERSON LIVING WITH SEVERE OBESITY

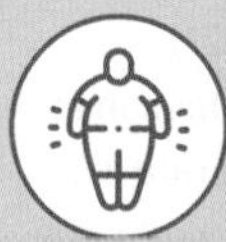

For people living with severe obesity (see **Clinical Skills 15 and 23** for a brief explanation), assessing their respirations is particularly important. Excess abdominal fat impinges on the diaphragmatic movement, making the severely obese person breathe more shallowly, causing reduced gas exchange. You will probably not be able to rest their arm on their chest to count respirations, so the person may be aware of and thus change their respiratory rate.

Count the respirations

As discussed, the person should be unaware when respirations are measured so that the rate and rhythm are unaffected by voluntary control. Adequate lighting helps you to see and count the person's respirations. Place the person's arm across their chest and count each inspiration–expiration cycle – this is one respiration.

Respiratory rate should be measured over a full 60 seconds, for accuracy, whether the person looks unwell or not (Palmer et al., 2022). The 15- or 30-second measurements often fail to identify deterioration in sick people (Rimbi et al., 2019). Thirty seconds would be the minimum time to count a healthy person's regular respiration pattern, but follow the policy of the facility if they have decided on one minute. Do not document an estimated rate or a 'normal' respiratory rate value (16, 18, 20) for expediency sake (Kallioinen et al., 2021).

Note any alteration of respirations from a normal rate, regular rhythm or easy, effortless and quiet respirations. Depth of respiration is the volume of air moving in and out of the lungs with each respiration. It is subjectively measured and recorded as shallow, normal or deep. Sighing is a single deep breath taken to open small airways and is normal. Assess the person for other physical signs and symptoms of respiratory dysfunction (e.g. dyspnoea, noisy breathing, tachypnoea, bradypnoea or apnoea).

Respiratory rate, depth and ease are indicators of ventilation. SpO_2 (see **Clinical Skill 12**) is NOT a substitute for respiratory rate count – it is a complementary assessment.

CLEAN, REPLACE AND DISPOSE OF EQUIPMENT

Dispose of probe covers and sheaths in the contaminated waste. If the probe cover fails to eject fully, use a gloved hand or a tissue to remove it. Clean electronic, digital, tympanic and temporal artery thermometers as per the manufacturer's recommendations. Replace the supply of probe covers or sheaths as necessary. The base should be plugged into a power source to ensure the batteries remain charged. Perform hand hygiene.

DOCUMENTATION

Temperature, pulse and respiration (TPR) are documented on the vital signs sheet of the person's chart or in the eHealth record. Note if the temperature reading was temporal, rectal or axillary, as oral or tympanic are the normal methods. Note if another pulse point than the radial was used. Document immediately after measuring so the reading will not be forgotten. Report abnormal readings in TPR (and associated symptoms) or trends to the shift coordinator so that further action can be promptly taken, if warranted. Brekke et al. (2019) demonstrated the importance of trends in identifying and predicting deterioration in a person's condition. The Australian Commission on Safety and Quality in Health Care (ACSQHC, 2021) suggests a 'Recognising and Responding to Acute Deterioration Standard' reporting, which includes the TPR observations among others, to alert staff of deterioration in a person. Examples of the vital signs and Adult Deterioration Detection System sheets will be available in your fundamentals text and in the laboratory for practice.

TPR are not assessed in isolation, but rather are analysed in conjunction with other signs (e.g. blood pressure) and symptoms (e.g. pain levels) and the person's ongoing health status.

CLINICAL SKILLS ASSESSMENT

Temperature, pulse and respiration measurement

Demonstrates the ability to effectively measure temperature, pulse and respiration. Incorporates the *National Safety and Quality Health Service Standards*: 2 Partnering with Consumers, 3 Preventing and Controlling Healthcare-Associated Infection, 5 Comprehensive Care, 6 Communicating for Safety, and 8 Recognising and Responding to Acute Deterioration (ACSQHC, 2021).

Performance criteria	1	2	3	4	5
(Numbers indicate NMBA *Registered Nurse Standards for Practice*)	**(Dependent)**	**(Marginal)**	**(Assisted)**	**(Supervised)**	**(Independent)**
1. Identifies indication (1.1, 3.3, 3.4)	☐	☐	☐	☐	☐
2. Evidence of therapeutic interaction with the person, e.g. gives the person a clear explanation of the procedure (1.4, 1.5, 2.1, 2.2, 3.2)	☐	☐	☐	☐	☐
3. Demonstrates clinical reasoning, e.g. prepares the environment, ensures sufficient light and quiet, provides for warmth and privacy (1.1, 1.2, 1.3, 4.2, 6.1)	☐	☐	☐	☐	☐
4. Gathers equipment (1.1, 5.5, 6.1): ■ thermometer (oral, electronic, tympanic, temporal artery or rectal) ■ tissues, alcowipes ■ sheath or probe covers ■ watch with a second hand ■ clean gloves	☐	☐	☐	☐	☐
5. Performs hand hygiene (1.1, 3.4, 6.1)	☐	☐	☐	☐	☐
6. Prepares the appropriate thermometer (1.1, 6.1)	☐	☐	☐	☐	☐
7. Assesses the person (4.1, 4.2, 4.3)	☐	☐	☐	☐	☐
8. Takes the temperature (1.1, 4.2, 6.1)	☐	☐	☐	☐	☐
9. Measures pulse rate, rhythm and quality (1.1, 4.1, 4.2, 6.1)	☐	☐	☐	☐	☐
10. Measures respiratory rate, depth, rhythm and quality (1.1, 4.1, 4.2, 6.1)	☐	☐	☐	☐	☐
11. Cleans, replaces and disposes of equipment appropriately (3.6, 6.1)	☐	☐	☐	☐	☐
12. Documents relevant information (1.1, 1.4, 1.6, 2.2, 2.7, 3.5, 3.7, 6.1, 6.2, 6.5, 7.3)	☐	☐	☐	☐	☐
13. Demonstrates the ability to link theory to practice (1.1, 3.3, 3.4, 3.5)	☐	☐	☐	☐	☐

Student:

Clinical facilitator: Date:

CHAPTER 11

BLOOD PRESSURE MEASUREMENT

INDICATIONS

The peripheral arterial blood pressure (BP) is obtained to:

- assess the haemodynamic health status of the person
- obtain a baseline measure of BP for subsequent comparison
- identify and monitor early changes in a person's status due to a disease process or medical therapy (Douglas et al., 2016).

A medical practitioner can order BP readings, nurses can initiate the assessment or they can be done for protocol reasons. Trends in BP readings over time are more significant than single readings. A single BP reading should never be used in isolation, because of the extreme variability due to the intrinsic dynamic nature of BP (Stergiou et al., 2022), but should be used as part of an overall clinical assessment. Nurses in general wards assess the BP non-invasively. Many facilities use observation units that incorporate BP, temperature, pulse and SpO_2 equipment.

EVIDENCE OF THERAPEUTIC INTERACTION

Communicating with the person you are caring for assists them to cooperate with the procedure and helps allay anxiety, which adversely affects the BP reading. However, refrain from speaking to the person during the BP reading and ask them not to speak, because these actions influence the reading. Conversation has been demonstrated to elevate BP by as much as 20 points (Padwal et al., 2019). Tell them the reading following the procedure (if they want to know) to develop trust.

DEMONSTRATE CLINICAL REASONING

Assess the person

Nurses are the front line in recognising and responding to deterioration of the person in their care and must take the responsibility of assessment seriously. Sit the person comfortably and allow them to rest quietly for five minutes. Observe them for physical signs and symptoms that may indicate altered BP, remembering that they may be asymptomatic.

LOOK for flushing, epistaxis, fatigue (hypertension), pallor or dusky skin colour (hypotension).

LISTEN for report of headache or fatigue (hypertension) or dizziness or confusion (hypotension).

FEEL for cool extremities, elevated pulse and respiratory rate (hypotension).

Consider factors that affect BP, such as activity, emotional stress, medications, bladder distension and recent ingestion of a meal, caffeine or nicotine (Padwal et al., 2019). Note other vital signs, such as pulse and respirations, and any previous readings, if available.

Be forewarned that diseases likely to affect BP include renal or cardiovascular disease, diabetes mellitus, blood-clotting disorders, toxaemia of pregnancy, acute or chronic pain and increased intracranial pressure. The postoperative situation, sitting with crossed legs, a full bladder, muscle tension, rapid intravenous (IV) infusion and a hot or cold environment will also alter the reading. If the person has eaten, smoked or exercised, the BP reading should be delayed (the National Heart Foundation [Gabb et al., 2016] recommends a two-hour delay following smoking or ingestion of caffeine), unless the situation is urgent. Unsworth, Tucker and Hindmarsh (2015) found the oscillometric (automatic) measurement of BP to be less accurate in people with many diseases. They suggest the growing reliance on the automated manometer is leading to a loss of skill in obtaining an accurate manual reading and suggest using the manual method on people with diabetes mellitus, arrhythmias, tremors and prolonged hypotension. Also, be aware that a large percentage of automatic sphygmomanometers marketed globally have not been clinically validated (Sharman et al., 2023a). Home BP readings with automated BP machines are used to confirm, manage and follow up hypertension. These machines provide multiple readings over the day in the person's usual environment.

A cuffless BP monitor (either a patch or a watch) noninvasively measuring changes at the skin surface in blood pressure, heart rate and oxygenation is now available, although their accuracy in tracking BP variations requires validation (Schutte, Kollias & Stergiou, 2022).

The person and their arm are assessed for contraindications to BP readings, such as: IV or blood therapy sites; arm or hand injury, surgery, disease or pain; arteriovenous shunt; current or previous breast, axillary or shoulder surgery; lymphadenopathy; casts or bulky bandages; or known vascular disease in that arm. The arm should be bare or only lightly clothed, as these readings are significantly lower than those taken below a rolled-up sleeve (Lins, 2023).

Use the contact time taken to obtain a BP to further assess the person for visual cues of an altered condition. Trends in the readings or a sharp change in a reading with concurrent changes in other vital signs indicate deterioration in the physiological functioning of an individual. The early warning allows rapid intervention to improve the person's safety and outcomes (Samani & Rattani, 2023). The change in BP reading is a later sign of deterioration as compensatory mechanisms fail. Holistically look, listen and feel for subtle changes that will alert you to impending deterioration.

Prepare the environment

Taking BP involves listening to very faint sounds and sound changes, so the surroundings should be as quiet as possible. You may need to turn off the radio or TV and ask visitors to be quiet. Temperature regulation is also an important consideration; for example, shivering alters the BP reading. Ask the person not to talk or use their phone. Do not talk to them during the procedure.

Position the person

The brachial artery in the upper arm, above the elbow, is most commonly used to obtain a BP measurement. This is the standard site for non-invasive BP measurement (Padwal et al., 2019). Take a BP reading with the person sitting with their feet flat on the floor. Support their arm with the midpoint of the upper arm at the level of the heart to improve accuracy (Sharma et al., 2023). Ask them to extend their elbow (firmly supported, e.g. on a table) with their palm upward. If necessary, the person can be in the supine position with the forearm extended, palm upward and supported on a pillow to prevent muscle contraction, which could increase the diastolic pressure by 10 per cent (Estes et al., 2020). The upper arm should be fully exposed so that the cuff can be properly applied.

Sometimes standing BP readings are required. These are taken after the 'lying' and 'sitting' BP readings, with the person being assisted to stand slowly.

?

If neither arm is available for obtaining a BP reading, use the leg. The person is placed in the prone position (if possible) and the appropriately sized cuff is snugly wrapped around the leg above the ankle. The posterior tibialis artery is palpated, then auscultated for the reading. Leg readings are higher than arm pressures. Note the use of the leg in the documentation.

Little empirical data has been published about the differences in BP in the arm and leg in the general population. Sheppard et al. (2020, p. 418) suggest 'a threshold of ≥155/90 mmHg … for diagnosing hypertension in routine practice when only ankle measurements are available'. These authors recommend the ankle rather than the thigh (cuff around lower leg) so the more easily palpated distal pulses are used.

ELDER CARE

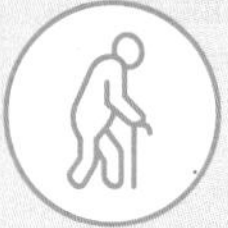

Knowing the baseline BP of elderly people is important in assessing their current BP. Their normal systolic readings may be high due to reduced compliance of the arteries and a 'normal' reading might then indicate shock (Mattu et al., 2016).

Arterial stiffness is associated with a widening pulse pressure (systolic BP minus diastolic BP). This, in turn, is associated with increased frailty, decreased functioning (Chuang et al., 2022) and increased sarcopenia (Rong et al., 2020). Sarcopenia is a decline in skeletal muscle mass and strength. Target systolic BP for those over 65 years is less than 130 mmHg with no recommendations made for a target diastolic BP (Flack & Adekola, 2020).

Hypertension is associated with ageing, with 79 per cent of those over 80 years old affected. Hypertension is asymptomatic, but has devastating effects on the cardiovascular, renal and neurological systems over time (Siedlinski et al., 2023).

Hypotension has also been linked to increased mortality in the elderly (Yamaguchi et al., 2023). Postural (also called orthostatic) hypotension is a significant contributor to falls in the elderly (Jones et al., 2023). Kubota et al. (2022) demonstrated the effectiveness of drinking cold/carbonated water in raising the BP in someone with postural hypotension in addition to repositioning.

THE PERSON LIVING WITH SEVERE OBESITY

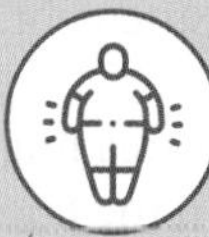

It is difficult to obtain an accurate BP reading on someone who is severely obese (see **Clinical Skills 15 and 23** for brief discussions of people living with severe obesity). The circumference of their upper arms often precludes the use of even the largest cuffs, and even large cuffs cannot accommodate the cone shape of the limb (Eley et al., 2019). The thick layer of tissue between the cuff/stethoscope and the artery muffle the pulse and make registering a BP difficult (Eley et al., 2019). As well, severely obese people usually have hypertension (due to increased circulating blood volume needed to oxygenate the excess tissue, plus increase in some hormones and possible kidney damage). You will need to obtain a sufficiently large conical-shaped cuff (a bariatric cuff – usually from central supply) and a Doppler to hear the pulse, or use an automated BP machine with a bariatric cuff, which is preferable.

GATHER EQUIPMENT

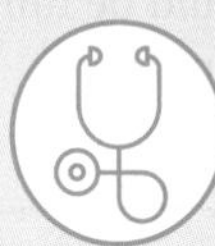

Gathering equipment is an organisational step that helps to create a positive environment for a successful interaction. It ensures that you have all needed material, boosts the person's confidence and trust in you, and increases your self-confidence. While gathering the equipment, you can familiarise yourself with any new equipment and mentally rehearse the procedure. Equipment may include the following items:

EQUIPMENT	EXPLANATION
Sphygmomanometer	Consists of a valved cuff with an inflatable bladder and a calibrated measuring unit (see below). When inflated, the cuff occludes the artery it surrounds (usually the brachial). During the measurement, the valve is released slowly and the artery below the cuff is listened to using the stethoscope
Manometer	*Manual auscultatory manometers* • Two basic types – the aneroid and the mercury manometer (the latter is being phased out due to safety and environmental concerns, and you will probably not use one) • An aneroid manometer consists of a calibrated dial that registers variations of pressure within the bladder of the cuff. A needle on the dial swings with the pressure variation. It requires frequent calibration (Padwal et al., 2019) *Automated digital BP measuring devices* • Frequently used and are accurate, effective and are the standard for measuring BP non-invasively (Sharman et al., 2023b) • Using an automated digital manometer does not allow you to monitor the quality or the rhythm of the pulse and is not precise in arrhythmias (Seidlerová et al., 2019). Some conditions increase the likelihood of measurement error (e.g. a weak, thready or irregular pulse or muscular tremors), in which case, use a manual BP measurement • Frequent readings are uncomfortable and do not allow the engorged vessels to empty • Lin et al. (2017) found new technological advances in non-invasive BP oscillometric equipment to be as accurate as invasive techniques
Cuff Sizes: Small adult – less than 26 cm Adult – 26–34 cm Large adult – 34–44cm Extra large adult – 44 cm + (Jackson et al., 2022)	• Made of occlusive cloth, which does not 'give' when the bladder is inflated, to ensure the pressure reading is accurate. The bladder is inflatable rubber that applies pressure to the arterial system • It should be chosen for the person (i.e. size, rather than age); the width must be 40 per cent of the arm circumference (see size list) to give accurate readings and the bladder should nearly encircle (80 per cent) the arm to prevent misapplication (Padwal et al., 2019) • Thigh cuffs are available for use on the thigh if arms are not suitable (i.e. obese, casts) • Readings from one area (e.g. the upper arm) are not interchangeable with those of another area (e.g. the forearm or the thigh). The arm gives the most accurate reading (Padwal et al., 2019)
Pressure valve	(On manual manometers only) holds in the air pumped by the bulb into the bladder. As the valve is released, the air leaves slowly so that changes in pressure can be measured
Stethoscope	• These are closed cylinders that conduct sounds from the body and do not allow sound to dissipate • It consists of earpieces, which should fit snugly and comfortably in your ear; binaurals, which are curved pieces of metal tubing that are angled to keep the earpieces comfortably in place; and plastic or rubber tubing (the shorter it is, within reason, the better the sound – 30 to 40 cm is ideal) to conduct sound; and the chest piece, with a diaphragm and a bell surface • The diaphragm side (flat surface) picks up high-pitched sounds best, like bowel and lung sounds. The bell (conical-shaped side) picks up lower-pitched sounds best, like heart and vascular sounds. Liu et al. (2016) found the choice of bell or diaphragm had only small influences on clinical BP readings and suggest using the diaphragm as it is easier to place over the artery
Alcowipes	Used to clean the stethoscope after use to reduce microorganisms

OBTAIN A BLOOD PRESSURE MEASUREMENT

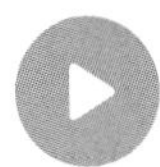

Blood pressure measurement is undertaken by nurses many times each day, but it should never become a habituated assessment – it is not routine. Each time you take a BP, attend closely to what you are doing, seeing and recording.

Hand hygiene

Hand hygiene (see **Clinical Skill 5**) removes microorganisms from your hands. It is the most effective preventative measure for cross-contamination, reducing incidences of nosocomial (i.e. hospital- or treatment-acquired) infection.

Blood pressure measurement

Apply the cuff

Place the fully deflated cuff over the brachial artery to ensure proper pressure is applied during inflation. Palpate the brachial artery to identify the placement. Wrap the cuff snugly around the arm about 2.5 cm above the antecubital space and secure (Padwal et al., 2019). Apply the cuff over bare skin (for a manual manometer) so the sounds heard through the stethoscope won't be muffled by clothing material (Ozone et al., 2016).

Automatic BP readings simply require you to apply the cuff, preset the upper systolic limit and press the start button. Manual readings require the remainder of these instructions.

Perform preliminary palpatory determination of systolic blood pressure

Preliminary palpatory determination is done on an initial BP reading to ascertain the accuracy of the systolic reading and that an auscultatory gap (an absence of Korotkoff sounds for a space of up to 30 to 40 mmHg when the cuff pressure is high), which occurs in some people with hypertension, does not interfere with accurate reading of the BP. The brachial artery (or radial artery if it is easier) is palpated with the fingertips of the non-dominant hand. With the (manual) manometer at eye level, close the pressure valve and inflate the bladder by squeezing the bulb repeatedly, until no pulse is discernible. Note this reading and deflate the cuff. The pressure reading on the sphygmomanometer gives an estimate of the maximum pressure required to determine the systolic pressure. Leave the arm for one to two minutes to allow the blood trapped in the veins to be released and returned to circulation.

Position the stethoscope

Tilt the binaurals forward, towards your face, so they follow the direction of your ear canal and sound is not muffled. The tubing should fall freely from the binaurals to the chest piece so that friction does not obliterate sounds. Turn the chest piece until the bell side is active (vascular sounds are low-pitched and are better picked up by the bell, although they can be heard using the diaphragm). Palpate the brachial artery in the antecubital fossa, place the bell over it and below the cuff, and maintain the position with the thumb and index finger of your non-dominant hand.

Auscultate the blood pressure

With your dominant hand, close the pressure valve and pump the bulb until the manometer registers 20 mmHg above the point where the brachial artery is occluded and the pulse disappears on palpation. Carefully release the valve so that the pressure falls slowly (2 to 3 mmHg/heartbeat [Padwal et al., 2019]) to reduce measurement errors. As the pressure falls, identify the Korotkoff sounds and note the pressure reading on the manometer when phases 1, 4 and 5 occur. The five phases are:

- *phase 1* – the first clear tapping sounds that gradually intensify (systolic sound)
- *phase 2* – the tapping sounds take on a swishing quality
- *phase 3* – the sounds become crisper and more intense
- *phase 4* – the sounds become muffled and have a soft, blowing quality (the diastolic sound in children and very active adults)
- *phase 5* – the sounds disappear (the diastolic sound in most adults) (Estes et al., 2020, p. 151).

Continue to listen for another 30 mmHg, then deflate the cuff rapidly and completely to decrease the person's discomfort. The systolic (phase 1) and the diastolic (phases 4 and/or 5) pressure should be immediately recorded, rounded off (upwards) to the nearest 2 mmHg.

Remove the cuff

Remove the cuff to allow the person to move their arm and restore circulation. Take more than one reading, especially if this is a baseline assessment. Wait two minutes between measurements to allow vessels to empty. If the readings vary by more than 5 mmHg, more readings should be taken.

The procedure is often repeated on the other arm to determine any difference in the two readings. A difference of 10 to 15 mmHg is not normal, and should be reported (Estes et al., 2020). Subsequent readings are taken on the arm with the higher reading (Padwal et al., 2019).

In summary

Strategies to obtain a valid BP measurement include:

- no caffeine, food, smoking or exercise 30 minutes prior
- empty bladder
- warm and quiet room
- sitting upright, back supported, feet flat on floor
- bare arm if possible
- arm supported on a flat surface at level of atrium
- no conversation or movement
- use a validated and calibrated BP machine

- choose an appropriate cuff size
- centre of cuff bladder over the brachial artery
- cuff edge 2 to 3 cm above antecubital fossa
- initial BP on both arms, subsequent BP on arm with highest initial reading (adapted from Cheung et al., 2022; Herrera et al., 2021; Loewy, 2023; Stergiou et al., 2021).

CLEAN, REPLACE AND DISPOSE OF EQUIPMENT

As a part of standard precautions, cleaning equipment reduces cross-contamination and fosters efficiency. Showlag et al. (2021) demonstrated the high bacterial load found on sphygmomanometers and cuffs (shared non-critical equipment). A non-disposable, plastic-coated sphygmomanometer is wiped down with antiseptic or alcowipes before use on another person to reduce the microbial load (Schroeder et al., 2022). If it has become grossly soiled, appropriate cleaning according to the manufacturer's recommendations is done. The stethoscope chest piece is wiped with an alcowipe to reduce microorganisms. The earpieces are also wiped with alcowipes unless the stethoscope is your personal one, in which case nothing is done to the earpieces.

DOCUMENTATION

The assessment data is recorded according to the facility's policy, usually on an observation sheet, although electronic recording is becoming more prevalent. BPs are generally recorded on the vital signs sheet. Often this is on a graph with inverted notches placed at the systolic reading point and upright notches denoting the diastolic reading. Note which arm or other site (thigh, wrist or ankle) was used. Also note this on the care plan.

In the hospital, individuals at risk of deterioration can often be detected through vital signs. The Australian Commission on Safety and Quality in Health Care (ACSQHC, 2021) advises the use of the Adult Deterioration Detection System (ADDS), a specialised observation sheet that incorporates the BP reading for people who are acutely or critically ill. These ADDS charts were designed to improve the recognition of deterioration using graphics, colour and scales to alert staff to a risk of critical change in the individual's condition (Cornish et al., 2019). (Examples will be supplied in laboratory sessions or can be found in fundamentals texts such as DeLaune et al., 2024.) Some populations (e.g. elderly) may deteriorate before there are objective changes in their vital signs, or a person may deteriorate further if there is a delay in escalating their care, resulting in increased morbidity and mortality. Thus the ADDS is an early warning system that has trigger points or mandatory criteria for escalating care (Fernando et al., 2019). Nurses must use holistic physical assessment as well as the vital signs and follow the algorithms to detect deterioration and promote the individual's safety (Wood, Chaboyer & Carr, 2019).

BP readings are documented as a fraction in written notes, with the systolic pressure over the diastolic pressure followed by mmHg (millimetres of mercury – the traditional measuring unit). All facilities use phase 1 sounds as the systolic recording. Some use phase 5 as the only diastolic reading, and some have a first diastolic (phase 4) and a second diastolic (phase 5); for example, you could have either 120/80 mmHg or 120/86/80 mmHg as BP readings.

Report any significant changes in a person's BP (e.g. systolic BP above 140 mmHg or below 100 mmHg or diastolic BP above 80 mmHg) or any significant shift within a number of readings (e.g. a drop in pressure from 180/90 mmHg to 150/80 mmHg within a short period) to the nurse in charge. Report trends in the readings, as these are most effective in detecting deterioration. Correlate the BP readings with other vital signs (temperature, pulse or respiration, pulse oximetry and pain assessments).

CLINICAL SKILLS ASSESSMENT

Blood pressure measurement

Demonstrates the ability to effectively measure blood pressure. Incorporates the *National Safety and Quality Health Service Standards*: 2 Partnering with Consumers, 3 Preventing and Controlling Healthcare-Associated Infection, 5 Comprehensive Care, 6 Communicating for Safety, and 8 Recognising and Responding to Acute Deterioration (ACSQHC, 2021).

Performance criteria	1	2	3	4	5
(Numbers indicate NMBA *Registered Nurse Standards for Practice*)	**(Dependent)**	**(Marginal)**	**(Assisted)**	**(Supervised)**	**(Independent)**
1. Identifies indication (1.1, 3.3, 3.4)	☐	☐	☐	☐	☐
2. Evidence of therapeutic interaction with the person, e.g. gives the person a clear explanation of the procedure (1.4, 1.5, 2.1, 2.2, 3.2)	☐	☐	☐	☐	☐
3. Demonstrates clinical reasoning abilities, e.g. assesses the person, prepares the environment, positions and prepares the person (1.1, 1.2, 1.3, 2.3, 4.1, 4.2, 4.3, 6.1)	☐	☐	☐	☐	☐
4. Gathers equipment (1.1, 5.5, 6.1): ■ sphygmomanometer (digital, aneroid or mercury manometer) and appropriately sized cuff ■ stethoscope ■ alcowipes	☐	☐	☐	☐	☐
5. Performs hand hygiene (1.1, 3.4, 6.1)	☐	☐	☐	☐	☐
6. Applies the cuff (1.1, 4.1, 4.2, 4.3, 6.1)	☐	☐	☐	☐	☐
7. Performs a preliminary palpatory systolic determination (1.1, 6.1)	☐	☐	☐	☐	☐
8. Positions the stethoscope appropriately (1.1, 6.1)	☐	☐	☐	☐	☐
9. Auscultates the person's blood pressure (1.1, 6.1)	☐	☐	☐	☐	☐
10. Removes the cuff (1.1, 6.1)	☐	☐	☐	☐	☐
11. Repeats the procedure on the other arm (1.1, 6.1)	☐	☐	☐	☐	☐
12. Cleans, replaces and disposes of equipment appropriately (3.6, 6.1)	☐	☐	☐	☐	☐
13. Documents relevant information (1.1, 1.4, 1.6, 2.2, 2.7, 3.5, 3.7, 6.1, 6.2, 6.5, 7.3)	☐	☐	☐	☐	☐
14. Demonstrates the ability to link theory to practice (1.1, 3.3, 3.4, 3.5)	☐	☐	☐	☐	☐

Student:

Clinical facilitator: Date:

CHAPTER 12

PULSE OXIMETRY – MEASURING OXYGEN SATURATION

INDICATIONS

Pulse oximetry is a simple assessment and non-invasive. It is an indirect approximation of arterial oxygenation (Pretto et al., 2014), which is also very complex and requires a good understanding of the physiology of respiration, oxygenation and circulation. Oxygen saturation is the amount of oxygen-saturated haemoglobin compared to the total haemoglobin in the blood (Kumar & Deo, 2019). A sensor (spectrographic technology) is used to detect the ratio of oxyhaemoglobin to deoxyhaemoglobin (Shinozaki et al., 2019). It emits light waves through the peripheral vascular bed (finger, earlobe). Both red light (which is preferentially absorbed by deoxygenated haemoglobin) and infrared light waves (which is preferentially absorbed by oxygenated haemoglobin) are then detected by the photo detector on the other side of the finger/earlobe. The ratio of the two light waves as they are detected is used by the pulse oximeter to compute the percentage of oxygen saturation of the peripheral blood.

Pulse oximetry detects hypoxia resulting from a deficiency of available oxygen in arterial blood and tissues (Karlen, 2019), reducing the need for arterial blood gas analysis and providing a basis for titrating oxygen supplementation (Pilcher et al., 2020). It is used to identify deterioration in physiologic function (cardiovascular and respiratory, especially) that may otherwise be missed, allowing the person to receive rapid treatment and avoid associated complications (Held, 2023).

Pulse oximetry is abbreviated to SpO_2 (**S**aturation of **P**eripheral arterial blood with **O**xygen). You will need a sound knowledge of respiratory anatomy and physiology, oxygen transport and the oxyhaemoglobin dissociation curve when interpreting SpO_2. (Please consult a nursing fundamentals text; for example, Delaune et al. [2024] or a physiology text for this information.) Very small changes in this curve can signal great physiologic and clinical changes. For example, an SpO_2 reading below 90 per cent saturation may indicate inadequate oxygen supply or excessive demand (Kumar & Deo, 2019). It is vital to evaluate the person's pulse oximetry readings in relation to their clinical status and history so that you can initiate appropriate clinical interventions.

EVIDENCE OF THERAPEUTIC INTERACTION

Introduce yourself and inform the person of your designation. Explain the procedure to the person. Clarify any immediate concerns to help allay fears and gain the person's cooperation. Pulse oximetry is a non-invasive procedure but involves electronic monitoring, which can be frightening to some people. Explanations should include the parameters within which their oxygen level should remain. Ensure the person is comfortable and warm enough.

DEMONSTRATE CLINICAL REASONING

Safety

Pulse oximeters are reliable when SaO_2 (arterial oxygen saturation measured by blood analysis) is 90 per cent or above, and accuracy deteriorates when SaO_2 falls to 80 per cent or less (Urden, Stacy & Long, 2017). Normal SpO_2 readings are between 95 and 100 per cent (DeLaune et al., 2024); however, oxygen therapy should be administered to achieve normal or near-normal SpO_2 of 94 to 98 per cent for all acutely ill people, and 89 to 92 per cent for those at risk of chronic hypercapnoeic respiratory failure (Buekers et al., 2019). When SpO_2 is abnormal, the arterial blood gases will provide vital information about ventilation, pulmonary gas exchange and acid/base status. Continuous SpO_2 monitoring is more effective at identifying clinical deterioration earlier than using intermittent SpO_2 readings. See TABLE 12.1 for an overview of pathophysiological and technical causes of unreliable SpO_2 readings. SpO_2 is NOT a substitute for respiratory rate count – it is a complementary assessment. Respiratory rate should be measured over a full 60 seconds, for accuracy, whether the person looks unwell or not (Palmer et al., 2022).

TABLE 12.1 Overview of pathophysiological and technical causes of unreliable SpO_2 readings

CAUSES OF UNRELIABLE SPO_2 READING	EFFECT ON PULSE OXIMETRY
Emergencies	
Cardiac arrest	Poor signal
Respiratory arrest	Poor signal
Sepsis and septic shock	Poor signal – falsely high or low reading
Physiological/Pathophysiological	
Dark skin pigmentation	No effect on accuracy when oxygen levels are normal; when arterial oxygen saturations are 90 per cent and below, SpO_2 may overestimate SaO_2 by approximately 2 per cent (Cabanas et al., 2022)
Anaemia	No interference; however, oxygen content reduced; potentially, tissue oxygen delivery is reduced
Low-perfusion state (e.g. peripheral vascular disease, smoking, coronary artery disease, poor peripheral circulation)	Inaccurate reading, low pulse signals, falsely low readings and poor signal
Presence of digital clubbing (from chronic respiratory failure)	Inaccurate reading, low reading on finger sensors – use earlobe sensor
Arteriovenous fistula	Poor signal
Injection of some intravenous dyes (methylene blue, indocyanine green, indigo carmine) used in imaging	Can lead to falsely low readings 20 minutes after administration
Dyshaemoglobinaemia	
Carboxyhaemoglobin (from carbon dioxide inhalation)	Similar light absorption to oxyhaemoglobin; unable to differentiate between oxyhaemoglobin, carboxyhaemoglobin and methaemoglobin, leading to falsely high readings
Methaemoglobinaemia (congenital or acquired through antibiotic use)	Similar light absorption to oxyhaemoglobin; unable to differentiate between oxyhaemoglobin, carboxyhaemoglobin and methaemoglobin, leading to falsely high readings
Environmental	
Nail polish and acrylic nails	Poor signal with brown, blue and black, falsely low reading; remove nail polish and acrylic nails
Bright light (particularly fluorescent), heat lamps or sunshine	False increase or decrease in signal, falsely high or low reading; cover probe with opaque barrier such as a washcloth
Movement artefact – shivering, tremors, rigors, motion	Poor signal, falsely low reading; keep person warm (if not contraindicated), encourage the person to minimise movement, use a less mobile monitoring site (e.g. earlobe). Some newer oximeters are motion tolerant
Mechanical barriers and/or obstructions to circulation (e.g. blood pressure cuff, tourniquet, arterial line)	Poor signal, falsely low reading
Poor probe positioning	Falsely high or low reading
Dirty sensor	Poor signal, falsely low reading

SOURCES: URDEN, STACY & LONG (2017). *CRITICAL CARE NURSING: DIAGNOSIS AND MANAGEMENT* (8TH ED.). ST LOUIS, MO: ELSEVIER; PILCHER ET AL. (2020). A MULTICENTRE PROSPECTIVE OBSERVATIONAL STUDY COMPARING ARTERIAL BLOOD GAS VALUES TO THOSE OBTAINED BY PULSE OXIMETERS USED IN ADULT PATIENTS ATTENDING AUSTRALIAN AND NEW ZEALAND HOSPITALS. *BMC PULMONARY MEDICINE, 20*(7). HTTPS://DOI.ORG/10.1186/S12890-019-1007-3; DEEP ET AL. (2019). COMPARATIVE STUDY OF PULSE OXIMETRY AND ANKLE-BRACHIAL INDEX AS A SCREENING TEST FOR ASYMPTOMATIC PERIPHERAL VASCULAR DISEASE IN TYPE 2 DIABETES MELLITUS AGAINST COLOR DOPPLER ULTRASONOGRAPHY AS REFERENCE STANDARD. *INTERNATIONAL JOURNAL OF ADVANCES IN MEDICINE, 6*(4), 1151–6.

ELDER CARE

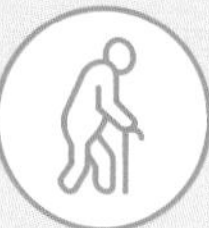

Cardoso, Pinheira and Carvalho (2023) found that SpO_2 values fall with advancing age, with average SpO_2 of 65- to 79-year-olds at 96.3 per cent and average SpO_2 of those older than 80 years at 94.6 per cent. Although age itself does not seem to affect SpO_2 readings, poor perfusion (from hypotension, vasoconstriction) and irregular heart rate are common in the elderly, and especially when they are ill, so low SpO_2 readings (below 95%) are significant.

PART 3

THE PERSON LIVING WITH SEVERE OBESITY

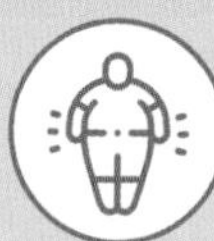

Kapur et al. (2013) found that people living with obesity consistently register a lower SpO_2 reading than those with normal weight/height ratios. They postulate that obesity restricts lung function and oxygen exchange. Xiong et al. (2022) found that in people with a >40 BMI, SpO_2 overestimates arterial oxygen saturation by 2.3 per cent, so the person could be hypoxic even if the SpO_2 reading was within the normal range.

GATHER EQUIPMENT

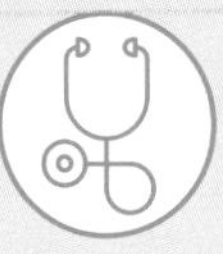

Gathering equipment is an organisational step that helps to create a positive environment for a successful interaction. Equipment may include the following items:

EQUIPMENT	EXPLANATION
Pulse oximeter/monitor	• Displays the readings of the sensor • Ensure the probe and equipment are clean and in working order • Follow the manufacturer's instructions to ensure the waveform and alarm limits are correctly set
Sensor probe and cord	• Most commonly used clinical oximeters are those in which the light emitter and the detector face each other, and the linear photo transmission is assessed through the tissues. Multi wavelength devices improve the accuracy if the person is hypoxic (Cabanas et al., 2022) • Are available and suitable for use on fingers, toes or earlobes in adults, and on neonates' feet (Pretto et al., 2014) • Reflectance oximetry uses an emitter adjacent to the detector, relying on signals being reflected or scattered through tissues on the person's forehead. Pretto et al. (2014, p. 42) suggest that these provide a more accurate reading because they are less sensitive to poor peripheral perfusion, reduced cardiac index, cold temperatures, and movement artefact, and respond more rapidly to central saturation changes • Probes can be spring-loaded clips or sensors that can be taped in place
Appropriately earthed electrical cable	• Provides electricity to operate the device • Batteries are usually also available to ensure measurement at all times • Cordless units are available
Alcowipes	Used (when indicated) to clean the finger or toe so the sensor can measure the oxygen levels

Determine the person's clinical need for pulse oximetry. Note the rate or percentage of any oxygen therapy administration. Assess the adequacy of blood supply to the selected finger, toe or earlobe. In a person with a low perfusion state (e.g. hypovolaemia, vasoconstriction, cardiac dysrhythmia, cold peripheries), an earlobe sensor is more accurate and rapid (Pertzov et al., 2019). Assess the person to determine the appropriate sensor size (i.e. a paediatric probe is adequate for a small adult).

Most people who are in hospital have their oxygen saturation assessed as a vital sign. All breathless and acutely ill people should have their oxygen saturation checked more frequently or continuously and documented using the Adult Deterioration Detection System (ADDS).

ASSESS AND EVALUATE OXYGENATION USING PULSE OXIMETRY

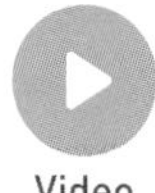

Video

Hand hygiene

Hand hygiene (see **Clinical Skill 5**) removes microorganisms from your hands. It is the most effective preventative measure for cross-contamination, reducing incidences of nosocomial (i.e. hospital- or treatment-acquired) infection.

Assess the person

Pay attention to the person – they are more important than the monitor (Alkhaqani & Ali, 2023). As you approach the person, assess them:

LOOK at them – observe their colour (both central and peripheral), assess their breathing (rate, rhythm and depth). Are they alert? Confused? Are they perspiring? Do they look comfortable?

LISTEN to what they tell you – are they short of breath? Is their breathing laboured or easy? Can they talk in sentences?

FEEL Do they have cool, damp peripheries? Hot, dry or damp skin? Rapid pulse?

Select and prepare the appropriate site

Select the site by checking that the person's pulse is adequate and has a good capillary refill in the selected limb. Do not take a blood pressure (BP) reading on the arm with the pulse oximeter probe as the pulse oximeter reading will be disrupted (World Health Organization [WHO], 2011). Check that the skin is not broken, oedematous or hypothermic, that it is clean and dry, and that nail polish has been removed.

Choose the appropriate probe to be applied to the forehead, earlobe or the bridge of the nose, if necessary (Hlavin & Varty, 2022).

> If the person has poor perfusion or a low-quality signal message is displayed, the oximeter probe needs to be moved to another site to obtain the best signal and most accurate reading (Pretto et al., 2014).

Attach the sensor probe

Use the manufacturer's instructions. Insert the digit fully – the emitters and detector are aligned opposite each other. Clip or tape the probe in place, taking care not to interfere with the circulation.

Ask the person to keep the finger that has the probe attached still, to reduce motion artefact, which compromises the accuracy of the pulse oximeter (Cabanas et al., 2022).

> If a low reading is detected, recheck the probe position and the perfusion of finger, toe or earlobe as well as the waveform.

Connect the probe to the oximeter monitor

Plug the cord into the appropriate outlet and turn on the oximeter. Leave the probe in situ long enough to get consistent readings. Correlate the oximeter pulse rate with the person's radial pulse to ensure reading accuracy (Dao Le, 2016). If these are not the same, check the probe placement.

Set alarms

The oximeter has preset alarm limits (e.g. SpO_2 set at high 100 per cent and low 85 per cent measurement and pulse high at 140 bpm and low 50 bpm). These need to be adjusted to levels appropriate for the person, according to their condition, the doctor's orders and the facility's policy. Alarm fatigue (desensitisation to the alarm sounds over time) is fostered by frequent, unnecessary alarms, so the alarm parameters need careful consideration (Berg et al., 2022). Follow the manufacturer's guidelines to adjust the alarm limits.

Appropriately monitor the person

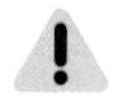
Safety

Monitor the person's SpO_2 readings as required. Take the SpO_2 reading, noting any supplementary oxygen administration. Evaluate the result with previous saturation levels, any changes in respiratory rate, oxygen therapy, pulse rate and your observations.

Inspect the sensor site frequently and rotate it according to the manufacturer's instructions. Generally, for continuous oximetry monitoring, check and rotate probe attachment sites every two hours to prevent pressure injury (Hlavin & Varty, 2022). Ensure the person is not lying on the probe lead (João et al., 2023).

Take care when removing a sensor to not injure the person in your care (e.g. careless removal of tape can tear fragile, elderly skin) or damage the sensor.

Care for equipment

An example of caring for equipment may be to replace batteries as necessary, silence alarms and alter the averaging mode, which averages the readings over a period of time (from two to 15 seconds).

Post-procedure

Assist the person to a comfortable position, replace the call bell and anything moved during the procedure so they are back within the person's reach. Perform hand hygiene.

CLEAN, REPLACE AND DISPOSE OF EQUIPMENT

Some sensors are disposable and changed every 24 hours (or as per the facility's policy). Others require cleaning according to the manufacturer's instructions. Clean and replace the oximeter, non-disposable probes and the leads and return these to the storage area. Plug the oximeter into a power source to recharge the battery, ensuring the equipment is ready for use when next required.

DOCUMENTATION

Use the ADDS chart to document SpO_2, any supplementary oxygen and other vital signs. Record in the progress notes the time, date and location of the sensor and condition of the skin. Document the person's response to any changes in oxygen therapy at frequent intervals, depending on the person's condition.

This chapter was kindly reviewed by Professor Malcolm Elliott, Senior Lecturer, Course Director, Master of Nursing Practice – Nursing & Midwifery, Monash University Member and past Chair Australian College of Critical Care Nurses Quality Advisory Panel.

PART 3

CLINICAL SKILLS ASSESSMENT

Monitoring pulse oximetry

Demonstrates the ability to effectively assess and evaluate a person's oxygenation using pulse oximetry. Incorporates the *National Safety and Quality Health Service Standards*: 2 Partnering with Consumers, 3 Preventing and Controlling Healthcare-Associated Infection, 5 Comprehensive Care, 6 Communicating for Safety, and 8 Recognising and Responding to Acute Deterioration (ACSQHC, 2021).

Performance criteria	1	2	3	4	5
(Numbers indicate NMBA *Registered Nurse Standards for Practice*)	(Dependent)	(Marginal)	(Assisted)	(Supervised)	(Independent)
1. Identifies indication (1.1, 3.3, 3.4)	☐	☐	☐	☐	☐
2. Evidence of therapeutic interaction with the person, e.g. gives person a clear explanation of procedure (1.4, 1.5, 2.1, 2.2, 3.2)	☐	☐	☐	☐	☐
3. Demonstrates clinical reasoning abilities, e.g. pulse oximeter precautions (1.1, 1.2, 1.3, 1.5, 4.1, 4.2, 4.3, 5.1, 6.1)	☐	☐	☐	☐	☐
4. Gathers equipment (1.1, 5.5, 6.1): ■ pulse oximeter/monitor ■ sensor probe and cord ■ earthed electrical cable ■ alcowipes ■ tape	☐	☐	☐	☐	☐
5. Performs hand hygiene (1.1, 3.4, 6.1)	☐	☐	☐	☐	☐
6. Selects and prepares an appropriate site (1.1, 4.1, 4.2, 4.3, 6.1)	☐	☐	☐	☐	☐
7. Attaches sensor probe (6.1)	☐	☐	☐	☐	☐
8. Connects the probe to the oximeter monitor (6.1)	☐	☐	☐	☐	☐
9. Sets alarms at levels appropriate for the person (6.1)	☐	☐	☐	☐	☐
10. Monitors the person appropriately (4.1, 4.2, 4.3, 6.1)	☐	☐	☐	☐	☐
11. Demonstrates the ability to care for the equipment, e.g. replaces batteries as necessary (3.4, 6.1)	☐	☐	☐	☐	☐
12. Assists the person to a comfortable position, replacing the call bell and things moved during the procedure to within their reach (2.3, 4.1, 4.2, 4.3, 6.1)	☐	☐	☐	☐	☐
13. Cleans, replaces and disposes of equipment appropriately (3.6, 6.1)	☐	☐	☐	☐	☐
14. Documents relevant information (1.1, 1.4, 1.6, 2.2, 2.7, 3.5, 3.7, 6.1, 6.2, 6.5, 7.3)	☐	☐	☐	☐	☐
15. Demonstrates the ability to link theory to practice (1.1, 3.3, 3.4, 3.5)	☐	☐	☐	☐	☐

Student:

Clinical facilitator: Date:

CHAPTER 13

PAIN ASSESSMENT

INDICATIONS

Pain itself is non-observable. Indications of pain range from blatant to invisible. Both reports of pain and non-verbal cues, such as grimacing, splinting or guarding an area, require a pain assessment. Accurate pain assessment is necessary for both effective pain management and to determine the response to treatment.

You should ask each person you care for if they are comfortable. There are many reasons that people do not volunteer a pain report. This may be due to:

- a wish to avoid increasing staff workload
- fear of being seen as weak, dependent or addicted
- fear that if the pain increases, medications used now will be ineffective
- worry about the costs of medications
- dislike of the adverse effects of the analgesia
- belief that pain is part of the recovery process or part of life.

Be aware, also, that many professionals are biased about pain. Disappointingly, Cousins et al. (2022) found that over the past 20 years, nursing students' knowledge about pain has not improved. They cited findings that students did not recognise a report of pain as being as valid an indicator as grimacing. Unfortunately, healthcare professionals may erroneously believe the persistent myths that the elderly (or newborns, children or cognitively impaired people) are less sensitive to pain. There may be gender bias (males are stoic, so their pain is assessed as more intense) (Earp et al., 2019). They may mistakenly believe that the use of opioid medications carries unacceptable risks or that pain is an inevitable consequence of ageing, surgery or other medical condition or treatment (DeLaune et al., 2024). Yang et al. (2023) demonstrated an underestimation of pain by nurses, risking persistent pain and post-surgical distress. Inadequately treated acute pain can potentially cause chronic pain through neurohormonal and neuronal mechanisms.

Pain may be chronic and unrelated to the reason for which the person has been hospitalised. Those who report acute pain require assessment frequently – every two hours, plus post-analgesia. People whose pain is stable or chronic should be monitored every four to eight hours and post-analgesia. Take care with the words you choose to inquire about pain. Using different terms such as 'discomfort', 'aches' or 'soreness' may make the person less reluctant to describe their pain.

Pain is considered a vital sign and should be assessed each time the other vital signs are done. Inadequate pain assessment can lead to both inadequate treatment and ongoing distress.

EVIDENCE OF THERAPEUTIC INTERACTION

Trust is established when you demonstrate your belief in the person's report of pain. When a person indicates that they are *not* comfortable, they have difficulty moving or they are unable to do effective postoperative exercises, further assessment is indicated. Tell the person of your intention to assess their pain. This knowledge fosters trust in you and creates a positive attitude that the pain will be addressed and alleviated. Advise people not to wait to be asked if they have pain and encourage them to tell you.

DEMONSTRATE CLINICAL REASONING

Providing privacy reduces distractions. Privacy encourages the person to disclose intimate information that they may otherwise be reluctant to discuss (e.g. if pain is felt in an embarrassing area or if there is reluctance to admit to pain).

People under-report pain because they are influenced by attitudes to pain based on age ('What can I expect at 77?') and gender (toughing it out). Sometimes specific questioning will help them to acknowledge the pain. Also consider the cultural context, because experience and expression of pain are mediated by culture (Givler & Maani-Fogelman, 2019).

Not only must pain be assessed, but some intervention to relieve the pain must be undertaken. Assessed pain needs to be addressed.

PART 3

ELDER CARE

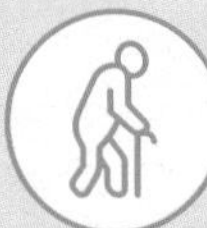

The elderly are a vulnerable group with specific needs (e.g. functional assistance) and limitations (e.g. deteriorating organ systems) whose pain level is often underestimated (Youngcharoen & Aree-Ue, 2023). Assessing pain in the elderly can be difficult due to many factors, such as sensory impairment (sight, hearing), cognitive impairment, polypharmacy, multiple comorbidities and frailty. More than 70 per cent of people over 85 years old have chronic pain (Atcherberg et al., 2013, cited in Scuteri et al., 2022). Choosing an appropriate pain assessment tool is critical to understanding and addressing the pain of the elderly person. Most pain scales do not assess the complexity of the pain experience, and therefore individualising your assessment and using situational awareness will assist in assessing the elderly person more appropriately.

THE PERSON LIVING WITH SEVERE OBESITY

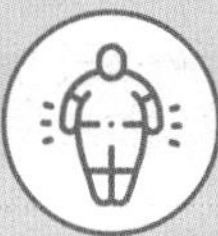

Obesity is strongly associated with chronic pain (Stokes et al., 2020). Osteoarthritis, lower back pain and diabetic neuropathy all contribute to the increasing incidence of pain for people living with obesity (Ewens et al., 2022). Pain assessments are crucial prior to and following moving a person living with severe obesity to ensure their comfort.

GATHER EQUIPMENT

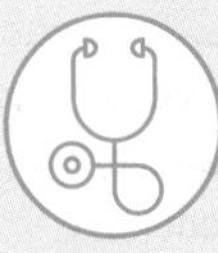

Gathering equipment is a time-management strategy. The tools needed for assessing pain are minimal, and include sphygmomanometer, stethoscope, thermometer and watch for vital sign assessment (temperature, pulse and respiration, blood pressure, pulse oximetry, level of consciousness), although fluctuations in the vital signs are not specific for pain detection (Freund & Bolick, 2019). The most important factors are your understanding of pain perception and your attitude to pain. You must understand pain physiology, including pain theories, structures of pain perception, the roles of pain centres in the brain and the roles of neuromodulators. These factors are discussed in medical-surgical textbooks.

The actual tools used range from simple scales such as visual analogue scales (VAS), numerical scales, colour scales and face scales, to more comprehensive tools that assess many facets of pain. The minimum pain assessment would be asking about presence of pain, and, if present, asking about location, intensity, quality, radiation, aggravating and relieving factors. (See further discussion below.) The type of pain being experienced directs the choice of pain tool. Generally, the VAS or the numerical rating scale, followed by the questions about location, quality, radiation, aggravating/relieving factors, and sometimes the Melzack tool or the McCaffery-Beibe form or a similar form, is adequate. The facility where you work will have a preferred tool.

CONDUCT THE PAIN ASSESSMENT

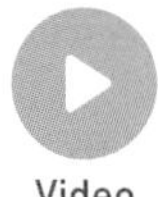

Video

Assess the person

Pain assessment is dependent on the situation and the individual. For everyone:

LOOK for signs of discomfort – grimaces, restlessness or stillness, protecting an area (e.g. cradling an arm or pressing on the abdomen), repetitive movements and swelling of an area.

LISTEN to reports of pain (pain is subjective – only the person experiencing it can know its impact) (Wideman et al., 2019), inarticulate sounds when moving, and moaning.

FEEL Skin texture is often clammy; tachycardia may be present.

Someone in severe acute pain would be asked a minimum number of assessment questions (location, intensity and quality) in order to establish a baseline before interventions are begun.

Although useful indicators of acute pain, vital signs are not valid pain indicators for people using opioid medications, those with an altered level of consciousness or on ventilation due to the changes in vital signs brought about by these conditions (Shahiri & Gélinas, 2023).

Obtain a history

The assessment continues with a history. As with any history, the person needs to be positioned as comfortably as possible and should be wearing any required aids, such as glasses, hearing aids and dentures. The history includes questions about the pain experience. The person should be given time and a sense of your belief in their pain so that they can describe it adequately. Background information helps you to understand their response to pain and affects the management of pain. Topics to cover include:

- the effect of pain on significant others
- the effect on the lifestyle of the person
- the effect on their activities of daily living and functioning (physical and social)
- any activities or remedies they have tried, either successfully or unsuccessfully
- how the person views their pain
- the disease process or underlying pathology causing the pain
- if the person feels they have control over their pain using any remedies
- what the person thinks causes the pain (this may be different from the disease process).

A good pain history will give clues as to the condition causing the pain and assist in making treatment choices. Document this well, so the person does not have to repeat this section of the pain assessment.

Difficulties may arise because of communication barriers, such as inability to speak English, deafness, aphasia/dysphasia, age (e.g. neonate, infant, paediatric), mental illness, dementia or intellectual disabilities, confusion, unconsciousness and sedation. Such communication barriers require different assessment approaches. A range of valid and reliable specialised assessment tools is available to assist in assessing the non-verbal person (Peters, 2017). Demographic factors are an important consideration.

The Faces Pain Scale has proved to be valid and reliable with many groups (e.g. children, the elderly, those who are cognitively impaired and many with communication difficulties). For preverbal children, pain assessment tools consist of pain-associated behaviours, plus (sometimes) the physiological markers of stress. Specific tools improve assessment for non-communicative people in areas such as intensive care (Phillips, Kuruvilla & Bailey, 2019). Determine which tool is used in the facility where you are located.

Establish pain parameters

It is important to establish pain parameters using the following guidelines. One dimensional pain assessment (i.e. intensity) is inadequate. Carefully assess all the dimensions of pain (Baamer et al., 2022). Determine these dimensions of the person's pain using a mnemonic such as OPQRST (onset, position and palliating factors, quality and quantity, radiation, setting and associated symptoms, and the timing and treatment [Estes et al., 2020]).

The following outlines the Brief Pain Inventory for initial assessment of a person's pain:

- Determine the location of the pain by asking the person to point to where it is located. A body diagram can be marked to record the location indicated. If the pain radiates, ask the person to touch the point of most severity and follow the pain along its path with their finger. Ask if there is more than one area or type of pain being experienced, then find out the following for each area of pain.
- Determine the intensity of the pain using a VAS or numerical rating scale. Using a pain rating scale requires careful explanation geared to the cognitive level of the person.
- Ask the person to describe the quality of the pain. This is often useful in diagnosing the cause. Using a list of pain descriptors, such as those on Melzack's pain tool, may assist if the person has difficulty in naming the quality of the pain. Peters (2017) suggests that for those from a different culture or language, adjectives, metaphors, cultural idioms or expressions to describe the pain can complement a verbal pain tool assessment. Wideman et al. (2019, p. 213) warn that 'failure to validate pain reports and show compassion can increase patient distress, degrade therapeutic alliance, and undermine hope for improvement', as well as make the person feel stigmatised and alienated.
- Ask the person to describe the onset of pain, including when it began and if there is a discernible pattern.
- Discuss the duration of the pain by asking if it is constant or episodic; of sudden or insidious onset; of short or long duration.
- Assess pain on both independent and nurse-initiated movement as well as at rest.
- Ask about the impact of the pain on their ability to function.

Finding out factors that induce the pain or precipitate its occurrence will help the person avoid these in the future. Similarly, note coping strategies and pain-control techniques (including medication) that have been used in the past, whether successfully or not. Explore the measures that the person uses to relieve the pain, such as rest, relaxation, distraction, over-the-counter medications, complementary therapies or any other interventions used. Note the time of the last dose of any analgesia.

Self-management of chronic pain using an artificial intelligence digital coach with behavioural approaches has been demonstrated to reduce pain interference in daily life, improve physical function and reduce anxiety, depression and pain catastrophising (Barreveld et al., 2023). The use of non-analgesic methods of pain control will need to be noted.

Psychological conditions may contribute to the pain experience. Discuss with the person any social, emotional and economic problems they may have.

Those who cannot verbally report pain (including people who are cognitively impaired and small children) should be monitored for non-verbal behavioural cues, such as restlessness, agitation, withdrawal, tense body language and any repetitive movement (rocking, rubbing), and a judgement should be made regarding the presence of pain. There are specialised tools to assess pain presence and intensity in those people who are non-verbal or have dementia (e.g. ABBEY Pain Scale, Pain Assessment in Advanced Dementia).

Although Freund and Bolick (2019) state that the physiological indicators of pain do not reliably distinguish between pain and stress, nevertheless the physiological effects of pain need to be observed and recorded. Acute pain can cause tachycardia, a change in blood pressure, pallor, grimacing, diaphoresis and hyperventilation/tachypnoea, and it may be accompanied by anxiety and apprehension. When associated with pain, the physiological signs wane over time.

Chronic pain may not alter vital signs, but may be observed by withdrawal, quiet demeanour, unwillingness to communicate, listlessness, fatigue, irritability and frustration.

Associated symptoms such as nausea, anorexia, dizziness, visual alterations and shortness of breath need to be determined. Explore the effects of any associated symptoms on activities of daily living.

Other assessment components include past pain experiences, the meaning of the pain to the person, coping strategies that were effective in the past and the affective response of the person. Pain affects mood, sleep patterns and physical and social functioning to reduce the quality of life (Peters, 2017).

Pain assessment tools (e.g. numeric rating scale, verbal rating scale, plus questions about location and quality) are used subsequent to the comprehensive assessment to determine changes in pain intensity levels.

Assessment of pain is not done in isolation. If pain is identified, nursing interventions and strategies must be implemented. Pain is assessed frequently to determine effectiveness of treatments and possible timing/intervals of pain episodes and return of ongoing pain. Usually the person is questioned about pain levels when the vital signs are taken, 20 to 30 minutes following analgesic or other treatments and whenever there are pain indicators.

Lee et al. (2020) found that pain assessment had a low priority in their study of juvenile arthritis, and even if pain was assessed, management depended on the healthcare professional's attitude to pain and the practical barriers (e.g. time constraints), leaving the children cared for in chronic pain. If the nursing interventions are insufficient to provide pain relief, the attending medical officer must be contacted for analgesia orders if necessary.

CLEAN, REPLACE AND DISPOSE OF EQUIPMENT

Cleaning equipment ensures safety and efficiency of time within the nursing unit. Cleaning and returning equipment is also a courtesy to colleagues. Wipe the ward stethoscope's earpieces and their bell/diaphragms with alcowipes before returning it to the storage place.

DOCUMENTATION

The person's response to treatment is monitored against the documented baseline of a pain assessment. An initial pain assessment also gives healthcare workers clues to the cause of the pain and to its management. Pain levels and quality (at least) should be documented within a half-hour after analgesic has been administered (DeLaune et al., 2024) and an assessment recorded every two to four hours for someone reporting acute pain.

CLINICAL SKILLS ASSESSMENT

Pain assessment

Demonstrates the ability to assess a person who is experiencing pain. Incorporates the *National Safety and Quality Health Service Standards*: 2 Partnering with Consumers, 3 Preventing and Controlling Healthcare-Associated Infection, 5 Comprehensive Care, 6 Communicating for Safety, and 8 Recognising and Responding to Acute Deterioration (ACSQHC, 2021).

Performance criteria	1	2	3	4	5
(Numbers indicate NMBA *Registered Nurse Standards for Practice*)	(Dependent)	(Marginal)	(Assisted)	(Supervised)	(Independent)
1. Identifies indication (1.1, 3.3, 3.4)	☐	☐	☐	☐	☐
2. Evidence of therapeutic interaction with the person, e.g. gives the person a clear explanation of the procedure (1.4, 1.5, 2.1. 2.2, 3.2)	☐	☐	☐	☐	☐
3. Demonstrates clinical reasoning abilities, e.g. provides privacy (1.1, 1.2, 1.3, 4.2, 6.1)	☐	☐	☐	☐	☐
4. Gathers equipment (5.5, 6.1): ■ pain assessment tools as required ■ sphygmomanometer, stethoscope, thermometer and watch	☐	☐	☐	☐	☐
5. Assesses the person's pain using the following guidelines (2.3, 4.1, 4.2, 4.3): ■ general assessment (look, listen, feel) ■ history of present pain ■ onset and duration ■ location ■ quality and character ■ intensity ■ aggravating or relieving factors ■ use of pain assessment tools ■ associated physical effects	☐	☐	☐	☐	☐
6. Cleans, replaces and disposes of equipment appropriately (3.4, 3.6, 6.1)	☐	☐	☐	☐	☐
7. Documents relevant information (1.4, 1.6, 2.2, 2.7, 3.5, 3.7, 6.2, 6.5, 7.3)	☐	☐	☐	☐	☐
8. Demonstrates the ability to link theory to practice (1.1, 3.3, 3.4, 3.5)	☐	☐	☐	☐	☐

Student:

Clinical facilitator: Date:

CHAPTER 14

BLOOD GLUCOSE MEASUREMENT

INDICATIONS

People with diabetes mellitus (DM) regularly measure their blood glucose level (BGL) to determine their real-time blood glucose levels (Antwi-Baffour et al., 2023). Blood glucose monitoring and regulation are crucial in preventing micro and macro-vascular complications in people living with diabetes (Antwi-Baffour et al., 2023). When a person is initially diagnosed with DM, a nurse determines the person's BGL to assess the effectiveness of the interventions (i.e. diet, exercise, oral medication or insulin) and teaches the person to monitor their BGL.

The first indication for measuring BGL is to assist the person in monitoring their DM. Hospitalisation tends to make it difficult for a person to control their BGL because of changes in daily routines (e.g. exercise levels, diet). People are generally hospitalised for an alteration in their health status and they may be too ill to determine their BGLs independently. Additionally, anxiety (a stressor that alters BGL) along with the stress of the condition or of surgery for which the person was hospitalised means these individuals often require blood glucose readings every four hours. The person who is newly diagnosed will require teaching so they can monitor their own BGLs.

The second indication is determination of hyper- or hypoglycaemia in a person with DM. Often, the initial signs and symptoms of these conditions are subtle, and the individual will need assessment to enable them/healthcare professionals to correct the BGL.

The third indication is determining the cause of loss of consciousness. People – either those known to have diabetes or those hospitalised for other reasons – who unexpectedly lose consciousness need to have their BGL measured. A BGL below 2 mmol/L causes loss of consciousness. Known diabetics have their BGL measured so that appropriate action can be taken. Others have their BGL measured so that a low BGL can be ruled out as a causative factor in their loss of consciousness, or so that they can be treated for hypoglycaemia.

Some facilities only allow nursing staff who have obtained a certificate of training in blood glucose monitoring to perform blood glucose assessment.

EVIDENCE OF THERAPEUTIC INTERACTION

Introduce yourself. Explain the assessment to the person to reduce their anxiety and gain their cooperation. This indicates tacit assent to the procedure. Good communication, genuine interest and honesty foster trust and enable you to build a working therapeutic relationship.

DEMONSTRATE CLINICAL REASONING

Determine frequency of monitoring

Review the doctor's order to determine frequency of monitoring. BGL is usually performed before a meal because ingestion of carbohydrates will increase the glucose level of the blood. Timing is crucial because insulin is prescribed according to the pre-prandial levels, and if the time lapse between testing and insulin injection is longer than 15 minutes, the insulin dose could be either inadequate or excessive (Haller et al., 2023) due to onset, peak or duration of insulin action. These authors suggest the BGL be retested if there is 30 minutes' discrepancy. A fourth test is often done at bedtime to ensure the person remains euglycaemic through the night. As well, some people need to have their BGL monitored following a meal (postprandial) – usually after two hours.

BGL may be elevated by hyperlipidaemia, dialysis treatment, some medications (e.g. high-dose steroids) or jaundice, and may be higher if the haematocrit level is below 35 per cent (Bao & Zhu, 2022; Gordon, 2019) or when there has been peripheral circulatory failure. In these cases, treatment should be based on laboratory measurements only. The blood sample taken from a finger prick may differ from venous or arterial samples.

ELDER CARE

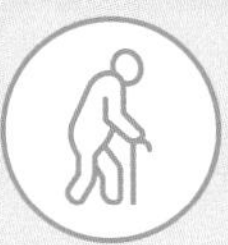

Elderly people are more vulnerable to the effects of hypoglycaemia and are less aware of the signals of hypoglycaemia. Acute changes in mental status, seizures, falls and resultant fractures and cardiac dysrhythmia can result from hypoglycaemia (Prately et al., 2020). Regular or continuous monitoring can ameliorate these problems.

THE PERSON LIVING WITH SEVERE OBESITY

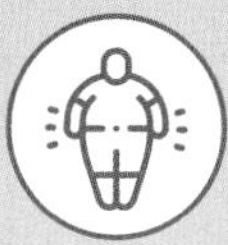

Obesity alters the body's use of insulin, resulting in higher levels of blood glucose and development of the metabolic syndrome (Sunil et al., 2023).

Monitor blood glucose level

Blood glucose meter technology is changing rapidly, and non-invasive systems are currently being used in Australia. One device is worn like a wristwatch and measures the blood glucose via interstitial fluid. Several non-invasive methods for obtaining blood glucose readings (e.g. near-infrared spectroscopy, similar to an oxygen saturation monitor or bio-impedance, which measures electrical changes that reflect the blood glucose concentration) are currently being developed and validated. These will eliminate the need for obtaining blood to test in the future (Premalatha & Prince, 2019).

Other invasive monitors are integral to insulin pumps and regulate the insulin according to the interstitial glucose level. Continuous glucose monitors (CGMs) test interstitial fluid every one to five minutes and send the results to a receiver. Caswell et al. (2020) demonstrated the accuracy of CGMs when used by both professional and lay persons. Use of CGMs showed reduced hypoglycaemia, hyperglycaemia and $HbA1_c$ (a measure of the control of the glucose level in the blood over time), demonstrating improved glycaemic control in children, teens, adults and the elderly (Beck et al., 2019). These authors warned that some CGMs require twice daily calibration with glucose levels obtained by blood glucose meter. These devices interface with smartphones to keep the physician or nurse practitioner or parents informed in real time.

Diabetes technologies are advancing rapidly and the National Diabetes Services Scheme subsidises people with diagnosed diabetes to obtain and use CGMs to manage their glycaemic control (Snaith & Holmes-Walker, 2021). CGM is currently undergoing accuracy and reliability testing for use in people who are hospitalised (BGLs become more erratic in people who are ill) (Wright et al., 2022).

All blood glucose meters require calibration frequently.

The remainder of this skill describes the use of intermittent BGL monitoring.

Assess the person

Determine whether the person is at risk of complications from specific conditions (e.g. bleeding disorders). Examine the site for broken skin, ecchymosis, rashes, lesions or other skin problems. Assess for compromised peripheral blood flow – fingertips should be warm and pinkish when the hand is gently massaged. Poor peripheral circulation or severe hypotension reduce the validity of the blood glucose measurement (Accu-Chek Inform II, 2019).

Assess the person's ability and willingness to learn the procedure, because they will need to perform the procedure independently.

Acutely ill people will need assessment of their level of consciousness and airway (hypoglycaemia causes confusion, disorientation and unconsciousness), breathing (those with ketoacidosis develop tachypnoea and Kussmaul breathing in an attempt to counter metabolic acidosis) and circulation (tachycardia and arrhythmias result from adrenaline and metabolic acidosis), as well as the vital signs (Palk, 2019).

GATHER EQUIPMENT

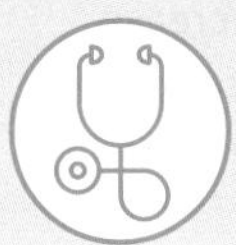

Gathering equipment is an organisational step that helps to create a positive environment for a successful interaction. It ensures that you have all needed material, boosts the person's confidence and trust in you, and increases your self-confidence. While gathering the equipment, you can mentally rehearse the procedure. The equipment required includes the following items:

EQUIPMENT	EXPLANATION
Blood glucometer or glucose meter (also known as a BG-Monitor)	• A battery-operated machine that accurately measures the level of glucose in whole blood • Range from very simple to those with options to manage data via a computer. Some measure ketones • Some read a chemical change on a reagent strip, while others use reflection to determine blood glucose in a sample • Errors may occur during calibration or sampling; develop the skills to calibrate and troubleshoot these problems • Master the blood glucose meter sample collection method used in the facility • Teach the person on the same glucometer that the person will use at home
Reagent strips for blood glucose	• Strips of paper impregnated with a chemical that reacts with glucose to change colour • Determine if they are needed for the blood glucose meter being used
Alcowipes or antiseptic swabs	• Should be avoided on individuals who require regular finger piercing because alcohol toughens skin (Dunning & Sinclair, 2020) • If not used in the facility, the person's hands should be washed with soap and warm water
Gauze squares	Used to provide pressure to stop bleeding once peripheral blood has been obtained
Autolet or lancet	• Peripheral blood access devices used to puncture the skin to capillary depth *Autolet* • Uses a spring that guarantees rapid and less-painful skin puncture • Comes in two parts: the spring device and a lancet that fits firmly into the spring device • Place perpendicular to the skin to puncture deeply enough to obtain capillary blood *Lancet* • May be used alone • Has a short, sharp end held in a plastic holder • You can use it or the person can use it themselves
Sharps container	A rigid container that holds used and contaminated sharps
Clean gloves	Protect you against contamination from the person's blood
Diabetic chart	Used to record BGL, medications, insulin and urinalysis results

OBTAIN A BLOOD GLUCOSE MEASUREMENT

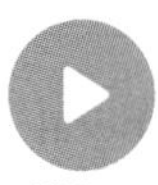
Video

To monitor BGL, you must select and prepare the site, access the blood droplet and correctly use the blood glucose meter.

Hand hygiene

Hand hygiene (see **Clinical Skill 5**) is an infection-control measure, removing transient microorganisms from your hands to prevent cross-contamination. Clean gloves are used to comply with standard precautions.

Position the person

Ask the person to sit or lie down. This is both for comfort and safety, in case the person feels faint. It is also easier for you to work with the hand that you will be drawing blood from.

Select the site

Usually the sides of the third and fourth fingers are used because it is less painful, there are fewer nerve endings and the sensitive pads are protected (Gordon, 2019). The fleshy part of the hand at the base of the thumb, the thigh, the forearm or the earlobe may be used if the person is in shock or if fingers are painful, callused or oedematous (Dunning & Sinclair, 2020). Alternative sites (a forearm or thigh) can be used for monitoring before meals, but the finger site is more accurate if BGL is changing rapidly, as there is up to 30 minutes lag in glucose levels in these alternative sites (Dunning & Sinclair, 2020). Owida et al. (2022) found the earlobe to be a valid substitute site to obtain blood, and Chan et al. (2016) found the earlobe to be significantly less painful, but less accurate if the person was hypoglycaemic. If an alternative site is used, it should be noted on the BGL sheet.

Rotate puncture sites to reduce the risk of infection from multiple stabbings, to prevent the area becoming toughened and to reduce pain (Gordon, 2019).

?

If you cannot obtain a drop of blood from the site, ask the person to keep the hand in a dependent position for a few minutes to slow venous return and increase blood available in the digits. Ask them to shake their hands for a few seconds as well. They can also try washing their hands in warm water, and shaking the hands from the wrists (Weinstock, 2023), which increases peripheral circulation due to vasodilatation, facilitating blood flow from the puncture site. Also, gentle massage starting at the palm to the base of the finger and stroking towards the puncture site, either by you or the person, increases ease of obtaining a blood drop (Gordon, 2019). A warm face washer over the site will increase vasodilatation as well. However, do not squeeze or apply pressure to the site.

Cleanse the site

Ask the person to wash their hands with soap and warm water. Handling food prior to BGL measurement results in significantly higher readings. If washing is not possible, the first drop of blood should be wiped away and a second drop of blood used for the test (Lima et al., 2016).

Hand hygiene with an alcohol-based cleanser is also used, but the hands must be allowed to dry thoroughly. The use of alcowipes to swab the site is contentious, and many facilities do not allow their use because the alcohol may toughen skin (Dunning & Sinclair, 2020). These authors found there was no interference with accuracy of the reading when alcowipes were used and allowed to dry thoroughly. Follow the facility's protocol.

Prepare the blood glucose meter

There are many different models of BGMs. Read the directions and understand them before you start. Follow the manufacturer's instructions and the following general principles.

BGMs need recalibration to ensure the accuracy of the result. Before taking the blood glucose meter to the person, check that the machine and the test strips have been calibrated together (they must match). If a new pack of strips is required, you will need to recalibrate the blood glucose meter as well as date the newly opened pack. Also ensure the high and low internal quality-control test has been carried out by checking the results in the log book. This is generally done daily (follow the institution's policy/manufacturer's guidelines). A personal blood glucose meter is generally calibrated monthly. Some blood glucose meters are accompanied by either a paddle or a solution used specifically for recalibration (follow the manufacturer's instructions).

If a reagent strip is used, check it is in date (the bottle is dated when opened) and has not been left exposed to light, air or extreme temperatures (Mathew, Zubair & Tadi, 2023). Do not touch the test pad: moisture or oils on your fingers may also alter the test results. Securely close the container so that the remaining reagent strips are not affected by moisture in the air. Follow the manufacturer's guidelines as to when the reagent strip is inserted into the machine. Generally, this is before blood is applied to the strip.

Some digital blood glucose monitors are used which deliver the results directly to the person's electronic medical record. Be sure to check the person's identification when you scan their armband (usually, hold the scan button down to display written information) to ensure accuracy.

Obtain peripheral blood

Perform hand hygiene and put on clean gloves.

Load the new lancet into the autolet (if used) and remove the cover. If the autolet has a depth setting, ensure it is correct for the person (most commonly in the middle). Ask the person which finger they would prefer to use. It is important to rotate sites to reduce the risk of infection from multiple stabbings, to prevent the area becoming toughened and to reduce pain (Krans, 2016). Place the finger on a sturdy surface to prevent pulling away (Craig, 2014). You may have to hold the finger in position with your non-dominant hand to help the person keep it still.

If the autolet is used, place the base firmly perpendicular to the side of the person's finger and press the release button. If a lancet is used, hold it perpendicular to the side of the finger and pierce the site quickly, to reduce discomfort. Wait a few seconds for blood to collect at the puncture site. Massage the skin gently from the palm towards the puncture site to obtain a large drop of blood. The finger should be held so that the blood drop is dependent (hanging downwards).

Time the process

Depending on the type of monitor, the procedure will differ. Allow the blood to drop onto the test pad of the reagent strip. The blood should cover the test pad completely. Do not smear it on, because either smearing or incomplete coverage of the test pad will result in an inaccurate reading. Some reagent strips are hydrophilic and fill from the side, not from a drop directly on top of the strip. Read the instructions and understand them before you start. Some facilities will require you to test for BGL on the second drop of blood after discarding the first. Check the procedure in the facility. Palese et al. (2016) found that the glucose level in the first drop of blood was adequate for clinical decision making. Conversely, however, Mathew, Zubair and Tadi (2023) recommend wiping away the first drop of blood as it may contain interstitial or intracellular fluid or be haemolysed.

Have the person apply pressure to the puncture site with the gauze square to stop the bleeding and prevent ecchymosis.

See the manufacturer's guidelines for the time period that gives the most accurate results (generally about 30 seconds). Most blood glucose meters display this in a digital readout. Read and document BGL. Abnormal BGL readings must be reported to the senior nurse or a medical officer for action.

Teach the person about blood glucose level

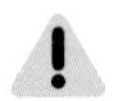
Safety

When teaching the person about BGL, emphasise the acquisition of self-care knowledge and skills (see **Clinical Skill 27**). These are essential for a person with DM. A collaborative approach is needed throughout the teaching process. Highlight the person's (and your) roles and responsibilities in self-managing the complexities of DM.

Through self-care practices, long- and short-term complications are reduced and the person is able to fully participate in their life (Gordon, 2019). Martos-Cabrera et al. (2020) demonstrated that the use of smartphone applications can assist people to manage their diabetes, but they must have a good understanding of the disease, its management and of the smartphone application.

CLEAN, REPLACE AND DISPOSE OF EQUIPMENT

If the blood glucose meter and reagent strips are the person's own, they are kept with them. The unit's blood glucose meter is to be cleaned and disinfected according to the manufacturer's instructions and returned to the usual storage place. If battery-operated, it will need to be recharged. The autolets and lancets are single-use only and once contaminated are disposed of in the sharps container. The used reagent strips and gloves are placed in the contaminated waste bin.

DOCUMENTATION

All BGLs are recorded on the diabetic chart so that trends are detectable. Error in transcription of the BGL either onto a paper chart or into the electronic record is an uncommon but potentially dangerous occurrence since insulin doses are based on the recorded BGL (Sowan et al., 2019). Many blood glucose meters and CGMs transmit the information to the person's electronic medical record automatically.

High or low BGLs are reported to the shift coordinator and may warrant a change in medication, diet or exercise. If the BGL is of concern, discuss it with medical staff. Any interventions (e.g. collecting a venous sample and sending it to pathology) and alterations to treatment are noted in the progress notes.

CLINICAL SKILLS ASSESSMENT

Blood glucose measurement

Demonstrates the ability to effectively measure and assess a person's blood glucose level. Incorporates the *National Safety and Quality Health Service Standards*: 2 Partnering with Consumers, 3 Preventing and Controlling Healthcare-Associated Infection, 5 Comprehensive Care, 6 Communicating for Safety, and 8 Recognising and Responding to Acute Deterioration (ACSQHC, 2021).

Performance criteria	1	2	3	4	5
(Numbers indicate NMBA *Registered Nurse Standards for Practice*)	**(Dependent)**	**(Marginal)**	**(Assisted)**	**(Supervised)**	**(Independent)**
1. Identifies indication (1.1, 3.3, 3.4)	☐	☐	☐	☐	☐
2. Evidence of therapeutic interaction with the person, e.g. gives the person a clear explanation of the procedure (1.4, 1.5, 2.1, 2.2, 3.2)	☐	☐	☐	☐	☐
3. Demonstrates clinical reasoning abilities; positions, selects a time and a site, assesses the person (1.1, 1.2, 1.3, 4.2, 6.1)	☐	☐	☐	☐	☐
4. Gathers equipment (1.1, 5.5, 6.1) ■ blood glucose meter ■ reagent strips for blood glucose ■ alcowipes or antiseptic swabs (if used in the facility) ■ gauze squares ■ peripheral blood access device ■ sharps container ■ clean gloves ■ diabetic chart	☐	☐	☐	☐	☐
5. Performs hand hygiene, encourages the person to wash their hands (1.1, 3.4, 6.1)	☐	☐	☐	☐	☐
6. Selects and cleans the site (1.1, 6.1)	☐	☐	☐	☐	☐
7. Prepares the blood glucose meter following the manufacturer's instructions (1.1, 6.1)	☐	☐	☐	☐	☐
8. Obtains peripheral blood (1.1, 6.1)	☐	☐	☐	☐	☐
9. Starts timing, and prepares the insert by applying blood and following the manufacturer's instructions (6.1)	☐	☐	☐	☐	☐
10. Times the process and reads the blood glucose meter (6.1)	☐	☐	☐	☐	☐
11. Teaches the person about blood sugar levels and how to use the blood glucose meter (2.3, 3.2, 3.4)	☐	☐	☐	☐	☐
12. Cleans, replaces and disposes of equipment appropriately (3.6, 6.1)	☐	☐	☐	☐	☐
13. Documents relevant information (1.1, 1.4, 1.6, 2.2, 2.7, 3.5, 3.7, 6.1, 6.2, 6.5, 7.3)	☐	☐	☐	☐	☐
14. Demonstrates the ability to link theory to practice (1.1, 3.3, 3.4, 3.5)	☐	☐	☐	☐	☐

Student:

Clinical facilitator: Date:

CHAPTER 15

PHYSICAL ASSESSMENT

INDICATIONS

Health history and physical assessment are fundamental to providing good nursing care. Comprehensive, holistic and culturally appropriate assessment is Standard 4 of the Nursing and Midwifery Board of Australia (NMBA) *Registered Nurse Standards for Practice* (2016). A sound knowledge of anatomy underpins competence in physical assessment (Ratero et al., 2020). The collection and organisation of the individual's information assists you to identify existing or potential healthcare problems, allowing you to make decisions to help the person return to a better state of health. Freeman and Kelly (2018) found that physically examining a person acts as a form of non-verbal communication to express care. This competency skill looks briefly at vigilant surveillance, the primary survey, and outlines the information needed to conduct a physical assessment.

Contact with a healthcare facility indicates that the person is concerned about their health, and they should be assessed accordingly. The initial contact is usually an admission procedure, which includes a structured core physical assessment. This should also be done any time the person's condition changes (Douglas et al., 2016), to allow you to report accurately and adequately to the other healthcare and medical staff and to improve your clinical decision making.

The purposes of a health history are to formulate a holistic database incorporating historical and current data, to establish a trusting professional relationship with the person (Estes et al., 2020), to provide information about their perception of their health concerns and to identify their learning needs. The physical assessment provides an opportunity to explore data obtained during the health history. To support a thorough health assessment, you must be aware of normal anatomy and physiology, and the impact of ageing on these, and of behavioural sciences. Practice is foundational to successfully learning the skill of physical assessment (Kardong-Edgren, Oermann & Rizzolo, 2019; Ma & Zhou, 2022).

BACKGROUND TO PHYSICAL ASSESSMENT

This outline is for a general physical assessment. It is dependent on the integration of several competencies (health history, assessment of the various systems and clinical documentation) and cannot be used in isolation. Discussion of a thorough, detailed health history and physical assessment is outside the scope of this Clinical Skill. If there are problems discovered or complaints that involve other systems than are discussed in this outline, please see the relevant fundamental and physical assessment textbooks, which describe health history and physical assessment in detail.

The scan

Beginning nurses need to be aware of the importance of briefly assessing (scanning) *each person* they are caring for at *each encounter*. Vigilant surveillance at both the individual and the system levels uncovers emerging problems so they can be addressed.

The scan (some facilities call it the head-to-toe assessment) consists of a quick **LOOK** at, **LISTEN** to and **FEEL** for the following:

- Airway, breathing and circulation (the ABCs):
  - *Airways* – LISTEN for an open airway (the presence of breathing, sounds of obstruction).
  - *Breathing* – LISTEN and LOOK for an inspiration/expiration cycle, the rate and ease of respirations, use of accessory muscles and ability to converse.
  - *Circulation* – LOOK at the person's colour, for obvious bleeding from surgical sites, FEEL for skin temperature and perspiration.
  - *Response* – LISTEN – assess the person's level of alertness (when awake). Are they able to converse? Are they confused? Has anything changed from previous encounters? Have they had sedation or pain medication?
- Tubes or monitors:
  - *Tubes* (e.g. catheters and intravenous [IV]) – LOOK – assess for patency, and note the level of IV fluids.
  - *Monitors* (e.g. cardiac monitors or pulse oximeters) – LOOK – assess their readings; are they within the person's normal range?

The *scan* folds into situational awareness, which is an important aspect of ongoing assessment to avert poor outcomes for people in our care. The process of situational awareness includes:

- **Anticipation** – being aware of the person's current illness and latest nursing/medical data and know what could go wrong with them.
- **Vigilance** – notice differences in the person since the last time you assessed them (or from reports), and actively look for differences that could indicate deterioration of their condition.
- **Use clinical reasoning** – identify key elements and look for supporting or refuting evidence of problems, and predict what might happen.
- **Address the problem** (within your scope of practice) or communicate your findings and suspicions to someone more experienced who can address the problem.

For example, Mr Stanley, who returned from abdominal surgery (anticipation) three hours ago, is pale and perspiring but denies much pain (vigilance). You take his vital signs and find both his respirations (22) and pulse rate elevated (108), and his blood pressure is 20 mmHg lower than a half-hour ago (actively look for key elements). You check his dressing and there is much more blood apparent since the last check (supporting evidence of a problem). You believe he might be going into shock from blood loss (prediction). You immediately tell the shift coordinator (communication), who alerts the surgeon. Mr Stanley is given blood and returned to theatre to find the cause of the bleeding.

The primary survey

A primary survey is used in *emergency* situations. It is a structured, systematic assessment of response, airway, breathing, circulation and disability used to identify life-threatening conditions in order to initiate necessary treatment without delay. Elbaih and Basyouni (2020) consider the primary survey approach as the first element in any initial healthcare assessment and especially in trauma situations. It has three major advantages:

- Data is collected according to clinical importance.
- Data is collected using the same framework as most organisations' rapid response system activation criteria.
- It acts as a safety checklist, thereby decreasing the risk of failure to recognise and respond to the person's deterioration.

The primary survey is more detailed than the scan and is not addressed further in this skill.

EVIDENCE OF THERAPEUTIC INTERACTION

Welcome the person, introduce yourself and give a clear explanation of the procedure, including the time it will take. Explanations are necessary to obtain (verbal or tacit) permission for the assessment; they allay fears, help gain the person's cooperation and initiate the therapeutic relationship. Thorough explanations of procedures to be undertaken and of hospital routines and regulations that affect the person, honest answers to questions and a sincere attitude to the person will foster an effective relationship. Explaining confidentiality will also assist in collecting information. By acknowledging the psychological and social needs of the person, you will facilitate holistic person-centred care, maintain the person's dignity and demonstrate respect for their individuality.

A relaxed person can provide more information, making the health history and physical assessment easier and more accurate. Most people are anxious on admission to hospital or other healthcare facilities. Reducing anxiety by establishing a therapeutic relationship with a newly admitted individual is a priority.

DEMONSTRATE CLINICAL REASONING

Prepare the environment. Ensure that the ambient temperature is comfortable without draughts and/or provide a blanket for warmth. Sufficient light and quiet are needed so you can examine the person. Close the room door, draw the curtains or speak quietly to provide privacy. Assist the person to maintain their dignity with the use of gowns and bath blankets. Provide toileting facilities and assistance if needed, so the examination will not be interrupted. Provide pain relief (as necessary and with orders) so the person can comply with the requirements of positioning and movement during the examination. Arrange for assistance from another nurse if the situation requires it. Familiarise yourself with the forms used by the facility prior to starting the health history.

ELDER CARE

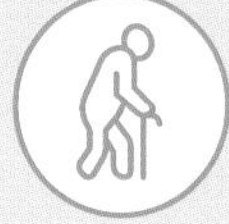

Be alert for signs of frailty (reduced physiological reserves and ability to compensate) in elderly people, as frailty has an effect on the outcome of an illness episode or a surgical intervention (Birkelbach et al., 2019). Look for weakened grip, slow, hesitant gait, and complaint of excessive or constant fatigue, and report these. Comorbidities and functional decline are also more common in the elderly and need to be recognised and documented to enhance care.

THE PERSON LIVING WITH SEVERE OBESITY

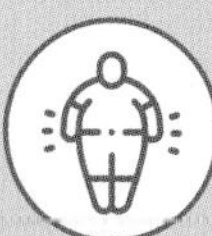

There is a growing minority of people who are living with severe obesity (100 kg over normal weight for height or a body mass index of 40+) being admitted to hospital. You may hear the term 'bariatric' (from '*baros*' meaning weight and '*iatros*' meaning doctor) issues. A person who is severely obese presents some nursing problems, including possible injury (to yourself, other staff or the person), the effects of excess adipose tissue on the various body systems, impaired circulation and relative immobility. Physical assessment is little different in the person living with severe obesity than any other adults. Each section in the assessment skills will suggest adaptations and equipment that will assist you.

Specialised hospital equipment will be needed. This includes a bariatrics bed (extra wide, weight capacity of 300 kg plus), appropriately sized linen and gowns, a lift with 450 kg capacity, an armchair and a wheelchair (85 cm wide and capacity of 300 kg plus) or a walker (again, for bariatric use), large floor-mounted toilet facilities or bedpan, and bed or lift scales and trolleys that all have to be capable of managing the weight. A private room enables staff and equipment to be used (1.6 m around the bed is required). Extra staff, time and lifting equipment with specific protocols are required for moving or mobilising the person living with severe obesity.

Be non-judgemental, even if you are uncomfortable discussing the person's weight for fear of offending them, or because you have been socialised into the false belief that the person is to blame for their obesity. Puhl (2016) cites decades of research into genetics, biological mechanisms and complexities of weight regulation that promote weight gain. Try to address any personal weight bias you may have and overcome any causal attributions so that you can provide excellent professional care.

Physical assessment of a person living with severe obesity will require extra time for reassurance, moving body parts, turning, specialised equipment (e.g. large conical blood pressure cuff, appropriate scales, Doppler for assessing pulses), lifting equipment to enable you to assess all areas, and other healthcare professionals to support limbs, assist with moving and hold excess tissue so you can assess the various body systems. Issues for people living with severe obesity are further addressed in **Clinical Skill 23** and are addressed in other skills where appropriate.

GATHER EQUIPMENT

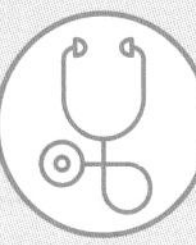

Gathering equipment is an organisational step that helps to create a positive environment for a successful interaction. Your eyes, ears, nose, sense of touch and an open mind are the most effective equipment you can use. You will also need the following equipment:

EQUIPMENT	EXPLANATION
Sphygmomanometer	For blood pressure measurement
Blood pressure cuff	In the appropriate size for the person
Stethoscope	To listen for blood pressure, heart, lung and abdominal sounds
Thermometer	Obtains a temperature measurement
Pulse oximeter	To determine peripheral oxygen saturation
Watch with a second hand	To calculate the pulse and respirations per minute
Height and weight scales, tape measure, body mass index chart	To determine weight and body mass index
Penlight	For pupil reactivity, and inspection of various areas (e.g. skin lesions, oral cavity)
Pupil measurement chart	To determine pupil size
Pen and paper/facility health assessment form	To record findings immediately

CONDUCT A PHYSICAL ASSESSMENT

Video

Physical assessment is a skill that requires practice. Initially, you will be slow and hesitant, but persistence and repetition will improve your comfort and efficiency.

Hand hygiene

Hand hygiene (see **Clinical Skill 5**) removes microorganisms from your hands. It is the most effective measure for preventing cross-contamination and reducing nosocomial (i.e. hospital- or treatment-acquired) infections.

Obtain a general health history

Unless the person is in acute distress (e.g. has severe pain or respiratory distress – see the 'If ... then' box below), the health history is taken first. The person is the primary informant; they can most accurately describe their symptoms, give their history and share their problems and perceptions. The information they give is subjective data; it is information only the person can supply, such as reports of pain, depression and other symptoms that are not verifiable by another person. If someone else, such as a parent or spouse, provides the information, they are considered a secondary source, and this should be noted during documentation.

The health history begins broadly with general information about the person, such as demographics and their general past health (see **TABLE 15.1**).

> If the person is in acute distress and is unable to answer questions, gather an abbreviated health history that focuses on the system involved and on the seven dimensions of the presenting problem (see later in this chapter), as well as any current medical problems, medications taken and allergies. You can gather any other information required either from secondary sources or from the person once the primary problem has been resolved or alleviated.

History specific to the presenting problem and body system

This outline is for a general physical assessment. It is dependent on the integration of several competencies (general and historical health history, specific health history of each system and physical assessment of the various systems followed by clinical documentation) and cannot be used in isolation. History of the presenting problem and the history specific to each of the body systems is addressed in the individual assessment skills (**Clinical Skills 17, 19, 20, 22 and 24**).

Gather data about the person (from observation) as well as from them during the interview. Note their level of anxiety, mood, level of discomfort, communication and intellectual ability. Interpersonal relationships, some idea of body image and self-concept can all be assessed from observation during the interview.

Begin the physical assessment during the interview. Inspect visible skin to assess colour (clues to cardiac perfusion or respiratory difficulties). Other diseases and conditions are sometimes readily visible in the face, hands, nails or hair. Personal hygiene, dress, eye contact, suitability of clothing, make-up and demeanour give insights into the mental status of the person. Observing the person while they are preparing for the physical assessment can provide a great deal of information. For example, their movements as they enter the room, change into the gown or get into the bed will give indications about their ability to balance, the general status of their health, their body build, posture, gait and any obvious disability or difficulty in moving (e.g. pain), body or breath odour, their range of movement, level of consciousness and level of cooperation. Odours can give you clues to the person's condition; for example, body odour, halitosis, alcohol or tobacco odours are all important information. Skin and nail assessment can provide valuable clues to underlying systemic pathological conditions, to self-concept and to their ability to self-care.

Observation and inspection are valuable tools that should be employed from the first moment of contact. It is extremely important to practise the other three skills of assessment – palpation (touch), percussion (tapping) and auscultation (listening) – until you are comfortable and confident in using them. Ensure adequate lighting, expose all areas for assessment, know normal variations, compare body areas (e.g. strength in each arm) and use an unhurried approach with attention to detail to gain information effectively. Assessment of the person does not stop when the physical assessment and the interview are complete. It is an ongoing process that continues to provide data until the person is discharged.

The seven dimensions of the presenting problem

Explore the presenting problem or chief complaint with the person. If there is more than one presenting

TABLE 15.1 Personal demographics and historical data

PERSONAL DEMOGRAPHICS INCLUDE:	HISTORICAL DATA INCLUDES:
• age and date of birth	• past events, such as experiences with previous hospitalisation and illness or medical conditions
• occupation	• previous experience of surgery or anaesthesia
• marital or family status	• allergies
• current medical problems	• blood transfusions
• medications, including over-the-counter and herbal supplements and vitamins, and illicit drugs, being taken and reasons for taking them	• exposure to infections
• allergies and reactions to the allergen	• history of childhood illnesses
• patterns of daily living	• family history
• other current data affecting the care given during hospitalisation	• history of medication or alcohol use (especially pertinent in older people) • social history • cultural background • any pertinent information that might impact on their nursing care (e.g. the person is the primary carer for their spouse)

problem, explore each in a systematic manner, starting with the symptoms the person finds most acute and distressing.

The seven dimensions are as follows:

- *Timing of the symptoms* – includes onset (when the symptom was first noticed), duration (how long the symptom lasts) and frequency (continuously, intermittently, regularly or irregularly, and how often it occurs).
- *Location of the pain or other symptoms* – ask the person to point at the area affected. Ask about radiation or movement of the pain to other parts of the body and ask them to point along the path that the radiation takes.
- *Quality of the pain or symptom* – ask them to describe the sensation (adjectives such as 'sharp', 'dull', 'burning' or whatever word fits the sensation).
- *Quantity or intensity of the symptom* – describes the extent of the symptom; for example, the number of times, amount or size, and how the symptom has altered the person's activities of daily living or interfered with their life (e.g. coughing, sputum production). Using a visual analogue scale or numerical rating scale can assist in quantifying pain.
- *Precipitating factors* – ask about the initial time the symptom occurred, what triggered the symptom and whether there are any activities that bring the symptom or sensation on (e.g. exercise-induced breathlessness).
- *Aggravating factors and alleviating factors* – anything that makes the symptom better or worse. Stress, activity, rest and medication are often noted.
- *Associated symptoms* – anything that happens in conjunction with the symptom (e.g. sharp chest pain with coughing).

There are various mnemonics that cover the same information, such as COLDSPA (character, onset, location, duration, severity, palliation, associated factors) or OPQRST (onset, position [location] or palliating factors, quality, radiation, severity [quantity], time [including duration] and treatment) (Estes et al., 2020).

The physical assessment

A systematic physical assessment of the person helps you to gather objective data through observation and inspection, and through additional information-gathering techniques such as palpation, percussion, auscultation and olfaction. The following is only a suggested systematic outline. It is a combination of the *head-to-toe* assessment and a *body systems* assessment. Other systematic assessment outlines can be used, as long as they are thorough and allow you to obtain effective data.

If there is an apparent problem, you may need to use the assessment tools available in the facility. These may include, but are not limited to, pain assessment scales, falls risk forms, oral assessment tools, pressure area assessments such as the Braden Scale, activities of daily living assessments and the Glasgow Coma Scale.

As well, the standard vital signs observation charts are required. The Adult Deterioration Detection System (ADDS; also known as an early warning system [EWS]) is designed to enable early recognition of deterioration and prompt intervention to stabilise the person and prevent adverse events (e.g. myocardial infarction [MI], respiratory arrest, ICU admission). However, its use as a track and trigger tool must not alter your responsibility to assess the person holistically and detect subtle cues NOT reflected in the vital signs (e.g. changes in mental status, pain or increased labour of breathing) (Azimirad et al., 2022; Chua et al., 2022).

Use observation, auscultation, percussion and palpation to:

- obtain vital signs – the blood pressure, pulse, temperature and respiratory status are assessed initially, in part to alleviate anxiety (see **Clinical Skills 10 and 11**)
- obtain height and weight (see **Clinical Skill 23**)
- assess the need for a mental status assessment – the entire assessment will not need to be undertaken for every person if you are confident that it is not necessary (see **Clinical Skill 16**)
- assess the neurological functioning (see **Clinical Skill 20**) – note the person's level of consciousness and orientation when you initiate contact with the person and during the interview
- assess the cardiovascular functioning (see **Clinical Skill 17**) – peripheral pulse checks and capillary refill can be done during the musculoskeletal assessment of the extremities, increasing the efficiency of the physical assessment
- assess the respiratory functioning (see **Clinical Skills 12 and 19**)
- assess the gastrointestinal functioning (see **Clinical Skill 22**)
- assess the genitourinary functioning – question the person about urinary activity and reproductive and sexual activity. Obtain a clean catch specimen for urinalysis (described in **Clinical Skill 36**). If there are urinary symptoms, it will be necessary to inspect the external genitalia and urinary meatus (see a physical assessment text for this assessment)
- assess the musculoskeletal system – assess muscle mass and tone and motor function; for instance, by raising limbs against gravity and resistance, assessing strength of handgrips bilaterally and assessing range of movement (see **Clinical Skill 24**).

Post-procedure

Once you have completed the health history, the physical assessment and the mental status assessment, reassure the person and ask them to relay any further information they can think of that would be of assistance in caring for them. Orientate them to the bed space and to the room and unit to increase their confidence. Inform them of any planned activities (laboratory tests, doctor's visits, meals and so on) and provide distraction (e.g. TV, magazines) if appropriate.

CLEAN, REPLACE AND DISPOSE OF EQUIPMENT

Cleaning and disinfecting equipment is an infection control measure. Returning clean equipment to its storage spot, plugging in batteries to recharge and restocking used materials also show respect for other staff members, increase efficiency in the unit and develop good organisational and work habits.

DOCUMENTATION

Documentation of the physical assessment and health history will be extensive. Many facilities will use electronic documentation, which will have a format for recording physical assessment. Some facilities have specific forms for most of the information; if no forms exist, document the data that you have gathered in a systematic manner. This will form a baseline from which deterioration or improvement can be tracked.

CLINICAL SKILLS ASSESSMENT

Physical assessment

Demonstrates the ability to effectively assess a person's physical status. Incorporates the *National Safety and Quality Health Service Standards*: 2 Partnering with Consumers, 3 Preventing and Controlling Healthcare-Associated Infection, 5 Comprehensive Care, 6 Communicating for Safety, and 8 Recognising and Responding to Acute Deterioration (ACSQHC, 2021).

Performance criteria	1	2	3	4	5
(Numbers indicate NMBA *Registered Nurse Standards for Practice*)	(Dependent)	(Marginal)	(Assisted)	(Supervised)	(Independent)
1. Identifies indication (1.1, 3.3, 3.4)	☐	☐	☐	☐	☐
2. Evidence of therapeutic interaction with the person, e.g. gives a clear explanation (1.4, 1.5, 2.1, 2.2, 3.2)	☐	☐	☐	☐	☐
3. Demonstrates clinical reasoning abilities, e.g. prepares the environment, ensures sufficient light and quiet, provides for warmth and privacy, assists with toileting if required, provides pain relief as required/ordered (1.1, 1.2, 1.3, 4.2, 6.1).	☐	☐	☐	☐	☐
4. Gathers equipment (1.1, 5.5, 6.1): ■ sphygmomanometer, stethoscope, cuff, thermometer, watch ■ height and weight scales, tape measure, body mass index chart ■ penlight, pupil measurement tape ■ pen and paper, forms	☐	☐	☐	☐	☐
5. Performs hand hygiene (1.1, 3.2, 3.4, 6.1)	☐	☐	☐	☐	☐
6. Obtains a focused health history (1.1, 2.1, 2.2, 2.3, 4.1, 4.2, 4.3)	☐	☐	☐	☐	☐
7. Explores the seven dimensions of the presenting problem (1.1, 2.1, 2.2, 2.3, 4.1, 4.2, 6.1)	☐	☐	☐	☐	☐
8. Conducts a systematic physical assessment (1.1, 2.1, 2.2, 2.3, 4.1, 4.2, 4.3, 6.1); obtains vital signs, height and weight, inspects throughout the physical assessment Assesses neurological, cardiac, respiratory, gastrointestinal, genitourinary and musculoskeletal functioning	☐	☐	☐	☐	☐
9. Gathers information for a mental status assessment during the physical assessment (1.1, 2.1, 2.2, 2.3, 4.1, 4.2, 4.3, 6.1)	☐	☐	☐	☐	☐
10. Cleans, replaces and disposes of equipment appropriately (1.1, 3.6, 6.1)	☐	☐	☐	☐	☐
11. Documents relevant information (1.4, 1.6, 2.2, 2.7, 3.5, 3.7, 6.2, 6.5, 7.3)	☐	☐	☐	☐	☐
12. Demonstrates the ability to link theory to practice (1.1, 3.3, 3.4, 3.5)	☐	☐	☐	☐	☐

Student:

Clinical facilitator: Date:

CHAPTER 16

MENTAL STATUS ASSESSMENT

INDICATIONS

A mental status assessment (MSA) is part of the overall mental health assessment of an individual, used to gather information to make an informed judgement about an individual's present mental state and possible need for care and to formulate clear treatment goals and plans for care (Hercelinskyj & Alexander, 2020). Most of the information for an MSA can be gathered during conversation with the person, careful listening and observation. The competency presented here is abbreviated, and abnormal findings demand a full mental health assessment, which is outside the scope of this skill. Please see a mental health text for a more in-depth discussion of this skill.

People who are admitted into the general part of the hospital are less likely to require a full MSA than those admitted to psychiatric care. However, if you observe during the physical assessment and history taking that the person has difficulty in some area, this assessment would be needed (DeLaune et al., 2024). One hospital area where MSA ability is important is the emergency unit.

EVIDENCE OF THERAPEUTIC INTERACTION

Introduce yourself and clearly explain the procedure to the person to gain their full cooperation and begin to establish the therapeutic relationship. Providing privacy and quiet can enhance engagement with the person and allow them to answer questions with less anxiety. Tell the person you will be taking notes to be able to accurately record the assessment in their case file. Some may be suspicious of your writing down their thoughts, so explanation before you begin helps to allay their anxiety (Hercelinskyj & Alexander, 2020).

DEMONSTRATE CLINICAL REASONING

Consider the person's age, culture and language when assessing mental status, since each of these impact the person's ability to process information and respond to your questions. For instance, educational level and attainment impact the person's vocabulary as well as their ability to process mathematical concepts. Having English as a second language may reduce a person's ability to display their knowledge or abstract reasoning and, in some cases, to adequately demonstrate reasoning and judgement. People who are refugees or victims of abuse may be very difficult to assess, and if you suspect there are problems in their mental state, you should refer them to a mental health professional. As well, a person who is in distress, is poorly nourished, is sleep deprived, has an intellectual disability, has a neurological condition or is medically ill may not be able to answer questions or participate in the assessment (Voss & Das, 2022).

When you suspect mental instability, undertaking a physical assessment of the person is important. While neglect of the physiological aspects of life occurs during mental illness, the risk of chronic physical disease is higher among those with severe mental illness than in the general population (Hercelinskyj & Alexander, 2020). As well, some physiological problems (e.g. dehydration, infection) can surface as mental instability (e.g. confusion, unwarranted belligerence). It is important to realise the MSA is not solely for admission proceedings. Any time you notice an alteration (e.g. confusion, memory disruptions) in a person, it is important to explore their mental status, and document it and report it to a senior healthcare professional.

PART 3

ELDER CARE

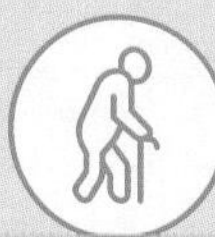

Davies (2023) suggests that ensuring the person has the appropriate aids, determining why they have come to the facility (e.g. were they coerced, or encouraged by their spouse or partner), taking time to permit the person to process the ideas and not rushing their responses will all improve the relationship and information gained.

Ask the person about their socialisation and activities of daily living to assess if they have a functional impairment. Be aware that older adults have many traumatic experiences (physical/traumatic injury, grief, retirement, body image/mobility changes, self-concept changes) that can alter their social support networks and contribute to changes in their mental health.

Up to 70 per cent of elderly people who are hospitalised will have some signs of delirium (Sillner et al., 2023). It is important to assess for, document and communicate these symptoms and any interventions used to ameliorate them (Sillner et al., 2023).

It is also important to note that, when assessing elderly people from various cultures (who may be illiterate, or have very low educational levels and speak another language at home), the use of a brief assessment tool (e.g. the Rowland Universal Dementia Assessment scale) to supplement the MSA can detect cognitive decline in elderly people (Goudsmit et al., 2018).

THE PERSON LIVING WITH SEVERE OBESITY

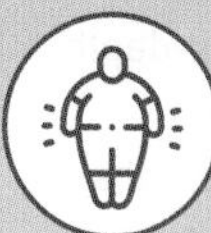

Meo et al. (2019) demonstrated impaired cognitive function, including reduction in attention, retention, intelligence and cognitive flexibility, in severely obese adolescents. Yıldırım, Eryılmaz & Aydın (2020) demonstrated a relationship between obesity and both depression and anxiety. Fulton et al. (2022) explained these findings relate to neuroinflammation associated with metabolic and vascular dysfunction occurring with severe obesity. Dobbie et al. (2023) added that eroded self-esteem also contributes to depression and anxiety. These findings may impact on the assessment of the severely obese adult in your care.

You may also need to take account of the effects of increased weight (e.g. on gait, speed of movement, level of personal hygiene and eye contact) on the various aspects of the general appearance category.

?

If you suspect that an elderly person has a mental health problem, even though the MSA is within normal parameters, it is your professional responsibility to make a referral to an experienced mental health professional.

CONDUCT A MENTAL STATUS ASSESSMENT

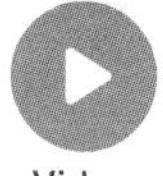

Video

An MSA is broken down here into key areas: general appearance, level of consciousness, orientation, mood, affect, knowledge and vocabulary, judgement and abstraction, memory, thought processes and content, language and speech, sensory and motor skills. However, when you do an MSA, the steps blur together as you gather data during conversation.

Assess each of the key areas to gather information and to form an understanding of a person's present mental state.

Assess general appearance

General appearance is defined by a combination of features notable during an initial encounter:

- *Appearance* – scars and needle tracks can attest to trauma, injury, self-harm or illicit drug use; tattoos can represent self-concept or perhaps gang affiliation.
- *A person's attire* – the way a person dresses can tell you a great deal; observe their dress for style, cleanliness, appropriateness and character.
- *Level of personal hygiene* – clean skin, hair and nails and minimal body odour are expectations of our culture; however, take the circumstances into consideration. For example, someone admitted to A&E straight from a work-related injury at a factory or construction site would not be expected to have that level of hygiene. Remember that illness often affects the person's ability for self-care. A woman's desire to apply make-up may reflect her self-concept. Again, be aware of culture.
- *Facial expression* – gives a clue about a person's mood. Is it alert, vacant, sad, pleasant, hostile or mask-like? For example, a scowl and frown may indicate an irritable mood or pain.
- *Posture and gait* – reflect self-concept, body image and self-esteem as well as physical conditions.
- *Motor activity* – speed of movement can hint at depression, other psychiatric conditions and medication side effects. Is it normal, retarded or agitated? For example, moving more slowly than expected for someone their age may indicate depression.
- *Mannerisms* – often reflect underlying emotions; for example, depression may be suggested by inertia, withdrawal and non-spontaneous communication; while wringing hands, picking at bedclothes and inappropriate laughter can alert you to anxiety.

- *Involuntary signs of emotion* – such as sweaty palms, sweaty brow or upper lip, and damp underarms indicate anxiety or fear.
- *Apparent age* – gives clues as to a person's self-concept and insight into both acute and chronic illness.
- *Eye contact* – is culturally determined, so be very aware of the person's culture when assessing this. Is the eye contact appropriate and comfortable for you?
- *Speech* – observe for pace; is it too fast, too slow, interrupted, does it skip from topic to topic, or does the person interrupt themselves or you? Observe the volume (moderate, too loud, inaudible), clarity (slurred, monosyllabic, pressured) and tone (moderate, calm, hostile).

Lastly, ascertain the person's response to the situation and to you.

Assess level of consciousness

The level of consciousness (LOC) is a person's awareness of and alertness to their surroundings. Initially, determine if the person is fully alert to their surroundings, whether they are able to sustain attention and their response to the environment. A fully alert person demonstrates clear and organised thoughts, clear articulation, appropriate flow of speech, prompt response to questions and no drifting of attention. The following descriptors of LOC are adapted from Vos and Das (2022) and Hercelinskyj and Alexander (2020).

- *Alertness* – whether the person is awake, attentive and appropriately responsive to stimuli, and oriented to person, place, situation and date.
- *Confusion* – the person's attention drifts; they are easily distracted, have decreased memory, are disoriented and have difficulty giving clear, appropriate answers to questions.
- *Lethargy* – the person is drowsy, falls asleep easily, but arouses easily to the sound of a voice.
- *Obtundation* – the person has moderately reduced alertness with diminished ability to consistently engage with the environment (i.e. drifting off).
- *Delirium* – the person is severely confused and has disordered perceptions (hears sounds and/or sees images others do not see; i.e. hallucinations), reacts inappropriately to stimuli, shows marked anxiety, motor and/or sensory excitement (agitation).
- *Stupor* – the person is only intermittently awake and is able to be aroused for only short periods, requires loud noise or painful stimuli for arousal, has limited awareness during response, responds with 'yes/no' or incoherently or with movement.
- *Coma* – the person is not able to be aroused, moves only involuntarily and assumes intermittent or fixed decerebrate posture in response to painful stimuli. In the decerebrate posture, the body is rigidly extended, the neck is arched, and the wrists, fingers and feet are flexed.

Assess orientation

To assess orientation, ask the person open-ended questions, including:

- 'What is your name?'; 'Where are you?'; also ask who significant people are, such as their wife/husband/partner, children or the current Prime Minister.
- 'What day/date is it?' Remember that it is common for people who are hospitalised to lose track of the exact date, or to be unaware of the room number or even the unit they are in. More general questions may be required.

People with English as a second language or who are from a different culture will require more considered questions to determine if they are oriented.

Assess mood

Mood is the person's own verbal description of their emotional state determined by asking the person how they feel. Descriptors might include happy, sad, euphoric, irritable, depressed, anxious, angry or fearful. Seek clarification (e.g. 'You say you feel depressed – what do you mean by that?'). Mood states can be labile (i.e. fluctuate between several moods in a short time). Hercelinskyj and Alexander (2020) suggest asking about libido, appetite and sleep, as these can be profoundly affected by mental disorder.

Assess affect

Affect is the quality or character of non-verbal emotional expression of mood, such as facial expression, posture and tone of voice. It is inferred from the person's conversation, appearance and behaviour. Affect can be described as:

- *full range* – normal variations in facial expressions, voice, tone and body language
- *blunted* – a low intensity in non-verbally expressed emotion
- *flat* – near absence of non-verbally expressed emotion; speaks in a monotone, one-word answers if any, no facial expression or eye contact, apathetic
- *labile* – great variation beyond normal expression; for instance, shifts from anger to depression to euphoria and back in a short time
- *incongruent* – non-verbal expression is not the same as stated emotion
- *inappropriate* – facial expression and behaviour that are opposite of what would be appropriate (e.g. laughing during a funeral)
- *restricted* – very little range in non-verbal expression.

Assess knowledge and vocabulary

Knowledge and vocabulary usually become apparent in the history taking and physical assessment of the person. If there is doubt about the person's cognitive ability, test their knowledge further by asking questions that would be within their frame of reference. Keep in mind that knowledge and vocabulary are dependent on culture, education and language spoken.

Assess judgement and abstraction

Generally, you gather sufficient data during the social history and physical assessment to assess judgement and abstraction. If you are concerned, ask questions to determine the person's judgement and ability to reason abstractly. Assess judgement by evaluating their ability to use appropriate thought processes to make decisions. Outline a specific situation and ask the person to make a judgement (e.g. 'What would you do if you were locked out of your home?'). Their answer should show an ability to consider a range of options and apply sound reasoning.

Assess memory

When taking the health history and conducting the physical assessment, the person's memory will be tested. If the person appears to have large gaps in their memory or is forgetful, formal evaluation is required. To gauge the memory, three tests are required.

- *Immediate recall* – recite a list of everyday items and ask the person to repeat them immediately.
- *Recent memory* – ask about something that happened today that is verifiable; for instance, what was eaten for the last meal. Asking the person about events in their past life can assess long-term or remote memory. Remember that you will need to be able to check these facts to decide if their memory is intact or not.
- *Mathematical calculation* – this requires both an intact memory and intact cognitive functioning as well as numeracy. Assess the person's ability to calculate by asking them to do a simple addition or subtraction exercise, such as counting backward from 100 by sevens, or forward from 50 by sixes without the use of paper and pencil.

Assess thought processes and content

Thinking should show logic, coherence and relevance. The individual's communication should make sense. Thought content is what the person is actually thinking about. Illogical or unrealistic thoughts and processes can be probed by asking about obsessive thoughts, guilt or feelings of being controlled, watched or followed by others. Illogical, unrealistic thinking and behaviour may indicate a mental disorder. Some terms used to indicate altered forms of thought are as follows:

- *autistic thinking* – individualised associations derived from within the self
- *blocking* – a sudden stop in speech and train of thought
- *circumstantiality* – the use of tedious and irrelevant details causing indirect progression of thoughts
- *confabulation* – imagined or fantasised experiences unconsciously filling in memory gaps
- *delusional* – holding a fixed false belief despite refuting evidence
- *flight of ideas* – a rapid verbal skipping from one idea to the next without relationship to preceding content
- *fragmentation* – disruption of thoughts resulting in an incomplete idea
- *hallucination* – false perception not seen, heard or experienced by others (e.g. hearing voices, seeing devils)
- *loose association* – disconnected associations between thoughts
- *neologism* – making up new words that symbolise ideas not understood by others
- *perseveration* – repetition of some verbal or motor response involuntarily
- *tangentiality* – thought digressions not related to preceding thoughts or ideas
- *word salad* – a mix of words or phrases that lack meaning.

Thought content should be assessed for destructive ideation (self-harm, suicide), somatic themes (physical symptoms) and ritualistic or repetitive thinking or behaviour. Defensive themes should also be assessed; these may include excessive ambivalence, distorted perceptions, religious or grandiose ideas, thought broadcasting, thought insertion, magical or nihilistic thinking or phobias.

Assess language and speech

Speech and the language used express thought content and processes. The person's speech should be clearly understood. Assess the rate, rhythm, volume and inflection. Slurred, extremely rapid, very slow or poorly intoned speech indicates neurological dysfunction or mental disorder. Be careful to determine that the person does not have a speech disorder (e.g. teeth or palate problems, a lisp or a stutter) or a hearing disorder (especially congenital) that may adversely affect speech.

Assess sensory and motor skills

Adults should be able to carry out all activities of daily living within their physical abilities. Inability to do so in some or all areas of activity may indicate neurological or mental disorder and requires further investigation. For instance, the inability to use familiar items such as a comb may indicate apraxia or severe depression. If you are in doubt about this assessment, ask the person to write their name or draw a circle or a square and observe for ease, speed, coordination, tremors and correctness. Again, culture, literacy and language will impact on the person's ability to accomplish the tasks.

DOCUMENTATION

An MSA requires formal documentation, including, in some instances, verbatim reports of what was said. An MSA is best recorded under the assessment headings in this chapter. Documenting an MSA will, of necessity, be more extensive in a psychiatric setting than in a general setting; however, any deviations from normal should be accurately recorded and reported. Electronic documentation will also follow the above conventions.

CLINICAL SKILLS ASSESSMENT

Mental status assessment

Demonstrates the ability to effectively assess a person's mental status. Incorporates the *National Safety and Quality Health Service Standards:* 2 Partnering with Consumers, 3 Preventing and Controlling Healthcare-Associated Infection, 5 Comprehensive Care, 6 Communicating for Safety, and 8 Recognising and Responding to Acute Deterioration (ACSQHC, 2021).

Performance criteria	1	2	3	4	5
(Numbers indicate NMBA *Registered Nurse Standards for Practice*)	**(Dependent)**	**(Marginal)**	**(Assisted)**	**(Supervised)**	**(Independent)**
1. Identifies indication (1.1, 3.3, 3.4)	☐	☐	☐	☐	☐
2. Evidence of therapeutic interaction with the person, e.g. gives the person a clear explanation of the procedure (1.4, 1.5, 2.1, 2.2, 3.2)	☐	☐	☐	☐	☐
3. Demonstrates clinical reasoning abilities, e.g. person's age, culture and language require consideration when assessing mental status (1.1, 1.2, 1.3, 2.3, 4.2, 6.1)	☐	☐	☐	☐	☐
4. Assesses each of the following (4.1, 4.2, 4.3, 6.1): ■ general appearance ■ level of consciousness ■ orientation ■ mood ■ affect ■ knowledge and vocabulary ■ judgement and abstraction ■ memory ■ thought processes and content ■ language and speech ■ sensory and motor assessment	☐	☐	☐	☐	☐
5. Documents relevant information (1.4, 1.6, 2.2, 2.7, 3.5, 3.7, 6.2, 6.5, 7.3)	☐	☐	☐	☐	☐
6. Demonstrates the ability to link theory to practice (1.1, 3.3, 3.5)	☐	☐	☐	☐	☐

Student:

Clinical facilitator: Date:

CHAPTER 17

FOCUSED CARDIOVASCULAR HEALTH HISTORY AND PHYSICAL ASSESSMENT

INDICATIONS

Cardiovascular assessment is carried out in a range of circumstances, from physical assessments during admission to monitoring the person's cardiovascular status following trauma or treatment or throughout a disease process. In this way, the person's individual needs are responded to appropriately.

EVIDENCE OF THERAPEUTIC INTERACTION

Explain the procedure to increase the person's compliance and reduce their anxiety, which affects heart rate and blood pressure (BP) readings. Advise the person that you are going to listen to their chest in several places and for extended periods, so you do not alarm them. Anxiety and fear of dying may make your assessment more difficult, so explanation and honest reassurance are important to anyone who has a history of cardiac disorder.

DEMONSTRATE CLINICAL REASONING

Consider the person's age and comfort levels during the assessment. Someone who is frail, elderly or in a great deal of pain may be unable to maintain a particular position. A thorough cardiovascular health history is fundamental to a cardiovascular assessment. A family history is taken because many cardiac disorders (e.g. coronary artery disease, systemic hypertension) have a heritable basis. Other risk factors are also explored (e.g. weight gain, smoking).

Do not expect to be able to do this assessment after one or two tries. It takes a lot of practice to become proficient in seeing, feeling and hearing the sometimes subtle cues that indicate normality and abnormality in the cardiovascular system.

ELDER CARE

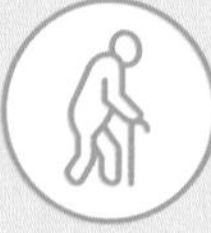

Elderly people have physiological alterations that affect their cardiovascular system. These include increased incidence of hypertension, increased arteriosclerosis leading to reduced distensibility of vessels, and an atypical presentation of myocardial infarction. Elderly people often have less intense pain of shorter duration than younger people, dyspnoea, confusion and failure to thrive (Jenkins & Winterbottom, 2019).

Frailty (due to advanced age, multimorbidities or disability) impacts negatively on cardiovascular health as well as on general health, morbidity and mortality. Assessing cardiovascular condition in elderly people should also include assessing for frailty. You can recognise frailty if the elderly person reports or demonstrates unintentional weight loss/sarcopenia, weakness, poor endurance/exhaustion, slowness and low physical activity level (Richter et al., 2022). If frailty is suspected, document your findings and report them to senior healthcare professionals.

THE PERSON LIVING WITH SEVERE OBESITY

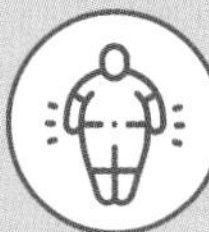

Obtaining a BP reading on a severely obese person can be difficult. An appropriately sized cuff may be available or a thigh cuff used (see **Clinical Skill 11**). Peripheral pulses may be difficult to find or distinguish due to altered landmarks (from excess adipose tissue) or excess tissue muffling the pulse. A Doppler may be needed to determine the pulses. Both heart rate and respiratory rate are often above normal (check the chart for a relative change from previous readings). Check for fluid balance by weighing daily, check for pitting oedema, measure the calf circumference to watch for deep vein thrombi and check nail beds for pallor/cyanosis. See also **Clinical Skills 15 and 23** for further explanations of issues affecting the person living with severe obesity.

?

If the person is obese, it may be necessary to sit them upright or slightly forward or on their left side (you may need to use the Doppler). These positions bring the cardiac structures close to the chest wall and render their sounds easier to hear.

Position the person

The supine position is well suited for assessing the anterior chest. The structures are easily accessible for inspection, palpation and auscultation. The supine position is comfortable for most people. Raising the head of the bed as high as 45 degrees is acceptable if the person has difficulty breathing.

Provide privacy and comfort

Privacy is essential to the person's feelings of self-worth. Privacy reduces feelings of embarrassment when clothing is removed from their torso. A warm ambient temperature is essential (removing clothing from half of the body exposes a large surface area and causes loss of heat through radiation, evaporation and convection). Assist the person to relax by starting the physical assessment with assessment of the BP, temperature, pulse and respiration, and pulse oximetry. These are part of the cardiac assessment, but are non-invasive and non-threatening, which helps put the person at ease. Ask the person (or assist them) to remove the clothing from their torso, including a woman's brassiere, since sounds are masked and altered if the stethoscope is used over clothing.

GATHER EQUIPMENT

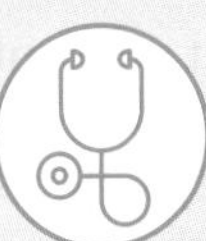

Gathering equipment ensures that you have all needed material, boosts the person's confidence and trust in you, increases your self-confidence and provides a time to mentally rehearse the procedure. You will need the following equipment:

EQUIPMENT	EXPLANATION
Sphygmomanometer or automatic BP machine	To obtain a blood pressure reading
Stethoscope	• Used for blood pressure readings and to listen to heart sounds • Consists of earpieces, binaurals, plastic or rubber tubing to conduct sound and the chest piece, with a diaphragm and a bell surface • The diaphragm side (flat surface) picks up high-pitched sounds best, like atrioventricular and lung sounds. Hold firmly in place for best effect • The bell (conical-shaped side) picks up softer, lower-pitched sounds best, like diastolic heart sounds and vascular sounds. Hold gently in place for best effect
Watch with a second hand	To calculate the pulse rate
A bath blanket (or similar)	Maintains warmth, privacy and dignity during assessment
Doppler ultrasonic flow meter (for use where peripheral pulse is not discernible)	Is able to discern the waveform and changes the ultrasound reading into an audible pulse

CONDUCT A FOCUSED CARDIOVASCULAR HEALTH HISTORY AND PHYSICAL ASSESSMENT

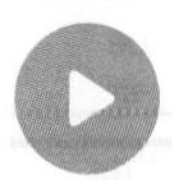
Video

The focused cardiovascular health history can provide cues and direction for the physical assessment. For example, with a history of previous deep vein thrombosis, you would measure the person's calf circumferences, temperature and colour of their lower limbs and ask about tenderness in the calf.

Hand hygiene

Hand hygiene (see **Clinical Skill 5**) removes microorganisms from your hands, preventing cross-contamination and reducing incidences of nosocomial (i.e. hospital- or treatment-acquired) infection.

Obtain a cardiovascular history

Gather a cardiac history, including information about the following:

- *age* – many cardiovascular disorders are found within specific age groups
- *gender* – some cardiovascular diseases are more prevalent in either males or females, or present differently
- *family history of cardiac problems* – to alert you to inheritable diseases
- *cardiovascular-specific conditions* – for example, claudication (leg cramps from poor peripheral circulation) or Reynaud's disease
- *chronic medical conditions* – alerts you to cardiac complications (e.g. diabetes, anaemia, cerebrovascular accident)
- *surgical history* – especially cardiac-related (e.g. cardiac catheterisation), response to anaesthesia
- allergies
- *medications* – include over-the-counter, herbal, natural medicines and illicit drugs
- *childhood illnesses or communicable illnesses* – for example, rheumatic fever
- *social history* – for example, smoking, alcohol use, illicit drug use, diet, exercise, sexual practices, stress, work and home environments, sleep difficulties (e.g. awakening at night due to shortness of breath, or to pass urine)
- weight and recent weight gain
- exercise tolerance
- cholesterol levels, if known.

Major cardiac symptoms include chest pain or discomfort (could be described as tightness or pressure), palpitations, weakness, fatigue, syncope, severe anxiety, extremity pains and oedema. These symptoms commonly occur in more than one cardiac condition and in non-cardiac disorders. Determine the OPQRST (onset, position and palliating factors, quality and quantity, radiation, setting and associated symptoms, and the timing and treatment [Estes et al., 2020]) of each of the chief complaints.

The chest pain of a myocardial infarct is usually in the central to left sternal area, and radiates to the jaw, neck, arm or shoulder, although women may have an atypical chest pain that does not radiate, or may be felt as back pain (Mechanic et al., 2022). If the person you are examining reports such chest pain, immediately report to a more senior healthcare professional (Lin & Buckley, 2019). As a beginning nurse, you need to be aware of your own limitations, but there are further assessments you can undertake (e.g. determining the seven dimensions of the pain [as above], taking the vital signs [see **Clinical Skills 10, 11, 12 and 13**]; and performing an electrocardiogram [ECG – see **Clinical Skill 18**).

Ask about any usual treatment of chest pain. Check the person's chart (ask or check their pocket or bag, with permission, for personal supply) for medication orders, such as glyceryl trinitrate or other antianginal medication, and administer a dose.

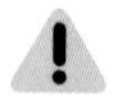
Safety

A complete examination of all systems is essential to detect peripheral and systemic effects of cardiac disorders and evidence of non-cardiac disorders, which may affect the heart. During physical assessment, take note of fever, hydration status (well hydrated or dehydrated – look at the oral membranes, skin turgor), recent intake of alcohol, nicotine, caffeine, other drugs, severe anxiety, recent physical exercise or intake of a heavy meal. These factors directly impact the cardiac perfusion, blood pressure and/or cardiac rhythm.

Assess the heart

Age considerations

The cardiovascular indicators are somewhat different in children and newborns than they are in adults. Innocent murmurs (with no other cardiac symptoms) develop in many children at some time in their lives (Estes et al., 2020). Heart rate is faster in younger children, slowing from approximately 120 to 150 bpm in a newborn to 80 to 130 bpm in a toddler, making apical pulse assessment necessary in these groups. Older school-aged children decrease from 70 to 110 bpm to the average adult rate of 60 to 100 bpm by the mid-teens. Consult a paediatric text for other findings.

Older adults generally maintain their heart rate between 60 and 100 bpm. Both bradycardia and tachycardia are more common in the older population.

Take the vital signs

Obtain a BP reading, temperature, pulse and respiratory rate and peripheral oxygen saturation (if not done earlier) to measure the functional aspects of the heart (see **Clinical Skills 10, 11 and 12**).

Inspect the anterior thorax

Identify landmarks such as the Angle of Louis, intercostal spaces (ICSs) and the midclavicular line (MCL). Look for an apical impulse (pulsations at the apex of the heart), indicating the position of the left ventricle – normally at the 5th ICS, medial to the left MCL. A visible pulsation at the mitral area is normal in about half the adult population (Estes et al., 2020). Visible pulsations in other areas of the precordium are not normal and are reported because they may indicate an aneurysm or enlarged ventricle.

Palpate the anterior chest

Use your finger pads to palpate the heart from base to apex for pulsations. Use the palm of your hand to palpate for thrills (vibrations) or heaves (lifts) of the cardiac area. Neither are normal findings and must be reported. Additional palpation may locate the exact location and timing in relation to the cardiac cycle.

Palpate the apical pulse

Use either your finger pad or the palm of your hand to locate the apical pulse, then pinpoint the pulse with one finger pad. This should disclose a light tap at the point of maximal impulse (apex of the heart: 5th ICS, medial to the left MCL). An unusually forceful or displaced apical pulse is not normal and must be reported.

Palpate the epigastric region just below the sternum for pulsations or masses. In a thin adult and in children, there is often a discernible pulsation. If strong pulsations are present, notify a senior nurse immediately, as this may indicate an aortic aneurysm.

Auscultate the apical pulse

Take care to keep the tubing of the stethoscope from rubbing on the person or bedclothes. Use the diaphragm of the stethoscope (warm it in your hand first) to assess the apical pulse for one minute for both rate and rhythm. If the heart rhythm is irregular, determine if there is a pattern to the irregularity. Report tachycardia, bradycardia and dysrhythmias for further assessment. Auscultate the high epigastric region just below the sternum. A bruit (a shooshing sound) at this position indicates an aortic aneurysm and must be immediately reported.

Auscultate the heart sounds

Identify each of the four cardiac auscultation sites. The opening and closing of the cardiac valves cause the heart sounds. The sites for auscultation are not directly over the corresponding valve but lie on the pathway the blood flow takes, located at the position where the sound from that valve is best transmitted. Listen to each auscultation site in sequence for several cycles.

The traditional cardiac landmarks (see FIGURE 17.1) are:

- *aortic area* – located at the 2nd ICS at the right sternal border (RSB)
- *pulmonic area* – located at the 2nd ICS at the left sternal border (LSB)
- *Erb's point* – located at the 3rd ICS at the LSB
- *tricuspid area* – located at the 5th ICS at the LSB
- *mitral area* – located at the 5th ICS at the MCL.

The diaphragm of the stethoscope should be inched in a Z pattern, from the base of the heart across and down to the apex (or use the reverse order – just be consistent). At each area, the heart sounds are auscultated for 10 to 15 seconds. Listen closely to the S_1 and S_2 sounds to become familiar with their rhythm.

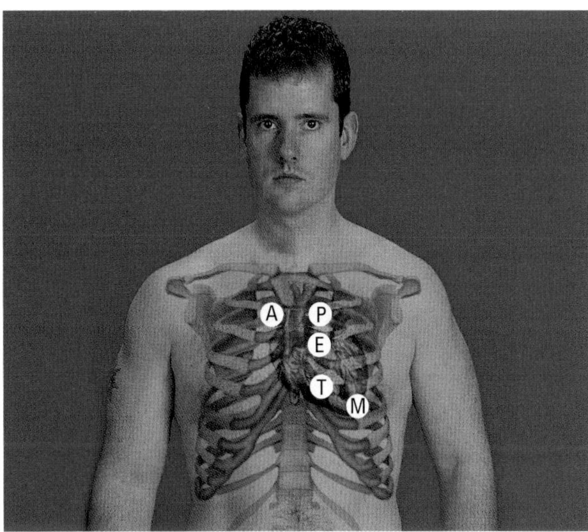

FIGURE 17.1 Location of traditional auscultation sites

Normal heart sounds last a fraction of a second, followed by a longer period of silence. To identify heart sounds:

- note the rate and rhythm
- identify S_1 (ventricular systole) and S_2 (beginning of diastole)
- assess S_1 and S_2 separately, using the diaphragm of the stethoscope
- listen with the bell of the stethoscope for extra heart sounds (e.g. S_3 and S_4)
- listen for murmurs or rubbing.

> If you are having trouble deciding which heart sound is S_1 (ventricular systole), palpate the carotid artery. The heart sound that correlates to the pulse wave is S_1.

Once you are familiar with normal heart sounds, you will recognise extra and abnormal sounds:

- S_1 sounds are heard at all sites and louder at the apical sites
- S_2 sounds are heard at all sites and louder at the base of the heart
- S_3 sounds are normal in children and young adults
- S_4 sounds are present in many older adults.

Murmurs are sounds created by turbulent blood flow and can occur at any time in the cardiac cycle; listen for timing within the cycle, quality, intensity and pattern.

When you identify abnormal sounds (S_3 or S_4 sounds in most adults, murmurs, ejection clicks, rubs, or normal heart sounds that are located in different areas or are louder than the others), inform a more experienced nurse or physician. Also, see a physical assessment text for more information on cardiac assessment.

Assess the vascular system

Assist the person to a position of comfort

Assist the person to a supine position with the head of the bed elevated to 30 to 45 degrees for carotid artery and jugular vein assessments. The remainder of the cardiovascular examination does not require any particular position, as long as all limbs are accessible for inspection and palpation.

Assess perfusion quality

Carotid arteries

Inspect the right carotid artery along the margin of the sternocleidomastoid muscle. Instruct the person to turn their head towards their right side. Place the finger pads of your index and middle fingers around the medial edge of the sternocleidomastoid muscle in the lower half of the neck (to avoid the carotid sinus).

Repeat on the left side. There should be no kinks or bulges and the pulse rate and rhythm should be equal.

Safety

The carotid arteries are never palpated simultaneously to avoid occluding the blood flow to the brain.

Instruct the person to hold their breath. Auscultate the carotid arteries, listening for bruits. There should be none.

Jugular veins

Assist the person to a supine position, with their head elevated to 45 degrees. Maintain their neck in a neutral position.

Inspect then palpate the right internal jugular vein. If the vein is distended, measure the vertical distance in centimetres from the angle of Louis to the top of the distension on the neck vein to obtain an indirect jugular venous pressure (1 to 2 cm is normal).

Repeat on the left side.

Peripheral pulses

Using bilateral simultaneous palpation of the pulses, assess volume, rate, rhythm and symmetry of peripheral pulses. Each pair should be equal. Usually radial, posterior tibialis and dorsalis pedis pulses are assessed, but the temporal, brachial, femoral and popliteal pulses can also be evaluated.

Reassess markedly diminished or absent pulses using a Doppler. Absent or diminished pulses indicate arterial occlusion and inadequate circulation.

Use of a common scale (e.g. 3 = bounding; 2 = normal; 1 = weak, thready, diminished; and 0 = absent) makes documentation of information consistent.

Assess tissue perfusion

Central perfusion (how well the vital organs are being perfused) is initially assessed by:

LOOK at the person's colour (pale, flushed, cyanotic), level of consciousness and urine output (>0.5 mL/kg/hour). Assess for cyanosis around the mouth, oral mucosa, sublingually and inside the cheeks.

LISTEN to their apical heart rate, rhythm and regularity.

FEEL their skin temperature, perspiration and pulse amplitude. Correlate these to the blood pressure.

Peripheral perfusion is assessed in the limbs and digits.

LOOK at both arms, hands and fingers; inspect both legs from groin and buttocks to feet and toes for indicators of poor perfusion. These include cyanotic or mottled digits; thickened toenails; shiny, hairless skin on lower legs and arms; and skin discolouration or ulcerations on lower legs. Note the presence of varicose veins, venous enlargement, redness or discolouration, and ulcers over saphenous veins.

FEEL for cool extremities, assess for oedema, warmth in a limb or area.

LISTEN to reports of tenderness or pain.

Assess each extremity

Look at the colour of the nail beds (pink is normal; pale, grey or bluish is not). The speed of capillary refill indicates the effectiveness of peripheral circulation. Firmly squeeze the nail beds of the fingers and toes and release them. Watch for colour change. The nail bed will initially blanch (turn white), but blood should return in less than three seconds. Assess several nail beds on each limb.

Inspect and assess peripheries, especially dependent areas, for oedema over bony areas. Press your finger firmly into the skin on the top of the foot or the inner ankle bone for five seconds. No depression should remain once your finger is removed. Description of the oedema includes whether there is 'pitting' (i.e. an imprint in the oedematous area remains when your finger is removed), the extent of the oedema, its location and whether it is bilateral.

Use a common scale for grading oedema to make documentation consistent, such as 1+ (2 mm), 2+ (4 mm), 3+ (6 mm), 4+ (8 mm). In a person with dependent oedema, the sacral area and buttocks should also be assessed for oedema.

CLEAN, REPLACE AND DISPOSE OF EQUIPMENT

Use alcowipes to wipe the bell and the diaphragm of personal stethoscopes, as well as the earpieces of ward stethoscopes to reduce the incidence of cross-contamination. If used, clean the Doppler according to manufacturer's directions.

DOCUMENTATION

As part of the physical assessment, document the cardiac assessment, noting the pulse rate, rhythm and amplitude, the BP, normal S_1 and S_2 heart sounds heard, any abnormalities seen in the chest (e.g. scars, heaves), the presence and strength of the peripheral pulses in all four extremities, and the capillary refill in all four extremities. Note any abnormal clinical manifestations (e.g. oedema, ulceration, increased jugular venous distension, clubbing of the fingers or abnormal heart sounds) and document these in the progress notes.
If you are using electronic documentation, take care to look at the trends and compare and analyse previous information to detect changes in the person's condition.

CLINICAL SKILLS ASSESSMENT

Focused cardiovascular health history and physical assessment

Demonstrates the ability to assess the cardiovascular system. Incorporates the *National Safety and Quality Health Service Standards*: 2 Partnering with Consumers, 3 Preventing and Controlling Healthcare-Associated Infection, 5 Comprehensive Care, 6 Communicating for Safety, and 8 Recognising and Responding to Acute Deterioration (ACSQHC, 2021).

Performance criteria	1	2	3	4	5
(Numbers indicate NMBA *Registered Nurse Standards for Practice*)	**(Dependent)**	**(Marginal)**	**(Assisted)**	**(Supervised)**	**(Independent)**
1. Identifies indication (1.1, 3.3, 3.4)	☐	☐	☐	☐	☐
2. Evidence of therapeutic interaction with the person, e.g. gives a clear explanation of the procedure (1.4, 1.5, 2.1, 2.2, 3.2)	☐	☐	☐	☐	☐
3. Demonstrates clinical reasoning abilities, e.g. provides privacy, comfort measures, analgesia if needed and warmth, positions the person supine or sitting upright (1.1, 1.2, 1.3, 3.2, 4.2, 6.1)	☐	☐	☐	☐	☐
4. Gathers equipment (5.5, 6.1): ■ sphygmomanometer ■ stethoscope ■ watch with a second hand ■ bath blanket ■ Doppler ultrasonic flow meter	☐	☐	☐	☐	☐
5. Performs hand hygiene (1.1, 3.4, 6.1)	☐	☐	☐	☐	☐
6. Obtains a cardiac history (2.1, 2.2, 2.3, 3.4, 4.1, 4.2, 5.1)	☐	☐	☐	☐	☐
7. Obtains a blood pressure reading (4.2, 6.1)	☐	☐	☐	☐	☐
8. Inspects the anterior chest (4.2, 6.1)	☐	☐	☐	☐	☐
9. Palpates the apical pulse (4.2, 6.1)	☐	☐	☐	☐	☐
10. Auscultates apical pulse; obtains rate and rhythm (4.2, 6.1)	☐	☐	☐	☐	☐
11. Identifies the cardiac auscultation sites; listens at each for several cardiac cycles (4.2, 6.1)	☐	☐	☐	☐	☐
12. Assists the person to a comfortable position (1.1, 6.1)	☐	☐	☐	☐	☐
13. Assesses peripheral pulses and perfusion of extremities – capillary refill, oedema, clubbing, varicosities (4.2, 6.1)	☐	☐	☐	☐	☐
14. Cleans, replaces and disposes of equipment appropriately (3.6, 6.1)	☐	☐	☐	☐	☐
15. Documents relevant information (1.4, 1.6, 2.2, 2.7, 3.5, 3.7, 6.2, 6.5, 7.3)	☐	☐	☐	☐	☐
16. Demonstrates the ability to link theory to practice (1.1, 3.3, 3.4, 3.5)	☐	☐	☐	☐	☐

Student:

Clinical facilitator: Date:

CHAPTER 18

12-LEAD ELECTROCARDIOGRAM

INDICATIONS

Electrical impulses, generated within the sinoatrial node of the heart, travel throughout the heart and are detectable on the surface of the skin. The electrocardiogram detects, measures and records this electrical activity into waveforms that represent the depolarisation and repolarisation of the cardiac muscle.

The 12-lead electrocardiogram (ECG) provides 12 different views of the heart's electrical activity. There are 12 distinct waveforms.

The six limb leads (three bipolar: I, II and III; three unipolar: $_aV_R$, $_aV_L$ and $_aV_F$) record electrical potential from the frontal plane, and the six unipolar chest leads (V_1, V_2, V_3, V_4, V_5 and V_6) record the electrical potential from the horizontal plane.

Each waveform represents the orientation of the lead to the wave of depolarisation passing through the heart. Normally, this depolarisation proceeds from right to left and base to apex – the normal electrical axis of the heart. In a healthy heart, depolarisation is initiated in the sinoatrial node and proceeds through the atria to the atrioventricular node and on through the ventricles. In an unhealthy or damaged heart, the electrical axis will vary as the electrical activity bypasses the area of damage or necrosis.

The indications for obtaining a 12-lead ECG include:

- identification of various pathological conditions, such as chest pain, myocardial infarction (MI), cardiac dysrhythmias, acute breathlessness or syncope
- following chest trauma, burns, envenomation, overdose, electrocution or successful cardiopulmonary resuscitation
- obtaining a baseline ECG for comparison prior to stressful interventions, such as surgery, anaesthesia or invasive diagnostic procedures
- ongoing comparison of the current electrical activity of the heart after a pathological condition has been identified
- for follow-up of irregularities detected using mobile or wearable cardiac monitoring (Marston et al., 2019).

EVIDENCE OF THERAPEUTIC INTERACTION

Introduce yourself, check the identification band, ask the person their name, and gain their verbal consent for the ECG. Explain the reason for the ECG. Although there are no sensations associated with the procedure, some people are fearful they may be shocked or they may be anxious about the findings. To help them relax, explain that the machine does not create electrical currents but only picks them up. Clearly explain the procedure to assist the person to comply with directions, such as lie still, do not talk and breathe slowly, because muscle movement interferes with the reading by increasing the amount of electrical activity picked up (Hadjiantoni, 2020). Teaching people about healthcare facts assists them to cooperate with the procedure and to make informed decisions. Smile – your relaxed attitude helps them to relax.

DEMONSTRATE CLINICAL REASONING

Know where the ECG machine is stored, that it is ready to use and how to use it, as it may be required in an urgent situation. Make yourself familiar with the model and lead attachments used in the facility.

Provide comfort measures (e.g. toilet, fluids) and analgesic, as necessary, to help the person tolerate the requirements of the assessment, including remaining still and relaxed throughout. At times, it will be impossible for the person to relax or be pain-free (e.g. during an acute episode of chest pain) when the ECG is needed to identify ischaemic changes. Help the person into a supine position with all four limbs supported. Damani et al. (2021) state that there is no evidence of difference between the supine position and a semi-recumbent position in the ECG recording, so position for comfort within these parameters. Support the person's head on one pillow. No muscular work should be used to maintain the position. Turn off the power to an electric bed to prevent electrical interference. Don't forget to turn it on again. Provide privacy to preserve the person's dignity. Remove clothing above the waist (including a woman's brassiere) to facilitate the location and attachment of leads. A chaperone may be required for women of some cultures (Menzies-Gow, 2018). Ensure the ambient temperature is warm so the person doesn't shiver (which increases muscular work). The hospital gown can be put back on for this brief diagnostic test. Jewellery (especially a wrist watch) should be removed so there is no electrical interference. Position the ECG machine on the person's left side, if possible, because most of the electrodes will be on that side. Raise the bed to a comfortable height for you.

If the person has difficulty breathing while supine, help them into a well-supported semi- to high Fowler's position (45 to 60 degrees). It is important to note this on the tracing so that subsequent readings are all taken in the same position; this is because the change in position will move the heart (Menzies-Gow, 2018).

CALIBRATE THE ELECTROCARDIOGRAM MACHINE

Use the manufacturer's instructions to calibrate and prepare the ECG machine to ensure the reading is as accurate as possible. Machines may be single-channel or multi-channel. You may need to use a filter (check with the medical officer, as filters may obscure some important details [Campbell et al., 2017]) if the baseline is thick to provide a better-quality tracing (Ricciardi et al., 2016). Familiarise yourself with the type of machine and its use to increase the accuracy of the recording and decrease stress for both the person and yourself.

ELDER CARE

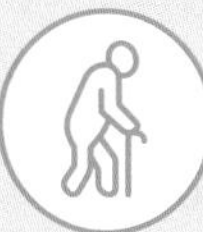

Be aware that up to 30 per cent of elderly women do not report chest pain as a symptom when they are experiencing a coronary event and report to an emergency department (Bunney et al., 2023). Therefore, using other coronary event symptoms (arm, neck pain, breathlessness, nausea and anxiety) plus age plus sex to decide to initiate an ECG may more accurately identify women who require treatment for some myocardial infarctions.

THE PERSON LIVING WITH SEVERE OBESITY

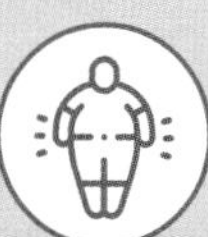

Obesity is a crucial determinant of cardiovascular disease risk, including hypertension, atherosclerotic disease and ischaemic heart disease (Dobbie et al., 2023). The electrode sites on a severely obese person may be very difficult to locate. You may require another nurse to assist you with positioning the person (often more upright because of breathing difficulties) and holding excess breast tissue out of the way, so you can apply the electrodes.

The person's skin will probably be damp with perspiration and will need washing and drying so the electrodes stick to the skin. Make sure you note the position of the person on the printout of the ECG.

GATHER EQUIPMENT

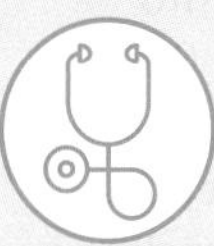

Gathering equipment ensures that you have all needed material, boosts the person's confidence and trust in you, increases your self-confidence, allows you to mentally rehearse the procedure and alerts you to anything that is missing or malfunctioning. The following equipment is required:

EQUIPMENT	EXPLANATION
ECG machine	• Records the electrical activity of the heart muscle and transcribes the waveforms onto a monitor or tracing paper • Make sure it is safe to use (has been checked and tagged by the facility's electrical department) and batteries are charged as applicable
ECG paper	Comes in sheets or on a roll, depending on the machine used
Electrodes	• Come in a variety of forms; most are now disposable, marked to indicate placement (limb leads may be colour coded), pre-gelled and adhesive, although some older varieties (suction bulbs, strap-on electrodes) are still used • Ensure the foil package (disposable) is intact and the gel in the centre of the electrode patch is moist • All contact the person's skin and pick up the electrical activity of the heart
Conduction gel	Only required if the electrodes are not pre-gelled
Gauze squares	Used to remove any conduction gel remaining on the skin
Scissors or a disposable razor	May be needed to clip or shave excess hair if the person is hirsute; electrodes do not conduct electrical impulses unless in direct contact with the skin
Paper towel and alcowipes	• Paper towel may be needed to gently abrade/exfoliate intact skin • Alcowipes may be required to remove oil from the skin to increase electrode contact (Campbell et al., 2017)

PERFORM A 12-LEAD ELECTROCARDIOGRAM

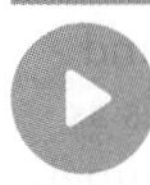
Video

This skill is generally quick to undertake, non-invasive and painless for the person.

Hand hygiene

Hand hygiene (see **Clinical Skill 5**) removes microorganisms from your hands. It is the most effective preventative measure for cross-contamination, reducing incidences of nosocomial (i.e. hospital- or treatment-acquired) infection.

Obtain the electrocardiogram reading

Attach the limb leads

Spread conduction gel on the electrodes (if not pre-gelled) to increase the conduction of the electrical impulses. Be sparing with the gel, because an excess interferes with the accuracy of the reading (Campbell et al., 2017). If the skin is unclean, oily or wet with perspiration, cleanse and dry the sites for electrode attachment using an alcowipe swab or soap and water. Dry thoroughly. Clean, dry skin ensures the best conduction of electrical impulses and reduces false readings (Royal Children's Hospital Melbourne [RCHM], 2020). Excess hair is clipped or shaved (with verbal consent), as it prevents adequate contact with the skin.

Attach the limb electrodes (marked with either colour codes, or with RA, LA, LL and RL) to clean, dry, hair-free areas on each of the four limbs equidistant from the heart. Choose areas over fleshy tissue, not bone, and on the forearm, proximal to the wrist and the lower leg, proximal to the ankle (Campbell et al., 2017). Placement is symmetrical on the arms and legs. If there is an amputation, place the contralateral limb lead in the same position bilaterally. The torso can be used rather than the limbs if necessary (shoulder and lower abdomen areas), but this causes distortion of the ECG structure and should be avoided if possible (Campbell et al., 2017). If an unusual position for the electrodes is necessary, note it on the documentation. Ensure that the lead wires are not taut, so they are not easily dislodged.

Position precordial electrodes

Precordial leads complement the limb leads to provide a complete view of the heart. These are colour-coded or identified by lead designations (V_1 to V_6) imprinted on the clips. Medani et al. (2018) found that V_1 and V_2 are commonly misplaced, leading to diagnostic errors. Hadjiantoni (2020) states the electrodes should be placed underneath the breast tissue in women and in very obese people to improve the accuracy of placement. Use the back of your hand to displace the breast tissue to reduce feelings of embarrassment. Attach chest electrodes with the centre of the electrode at each carefully located, clean, dry, hair-free site. Finding the placement of V_1 and V_2 starts with identifying the Angle of Louis (a surface landmark – the joint between the manubrium and body of the sternum, located about 5 cm below the sternal notch in adults), where the 2nd intercostal space (ICS) is located. Correct placement of these two leads is essential to obtain an accurate ECG reading (Gregory et al., 2021).

Remember: the ICS are named for the number of the rib above them. 'Walk' your fingers down from there to the 4th ICS. The chest leads (electrodes) are placed in the following way:

- V_1 – 4th ICS, right sternal border
- V_2 – 4th ICS, left sternal border
- V_3 – 5th ICS, left sternal border *or* midway between V_2 and V_4 (use the facility's protocol or the diagram provided with the ECG machine)
- V_4 – 5th ICS, left midclavicular line
- V_5 – 5th ICS, left anterior axillary line (same level as V_4)
- V_6 – 5th ICS, left midaxillary line (same level as V_4) (Campbell et al., 2017).

Place the electrodes accurately, since errors in diagnosis occur if they are incorrectly placed (Bickerton & Pooler, 2019; RCHM, 2020). Hadjiantoni (2020) found that distortion of the waveform occurred if leads were displaced by 2 cm. Disposable electrodes come already attached to leads; however, if not, attach the electrodes to the lead wires so the electrical activity is conducted to the ECG machine. Do not place pressure on the chest wall when attaching the lead wires to the electrodes. Especially following chest surgery, lead wires must be attached to the electrodes prior to placing the electrode.

Take the reading

Once you are satisfied that the electrodes are correctly placed, activate the machine. Some machines require only the initial activation. Others require you to change channels to obtain a tracing from each lead.

Put the person's details, time and date into the ECG machine (for those provided with this convenience). Take the recording. On some machines, you will need to use the 'print' button. Check that all 12 views of the ECG are clear and the baseline is stable (a fuzzy recording or an undulating baseline indicate poor electrode contact or excessive muscle movement [Chatterjee et al., 2020]) on the printout of the recording. You may need to check the electrodes and re-record the ECG. Note the person's details, time and date on the printout of the recording if not done by the machine.

It is important to remember that ECGs show the electrical activity of the heart. Observe the person to assess their cardiac output and their general condition. Determine if the person requires serial tracings. If so, leave the electrodes in situ if possible. If they must be removed, mark the placement of each one with a waterproof pen so that subsequent readings are reproducible and are taken from the same electrode placements.

> If you accidentally press any button other than the 'print' button (e.g. 'copy'), you may print another, previously stored ECG recording. It will be labelled with another person's details. You must check and confirm that the 12-lead ECG recording is labelled correctly with the information of the person you just took the recording from (McStay, 2019, p. 7).

Show each tracing to an experienced RN

Lack of experience and ability in interpreting an ECG recording might lead you to overlook significant changes. Demonstrate knowledge of your own limitations by consulting with someone more experienced. McStay (2019) stresses that the 12-lead ECG recording must be interpreted without delay by a suitably qualified healthcare professional and any abnormal findings acted upon in a timely and effective manner.

Post-procedure

Carefully and gently remove the electrodes and wipe off the conduction gel to increase the person's comfort. Electrode gel is removed with dry gauze squares or with a damp washcloth. Assist the person to dress and reposition. Although the supine position is generally comfortable, moving to a different position following enforced stillness will be more comfortable for the person. Provide them with the call bell, and personal items as desired.

CLEAN, REPLACE AND DISPOSE OF EQUIPMENT

Clean the ECG machine and its lead wires and appropriately dispose of used material (gauze squares, disposable electrodes into clinical waste and razor blade into the sharps container). Replenish ECG paper, gauze, alcowipes and conduction gel as needed. Coil the lead wires to prevent tangling. Plug the machine into an electrical source to recharge batteries if appropriate. Ensuring the equipment is replaced and the machine is charged is a courtesy to other staff and a safety measure when the ECG machine is required in an urgent situation.

DOCUMENTATION

Documenting the ECG includes attaching the actual recording to the progress notes. Check that the printed recording is correctly identified with the person's name, date of birth and hospital or unit registration number, doctor, date and time (if not done by the machine), and lead numbers (if not done by the machine) on the tracing (Campbell et al., 2017). Some facilities will have digital recording of the ECG for the electronic medical record. If this is the case, check that the above information is included on the recording.

ECG readings are numbered sequentially commencing with the first one taken during that admission, usually in the emergency department. Record who reviewed the ECG and what time it was reviewed, whether it was normal or not and what action, if any, was taken (Damani et al., 2021). Any symptoms exhibited or any difficulty experienced by the person, and subsequent nursing interventions carried out, are recorded in the progress notes and on a chest pain chart (if using). If the person was experiencing chest pain when the ECG was taken, note this on the ECG. Some facilities require you to sign the ECG and have it countersigned by the shift coordinator or the person who reviewed the ECG.

CLINICAL SKILLS ASSESSMENT

12-lead electrocardiogram

Demonstrates the ability to obtain a recording from a 12-lead electrocardiogram. Incorporates the *National Safety and Quality Health Service Standards*: 2 Partnering with Consumers, 3 Preventing and Controlling Healthcare-Associated Infection, 5 Comprehensive Care, 6 Communicating for Safety, and 8 Recognising and Responding to Acute Deterioration (ACSQHC, 2021).

Performance criteria	1	2	3	4	5
(Numbers indicate NMBA *Registered Nurse Standards for Practice*)	**(Dependent)**	**(Marginal)**	**(Assisted)**	**(Supervised)**	**(Independent)**
1. Identifies indication (1.1, 3.3, 3.4)	☐	☐	☐	☐	☐
2. Evidence of therapeutic interaction with the person, e.g. gives the person a clear explanation of the procedure (1.4, 1.5, 2.1, 2.2, 3.2)	☐	☐	☐	☐	☐
3. Demonstrates clinical reasoning abilities, e.g. provides privacy, comfort measures and pain relief, and positions the person (1.1, 1.2, 1.3, 4.2, 6.1)	☐	☐	☐	☐	☐
4. Gathers equipment (1.1, 5.5, 6.1): ■ ECG machine ■ ECG paper ■ electrodes: pre-gelled disposable or gel, suction bulb electrodes, strap electrodes, straps ■ gauze squares ■ scissors or razor, if necessary ■ paper towel and alcowipes	☐	☐	☐	☐	☐
5. Performs hand hygiene (1.1, 3.4, 6.1)	☐	☐	☐	☐	☐
6. Attaches limb electrodes to clean, dry, hair-free sites on the person's arms and legs (1.1, 6.1)	☐	☐	☐	☐	☐
7. Determines chest sites and attaches electrodes to clean, dry, hair-free sites (1.1, 6.1)	☐	☐	☐	☐	☐
8. Attaches lead wires to electrodes (1.1, 6.1)					
9. Sets ECG paper speed and calibrates the ECG machine according to the manufacturer's instructions (1.1, 6.1)					
10. Records ECG, checks with an RN regarding the significance of the tracing (1.1, 1.4, 2.7, 3.3, 3.4, 3.5, 6.1, 6.2, 6.5)					
11. Removes electrodes and cleans the gel residue; positions the person comfortably after the procedure (1.1, 6.1)					
12. Cleans, replaces and disposes of equipment appropriately (3.6, 6.1)					
13. Documents relevant information (1.1, 1.4, 1.6, 2.2, 2.7, 3.5, 3.7, 6.1, 6.2, 6.5, 7.3)					
14. Demonstrates the ability to link theory to practice (1.1, 3.3, 3.4, 3.5)	☐	☐	☐	☐	☐

Student:

Clinical facilitator: Date:

CHAPTER 19

FOCUSED RESPIRATORY HEALTH HISTORY AND PHYSICAL ASSESSMENT

INDICATIONS

Respiratory assessment is done:

- as part of a physical examination
- to assess for infections (e.g. pneumonia, influenza) or ongoing medical conditions (e.g. chronic obstructive pulmonary disease, asthma)
- before and after medical or surgical interventions (e.g. anaesthesia, surgery or treatment of trauma to the respiratory tract or thorax)
- when subjective or objective symptoms indicate a change in the person's condition.

If the person is in acute respiratory distress, limit the health history to a few closed questions about their chief complaint, perception of the problem and precipitating events, current medications and any allergies. More detail can be obtained when their distress is relieved. Any combination of signs and symptoms constitutes respiratory distress, including retraction, air hunger, use of accessory muscles, inability to speak in sentences or to lie flat, diaphoresis, restlessness, agitation or altered level of consciousness. The inability to talk in full sentences is clinically significant and in asthma it is considered severe or life-threatening (Hunter et al., 2019). Prompt action to relieve the respiratory distress is necessary (sit upright, oxygen administration). Inform the shift coordinator and medical staff.

EVIDENCE OF THERAPEUTIC INTERACTION

If the person has a respiratory disease, they may be hypoxic and very anxious. Give them plenty of time to answer questions, as dyspnoea causes speech patterns to change with more frequent and longer pauses in their sentences (Nathan et al., 2019). Thoroughly explain each step to the person to reduce their anxiety and to foster a cooperative attitude. Explain positioning and other requirements, such as breathing through an open mouth (to reduce extraneous sounds in the upper airway). Also, explaining the reasoning behind not speaking unless you request them to do so (since voice sounds interfere with your ability to hear the breath sounds) helps them comply. Instruct them to take reasonably deep and slow breaths, but to tell you if they feel light-headed or dizzy (hyperventilation). If this happens, ask the person to resume their normal breathing pattern. Try to remain calm, as your anxiety will escalate their feelings of breathlessness. Try asking them to breathe with you as you consciously slow and deepen your breathing.

DEMONSTRATE CLINICAL REASONING

An initial requirement for assessing the respiratory system is a thorough understanding of the anatomy of the thorax and the anatomy and physiology of the respiratory system (Majder et al., 2020). Provide comfort during a respiratory assessment. Warmth is necessary because the person's torso is often bared for a considerable length of time. Privacy is important, as many people, especially women, are embarrassed to have their torso exposed. Consider asking women of some cultures if they want a chaperone. Remove clothing to prevent the sound of friction from clothing on the stethoscope. Privacy also implies less noise, and quiet is necessary to hear the slight differences that may occur in the breath sounds. To ensure quiet, close the door, shut windows, turn off the radio, TV, oxygen humidifier or suction machine (if appropriate), and ask visitors to wait outside the room. A well-lit room allows easier inspection of the thorax.

Other comfort measures (e.g. assisting them to toilet) before the examination help the person to more easily cope with the procedure. Pain relief, if necessary, given half an hour prior to assessing the respiratory system, helps the person change position more readily, breathe deeply on request and remain still when required.

ELDER CARE

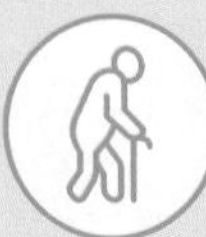

Older adults have fewer cilia, making them more prone to respiratory infections. Their ribcages are stiffer and the intercostal muscles weaker, reducing their ability to expand their lungs. This leads to a lower arterial oxygen saturation.

THE PERSON LIVING WITH SEVERE OBESITY

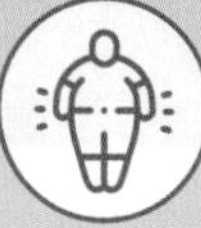

Obstructive sleep apnoea (OSA) is a common finding, as is obesity-related hypoventilation (Dobbie et al., 2023). Assess for decreased peripheral arterial oxygen levels (SpO_2), dyspnoea, increased work of breathing and the symptoms of OSA (snoring, daytime sleepiness). The breath sounds of a severely obese person are muffled. You may require another nurse to assist you with positioning the person and holding excess tissue out of the way so that you can listen to the various areas of the lungs. Assess the respiratory rate and depth, watch for accessory muscle use and how much effort is required to breathe. Note the position the person assumes to breathe comfortably. Monitor the pulse oximetry reading. See **Clinical Skills 15 and 23** for further information on issues related to caring for people living with severe obesity.

GATHER EQUIPMENT

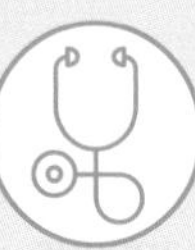

Gathering equipment is an organisational step that helps to create a positive environment for a successful interaction. While gathering the equipment, you can mentally rehearse the procedure. The following items are required:

EQUIPMENT	EXPLANATION
Stethoscope	• Consists of earpieces, binaurals, plastic or rubber tubing to conduct sound and the chest piece, with a diaphragm and a bell surface • Ensure the diaphragm side is operative and warm (use your hand or put it in your pocket) to avoid discomfort of the cold disc on the person's skin • Keep the tube of the stethoscope from rubbing on the person or bedclothes
Pulse oximeter	Displays the pulse rate and the SpO_2 level (see **Clinical Skill 12**)
Watch with a second hand	To calculate respirations per minute

FOCUSED RESPIRATORY HEALTH HISTORY AND ASSESSMENT

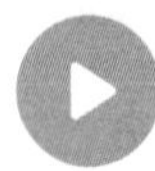

Video

The focused respiratory health history provides you with information that may guide your physical assessment of the thorax and lungs (e.g. report of smoking heavily should alert you to possible alteration in lung sounds). You will also be observing the person for signs and symptoms of respiratory problems (e.g. wheezing, inability to talk for reasonable periods) during the health history.

Hand hygiene

Hand hygiene (see **Clinical Skill 5**) removes microorganisms from your hands. It is the most effective preventative measure for cross-contamination, reducing incidences of nosocomial (i.e. hospital- or treatment-acquired) infection.

Obtain a respiratory health history

History about respiratory health can establish whether the symptoms of dyspnoea, chest pain, wheezing, stridor and cough are likely to be of respiratory origin. Where possible, the respiratory health history should be conducted before the physical assessment to guide it. The respiratory history focuses on the primary symptom when more than one symptom occurs (e.g. dyspnoea and productive cough). Determine other symptoms (e.g. fever, weight loss, night sweats).

For someone who is not in obvious respiratory distress, the history should focus on the review of:

- age and sex, because some respiratory conditions are more likely at specific ages and in either males or females
- their present illness and chief complaint (e.g. dyspnoea, cough, sputum production, chest pain, associated symptoms like vomiting)
- an overview of their general respiratory status
- their general health status.

The information gained will alert you to possible abnormalities in the individual's thoracic or respiratory status. Many factors can significantly affect respiratory function. These can be grouped under:

- *Surgical history* – for example, lobectomy, tracheostomy or chest tube insertion.

- *Medical history:*
  - infectious respiratory diseases, such as COVID-19 virus or pneumonia
  - previous diagnosis of respiratory disorders (e.g. asthma, cystic fibrosis and lung cancer)
  - previous test results (e.g. lung function studies, tuberculin skin tests or chest X-rays)
  - hospitalisations
  - other chronic disorders (e.g. congestive cardiac failure, renal disease, sleep apnoea).
- *Social history:*
  - tobacco use (present and past) and types (cigarettes, cigar, pipe), duration of habit and amount smoked per day, any efforts to quit. Remain non-judgemental, so the person continues to be at ease and offers information
  - recreational drug use (including vaping)
  - travel history (Chow, Uyeki & Chu, 2023) (e.g. COVID-19 virus)
  - family history (e.g. asthma) and contact history (e.g. tuberculosis [TB], bronchitis).
- *Work environment:*
  - type of work and environmental hazards (e.g. chemicals, dust). Repeated workplace exposure can create respiratory complications ranging from minor to life-threatening (e.g. silicosis – glass makers, cement workers; occupational asthma – bakers, painters; chronic bronchitis – welders, firefighters).
  - stress – can exacerbate asthma
  - use of protective devices (e.g. masks, air scrubbers).
- *Home environment:*
  - location, crowding (ideal condition for contracting TB)
  - air pollution
  - cigarette smoke
  - wood-burning, gas stoves or kerosene heaters or recent bushfire exposure
  - possible allergens (e.g. pets, houseplants, plants, trees outside the home)
  - other environmental hazards or stairs to climb.
- *Hobbies and leisure activities* (e.g. bird breeding – bird breeder's lung; woodwork– fibrotic changes; scuba diving – oxygen toxicity, decompression sickness).

During the respiratory history, observe for any signs of respiratory difficulty. Rapid and/or dyspnoeic breathing, use of accessory muscles to breathe, inability to talk in full sentences and altered neurological state (e.g. restlessness, confusion, irritability) all indicate suboptimal oxygenation. Changes in skin colour are not very reliable. Cyanosis is both a late and unreliable sign of hypoxaemia (e.g. it can occur with anaemia without hypoxaemia, or it might not occur with polycythaemia even with hypoxia [Estes et al., 2020]).

Obtain a pulse oximeter reading and note the readings (see **Clinical Skill 12**). Oxygen saturation via pulse oximetry is an essential part of respiratory assessment and is comparable to arterial oxygen measurement (Hlavin & Varty, 2022).

Position the person for assessing the thorax

Help the person to remove their clothing (including the woman's brassiere) and drape well for privacy. Assess the posterior thorax first (the person is less fatigued and able to sit forward more easily than they will be towards the end of the examination). Ask them to sit forward with their arms across their chest (to separate scapulae) and their head bent down for you to inspect, palpate, percuss and auscultate the posterior thorax. The person may need to rest their forearms on an over-bed table, or another nurse may be needed to help them lean forward and maintain a comfortable position while you assess the posterior thorax. The lateral thorax is also assessed at this time. Then ask them to sit up with the thorax exposed, to allow you to inspect the entire anterior thorax. The person can relax against the chair or into a Fowler's position, if necessary, for the remainder of the assessment.

Raise the bed to a comfortable height for you and use good body mechanics during the procedure to avoid straining your own muscles.

> ?
>
> If the person you are assessing is dyspnoeic and tachypnoeic during the examination, help them into a 'tripod' position to assess the posterior thorax – sitting with their arms forward, elbows bent, wrists crossed and with their arms resting on a pillow on an over-bed table. This position expands the ribcage and allows the diaphragm more movement.

Assess the respiratory system

Overview

The physical assessment of the respiratory system is comprised of observation (initial survey), inspection, palpation, percussion and auscultation. Each of these is discussed below.

Observation (initial survey)

Normal respiratory function is effortless and almost unconscious. The person can eat, drink and speak in full sentences without appearing breathless. The essential first step in a respiratory assessment is to observe the person's breathing for the following:

- ease and comfort
- rate and depth (e.g. shallow and rapid; deep and slow)
- pattern of respirations (e.g. long periods of apnoea)
- position the person has adopted to breathe effectively (e.g. lying, sitting upright, tripod position)
- rate and ease of breathing while speaking or moving – inability to speak in sentences is a sign of extreme respiratory distress and signals an emergency

- mode of breathing – whether mouth or nose breathers, and when in the respiratory cycle; note pursed lip breathing
- general colour and appearance (e.g. cyanosis, pallor, sweating)
- additional audible breath sounds (e.g. wheezing, stridor).

Do this rapid assessment during the respiratory health history.

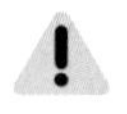
Safety

The respiratory rate is one of the first indicators of clinical deterioration, and as such is a valuable tool. SpO_2 (see **Clinical Skill 12**) is NOT a substitute for respiratory rate count – it is a complementary assessment. The respiratory rate should be measured over a full 60 seconds, for accuracy, whether the person looks unwell or not (Palmer et al., 2022). Do not document an estimated rate or a 'normal' respiratory rate value (16, 18, 20) for expediency sake.

Complete the inspection, palpation, percussion and auscultation of the thorax first on the posterior, then anterior chest to avoid tiring the person rather than asking them to sit forward and then sit backward several times.

Posterior thorax

Inspect the thorax

Note the contour of the thorax, which is normally fairly symmetrical and oval-shaped. Estimate the anteroposterior diameter (smaller than the transverse diameter, resulting in an oval-shaped thorax in cross-section). Increased anteroposterior diameter (i.e. barrel chest) can be a result of chronic obstructive pulmonary disease. Note any scars (e.g. from thoracic surgery).

Respiratory rate should be between 12 and 20 breaths per minute. Time the rate for a full minute if it is regular, and for two minutes or more if it is irregular, to establish if there is a pattern present. Extreme tachypnoea (30+ breaths per minute in an adult), bradypnoea and apnoea constitute medical emergencies requiring immediate intervention (Estes et al., 2020).

Inspect for symmetry. Are the scapulae at the same height? One scapula higher than the other indicates scoliosis. Look for the slope of the ribs at the costovertebral angle (downward sloping) and for musculoskeletal deformities. Watch for impaired respiratory movement (which indicates diseases of the lungs or pleurae).

Palpate the thorax

Lightly place the palms of both hands flat on the person's posterior chest. Gently palpate the musculature for tenderness (e.g. indicating bruising, superficial skin lesions, tumours or musculoskeletal injuries such as cracked ribs, strained muscles or inflammation). Determine respiratory excursion. Place your thumbs lightly at right angles to the spine at the level of the 10th rib (Staines, Sheridan & Pickering, 2020), thumb tips touching, and allow your hands to move with each inspiration and expiration. They should move symmetrically out and in by 3 to 5 cm with each cycle (see FIGURE 19.1).

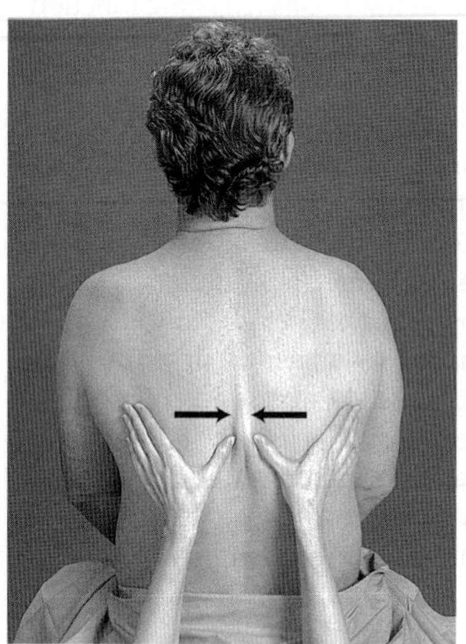

FIGURE 19.1 Palpating posterior thoracic expansion

Palpate for tactile and vocal fremitus

Assess for tactile fremitus with the ulnar aspect of your open hand. Place it on each location shown in FIGURE 19.2 in sequence. Ask the person to say 'Ninety-nine' with the same intensity every time your hand is placed on their back. Feel for vibrations created by the sound waves. Note areas of increased or decreased fremitus (vibration).

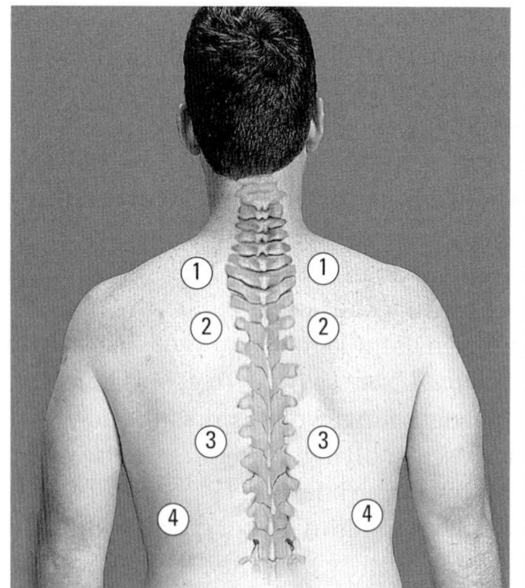

FIGURE 19.2 Palpation pattern for tactile fremitus – posterior thorax

Voice sounds can be used to determine the density of the lung contents. Normally, in an air-filled lung, voice sounds are faint and indistinct. However, when transmitted through secretions and fluid, voice sounds are heard loudly and clearly. Ask the person to whisper 'Ninety-nine' as you listen to the lung fields. If the words are loud and clear, the person is exhibiting bronchophony and this indicates secretions and consolidation. An absence of sound transmission would indicate more air than usual (i.e. pneumothorax).

Percussion

Lay your pleximeter finger (the middle finger of your non-dominant hand) flat on the chest wall (keep the other fingers up off the chest wall) and tap the pleximeter finger (and through it the chest wall) with the index and middle finger of the dominant hand. Place your pleximeter finger on intercostal spaces (ICSs) only.

Listen for resonance, which is the sound made by lung tissue filled with air. Lung tissue filled with fluid sounds dull, and if bone is struck the sound is flat. Percuss the thorax in a systematic pattern so that no area is neglected.

Percuss the posterior thorax

Start at lung apices and move hands from side to side across the top of each shoulder. Note sound produced from each percussion strike and compare with contralateral sound. Continue downward in lateral movements, percussing over every other ICS (see FIGURE 19.3). Avoid percussing over vertebrae and scapulae. Note the intensity, pitch, duration and quality of percussion.

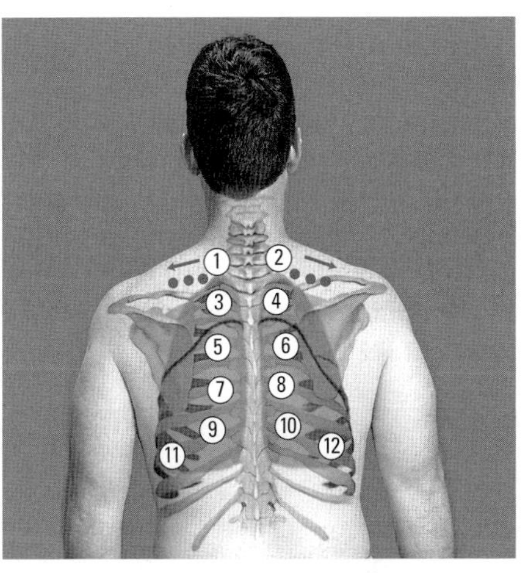

FIGURE 19.3 Percussion and auscultation pattern of posterior thorax

Auscultate for breath sounds

Ask the person to lean forward with their arms crossed in front of their chest (this spreads the scapulae further apart). Ask them to breathe a little deeper than usual through an open mouth. Respiratory auscultation is performed to identify the presence of normal breath sounds and adventitious (additional or abnormal) lung and pleural sounds (Estes et al., 2020). Listen for one complete inhalation and expiration at each position. Adventitious breath sounds may be identified by location, sound, rhythm and occurrence during the respiratory cycle. Use the flat diaphragm of your stethoscope and auscultate all areas of the lungs in a systematic sequence: side-to-side, top-to-bottom, posteriorly, laterally and anteriorly (as shown in FIGURE 19.3). For comparison, this is done bilaterally in a zigzag pattern across the chest. Listen to both the left and right side at each of the landmarks for one entire respiratory cycle – do not miss any areas.

FIGURE 19.4 shows the location of normal breath sounds (for a more detailed discussion of the various breath sounds, see a physical assessment or fundamentals textbook). Normal breath sounds are characterised as:

- *bronchial sounds* – high-pitched, loud, blowing expiratory sounds over the trachea
- *bronchovesicular* – moderately loud and medium-pitched sounds on inspiration and expiration heard between the scapulae and over the 1st and 2nd ICS near the sternum
- *vesicular* – gentle rustling or breezy sounds over the peripheral lung fields.

Extra or abnormal sounds are called adventitious; they consist of the following:

- *fine crackles on inspiration* – these sound like rolling a few strands of hair between your fingers near your ear
- *coarse crackles* – lower pitched than the fine crackles and sound moist; may clear with a cough

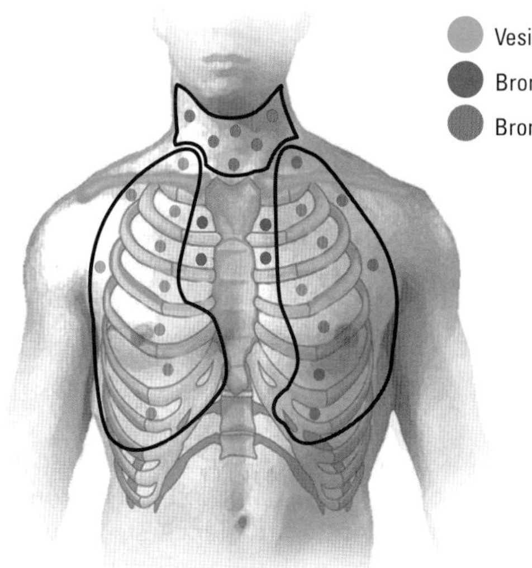

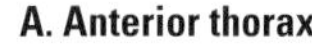

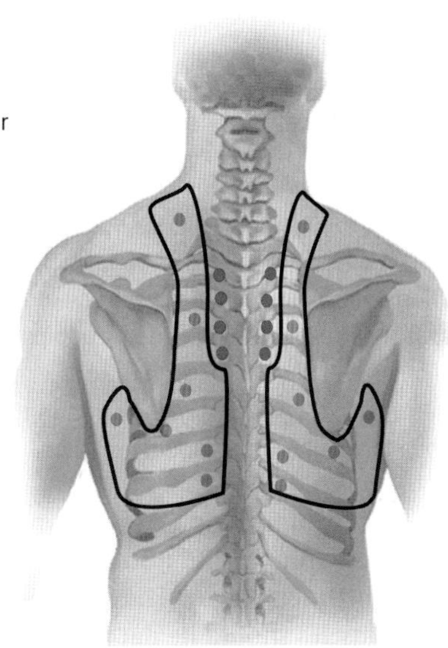

FIGURE 19.4 Location for normal breath sound

- *sibilant and sonorous wheezes* – musical sounds caused by narrowing of the large airways; may be high-pitched or have a snoring quality
- *pleural friction rub* – a creaking, grating sound produced by inflammation of the pleura
- *stridor* – an inspiratory crowing sound caused by partial obstruction of the larynx/trachea (Estes et al., 2020).

Auscultate the posterior lung fields

Be sure to note where the scapulae lie so that you do not listen over the bone. Instruct the person to inhale and exhale deeply and slowly through their mouth when the stethoscope is felt on their back (see FIGURE 19.3 for the posterior auscultation locations). Starting at the apex of the right lung at C7, move the stethoscope inferiorly about 5 cm (or to every second ICS) until you reach the bases at T10. Listen on the contralateral side at each site and compare the sounds. Continue to move inferiorly until the entire posterior lung has been auscultated. Listen to the breath sounds.

Lateral chest

The lateral chest is auscultated at four places; you may auscultate either the right and left lateral thorax independently or auscultate the areas alternately to compare, side to side. Ask the person to raise their arms above their head (if possible) and place your stethoscope directly below the axilla. Note the sound and again move the stethoscope inferiorly about 5 cm or to every second ICS. (Each of the four positions created by moving your stethoscope is referred to as a 'site' here.) On the right side, place the stethoscope posterior to the midaxillary line at sites 1, 2 and 4. Site 3, which is used to listen to the tail of the right middle lobe, is anterior to the midaxillary line. On the left side, sites 1, 2 and 3 are on the midaxillary line, and site 4 is posterior to the midaxillary line.

Anterior thorax

Inspect the anterior thorax

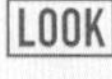

for the shape of the chest (e.g. barrel shaped, normal or symmetrical), costal angle (normal is less than 90 degrees during exhalation [Estes et al., 2020]), intercostal spaces (note bulging), and any visible veins, scars or bruises. Observe the respirations (do not tell the person you are doing this, as their respiratory rate, depth and pattern may change if they are aware). Note rate, depth, pattern, symmetry, audibility, their position and if/when they are nose or mouth breathers.

Respiratory excursion should be even, symmetrical and appear effortless. You should not be able to hear them breathe from 1 metre away. The intercostal and other accessory muscles should lie flat throughout the respiratory cycle. The thorax should rise and fall in unison with the respiratory cycle. The ribs should slope across and downward, without movement or bulging in the ICS.

Palpate the anterior thorax

Place your finger pads on the right lung apex, above the clavicle. Move downward to each rib and ICS (see FIGURE 19.5). Note tenderness, pulsation, masses and crepitus (a grating, crackling sensation caused by two rough surfaces rubbing together). Repeat on the left side.

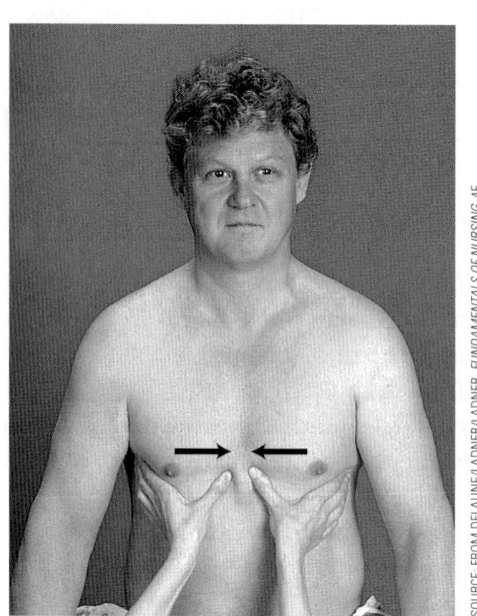

FIGURE 19.5 Palpating anterior thoracic expansion

Assess respiratory expansion. Place your thumbs along each costal margin at the xiphoid sternum with your hands on the lateral ribcage. Instruct the person to inhale deeply. Note divergence of your thumbs on expansion (normal is 3 to 5 cm). Feel the range and symmetry of respiratory movement. Palpate for tactile fremitus (see FIGURE 19.6).

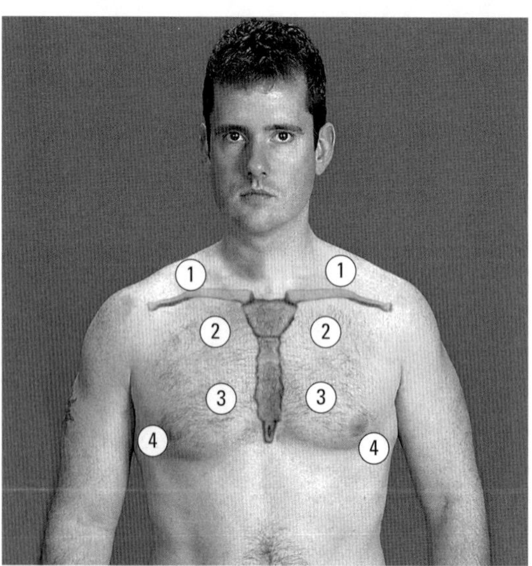

FIGURE 19.6 Palpation pattern for tactile fremitus – anterior thorax

Ask females (and obese males) to displace their breast tissue during palpation, percussion and auscultation of the anterior chest, because the extra tissue interferes with the assessment of the underlying structures (Estes et al., 2020, p. 396). If you must displace the breast tissue, use the back of your hand to gently do so (as it feels less intimate).

Palpate for vocal fremitus

The method of assessing for vocal fremitus is the same as that described for the posterior thorax; the anterior locations are depicted in FIGURE 19.6. Increased tactile fremitus should be noted in the documentation.

Percuss the anterior thorax

Percuss symmetrically; two to three strikes along the right lung apex, above the clavicles, then repeat on the left lung apex (see FIGURE 19.7). Proceed downward and percuss in every other ICS (right to left in same position) on both sides. In each thoracic area, assess for:

- resonant lung field
- cardiac dullness – 3rd to 5th ICS left of sternum
- liver dullness – place pleximeter finger above and parallel to the expected upper border of the liver in the right midclavicular line; percuss downward
- gastric air bubble – repeat procedure performed for liver dullness on the left side.

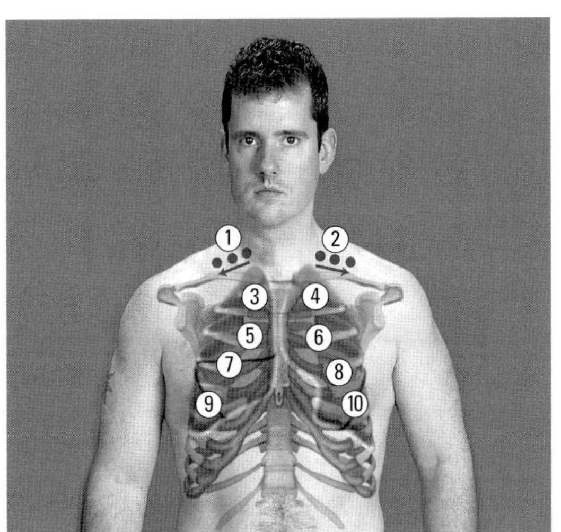

FIGURE 19.7 Percussion and auscultation pattern for anterior thorax

Auscultate the anterior lung fields

Ask the person to cough (to clear the airways). Instruct the person to breathe through their mouth (to reduce the sounds of air turbulence through the nasopharynx), a little more deeply and slowly than normal.

Auscultate the anterior chest by starting slightly above the clavicles at the apex of the lung. Note the breath sound during one complete inspiration and expiration. Move your stethoscope to the contralateral side. Compare the sounds. Continue to move your stethoscope down approximately 5 cm to every second ICS until the base of the lungs at the sixth rib, again comparing the contralateral sides at each site to compare the breath sounds. Listen to the breath sounds; note the intensity and identify abnormal variations. See FIGURE 19.7 for locations of anterior chest auscultation. (FIGURE 19.4 shows the locations for normal breath sounds, auscultation and percussion.)

Check the junction between the fingers and fingernails for clubbing (a reduced, flattened angle between the nail and the nail bed), which indicates long-term oxygenation deficiencies.

Post-procedure

Assist the person to re-dress, return their bed to a normal height and provide them with their call bell, water and any material or belongings that were moved. Tell them your findings if they are interested. Ask if there is any more information about their breathing that they can recall.

CLEAN, REPLACE AND DISPOSE OF EQUIPMENT

Wipe the bell and diaphragm of your own or the unit's stethoscope with an alcowipe. Having your own stethoscope is an infection control measure as well as a convenience. Wipe the unit's stethoscope earpieces with alcowipes to thoroughly decontaminate them.

DOCUMENTATION

Relevant information about the respiratory condition provides healthcare workers with a baseline assessment and a record of ongoing changes in a person's condition. Document the health history using the facility's form, if available. The respiratory rate is noted on the vital signs sheet and the Adult Deterioration Detection System (ADDS), if used. Changes or trends in the respiratory rate should be brought to the notice of a senior healthcare professional. Documentation of physical findings should include time and date, and objective findings, including those from inspection, palpation, percussion and auscultation and the anatomical location (use the landmarks and distances in centimetres, or note specific lung lobes) of any abnormalities. Document any part of the procedure that was omitted (e.g. Mrs Green was unable to comply with raising her arms, so lateral auscultation of the lungs was not done). If you are recording an initial assessment or if there are changes from previous assessments, include the person's subjective description.

PART 3

CLINICAL SKILLS ASSESSMENT

Focused respiratory health history and physical assessment

Demonstrates the ability to assess the thorax and lungs. Incorporates the *National Safety and Quality Health Service Standards*: 2 Partnering with Consumers, 3 Preventing and Controlling Healthcare-Associated Infection, 5 Comprehensive Care, 6 Communicating for Safety, and 8 Recognising and Responding to Acute Deterioration (ACSQHC, 2021).

Performance criteria	1	2	3	4	5
(Numbers indicate NMBA *Registered Nurse Standards for Practice*)	(Dependent)	(Marginal)	(Assisted)	(Supervised)	(Independent)
1. Identifies indication (1.1, 3.3, 3.4)	☐	☐	☐	☐	☐
2. Evidence of therapeutic interaction with the person, e.g. provides a clear explanation of the procedure (1.4, 1.5, 2.1, 2.2, 3.2)	☐	☐	☐	☐	☐
3. Demonstrates clinical reasoning abilities, e.g. provides privacy, comfort measures and pain relief if necessary. Obtains a respiratory history. Positions the person – sitting if possible (1.1, 1.2, 1.3, 4.2, 6.1)	☐	☐	☐	☐	☐
4. Gathers equipment (5.5, 6.1): ■ stethoscope ■ pulse oximeter ■ watch with a second hand	☐	☐	☐	☐	☐
5. Performs hand hygiene (1.1, 3.4, 6.1)	☐	☐	☐	☐	☐
6. Observes general appearance, thoracic symmetry, respiratory rate, pattern, use of accessory muscles or supraclavicular retraction (4.2, 6.1)	☐	☐	☐	☐	☐
7. Palpates anterior and posterior chest, and percusses thorax and lung fields (4.2, 6.1)	☐	☐	☐	☐	☐
8. Auscultates the lungs, and identifies normal and adventitious breath sounds (4.2, 6.1)	☐	☐	☐	☐	☐
9. Cleans, replaces and disposes of equipment appropriately (3.6, 6.1)	☐	☐	☐	☐	☐
10. Documents relevant information (1.4, 1.6, 2.2, 2.7, 3.5, 3.7, 6.2, 6.5, 7.3)	☐	☐	☐	☐	☐
11. Demonstrates the ability to link theory to practice (1.1, 3.3, 3.4, 3.5)	☐	☐	☐	☐	☐

Student:

Clinical facilitator: Date:

CHAPTER 20

FOCUSED NEUROLOGICAL HEALTH HISTORY AND PHYSICAL ASSESSMENT

INDICATIONS

Neurological assessment is a combination of assessments that indicate functioning of the autonomic and peripheral nervous systems. The complete assessment includes assessment of mental status (see **Clinical Skill 16**), cranial nerve, cerebellar function and motor function as well as reflexes. This Clinical Skill addresses the neurological assessment and the Glasgow Coma Scale (GCS) assessment; however, the complete suite of these assessments is not within the scope of this competency. For the complete assessment guide, refer to a physical assessment textbook (e.g. Estes et al., 2020).

Neurological assessment and then observations (i.e. GCS) are done on any person in danger of deterioration in central nervous system (CNS) functioning. The observations are done frequently on those with an acute or rapidly changing status (i.e. 15 minutes to hourly). Subtle alterations alert you to neurological complications early so that intervention can begin, to prevent further deterioration of neurological functioning and irreversible damage (e.g. hemiparesis or impaired cognitive function). Neurological assessment and the GCS are done for those with:

- head trauma
- cerebrovascular accidents
- pre- and post-neurological surgery
- brain tumours
- cerebral infections
- decreased level of consciousness (LOC) (e.g. post-CPR, post seizure, post-hypoglycaemic coma, severe hyper- or hypothermia).

Neurological assessment

It is important not to take any aspect of the neurological assessment in isolation. The following are assessed during an admission neurological assessment:

- *Mental status* – note general appearance, affect, speech content, memory, logic, judgement and speech patterns. If abnormal, conduct a full mental status assessment.
- *Level of consciousness* – note arousal and awareness. If the person is not fully conscious, perform a GCS, motor assessment and pupil assessment.
- *Sensation* – during both admission and assessment of peripheries, watch for abnormal responses to touch, heat or cold, or to minor pain if you are concerned.
- *Cranial nerves (CN)* – during conversation watch for facial expression (CN vii), gross hearing (CN viii), tongue movement, voice (CN ix, x, xii). Ask about visual acuity and visual fields, test for pupillary actions (CN ii and iii) and test the cardinal fields of gaze (CN iv).
- *Motor system* – assess muscle tone and strength, abnormal movements and grasps. The person should be able to move against resistance with their dominant side a bit stronger than their non-dominant side.
- *Cerebellar function* – during admission, observe the person's gait and their ability to stand and sit upright without support. If there is a difficulty, ask them to do heel-to-toe walking and shallow knee bends. Normally, these are easily done.

Reflexes are either deep tendon reflexes or superficial reflexes. Beginning nurses seldom assess these. They require a patellar hammer and a very good knowledge of anatomy so that the tendons are struck squarely, adequately and briskly.

EVIDENCE OF THERAPEUTIC INTERACTION

Warmly greet the person and verify their identity. A clear explanation of the procedure will both elicit cooperation from the person and help to reduce frustration, anger or embarrassment if they are unable to answer questions or comply with requests during a neurological assessment. An explanation about why the questions are being asked and what you are assessing will allay fears in most people. If the person is confused or their LOC is decreased, the explanation may need to be given at each encounter. If they are confused or with decreased LOC, use their name frequently in the assessment (after you have established their orientation). When using the GCS, offer explanations following the initial observation for eye opening.

DEMONSTRATE CLINICAL REASONING

Ensure the person is comfortable, preferably in an upright or high Fowler's position unless there are contraindications (e.g. brain injury). The room should be private (for confidentiality), warm and well lit.

Consider the person's age, culture and existing physical conditions, and modify the questions you ask to establish orientation (awareness of self and of the environment).

Think carefully about what questions can establish a young child's orientation; recognition of a parent, sibling or toy will be more telling than their inability to tell you what day it is or where they are.

Cultural difficulties may arise; for example, your gender may interfere with the person's ability to respond, or you may misjudge the person's response because of your own cultural biases.

Other conditions and characteristics will alter the ease with which a neurological assessment can be made. The following should be noted:

- If the person does not speak English (but is physically able to speak), commands to determine orientation and motor response cannot be followed without the assistance of an interpreter.
- If the person is blind, eye opening as a response is not reasonable.
- If the person has facial trauma and the eyes are affected or swollen shut, pupil response cannot be obtained.
- If the person is aphasic, intubated or unable to physically speak for any reason, orientation cannot be assessed.
- Opiate use (and other drugs used both medically and illicitly) may make the pupils pinpoint, while parasympathetic medications such as atropine or scopolamine may enlarge pupils.

Any deterioration from baseline must be reported to the shift coordinator and the medical officer. Serial assessments of neurological status detect deterioration, and their communication and documentation ensure rapid response to the person's changing condition.

Warning postures are late indicators of deterioration of the CNS. *Posturing* is non-purposeful movement that indicates damage to the corticospinal system. *Decorticate posturing* is recognised by extreme flexion of the upper extremities – arms are flexed onto the chest, and fingers and wrists are tightly flexed. There is plantar flexion, but the legs are extended and internally rotated. *Decerebrate posturing* is the abnormal extension of the arms with the wrists extended and pronated, and the fingers flexed. The legs are extended with the feet in plantar flexion. (Consult your medical surgical text for visual examples.)

ELDER CARE

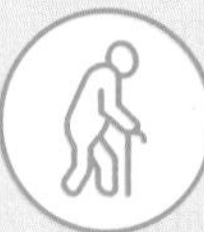

An elderly person with a hearing deficit may be unable to understand what is expected of them. Some elderly individuals may respond slowly because their processing abilities are slower than those of a younger adult, or there may be an established dementia that interferes with assessment of recent or current changes in their LOC. The incidence of dementias increases with age. Take care to ask about sleep–wake cycles as alterations in these can result in mental or neurological symptoms in the elderly (Bell et al., 2021).

THE PERSON LIVING WITH SEVERE OBESITY

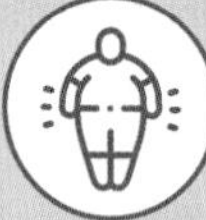

Meo et al. (2019) demonstrated impaired cognitive function, including reduction in attention, retention, intelligence and cognitive flexibility, in severely obese adolescents. Balasubramanian et al. (2021) found obesity in ageing promotes cognitive impairment and dementia. Fulton et al. (2022) found neuroinflammation arising from metabolic and vascular dysfunction related to severe obesity resulted in both anxiety and depression. These findings may impact on the neurological assessment of the severely obese adult in your care.

GATHER EQUIPMENT

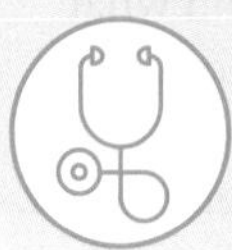

Gathering equipment is an organisational step that helps to create a positive environment for a successful interaction. It ensures that you have all needed material, boosts the person's confidence and trust in you, and increases your self-confidence. While gathering the equipment, you can mentally rehearse the procedure. The following equipment is needed:

EQUIPMENT	EXPLANATION
Sphygmomanometer and stethoscope	Used to assess blood pressure
Thermometer and watch with a second hand	• Used to determine body temperature, pulse and respiratory rate • Oral thermometers are not used in people with an altered LOC; tympanic thermometers are the most efficient • Axillary temperatures are obtained if there is no alternative available
Pulse oximeter	Determines oxygen saturation of the blood and therefore the oxygen available to the brain
Penlight and pupil gauge	Used to determine the size of the pupils and their responsiveness to light
Neurological assessment sheet	• Used to record various assessments for comparison • Vary between facilities, but most contain the GCS (eye opening, motor response and verbal response), pupillary size and response, vital signs and motor function or limb movement

CONDUCT A NEUROLOGICAL ASSESSMENT

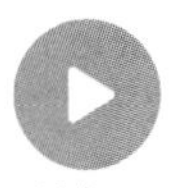
Video

Neurological assessment begins when the person enters the room. Observation of their gait, coordination, alertness and engagement with you and the environment will give you initial clues as to their neurological condition.

Hand hygiene

Hand hygiene (see **Clinical Skill 5**) removes microorganisms from your hands. It is the most effective preventative measure for cross-contamination, reducing incidences of nosocomial (i.e. hospital- or treatment-acquired) infection.

Neurological health history

The neurological health history is an important aspect of the neurological assessment. The person should be put at ease and allowed to tell their story in their own words. At times, a family member (note as a secondary source in documentation) may need to be interviewed to obtain a reliable history. Specific questions clarify the quantity, intensity, distribution, duration and frequency of each symptom.

Explore the chief complaint (headache, seizure, syncope, tremors, paraesthesia, vertigo, disturbances in memory, gait, swallowing or speech are the most common) using questions about precipitating and palliating factors, quality, quantity, region (location) and radiation, associated symptoms, and setting and timing for each complaint.

Disabilities should be described quantitatively (e.g. headache every third or fourth day lasting about 18 hours each time, intensity is 9/10 most of those days) and the effects on the person's daily routine (e.g. I have to stay in a quiet dark room and cannot look after the children, do my chores, read, watch TV or go to work).

Past medical history and a complete health review are essential because neurological complications are common in other disorders (e.g. diabetes mellitus, vascular disorders, HIV infections) as well as neurological-specific problems (e.g. Parkinson's disease, migraine, childhood seizures). Medications (e.g. antidepressants, anxiolytics, antipsychotics) can also be linked to neurological problems. Communicable diseases like encephalitis or poliomyelitis, and accidents involving injuries like closed head injury and concussion, should be noted.

Family history is important, because migraine and many metabolic, nerve and neurodegenerative disorders have a genetic component. There are also several neurodegenerative disorders that can appear together within a family (Estes et al., 2020).

Taking information regarding the person's social, occupational and travel history provides information about exposure to such things as stress, drugs and alcohol, toxins, parasites and unusual infections.

Gather information for a mental status assessment during the health history and physical assessment. If there are any indications that the person requires further assessment of their mental status, a complete mental status assessment should be carried out (see **Clinical Skill 16**).

Assess level of consciousness

LOC is the most sensitive of the assessments in demonstrating early deterioration of brain function. The LOC of most people will be 'alert', meaning they are awake, meet your gaze or respond to your questions. They are oriented to person, place and time and are able to interact with you and the environment, provide you with their health information and discuss their health problems. If this is the case, continue on to the pupillary activity, muscle tone and strength and vital signs.

Decreased levels of consciousness require a different assessment, such as the GCS.

Glasgow Coma Scale

The GCS is used to assess neurological functioning when there has been a brain injury (Geethvani & Youtham, 2022). Originally developed as a research tool, it has been widely adopted in clinical settings to objectively measure and identify trends in a person's LOC (Estes et al., 2020; Mehta & Chinthapalli, 2019). Please use this discussion in conjunction with the neurological assessment chart or the GCS chart supplied in your laboratory or in your nursing fundamentals textbook.

The GCS is a numerical scale where a summed score out of 15 indicates the person:

- opens their eyes spontaneously (4 points)
- is oriented (verbal response – 5 points)
- obeys commands (motor response – 6 points).

A GCS score of 7 or less indicates coma, and a score of 3 (the lowest possible) indicates the person is not able to open their eyes, verbalise at all or respond to pain. However, it is most useful to report the scores in *each of the three sections* – eye opening, verbal and motor response – rather than the overall score (Mehta & Chinthapalli, 2019).

Serial recordings of the responses and scores in each section demonstrate the changing clinical condition of the person with altered consciousness (Ahmed, Adley & Hassan, 2019). Mehta and Chinthapalli (2019) found that a reduction in the GCS predicted an adverse event and that a drop of 2 or more is a significant predictor of a major adverse event.

For serial assessment, the GCS provides data about the LOC *only*. It is not:

- a complete neurological examination
- a sensitive tool for evaluation of altered sensorium
- able to account for possible aphasia
- a good indicator of lateralisation (e.g. decreasing motor response on one side or unilateral changes in pupillary reaction).

A baseline assessment is done and changes are tracked from admission. Your assessment must be consistent with that of other nurses, otherwise the tracking system will not be useful. Initially when you begin to care for the person, you and the nurse who previously cared for the person will assess them together so that your assessments are comparable. Accurate and consistent assessment of LOC and GCS are dependent on knowledge and experience (Mehta & Chinthapalli, 2019); therefore, it is professionally sound to seek mentorship.

The AVPU scale (DeLaune et al., 2024) outlined below is a quick assessment (rather than the GCS) used on contact with a person at any time, based on their best level of response:

- *alert* – spontaneous eye opening and interaction without prompting
- *voice* – verbal interaction (e.g. calling their name) is needed to gain a response
- *pain* – painful stimulus (e.g. trapezius squeeze) is required to gain a response
- *unresponsive* – the person does not respond despite the application of a painful stimulus.

Anyone with a changed category or who scores a P or U (who was previously alert) requires immediate medical review.

Level of consciousness

LOC indicates arousal and awareness and is a measure of brain function or failure. The GCS assesses three aspects of consciousness: eye opening, verbal response and motor response. Eye opening is categorised (scored) as:

- spontaneous (4)
- to speech (3)
- to pain (2)
- none (1).

Eye opening (as part of LOC) is assessed by initially (carefully and without speaking and assuming they are awake) observing the person for spontaneous eye opening (note also their body position and movement, or verbalisation). If no response is noted, call the person's name, at first in a normal tone, then more loudly. You may need to shout. Response is opening of the eyes (and/or a verbal response).

If the person has not responded to firm and clear auditory stimulation and then to touch and then to a gentle shake, employ painful/noxious stimulation techniques to elicit their arousal. Use the least amount of pressure to stimulate a response to avoid bruising or pain. The brain responds to central stimulation and the spine responds first to peripheral stimulation (Schick, 2023).

Follow the facility's policy and procedure for the painful stimulation technique used for LOC assessment and use that technique consistently. Apply *central stimulation* by squeezing the trapezius muscle using the thumb and two fingers to hold 5 cm of the muscle where the neck meets the shoulder and twisting the muscle. Another pain stimulation point is supraorbital notch pressure (run your finger along the supraorbital margin and you will feel a notch). This method is not used if the facial or cranial bones are fractured or unstable, or after facial surgery. These are the preferred methods. A sternal rub uses the knuckles of your clenched fist to apply pressure to the centre of the sternum. This method is not used for repeated assessment because the sternal tissue is tender and bruises easily.

Apply *peripheral stimulation* by placing a pen alongside the person's 3rd or 4th interphalangeal joint and applying increasing pressure, or by placing the fingernail bed between your finger and a pencil or a pen (nailbed pressure). Gradually increase pressure over 10 to 15 seconds until the slightest response is seen. Any finger can be used, although the third and fourth fingers are often the most sensitive (Estes et al., 2020). This is extremely painful so use it only if necessary (i.e. no response to a trapesius pinch) and only until the slightest response occurs.

When applying pain, watch all three categories – eye opening, verbal response and motor movement to the pressure, so the pain is applied only once per assessment. The amount of stimulation required for a response is recorded in the baseline assessment. Some people may need a lot of stimulation to maintain their concentration to answer questions, even though they can answer them correctly.

Best verbal response – orientation

The second aspect of the GCS is 'best verbal response', determined by orientation and scored out of a possible 5. Orientation is the awareness of self and of the environment. If the person is able to respond, ask them for the following to determine their orientation: to identify themselves, the day, the month, the year and where they are. Note that some questions cannot be answered easily even by individuals who have full cognitive ability after they have been hospitalised for a while, so you may need to reorientate them to the day and date. Sometimes they are able to memorise the right answer, so vary your questions occasionally and ask their home address or their children's names. You must know the correct answers to these questions.

If the person is not oriented to person, time and place, ascertain their best verbal response. The categories are:

- oriented (scored as 5)
- confused (uses sentences, but unable to tell you the time, place or even their name, scored as 4)
- inappropriate (random often inaudible words that have no logic, scored as 3)
- incomprehensible (mumbles or groans, scored as 2)
- none (no response, scored as 1).

Motor response

This is the third aspect of the GCS. It is scored out of 6. Give the person single-response commands requiring a motor response, such as 'touch your nose' or 'wiggle your toes'. Allow time to comply. Asking the person to 'grasp my hand' while touching their palm may elicit a reflex response even if the person is not able to obey commands. Asking them to 'let go of my hand' will determine if they can obey commands. If they are unable to obey commands, apply a pressure stimulus (pressure on a finger and toe on each extremity) and watch the response. They may try to localise (i.e. push the stimulus away) or withdraw (move their hand or foot away from the pressure) or assume an unusual posture. Compare the right and left sides and upper and lower extremities. The *best response* is recorded for the GCS. The categories for best motor response are:

- obeys commands (scored as 6)
- localises pain (tries to push your hand away, scored as 5)
- withdrawal (flexes or extends away from the pain, scored as 4)
- flexion abnormal (also called decorticate posturing, scored as 3)
- extension to pain (also called decerebrate posturing, scored as 2)
- none (scored as 1).

Neurological charts incorporate an assessment of limb movements where you are able to document separately the response of each limb if there are differences. Also note any abnormality that indicates altered function in any extremity.

Remember, the GCS is used if there is suspected or established injury to the brain. It is not necessary to 'score' anyone if they are alert, chatting appropriately with you and moving all their limbs appropriately. If this is the case, the remainder of a neurological assessment is done as follows. **The GSC is only one part of the neurological examination and is more meaningful if examined along with vital signs, pupil size and reaction and is watched for trends.**

Assess vital signs

Vital signs (VS) are done as part of any physical assessment. Changes in the VS of people with brain injury/disease are late signs of brain deterioration. Initially, VS are monitored every 15 minutes until they are stable, then hourly depending on the person's condition. In some facilities, nursing staff are unable to decrease the frequency of neurological assessment without a doctor's order. The VS should be checked in the following order (and especially so if there are GCS alterations from normal):

- *Respiratory pattern* – provides the clearest indication of brain function due to the complex process of respiration involving different areas of the brain. Record pattern of respirations as well as rate and depth because they give clues about damaged areas of the brain. Note Cheyne-Stokes, rapid, irregular, clustered, gasping or ataxic breathing, and, of course, apnoea (see **Clinical Skill 19**).
- *Temperature alterations* – may indicate dysfunction of the hypothalamus or brain stem. CNS function is affected by alterations in body temperature above or below normal. Hyperthermia may also be caused by infection. Hyperthermia increases the metabolic rate and therefore the cerebral metabolism, increasing the brain's need for glucose and oxygen. Hypothermia decreases the metabolic rate, thereby decreasing the cerebral blood flow and oxygen concentration of the brain (see **Clinical Skill 10**).
- *Blood pressure* – increases with increased intracranial pressure as a compensatory mechanism. Increased intracranial pressure exerts pressure on the vessels in the brain and ischaemia of the tissue results (see **Clinical Skill 11**).
- *Pulse rate* – initially rises as a compensatory mechanism, and then slows in instances of increased intracranial pressure due to vagal stimulation from increased blood pressure (see **Clinical Skill 10**).

Consult a medical-surgical text for a detailed explanation of increased intracranial pressure and its effects on the VS.

Assess pupillary activity

Pupillary activity, found on the neurological assessment sheet, assesses CN iii. These are not part of the GCS but are part of the neurological assessment.

Pupil size is controlled by the integration of the sympathetic and parasympathetic nervous systems. It is assessed in each eye, before the light reflex is tested, and against a pupil gauge measured in millimetres (see FIGURE 20.1). Hold the pupil gauge close to each eye for comparison. Rest your fingers on the person's temple or cheekbone (assuming no injury in that area) so the gauge is held as close as possible to the pupils for comparison. Note anisocoria (unequal pupil size), which occurs in about 17 per cent of the population.

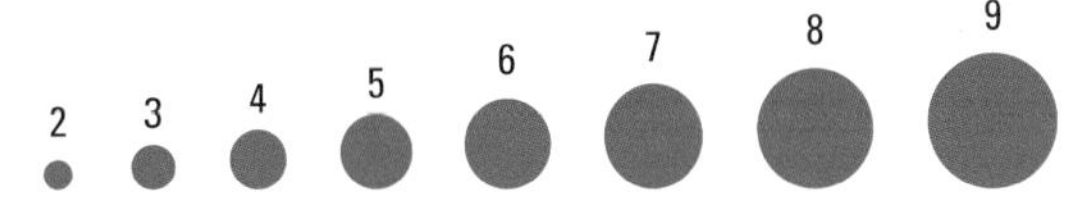

FIGURE 20.1 Pupil sizes in millimetres

SOURCE: FROM DELAUNE/LADNER/LADNER. *FUNDAMENTALS OF NURSING*, 4E. © 2011 DELMAR LEARNING, A PART OF CENGAGE LEARNING, INC. REPRODUCED BY PERMISSION. WWW.CENGAGE.COM/PERMISSIONS

Determine the *pupil shape* and record it as round or draw the shape to indicate an abnormality (e.g. following surgery for glaucoma).

Assess *pupil reactivity* to light by bringing the light from the penlight across from the lateral side of the person's head towards the nose. Do not cross the nose with the light. Observe the pupil for constriction (it should be brisk) and repeat, observing the opposite pupil for constriction to indirect light (i.e. consensual constriction). Repeat with the other eye. Do not confuse a prosthetic eye with a fixed pupil. Responses are usually recorded as equal or not, and brisk, sluggish or fixed (i.e. no response). Inform the senior nurse if the person's pupils become unequal or if one pupil becomes more sluggish than the other; these are early signs of increasing intracranial pressure and the person's condition needs to be reviewed promptly.

Assess for *accommodation* by asking the person to focus their gaze on a distant object for approximately 30 seconds and then look back at your finger or a pen held approximately 10 cm away from them. Note the reaction and size of the pupil. Accommodation occurs when pupils constrict and converge to focus on an object at close range. Pupils are recorded as reactive to accommodation. You will see 'PERRLA' recorded. This means the **P**upils are **E**qual, **R**ound, **R**eactive to **L**ight and **A**ccommodation. Use this if it is an approved term in the facility where you are working.

Extraocular movements (EOMs, the cardinal fields of gaze) assess the oculomotor, trochlear and abducens (iii, iv, vi) cranial nerves. They are included in the neurological assessment. Ask the person to follow the tip of the penlight or your finger with their eyes only, without moving their head. Hold the penlight/finger 25 to 40 cm in front of them and move it slowly upward, downward, laterally and obliquely, watching the pupil movement as it tracks the object. The eye's movements should be smooth and symmetrical. The EOMs are recorded as symmetrical. Any abnormalities in tracking (lag, nystagmus) are noted.

The *oculocephalic reflex* is tested in an unconscious person (if there is no spinal injury). With the person lying flat, without a pillow, stand beside their head, place one hand on their forehead and hold both eyes open. Quickly, but gently, turn their head from one side to the other and watch their pupil movements. If the reflex is intact, their eyes will move in the opposite direction to the side to which you turned their head. If the person does not have intact reflexes, their eyes will move slowly from side to side, or not at all (i.e. they will move with the head).

Assess muscle strength and tone

Each extremity is tested unless there is a physical injury or other problem in the limb. Ask the person to move each limb. Compare the opposite sides. Ensure your instructions are clear and contain only one command. Ask the person to:

- grasp your fingers with both hands simultaneously to assess for strength (use only two or three fingers to avoid being inadvertently hurt). The grasp of the dominant hand is usually stronger
- put their fist on their chest while you provide resistance (hold the arm) to test arm strength
- raise their arms (to assess movement against gravity)
- raise their arms again (now apply downward pressure on their forearm [resistance] to test for strength)
- raise their legs (both against gravity and resistance)
- plantar flex and dorsiflex their feet, again with and without resistance, to assess their feet.

The limb movement categories on the neurological chart are usually 'normal power', 'mild weakness', 'severe weakness', 'flexion', 'extension' and 'no movement'. Any flicker of movement is recorded.

Changes in motor strength, especially between right and left sides, may indicate imminent neurological failure and are to be reported immediately to the shift coordinator and medical staff. If the person is unable to follow commands, watch for movement in each of the limbs for a *localised* (moves the other hand to the site of the stimulus), *flexion* (flexes away from the pain), *extension* (the person's limb extends from pain) or *flaccid* (no motor response at all) response to painful stimulus. Motor response is recorded as symmetrical, equal with normal strength unless there is an abnormality.

CLEAN, REPLACE AND DISPOSE OF EQUIPMENT

If a person requires regular neurological observation, the equipment will remain at the bedside. Otherwise, clean the stethoscope (diaphragm/bell plus earpieces) and penlight with alcohol swabs, discard the thermometer sheath and return the unit's equipment to its storage area.

DOCUMENTATION

Accurate serial documentation of comprehensive assessments prompt referral and further assessment when deterioration occurs improves survival following traumatic brain injuries and strokes, and reduces the incidences of further injury (Mikkelsen et al., 2020). The information gathered is promptly recorded on the GCS or neurological observation chart. In the progress notes, document exactly what stimulus was used, where it was applied, the pressure needed to elicit the response, and the person's response. Avoid vague terms because these can be misinterpreted.

If there are no abnormalities, the documentation would be something like: Alert, oriented × 3, PERRLA; EOMs symmetrical, no abnormalities; motor movement symmetrical (or equal) and strong. Vital signs would be charted on the VS sheet.

CLINICAL SKILLS ASSESSMENT

Focused neurological health history and physical assessment

Demonstrates the ability to effectively assess the neurological status of the person. Incorporates the *National Safety and Quality Health Service Standards*: 2 Partnering with Consumers, 3 Preventing and Controlling Healthcare-Associated Infection, 5 Comprehensive Care, 6 Communicating for Safety, and 8 Recognising and Responding to Acute Deterioration (ACSQHC, 2021).

Performance criteria	1	2	3	4	5
(Numbers indicate NMBA *Registered Nurse Standards for Practice*)	(Dependent)	(Marginal)	(Assisted)	(Supervised)	(Independent)
1. Identifies indication (1.1, 3.3, 3.4)	☐	☐	☐	☐	☐
2. Demonstrates clinical reasoning abilities, e.g. modifies questions with regard to age, culture and existing physical conditions; can describe warning signs of increasing cerebral pressure (1.1, 1.2, 1.3, 4.1, 4.2, 6.1)	☐	☐	☐	☐	☐
3. Evidence of therapeutic interaction with the person, e.g. gives a clear explanation of procedure (1.4, 1.5, 2.1, 2.2, 3.2)	☐	☐	☐	☐	☐
4. Gathers equipment (1.1, 5.5, 6.1): ■ sphygmomanometer, stethoscope ■ thermometer, watch with a second hand ■ penlight, pupil gauge ■ neurological assessment sheet	☐	☐	☐	☐	☐
5. Performs hand hygiene (1.1, 3.4, 6.1)	☐	☐	☐	☐	☐
6. Assesses level of consciousness (4.1, 4.2, 4.3)	☐	☐	☐	☐	☐
7. Assesses orientation of the person (4.1, 4.2, 4.3)	☐	☐	☐	☐	☐
8. Assesses pupillary activity, vital signs, motor response and muscle strength and tone (4.1, 4.2, 4.3)	☐	☐	☐	☐	☐
9. Cleans, replaces and disposes of equipment appropriately (3.6, 6.1)	☐	☐	☐	☐	☐
10. Documents relevant information (1.4, 1.6, 2.2, 2.7, 3.5, 3.7, 6.2, 6.5, 7.3)	☐	☐	☐	☐	☐
11. Demonstrates ability to link theory to practice (1.1, 3.3, 3.5)	☐	☐	☐	☐	☐

Student:

Clinical facilitator: Date:

CHAPTER 21

NEUROVASCULAR OBSERVATIONS

INDICATIONS

Neurovascular observations combine repeatedly assessing the peripheral pulse(s) and perfusion of the limbs and the neurological functioning of the limbs to detect pressure on the nerves or vascular supply. Neurovascular status is assessed to:

- obtain a baseline prior to surgery on a limb or phalange and to monitor after surgery (orthopaedic, vascular, spinal, plastic) and procedures that may cause thrombi (e.g. cardiac catheterisation). Make sure there is an assessable pulse in each limb; 12 to 17 per cent of people do not have an assessable dorsalis pedis pulse (Thunyacharoen et al., 2022) or have other injuries or conditions that alter perfusion, movement or sensation
- assess the status of the vasculature and nerve supply to a traumatised limb (fractures, crush injuries, envenomations, bites, soft tissue injuries, circumferential burns, infection, prolonged limb compression due to an altered level of consciousness), from treatment (casts, traction, restrictive dressing, tourniquet) or those with bleeding disorders.

Monitor this status over time so permanent damage or complications to the limb are avoided (Royal Children's Hospital Melbourne [RCHM], 2019).

The sequelae of neurovascular compromise include:

- permanent deficits or loss of function in the limb (paralysis)
- cardiac arrhythmias
- rhabdomyolysis
- amputation
- death.

Neurovascular observation helps to prevent these complications by identifying changes or problems early to enable early intervention. The major complication to the vessels and nerves in a limb is compartment syndrome. Compartment syndrome is an array of symptoms of muscle, nerve and bone ischaemia caused by pressure build-up in an enclosed space (e.g. within a fascial sheath, cast, bandage or eschar). Tissue perfusion is reduced to below what is needed for viability. The muscle and nerve tissues become ischaemic with irreparable damage within four hours if the pressure is not relieved. Compartment syndrome (of limbs) most commonly occurs in fractures of the tibial shaft when there is soft-tissue injury to the limb following high-energy trauma (Guo et al., 2019) in elbow/forearm fractures, and in males aged between 12 and 29 (Sonawane et al., 2022).

EVIDENCE OF THERAPEUTIC INTERACTION

Determine the person's level of understanding so they are not given information they already understand. Clearly explain the assessment and answer any questions to involve them as an active participant in their care. If they understand the rationale for the assessment and the changes to look for, they will be able to identify any deterioration and will know to alert you to early changes. Informing the person of repetitive assessments also reduces anxiety, as otherwise it can lead them to believe their condition is deteriorating.

DEMONSTRATE CLINICAL REASONING

Providing privacy to the person permits fuller disclosure of symptoms, fears and worries that they may be reluctant to make publicly. Privacy also reduces the embarrassment the person feels and supports their dignity when body areas may need to be exposed. Make sure there is good, consistent lighting to enable comparisons of colour or pallor.

Providing comfort measures and pain relief increases the person's physical comfort and also increases their trust and confidence in caregivers. Nursing interventions to minimise compromise to the peripheral circulation include supported elevation of the person's affected limb at the level of the heart. This enhances venous return and lymph drainage, decreasing peripheral oedema. An active (wriggling their fingers or toes regularly) or passive range of movements help reduce oedema and should be encouraged, unless contraindicated. Check that the person has not put their rings/watches back onto the affected limb, in case swelling occurs.

ELDER CARE

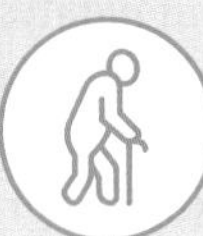

Soft tissue injury without fracture is common in older people, as is the need for anticoagulant medication. Both of these contribute to acute compartment syndrome. Be vigilant when assessing an older person because these conditions may not be recognised causes of this complication. Physiological vulnerability in the aged population means complications such as acute compartment syndrome become independent risk factors for mortality (Stonko et al., 2021).

THE PERSON LIVING WITH SEVERE OBESITY

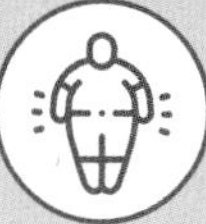

Severe obesity predisposes to and increases the risk of an individual to suffer knee dislocation with vascular injury, even with minimal trauma (e.g. tripping and falling to the ground) (Mirajkar et al., 2022). Although rare, acute compartment syndrome may develop in the popliteal space. Be vigilant with neurovascular observations if someone living with severe obesity is admitted with this diagnosis.

GATHER EQUIPMENT

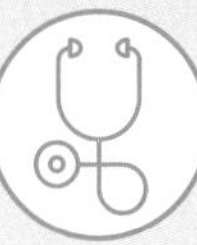

Gathering equipment is an organisational step that helps to create a positive environment for a successful interaction. In this case, you carry the essential tools with you – your observation skills. You will also need:

EQUIPMENT	EXPLANATION
Neurovascular assessment chart	• This is left at the bedside • Using the same chart over time aids in recognition of change despite different nurses conducting the individual assessments and promotes accurate inter-staff communication
Torch or portable light source	Ensure that light is consistent to determine skin colour
Indelible pen	This may be needed to mark position of pulses

If two or more limbs are involved, a neurovascular observation chart will be required for each limb. Ensure that each set of observations for each limb is recorded on the appropriate form.

CONDUCT A NEUROVASCULAR OBSERVATION

Hand hygiene

Hand hygiene (see **Clinical Skill 5**) removes microorganisms from your hands. It is the most effective preventative measure for cross-contamination, reducing incidences of nosocomial (i.e. hospital- or treatment-acquired) infection.

Assess the person

Safety

The aim of neurovascular observations is the early identification of decreased peripheral tissue perfusion, so that measures preventing compartment syndrome or providing prompt treatment of it can occur. Initial signs of compartment syndrome are subtle, and the warning signs are only elicited from a conscious person.

?

If a person is unconscious and unable to, or for any other reason cannot, communicate pain and paraesthesia, they need to be closely monitored (Hak, 2019). Watch for restlessness, diaphoresis, grimacing, moaning, guarding, tachycardia, tachypnoea and hypotension. Suspect a problem and actively look for it.

Neurovascular assessments are usually done from 15-minute intervals (e.g. cardiac catheterisation) to hourly (RCHM, 2019). The observations can be more frequent if you are concerned with the assessment. Hourly observations continue for up to 24 hours. If stable, the limbs are assessed every four hours for a further 48 hours. If not stable, they are continued every one to four hours, depending on severity, until they are stable. Compartment syndrome can occur within eight hours of injury/surgery (Sonawane et al., 2022). Hak (2019) found it could occur much later than immediately following the injury, especially in children – from two to 72 hours after injury.

If a person is in either skin or skeletal traction, after the initial 24 hours, neurovascular assessment is done one hour following washing and/or rebandaging of the limb(s). Occasionally, half-hourly observations are ordered if there is concern. When a plaster cast is replaced, an hourly observation for four hours is usually sufficient.

Assess the contralateral limb first to establish a 'normal' finding. Assess and compare the findings from the affected limb at the same assessment pulse point (Olinic et al., 2019) distal to the injury or site of injury/surgery to determine compromised vascular or neurological function. Nerve assessment includes checking for sensation and movement. Vascular assessment includes assessing for colour, temperature, capillary refill and pulses. The major peripheral pulse points are brachial, radial, ulnar, femoral, popliteal, posterior tibialis and dorsalis pedis.

A high level of suspicion is required – the physical signs and symptoms of compartment syndrome are late developments and often very subtle. Both limbs are assessed for the following indicators, often referred to as the '6 Ps' – pain, pallor, polar, pulses, paraesthesia, paralysis. Jakob, Benjamin and Demetriades (2023) add 'pressure' caused by oedema to this list. These authors state that 'pain out of proportion', paraesthesia and a tense compartment are the most common symptoms.

- *P = Pain level* – pain is caused by tissue ischaemia and is the most reliable and earliest of the symptoms. Ask the person about pain at the site of injury/surgery. Use a visual analogue scale or numerical rating scale for comparison and use a Faces scale for children (RCHM, 2019). Ask about pain on movement. Passively move the limb, fingers or toes and assess for pain (pain on passive stretch is an important indicator). Find out about location, radiation and characteristics. Compartment syndrome pain is typically a deep, burning ache (Sonawane, 2022). Moderate pain controllable with opioid analgesia is normal. However, intense pain disproportionate to the injury, unrelieved by repositioning, elevation or by opioid analgesic, and exacerbated by passive movement and elevation above heart level is a cardinal symptom of compartment syndrome (Ohns, Walsh & Douglas, 2019). A person with this intense pain, paraesthesia (see below) and paralysis of the limb requires intervention within four hours to prevent permanent damage. Immediately report severe or unrelieved pain to the shift coordinator and medical staff.
- *P = Paraesthesia* – a tingling, burning in the skin. Paraesthesia may occur earlier than the other signs and symptoms (Sonawane, 2022). Sensation is assessed in the distal digits. Ask the person about any alteration in sensation in the limb, such as numbness, pins and needles, pressure, tightness, tingling, burning or any other sensation. These are symptoms of nerve compression. Then ask them to close their eyes and identify touches (sharp – pen end; soft – cotton wisp) along different dermatomes. Diagrams of assessment sites are available on the reverse of most neurovascular assessment charts (see FIGURE 21.1). Make sure to thoroughly assess all dermatomes because different nerves pass through different compartments. Paraesthesia, initially affecting two-point discrimination (i.e. the person is unable to discriminate between two touches that are close together), is the earliest sign of neurological compromise. Be aware of lingering regional or spinal anaesthetic causing paraesthesia – check the anaesthetic record.

The other 'Ps' are both less reliable and occur later in the development of compartment syndrome; however, they become important if the person cannot report pain (Limbert & Santy-Tomlinson, 2017).

- *P = Pressure* – oedema causes tenseness (skin looks stretched, shiny and full) in the distal limb, and swelling may be visible. The tissue will feel firm. Agrawal et al. (2023) recommend measuring the limb circumference using a measuring tape (if possible – e.g. leave a tape measure within the splint) and comparing it with both the initial measurement and the unaffected limb to assess for pressure.
- *P = Pallor* – colour in both limbs should be a healthy, well-perfused pink in Caucasians. The palms, soles and nail beds of people with darker

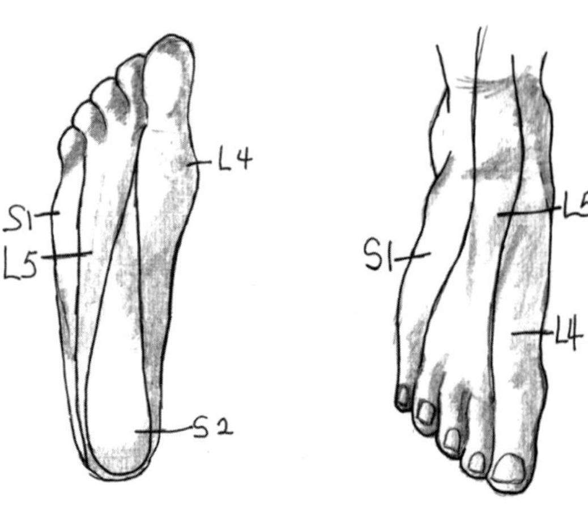

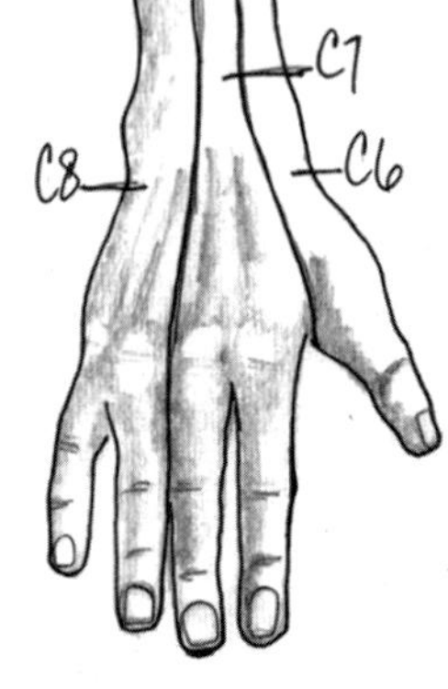

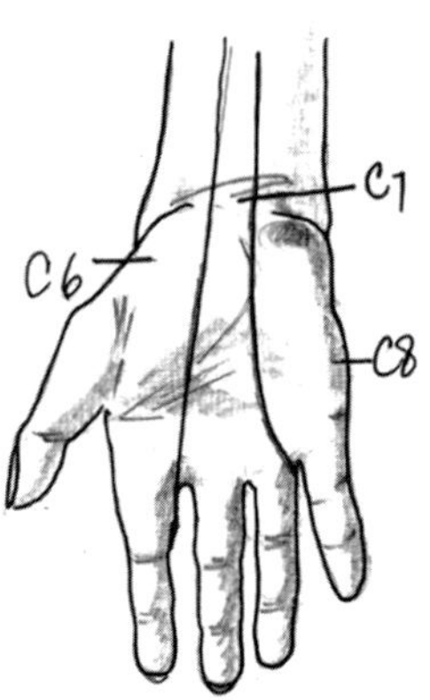

FIGURE 21.1 Assess each of the dermatome areas separately

skin are pink. Skin must be cleansed of blood, dirt and Betadine before you assess colour. Wear gloves to clean any blood to comply with standard precautions. Compartment syndrome usually causes pallor in arterial insufficiency or redness or cyanosis if there is venous compromise.

- *P = Polar* – the limb should be warm to the touch or of a similar temperature to the unaffected limb. Use the back of your hand to assess temperature. If compartment syndrome is occurring, the affected limb will most likely be cold to your touch and cooler than the other limb.
- *P = Pulses* – should be at the same rate as and volume of the same pulse point on the unaffected limb. Mark pulse points that are hard to find with an indelible pen to ensure consistency among staff or use a Doppler if the pulse is faint (Schreiber, 2016). Use a four-point scale where 3 is bounding, 2 is normal, 1 is weak and 0 is absent. If pulse points are inaccessible (e.g. under casts), assess the capillary refill on several digits (press on the digit for five seconds). Capillary refill should be less than two to three seconds. Pulses and capillary refill may be absent or may remain normal until very late in compartment syndrome.
- *P = Paralysis* – assess motor function. Ask the person to move their distal joints through a full range of motion; for example, plantar flex and extend the foot, dorsiflex the foot, spread the toes; or, dorsiflex and extend the hand, make an 'L' with thumb and first finger, touch the thumb and little finger together, make an OK sign with thumb and first finger, spread and stretch all the fingers wide. Movement may be restricted by a cast or splint. Muscle weakness or inability to flex or extend digits are late symptoms of compartment syndrome. Exceptions to assessing movement in the joints include anyone who has had microsurgery or repairs to tendons, arteries or nerves. Movement can cause sutures on these tissues to break free and retract damaged parts further into the tissues.

Blood loss must also be assessed. Check the dressing or cast over the injury/surgical site for visible ooze. Check under the cast – blood may have trickled down the limb and collected and oozed through the bottom of the cast or dressing. If a wound drainage system (e.g. Bellovac) is in situ, ensure it is patent and draining the anticipated amount for the surgery performed. Check that it is not clamped, and notify the shift coordinator if it is open but has no drainage. Check the puncture point of a cardiac catheterisation (usually the femoral artery). There should be no leakage.

> ?
> If you are caring for a child in a cast, assess them for 3 As – increased **A**nalgesic requirement (unremitting pain), **A**nxiety and **A**gitation (Ohns, Walsh & Douglas, 2019). Children who develop compartment syndrome present differently to adults and often do not demonstrate any of the signs other than pain. If you are suspicious, remove bandages or split the cast, leaving it in situ, and assess the limb for swelling. Notify the doctor urgently.

Responsibilities

It is your responsibility to immediately alert the shift coordinator if abnormal changes are noted. A colour-coded track and trigger observation sheet may be helpful. The registered nurse (RN) assesses the person and notifies the medical officer.

The extremity is kept at heart level (not elevated) and the person is given supplemental oxygen. Intravenous therapy is commenced to maintain hydration, reducing the effects of myoglobin released when skeletal muscle cells break down. Monitor the person for diminished urine output and dark, tea-coloured urine suggesting myoglobinuria; this can lead to the development of renal failure and should be reported to the shift coordinator and medical staff (Burgess, 2022). The neurovascular observations are increased to every 15 minutes.

Treatment for compartment syndrome is based on relieving the pressure within the enclosed space. Bandages are removed; casts need bivalving and spreading (but are left on), and the padding under the cast may need loosening or removal; splints are loosened and, if required, they are removed; drainage systems (Bellovacs) are checked to ensure they are patent and draining. The orthopaedic specialist will assess the limb and measure the intracompartment pressure directly. The person may be taken to theatre to have a fasciotomy performed (an incision through the fascia to relieve the pressure within the fascial compartment).

A delayed notification of compartment syndrome to the medical officer results in delayed treatment, which in turn can result in permanent muscle/nerve damage or even necrosis, which may then result in amputation (Sonawane, 2022).

DOCUMENTATION

Serial observations and documentation are vital to quickly identify deterioration and escalate care (Faraz et al., 2022). The observations are recorded on the neurovascular observation sheet. Neurovascular status is noted on the clinical notes once per shift. Any deterioration in neurovascular status and nursing interventions to address this are noted in the clinical notes.

PART 3

CLINICAL SKILLS ASSESSMENT

Neurovascular observations

Demonstrates the ability to assess the neurovascular status of a person. Incorporates the *National Safety and Quality Health Service Standards*: 2 Partnering with Consumers, 3 Preventing and Controlling Healthcare-Associated Infection, 5 Comprehensive Care, 6 Communicating for Safety, and 8 Recognising and Responding to Acute Deterioration (ACSQHC, 2021).

Performance criteria	1	2	3	4	5
(Numbers indicate NMBA *Registered Nurse Standards for Practice*)	(Dependent)	(Marginal)	(Assisted)	(Supervised)	(Independent)
1. Identifies indication (1.1, 3.3, 3.4)	☐	☐	☐	☐	☐
2. Evidence of therapeutic interaction with the person, e.g. gives the person a clear explanation of the procedure and answers questions appropriately (1.4, 1.5, 2.1, 2.2, 3.2)	☐	☐	☐	☐	☐
3. Demonstrates clinical reasoning abilities, e.g. provides privacy, comfort measures and pain relief as necessary; identifies early and late signs of compartment syndrome (1.1, 1.2, 1.3, 4.2, 6.1)	☐	☐	☐	☐	☐
4. Gathers equipment (1.1, 5.5, 6.1): ■ neurovascular assessment chart ■ torch	☐	☐	☐	☐	☐
5. Performs hand hygiene (1.1, 3.4, 6.1)	☐	☐	☐	☐	☐
6. Assesses the limb distal to the injury/surgery. Compares the affected limb with the unaffected limb. Assesses both limbs for the following: colour, oedema, temperature, pulses, sensation and motor function. Assesses the person's pain level and location (1.1, 4.1, 4.2, 4.3, 6.1)	☐	☐	☐	☐	☐
7. Outlines responsibilities (1.1, 6.1)	☐	☐	☐	☐	☐
8. Documents relevant information as appropriate (1.1, 1.4, 1.6, 2.2, 2.7, 3.5, 3.7, 6.1, 6.2, 6.5, 7.3)	☐	☐	☐	☐	☐
9. Demonstrates the ability to link theory to practice (1.1, 3.3, 3.4, 3.5)	☐	☐	☐	☐	☐

Student:

Clinical facilitator: Date:

CHAPTER 22

FOCUSED GASTROINTESTINAL HEALTH HISTORY AND ABDOMINAL PHYSICAL ASSESSMENT

INDICATIONS

Abdominal assessment is conducted in routine admission physical assessments to monitor a person's status following trauma, treatment or through a disease process, in order to respond appropriately to each individual's needs. Nurses inspect, auscultate, percuss and lightly palpate the abdomen to determine visible abnormalities, bowel sounds and softness/tenderness. (Note the altered order of assessment – palpation is undertaken last to prevent stimulating bowel activity.) Deep palpation to detect organomegaly and rebound tenderness is undertaken as indicated, usually by more experienced nurses.

EVIDENCE OF THERAPEUTIC INTERACTION

Explain the procedure to increase the person's compliance, to reduce their anxiety and to make the examination easier. Avoid stigmatising language (e.g. fat, skinny) (Dobbie et al., 2023) so that the person will feel more comfortable talking about their gastrointestinal (GI) problems. To prevent alarm, tell the person that you will listen in several places on their abdomen and for extended periods of time.

OBTAIN A GASTROINTESTINAL HISTORY

During the interview for the health history, the person can be in any position that is comfortable for them. Ensure privacy. Observe them for comfort, guarding and any indications of pain. A comprehensive abdominal health history usually assists in directing the physical assessment.

- Explore the chief complaint using questions about provoking and palliating factors, quality and quantity of the problem, region and radiation, setting and associated symptoms and timing of the complaint. The most common complaints are pain, nausea and vomiting, diarrhoea or constipation, increased eructation or flatulence, weight gain or loss, anorexia or dysphagia. Of particular importance is the location (and radiation) of pain, its characteristics (precipitating/palliating factors, onset, intensity, quality and duration), history of similar pain, fluctuations in the pain (and the worry it causes) and any associated symptoms. Reports of symptoms such as gastro-oesophageal reflux, eructation (burping) nausea, vomiting, diarrhoea, flatulence, changes to bowel motions (consistency, frequency) constipation, jaundice, melaena, weight loss and mucus or blood in the stool can help direct the physical assessment.
- Known medical conditions and previous abdominal surgeries are important. Abdomen-specific disorders (e.g. malignancies, Crohn's disease, gall stones or gastro-oesophageal reflux) or general history (e.g. allergies, diabetes mellitus, nutritional disorders and previous surgeries) can provide clues. Note communicable diseases like hepatitis and injuries.
- Many medications cause gastrointestinal (GI) upsets; for example, immunosuppressants can cause gastric erosion, and anticoagulants increase the chances of bleeding and haematoma formation. Ask specifically about over-the-counter medications (e.g. antacids, laxatives, stool softeners) and herbal preparation (e.g. ginger, peppermint), as many people do not consider these medications since they are not ordered by the physician.
- Social history, including alcohol, tobacco and illicit drug use, and travel, work and home environment, may have implications for GI problems. Alcohol intake can predispose some people to pancreatitis. Travellers may return home with a GI infection or parasite, and poor sanitation may lead to infections.
- Ask about diet and usual and current appetite. Assess nutritional status (poor nutrition is evident in either weight gain or loss, but it affects most of the body's systems – consult a health assessment text for further information). Ask about sleep difficulties (e.g. awakening at night with heartburn).
- Women of childbearing age should be asked about their menstrual cycle and pregnancy status.

ELDER CARE

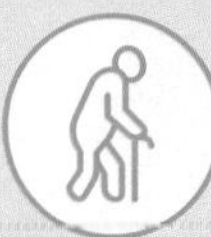

Be sure to ask about frequency and consistency of bowel movements, because constipation is one of the most common problems for the elderly (Roberts et al., 2019). You may be able to palpate a mass in the left lower quadrant if the person is constipated. Both obesity and underweight increase the risks of frailty in the aged population (Yuan, Chang & Wang, 2021), so be vigilant during the assessment for the signs of frailty (unintentional weight loss/sarcopenia, weakness, poor endurance/exhaustion, slowness in moving and a low physical activity level [Richter et al., 2022]). If frailty is suspected, document your findings and report them to senior healthcare professionals.

THE PERSON LIVING WITH SEVERE OBESITY

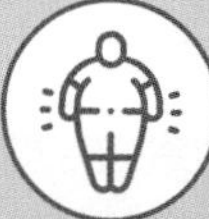

Take care to use destigmatising language (e.g. use 'extra weight' or 'adipose tissue' rather than 'fat'). During the history taking, ask about current and previous alcohol intake, acid reflux symptoms (burning sensation along the oesophageal track) and any right upper quadrant abdominal pain (which may indicate gallbladder/liver disease) (Dobbie et al., 2023).

Assess the bowel sounds, if possible. It may be very difficult to identify landmarks, and the bowel sounds will be muffled by the excess tissue. Monitor the frequency and characteristics of the stools. Faecal incontinence may occur due to the increased pressure of an enlarged abdomen on the bowel as well as decreased mobility. See **Clinical Skills 15 and 23** for more information on issues that people living with severe obesity encounter.

GATHER EQUIPMENT

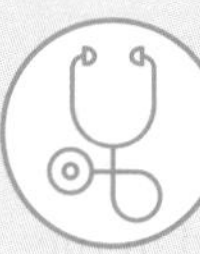

Gathering equipment is an organisational step that helps to create a positive environment for a successful interaction. It ensures that you have all needed material, boosts the person's confidence and trust in you, and increases your self-confidence. While gathering the equipment, you can mentally rehearse the procedure. Take the following to the bedside:

EQUIPMENT	EXPLANATION
Stethoscope	• Diaphragm side (flat surface) down, held firmly, is best to hear high-pitched sounds, such as the bowel sounds • The bell, held lightly on the skin, is best to listen for bruits over arteries
Bath blanket (or similar)	• Maintains warmth, privacy and dignity during the assessment

DEMONSTRATE CLINICAL REASONING

Positioning, privacy, warmth and being able to find landmarks will assist you to gain the most information about the GI system with the least discomfort for the person.

Position the person

Assist the person into a supine position so the abdominal structures are easily accessible to inspect, auscultate, percuss and palpate. The supine position with the head supported on a flat pillow is generally comfortable and the abdominal musculature is relaxed. Placing a small pillow under the person's knees helps relax the abdominal muscles. The person may keep their arms loosely at their sides or with their hands folded up on their chest.

Provide privacy, warmth and comfort

Ask (or assist) the person to empty their bladder before the assessment. It is very uncomfortable to have one's lower abdomen palpated when the bladder is full.

Privacy is essential to the person's feelings of self-worth. Close the door and the curtain. Put up a 'Do not disturb' sign. Remove the person's clothing from above the costal margin to the level of the symphysis pubis. Drape well to reduce embarrassment.

Warmth is essential. The person will experience heat loss from radiation, evaporation and convection when a large surface area is exposed. Ask or assist the person to reposition or remove their clothing or bedding to the level of the symphysis pubis. Inspection requires full exposure. Sounds are masked or altered if the stethoscope is used over clothing. Cover the person's torso with a drape or bath blanket to provide warmth and reduce exposure.

Warm your hands and the stethoscope if they are cold.

Identify landmarks

Identify each of the four anterior quadrants on the bared abdomen by mentally dividing it into four, using the umbilicus as the centre point. It is easier for you to identify both normal and abnormal findings if you can visualise the organs (study your anatomy texts) underlying the abdominal muscles and skin. There are more methods of dividing the abdomen for examination. This is the simplest and is very useful, until you need more precise descriptions (e.g. working in a gastrointestinal surgery unit).

Conduct the abdominal physical assessment

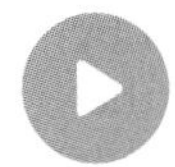

After you have obtained the GI health history, you are ready to assess the abdomen, using inspection, auscultation, percussion and palpation.

Hand hygiene

Hand hygiene (see **Clinical Skill 5**) removes microorganisms from your hands. It is the most effective preventative measure for cross-contamination, reducing incidences of nosocomial (i.e. hospital- or treatment-acquired) infection.

Inspect the abdomen

Good lighting is necessary to see subtle changes. Identify landmarks such as the umbilicus, the symphysis pubis and the xiphoid process of the sternum. Mentally divide the abdomen into quarters. Inspect from the rib margin to the symphysis pubis. Look at the general contour and symmetry of the abdomen (Estes et al., 2020):

- Is it concave or convex? Normally, the contour is flat or rounded and bilaterally symmetrical.
- Is it smooth or are there protrusions or distension (i.e. is the abdominal skin taut and displaced outward)?
- Are the abdominal muscles relaxed or can you see their outlines? Ask the person to raise their head – does the muscle contour change? (Hernias and muscle separation will become apparent.) Can they lie flat? Note scars, bruises, altered colour, lesions, rashes, hair distribution, striae or fine veins. If there are scars, ask about the cause (if the person has not mentioned abdominal surgery before). If female, is there a linea nigra? Observe abdominal movement during respiration. Normally, it rises with inhalation and falls with exhalation.
- Can you see the bowel activity (peristalsis) in a slender person? Visible peristalsis slowly traverses the abdomen in a downward-slanting movement. Is there a pulsation near the xiphoid sternum? Abdominal aorta pulsations are visible in many slim people.
- Observe the umbilicus for abnormalities (colour, contour, discharge, protuberance) – it is usually midline, depressed beneath the abdominal surface (an 'innie'). 'Outies' are also normal, but not so common. They are very small stable hernias and protrude up to 2 cm above the abdominal surface (Reinhorn, 2020). A larger protrusion or one that occurs when the person performs the Valsalva manoeuvre is not normal, and needs to be reported.

Auscultate the abdominal quadrants

Ask the person not to talk during this part of the assessment, as quiet is required to hear many of the faint sounds in the abdomen. Watch the person's face while auscultating, percussing and palpating to detect discomfort. Auscultate quadrants in sequence, for several minutes if necessary. Do this systematically, first listening with the diaphragm of the stethoscope to the right lower quadrant (RLQ), right upper quadrant (RUQ), left upper quadrant (LUQ) and left lower quadrant (LLQ). This follows the anatomical lie of the large intestine and reduces the possibility of missing a quadrant. Listen over the ileocaecal valve. Bowel sounds should be audible. Familiarity with the frequency, pitch and intensity of the normal bowel sounds enables you to recognise abnormal sounds. Listen to each quadrant for a full minute to recognise the character and frequency of the bowel sounds (high-pitched gurgles, clicks and other soft sounds occurring from five to 30 times per minute). Borborygmi are hyperactive loud bowel sounds (stomach growls) due to hyperactive peristalsis or flatus in the intestines. They are normal (Estes et al., 2020). If bowel sounds are not heard immediately, continue to listen for up to five minutes before deciding that they are absent. When you identify absence of bowel sounds or abnormal sounds, inform a more experienced nurse or physician.

Use the bell of your stethoscope to listen for vascular bruits (low-pitched murmuring sounds) in the epigastric region (aorta, renal arteries) and the lower quadrants (femoral arteries). Vascular sounds are generally abnormal and need to be reported.

Percuss the abdomen

Percuss all four quadrants in a systematic fashion (see **FIGURE 22.1**).

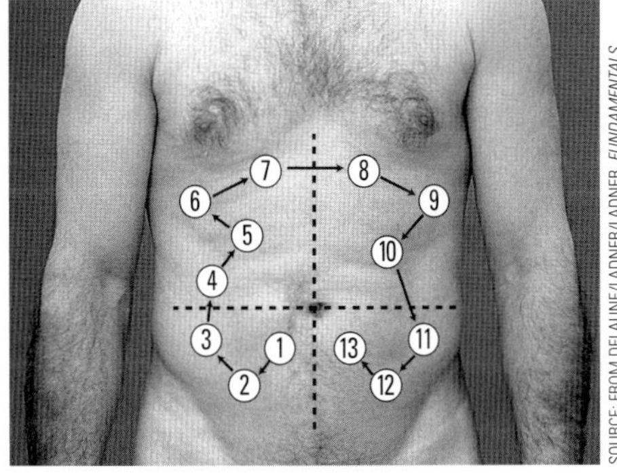

FIGURE 22.1 Directional pattern of abdominal percussion

Generally, you begin percussion in the RLQ (again, following the anatomical lie of the large intestine), move up to the RUQ, cross over to the LUQ, and move down to the LLQ. If the person has pain in any quadrant, leave that one until the end of your percussion. Listen for tympany (a musical drum-like sound heard over hollow organs) over the stomach and intestines because of the gases in these organs. Dullness (a flat, muffled thudding sound) is normally heard over solid organs (e.g. the liver, the spleen or a full bladder). Percussion is useful to distinguish between gas and fluid in the abdominal organs.

Palpate the abdomen

Use light palpation to determine any areas of tenderness, abnormal masses or distension. Note the texture and consistency of underlying tissues. Use the palmar surface of your straight fingers held horizontal to the abdomen to gently palpate (indenting the surface by 2 cm) the abdomen through all four quadrants (see FIGURE 22.1). Never palpate over areas where bruits were auscultated.

> If light palpation elicits a tickling response, then ask the person to put their hand on their abdomen, and palpate through their hand, slowly moving your hand off theirs until you are able to palpate without their hand under yours.

If the person has pain (ask them to cough, which elicits abdominal pain), commence palpation in the quadrant furthest away from the pain. If tenderness is found, palpate that area last.

Deep palpation is only possible when the person is relaxed. It is a skill requiring experience and advanced training. With deep palpation, the examining hand is pressed from 2.5 to 6 cm into the abdomen, to feel the deeper structures and to determine size and consistency of any masses found. With direct supervision, you may be guided to palpate for the edge of the liver and for rebound tenderness by a more experienced healthcare professional.

The liver's lower edge can be felt (usually if it is enlarged, but some normal livers have a palpable edge) by using deep palpation. With the fingers of the right hand on the person's RUQ just below their costal margin, palpate deeply. Ask them to take a deep breath, which pushes the liver against your hand. You might need to support their back with your left hand, lifting under the RUQ (posterior) to bring the liver closer to your examining hand. Normal livers are non-tender, feel solid and have a regular and sharp lower edge. Determine the upper edge of the liver by percussing the right midclavicular line (MCL) of the chest downwards until the lung's resonant sound gives way to the liver's dull sound.

Rebound tenderness indicates an inflamed peritoneum. Press slowly and deeply into the painful area, then quickly withdraw your hand. Increased pain means the test is positive.

Post-procedure

Assist the person into a comfortable position and adjust their clothing to complete the procedure. The most comfortable positions for individuals with abdominal pain are side-lying or semi-Fowler's position with knees elevated. Replace any personal items and ensure the call bell is within reach.

CLEAN, REPLACE AND DISPOSE OF EQUIPMENT

Wipe the bell and diaphragm of personal stethoscopes with an alcowipe. Unit stethoscopes should also have the earpieces wiped with alcowipes and be returned to the appropriate storage area.

DOCUMENTATION

Document the abdominal assessment in the progress notes. Note the presence of pain, softness or rigidity of the abdomen, bowel sounds (absent, present, active or hyperactive) and any abnormalities detected during the assessment.

CLINICAL SKILLS ASSESSMENT

Focused gastrointestinal health history and abdominal physical assessment

Demonstrates the ability to assess the abdomen. Incorporates the *National Safety and Quality Health Service Standards*: 2 Partnering with Consumers, 3 Preventing and Controlling Healthcare-Associated Infection, 5 Comprehensive Care, 6 Communicating for Safety, and 8 Recognising and Responding to Acute Deterioration (ACSQHC, 2021).

Performance criteria	1	2	3	4	5
(Numbers indicate NMBA *Registered Nurse Standards for Practice*)	(Dependent)	(Marginal)	(Assisted)	(Supervised)	(Independent)
1. Identifies indication (1.1, 3.3, 3.4)	☐	☐	☐	☐	☐
2. Evidence of therapeutic interaction with the person, e.g. gives a clear explanation of the procedure (1.4, 1.5, 2.1, 2.2, 3.2)	☐	☐	☐	☐	☐
3. Demonstrates clinical reasoning abilities, e.g. positions the person supine, provides privacy, comfort measures, analgesia if needed and warmth (1.1, 1.2, 1.3, 3.2, 4.2, 6.1)	☐	☐	☐	☐	☐
4. Gathers equipment (5.5, 6.1): ■ stethoscope ■ bath blanket	☐	☐	☐	☐	☐
5. Performs hand hygiene (1.1, 3.4, 6.1)	☐	☐	☐	☐	☐
6. Takes a gastrointestinal history (2.1, 2.2, 3.4, 4.1, 4.2, 4.3)	☐	☐	☐	☐	☐
7. Inspects the abdomen (3.2, 4.2, 6.1)	☐	☐	☐	☐	☐
8. Auscultates the abdominal quadrants (3.2, 4.2, 6.1)	☐	☐	☐	☐	☐
9. Percusses and palpates the abdomen (3.2, 4.2, 6.1)	☐	☐	☐	☐	☐
10. Assists the person to a position of comfort (3.2, 4.2, 6.1)	☐	☐	☐	☐	☐
11. Cleans, replaces and disposes of equipment appropriately (3.4, 3.6, 6.1)	☐	☐	☐	☐	☐
12. Documents relevant information (1.4, 1.6, 2.2, 2.7, 3.5, 3.7, 6.2, 6.5, 7.3)	☐	☐	☐	☐	☐
13. Demonstrates the ability to link theory to practice (1.1, 3.3, 3.4, 3.5)	☐	☐	☐	☐	☐

Student:

Clinical facilitator: Date:

CHAPTER 23

HEIGHT, WEIGHT AND WAIST CIRCUMFERENCE MEASUREMENTS

INDICATIONS

Height, weight and waist circumference measurements are integral to the initial assessment of any person entering the healthcare system. They give a baseline for:

- monitoring the individual's hydration and nutritional status
- determining alterations during care and treatment
- assessing cardiometabolic risk
- providing essential information for the physician to use when prescribing medications and intravenous fluids.

They also provide information for selecting supportive equipment, such as pressure-relieving devices, chairs and so on (National Nurses Nutrition Group, 2017). People at risk for nutritional deficiency (e.g. those with cancer, dementia, chronic pulmonary diseases) require regular weight assessment during hospitalisation to assess their nutritional status (Estes et al., 2020). In children, height and weight are used to determine physical development and provide a basis for determining medication dosages.

One measure of nutritional status and cardiometabolic risk is the body mass index (BMI). It is an approximate measure of body fat and an effective measure for risk in population wide obesity, but limited in its use on an individual level since it varies with age, ethnicity, body frame and muscle mass (Laine & Wee, 2023).

Waist circumference measurement is another method of determining cardiometabolic risk, with a larger waist circumference indicating a greater risk (Australian Institute of Health and Welfare [AIHW], 2019). The waist measurement indicates the level of internal fat deposited around the heart, kidneys, liver, digestive organs and pancreas. These fat deposits can increase the risk of heart disease and stroke (Heart Foundation, n.d.).

The waist to height ratio, in addition to the BMI, helps to estimate central adiposity and therefore health risks more effectively than waist circumference or BMI alone (Dobbie, 2023; Rahimi et al., 2022; Zoler, 2023).

More information on assessing nutritional status, the BMI and other cardiometabolic risk factors will be found in your medical-surgical texts. Paediatric texts should be consulted for discussions of height and weight in children.

ELDER CARE

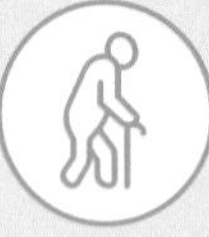

Although older people have a decreased need for kilojoules, poor nutrition is commonly found in elderly people for a number of reasons:

- functional – inability to obtain or prepare food
- social – grieving, isolation, reluctance to eat by themselves
- economic – inability to afford food
- physiological – inability to chew, taste, swallow or digest their food, illness, low mood.

Assessment of the nutritional status using a validated assessment tool (as used in the facility) is important. Assess also for sarcopenia (loss of muscle mass and strength) and frailty (a syndrome characterised by a decline of physical and cognitive reserves that leads to increased vulnerability, morbidity and mortality [Health Victoria, 2021]).

EVIDENCE OF THERAPEUTIC INTERACTION

Explain to the person the reason for the procedure and what it entails. Many people are embarrassed about their height or weight, so remain non-judgemental and do not comment on the findings unless the person asks about it. If they do ask, answer in a matter-of-fact tone and use neutral words, but be honest with them. Waist circumference measurement may be a new assessment to many people. Discuss the use of waist circumference measurement in relation to their cardiometabolic risk assessment.

DEMONSTRATE CLINICAL REASONING

THE PERSON LIVING WITH SEVERE OBESITY

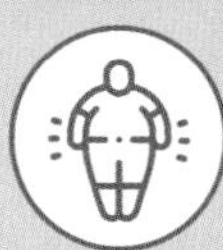

'Obesity is a disease you wear' (Dr Fatima Stanford, cited in Shear, 2023).

People who are severely obese, and whose obesity interferes with their normal body functions (National Center for Chronic Disease Prevention and Health Promotion, 2020) and impairs health, have functional, social and health issues that interfere with their lives. Severely obese people have in excess of 100 kg of body weight over the ideal for their height, or a BMI of 40 or more (see the explanation of BMI on page 129). Obesity is a chronic disease that is prevalent, complex, progressive and relapsing. There is substantial bias, even from healthcare professionals. People living with obesity are burdened with fat stigma, which influences both their experience of the disease and their life expectancy, independent of their weight or BMI. Internalisation of the weight bias experienced over a long period impairs both the individual's quality of life and their medical care (Nadolsky et al., 2023). Using sensitivity and a consultative approach can gain more information and assist the person to adhere to treatment programs (Dobbie et al., 2023). Weight loss alone is not effective, and the epidemiology, determinants, pathophysiology, assessment, prevention and treatment of obesity demonstrate that obesity management should focus on person-centred health improvement. Evidence-based principles of chronic disease management, validation of the person's experiences and access to evidence-informed interventions, including medical nutrition therapy, physical activity, psychological interventions, pharmacotherapy and surgery, are ideally employed in the care of the person living with obesity (Wharton et al., 2020).

People living with severe obesity have many additional difficulties during the processes of health care in addition to the health problem that brought them to a clinic or hospital. The excess weight adds burdens to many of the organ systems as well as an increased risk of psychological morbidity to the individual, making it imperative for nurses to be aware of the specialised care required during nearly any encounter. Bariatric surgery (e.g. gastric banding, stapling) is only done after the person has unsuccessfully undergone a supervised weight management program for several years. Therefore, you may need to care for a severely obese person on any hospital unit or in the community.

Caring for a person living with severe obesity can cause injuries to nurses and other healthcare staff, so learning about the specialised care of these people is imperative.

Severe obesity impacts negatively on all body systems. Even being overweight can hamper the ability to control or manage chronic disorders, and people who are overweight or obese have higher rates of death (AIHW, 2019). People have difficulties with ventilation (excess abdominal tissue interferes with breathing, can crush alveoli), an inhibition of muscle use of glucose (leading to greater fat deposits, muscle weakness), and impaired perfusion (cardiac, skin, vital organs). Severe obesity is a chronic disease with a high incidence of associated conditions, including hypertension, type 2 diabetes, obstructive sleep apnoea, stroke, cardiovascular disease and some cancers (Hohol, Gilbert & Johnston, 2019). Some additional common health problems encountered by the severely obese person are joint degeneration and pain, asthma, acid reflux and depression, low self-esteem and distorted body image. People with severe obesity are likely to endure longer hospitalisation, feelings of shame, guilt and stigmatisation, relative immobility and polypharmacy as well as the current condition reducing their quality of life.

A severely obese person is too heavy to use the mainstream hospital equipment such as beds, scales, trolleys, lifting equipment, chairs or walkers safely. When someone is admitted to a unit for care, every piece of equipment that might be used while caring for them has to be vetted for their weight. Most facilities will have specific equipment available, although it may need to be ordered and brought to the unit from a storage area or shared between units. There will be lifting protocols that outline the minimum number of staff needed to assist with any lift or movement (e.g. turning over, moving up in bed, moving from a lying to a sitting position). Often, the person cannot assist and may become panic-stricken if moves are not well explained and coordinated. They will be cared for in a private room because there is more space for equipment and for extra personnel. Keep in mind that hospital gowns and thromboembolism deterrent (TED) stockings will need to be especially ordered from stores for the severely obese person.

A severely obese person will need assistance to turn, get out of bed, mobilise, go to the toilet (often requiring incontinence [bariatric briefs] assistance), dress and undertake personal hygiene. Several nurses may be needed to provide the level of assistance required. Techniques for moving the severely obese individual involve specialised lifts and hoists that are engineered to take the additional weight. Often, the person cannot move their limbs freely and/or with the body; nursing staff need to be aware and take precautions to keep the body aligned. When the person is transferring to another unit (e.g. X-ray), they may need to be taken on their extra large bed and someone will need to 'scout' the path to ensure there is no equipment in the hallways, that the elevator is large enough for the person and their bed, that there is sufficient room to manoeuvre around corners and through doorways.

The person will be on a supervised weight loss program, although, if acutely ill, Starr et al. (2016) suggest that restricting calories in the older adult does not improve morbidity. Agarwal et al. (2019) demonstrated that, although malnourished obese people in hospital had significantly more morbidity than normal weight people, they were less likely to receive additional and appropriate nutritional support to enhance healing. The severely obese person facing surgery will need to undergo more testing than someone of normal weight (e.g. lung function studies, metabolic screening) and is at greater risk post-surgically for many complications, including respiratory infections, deep vein thrombosis and urinary tract infections. Their skin is under constant pressure and pressure injuries are quick to form (see **Clinical Skill 59**). As well, intertrigo (rash, then excoriation in skin folds in perineal area, between buttocks, under breast tissue, under the abdominal 'apron' and in the axilla as well as in unusual places, such as above the elbows or knees) can easily occur due to the large skin folds, moisture from increased perspiration, friction and decreased ventilation in these areas (Hohol, Gilbert & Johnston, 2019).

The most valuable nursing tool you have is a non-judgemental attitude towards the individual. Many of us are not comfortable working with and speaking to severely obese people because we do not want to offend or hurt them by talking about or referring to their weight. This attitude has a downside – the person will not feel comfortable raising any obesity-related concerns. As well, our own mainstream socialisation has moulded us to treat obese people differently and it has been found that most instances of 'seepage of negative feelings' (derogatory remarks) towards obesity were not directed at the person but were shared among the staff (e.g. in the operating theatre) out of the hearing of the obese individual (Burdette et al., 2023). Implicit weight bias impacts the professional relationship with the person living with obesity, reducing engagement, discouraging health-seeking behaviours and fostering poorer health outcomes (Abbott et al., 2023). Often the obese person, in order to avoid humiliation and reduce social awkwardness, enters into a more comfortable 'mutual pretence' with the staff where the obesity is not mentioned.

Societal stereotypes and causal attributions (e.g. laziness, gluttony) promote personal blame for obesity. Such assumptions disregard and oversimplify decades of substantial, sound science demonstrating the complexities of body weight regulation, including biological and genetic mechanisms that promote weight gain, social factors, economic factors and obesity-promoting environments. Our genetically determined physiology has not evolved to deal with our current lifestyles, diets and obesity's numerous associated maladaptations, such as massive adipocyte hypertrophy (excess quantity and dysfunction of white adipose tissue, particularly visceral adipose depots) (Valenzuela et al., 2023). Towell-Barnard (2019) adds the effects of childhood abuse and neglect and other mental health issues as contributing to people developing excess weight problems.

Healthcare professionals often exacerbate the problems by victim blaming and disrespecting individuals, thus causing increased vulnerability and feelings of inadequacy (which lead to excess intake). We need to consciously address our personal views about fat stigma and develop more appropriate professional practices to deliver excellent care.

GATHER EQUIPMENT

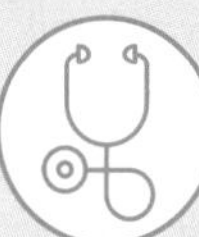

Gathering equipment ensures that you have all needed material, boosts the person's confidence and trust in you, and increases your self-confidence. Equipment required for measurement of height, weight and waist circumference includes:

EQUIPMENT	EXPLANATION
Height	
Stadiometer	This is the bar and level attached to the floor scales. If not available, substitute a piece of paper taped to the lintel of a door at about the person's head height, a marker pen, straight edge and a tape measure
Tape measure	This is used as an alternative method of measuring height for a person who is bed- or chairbound
Weight	
Scales	*Floor scales* • Usually located in a convenient spot on the unit (or physician's surgery) and the person is brought to the scale • Needs to be calibrated each time it is used *Portable scales* • Can be carried into the person's room, similar to domestic bathroom scales, and are often used for convenience • Place on a hard surface (not carpet) to ensure accuracy *Chair or lift scales* • Can be used for anyone unable to stand • Some manual lifts now have attachments that can measure the person's weight while they are being lifted into or out of a bed or chair
	Bed scales • Weighs a person who cannot sit or stand • The person needs to be lifted onto the bed scale and back into their bed afterwards • Some specialised care beds have built-in scales so weight can be measured at any time and fluctuations noted
Paper towel or waterproof pad	• *Paper towel* can be placed on the platform of the scales • *Waterproof pad* can be placed on the seat of the chair scales
Waist circumference	
Tape measure	• Used to determine the circumference of the waist and hip • Must be made of non-stretch material
Water-soluble marker	• Used to mark the level of the waist/hip in order to place the tape

CONDUCT A HEIGHT, WEIGHT AND WAIST CIRCUMFERENCE ASSESSMENT

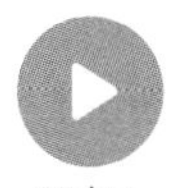

Hand hygiene

Hand hygiene (see **Clinical Skill 5**) removes microorganisms from your hands. It is the most effective preventative measure for cross-contamination, reducing incidences of nosocomial (i.e. hospital- or treatment-acquired) infection.

Measure weight

Most people, if asked, underestimate their weight (Wilson et al., 2019). Weight assessment begins by calibrating the scales. For most scales, this simply means setting the balance arm or indicator reading to '0' before the person steps onto the scales platform. The person should be naked or lightly clad. If the weight measurement is a serial one (e.g. daily or weekly weights), the person should be wearing the same type of clothes, such as a hospital gown, and the weight obtained at the same time of day as previous readings. Before weighing, ask the person to use the toilet.

Place a paper towel on the platform of the scales or a waterproof pad on the seat of the chair scales (remember to use a similar pad every time if the reading is a serial one). Help the person as needed to stand on the scales facing the balance arm or to sit on the chair scales. Once the person is stable on the scales, settled and still, adjust the arm until balanced. Read the weight to the nearest 100 g (Estes et al., 2020). Record it on the care plan (along with the clothes worn and the time of day), the vital signs sheet and sometimes on the medication administration sheet.

Lift (or hoist) scales only need be turned on and the recording read when the digital mechanism signals; bed scales are similar. Assist the person onto and off the scales and help them to return to their bed or previous activity. Clean the scales surfaces following the hygiene protocols of the facility.

Measure height

Most people, if asked, overestimate their height (Wilson et al., 2019). Ask the person to remove their shoes. While they are doing this, raise the level measurement bar well above the estimated height of the person. Place a paper towel on the platform of the scales. Help them to stand on the platform. Then ask them to stand straight with their back and buttocks against the measuring stick, and with their heels together and against the bar. They should be looking straight ahead with their head level. You then lower the level bar until it is resting on top of their head (make sure the level is on the head, not resting on raised hair). Read the measurement to (usually) the nearest centimetre.

If you are too short to read the measurement at eye level, you will need to stand on a stool so you can read the measurement accurately.

The height of someone unable to stand is obtained using a non-stretch but pliable measuring tape to measure the body from heel to knee, knee to hip, hip to shoulder, and shoulder to top of head. The measurements added give the height of the person (Cirillo et al., 2018), although Lima et al. (2018) warn that the accuracy of this method depends on the age and race of the individual. Take care when measuring someone with contractures, large fat deposits on their back, scoliosis, arthritis or pulmonary disease, because these will distort the measurements, especially the hip-to-shoulder measurement. For those who are bed-bound, the demi-span (mid-sternal notch to the web between the middle and ring fingers along an outstretched arm) measurement, although requiring a formula to calculate, is the closest approximation to measured standing height. However, Silva and Figuera (2017) found estimations of height from various non-standing measurements to be inaccurate for use in calculating BMI.

Height assessment of children and babies is similar, using a stadiometer for children who are walking/standing and a tape measure for babies. Refer to a paediatric textbook for more on this skill.

BMI

The BMI formula divides the weight (kg) of the person by the square of their height (m) (i.e. kg/m^2). Someone who is 1.74 m tall and weighing 86 kg would have a BMI of (86/1.742) = 27, which is overweight. The categories are:

- under 20: underweight
- 20–24.9: ideal weight
- 25–29.9: overweight
- 30–39.9: obese
- 40+: severely obese.

BMI conversion charts are available and convenient.

Measure waist circumference

Ask the person to stand with their feet at shoulder width and their arms crossed over their chest with their midriff and abdominal region bare. Palpate the top of the iliac crest and the lower rib and mark the midway point between them (Heart Foundation, n.d.). For use with BMI for calculating cardiometabolic risk, these authors found measuring the waist circumference just below the lowest rib to be easier to use and the better method.

Encircle the abdomen with the tape. Place the bottom edge of the tape on the mark. Straighten the tape so it is in line with the mark. Gently tighten the tape, ensuring that the skin is not depressed. Ask the person to breathe normally and, at the end of a normal expiration, measure from the '0' line on the tape to the nearest millimetre.

Abdominal girth is obtained for some medical conditions (e.g. ascites). It is serial and usually frequent (daily). The person lies supine and their widest abdominal measurement is determined using a tape measure. That point is marked with an *indelible* marker. The mark is used in subsequent measurements to determine the effectiveness of treatment.

Measure hip circumference

Ask the person to stand with their feet together and their arms crossed over their chest with their hip region bare or lightly (underwear) clad. Place the measuring tape (level with the floor) snugly around the largest circumference of the hips and buttocks. Do not twist or pull the tape tight. Note the measure in centimetres and millimetres.

Waist to hip ratio

Divide the waist measurement by the hip measurement to obtain the waist to hip ratio (WHR). Males who are of a healthy body composition have a WHR or 0.9 or less and females have a WHR of 0.85 or less.

CLEAN, REPLACE AND DISPOSE OF EQUIPMENT

Remove and dispose of the paper towel or waterproof pad into the normal waste bin. Disinfect the scales platform if you have forgotten to use one of these. Wipe the tape measure if it is soiled. Some facilities have disposable tape measures. If so, they are placed in the normal waste if they are not contaminated with body fluids.

DOCUMENTATION

Height, weight and waist circumference and waist to hip ratio (if done) are to be noted on the admission notes and the vital signs sheet. There may also be a notation in the care plan. Report any abnormal or unusual changes and trends in weight gain or loss to senior staff.

CLINICAL SKILLS ASSESSMENT

Height, weight and waist circumference measurements

Demonstrates the ability to effectively measure height, weight and waist circumference. Incorporates the *National Safety and Quality Health Service Standards*: 2 Partnering with Consumers, 3 Preventing and Controlling Healthcare-Associated Infection, 5 Comprehensive Care, 6 Communicating for Safety, and 8 Recognising and Responding to Acute Deterioration (ACSQHC, 2021).

Performance criteria	1	2	3	4	5
(Numbers indicate NMBA *Registered Nurse Standards for Practice*)	(Dependent)	(Marginal)	(Assisted)	(Supervised)	(Independent)
1. Identifies indication (1.1, 3.3, 3.4)	☐	☐	☐	☐	☐
2. Evidence of therapeutic interaction with the person, e.g. gives the person a clear explanation of the procedure (1.4, 1.5, 2.1, 2.2, 3.2)	☐	☐	☐	☐	☐
3. Demonstrates clinical reasoning, e.g. understands how to care for a severely obese person, including use of special equipment, when assistance of colleagues is required and what the unit protocols for care are, and employs a non-judgemental attitude (1.1, 1.2, 1.3, 3.2, 4.2, 6.1)	☐	☐	☐	☐	☐
4. Gathers equipment (1.1, 5.5, 6.1): ■ stadiometer ■ tape measure ■ scales ■ paper towel or waterproof pad ■ water-soluble marker	☐	☐	☐	☐	☐
5. Performs hand hygiene (1.1, 3.4, 6.1)	☐	☐	☐	☐	☐
6. Prepares the scales and the stadiometer (1.1, 6.1)	☐	☐	☐	☐	☐
7. Measures the weight (1.1, 4.1, 4.2, 6.1)	☐	☐	☐	☐	☐
8. Measures the height (1.1, 4.1, 4.2, 6.1)	☐	☐	☐	☐	☐
9. Measures the waist circumference (1.1, 4.1, 4.2, 6.1)	☐	☐	☐	☐	☐
10. Cleans, replaces and disposes of equipment appropriately (3.6, 6.1)	☐	☐	☐	☐	☐
11. Documents relevant information (1.1, 1.4, 1.6, 2.2, 2.7, 3.5, 3.7, 6.1, 6.2, 6.5, 7.3)	☐	☐	☐	☐	☐
12. Demonstrates the ability to link theory to practice (1.1, 3.3, 3.4, 3.5)	☐	☐	☐	☐	☐

Student:

Clinical facilitator: Date:

CHAPTER 24

FOCUSED MUSCULOSKELETAL HEALTH HISTORY AND PHYSICAL ASSESSMENT AND RANGE OF MOTION EXERCISES

INDICATIONS

Musculoskeletal assessment
Musculoskeletal assessment is undertaken whenever a person seeks health care. Often, you do this unconsciously. Whenever the person has a visible musculoskeletal problem or complaint of discomfort, tingling or paraesthesia in an area, a formal musculoskeletal assessment needs to be done. To complete a thorough nursing assessment, you will need to inspect and palpate muscles and joints, assess the range of motion (ROM) of each joint, and document your findings. Musculoskeletal assessment assists you to determine the person's position on the dependence/independence continuum and how much assistance they will require. It allows you to identify current and future needs (Toney-Butler & Unison-Pace, 2019) and potential risks.

Range of motion exercises
Inactive people do not move their joints through the entire ROM because of reduced activity. Impaired physical mobility may be due to unconsciousness, a stroke or paralysis, postoperative discomfort (or limitations due to such things as mastectomy, drains), brain damage or pain. Over time, the range of joint movements reduces due to a shortening of ligaments and tendons. The result is a non-functional joint and eventually a contracture of that joint. Knowledge of the diagnosis helps to determine the exercises needed and those that are contraindicated. Regularly exercising the joints prevents spasticity, muscle wasting and contracture development.

EVIDENCE OF THERAPEUTIC INTERACTION

Introduce yourself and give the person a clear explanation of the musculoskeletal assessment, the ROM exercises and the reasons for undertaking them. This will gain the person's consent and cooperation and alleviate their anxiety.

DEMONSTRATE CLINICAL REASONING

ELDER CARE

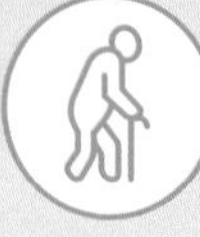

Osteoarthritis, osteoporosis and osteopenia are all commonly found in the elderly. Ask about independent functioning and falls and quality of life. Sarcopenia (the accelerated loss of muscle mass, and thus function, often associated with ageing) results in increased numbers of falls, functional decline and frailty (Dobbie et al., 2023).

THE PERSON LIVING WITH SEVERE OBESITY

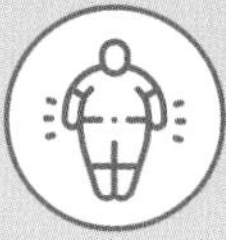

For anyone living with severe obesity, you will need to assess the their ability to move. Many severely obese people sit in an upright position in order to breathe more effectively. They often have a very low activity tolerance and can move only short distances before tiring. Both assessment and ROM exercises may need to be done over an extended period to allow for rest periods. Disuse of muscles can produce atrophy and muscle weakness, and bones may become decalcified due to immobility. Joints are prone to deformity, immobility, osteoarthritis, gout and pain. The knees are particularly vulnerable. Assessing joints requires palpation, as often the joint is obscured by excess tissue. ROM exercises are encouraged. Passive ROM exercises are often necessary. Assess the person's ability to rise from a chair, climb stairs, transfer their weight and maintain their balance (Estes et al., 2020). Assist with ambulation, if possible, using equipment such as walkers. Ask about their functional levels – standing, walking independently – and how it affects their quality of life. For more information on issues of people living with severe obesity, see **Clinical Skills 15 and 23**.

Safety

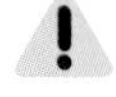
Safety

Assess the person for their ability to move and to help you to move them. Ask for assistance if you think you will need it (especially for someone with severe obesity or who has severely limited ROM). Falls injure people, cause pain and suffering, increase hospital stays and impact medical and financial resources (Satoh, Miura & Shimada, 2023). Use a valid falls risk-assessment tool (most facilities will consistently use one, but a FRAT is available from the Victorian Government Health website if needed [see Victorian Government, 2015]) if you are at all concerned about the person's psychological status (e.g. depression, agitation), a history of recent falls, their current medications (e.g. sedatives, hypnotics, antihypertensives), visual problems or incontinence, or if they seem frail or weak. Satoh, Miura and Shimada (2023) add age, impaired extremities, muscle weakness requiring mobilisation assistance and/or an unstable gait, which all increase risk of falls. This demonstrates good clinical judgement. Follow the facility's protocols regarding manual handling as musculoskeletal injury to healthcare workers is a significant risk (McClean, Cross & Reed, 2021). See also **Clinical Skill 57** for information on assisting a person to reposition.

Position the person and the bed

After the initial observations, both the assessment and the upper-body ROM exercises are most effective if the person is in a sitting position. They should be well supported with their feet flat on the floor. Any painful area is supported on pillows. If the person is unable to sit, they should be positioned in the supine position with heels close together and arms resting at their sides. Painful limbs/joints should be supported on pillows.

The prone position is used for some extension and flexion exercises. If the person is unable to assume a prone position, left and right side-lying positions are used. The person must be fully supported in the side-lying positions so that when the joints are moved the person is not pulled out of the position.

Position the bed at waist level to keep activity near your centre of gravity, thereby minimising stress on your muscles, and reducing your energy expenditure and friction and shearing forces on the person's skin.

Range of motion exercises

Comfort

ROM exercises should be carried out within the pain-free range; this can be extended by judicious use of analgesia. Watch the person for non-verbal expressions of pain during the exercise: facial grimaces, withdrawal of the limb or tensing the body indicate pain. If a joint movement is painful, consult a physiotherapist. Physiotherapists have the training and experience to stretch tight joints and release contractures. The increased exercise level involved in ROM exercises will cause fatigue for many people. Do not continue the exercises to the point of exhaustion.

Choose the appropriate type of exercise

There is no need to do ROM exercises on a joint that is moving adequately and as part of the activities of daily living. If a joint is weak or immobile, the person must commence a regimen to improve movement. The various types of ROM exercises are:

- *Passive ROM exercises* – move each of the person's joints through its full ROM with little or no input from the person. These exercises only maintain joint mobility and assume you know each joint's ROM.
- *Active ROM exercises* – the person moves their own joints through the full ROM. They must be motivated to be actively involved. People can be taught to do active ROM exercises on weak or inactive joints. They use adjacent muscles to move a joint through its entire range. These exercises maintain/increase muscle strength, endurance and cardiorespiratory function in an immobile person.
- *Active assisted ROM exercises* – the person uses one part of the body to move another joint in their body through its ROM. An example of this would be someone who has had a cerebrovascular accident, and uses the stronger arm and leg to move the weaker ones through their ROM.

PART 3

GATHER EQUIPMENT

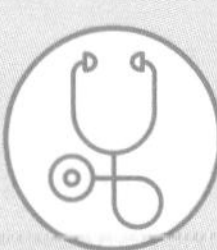

Gathering the required equipment helps you to complete the procedure efficiently.

The equipment required includes the following items:

EQUIPMENT	EXPLANATION
Slide sheets	Used to assist in repositioning the person
Lifts or hoists	• McClean, Cross and Reed (2021) warn that the risks of work-related musculoskeletal injuries to nurses increase when working with obese people and recommend safe moving practices, including lifting devices and ergonomic assessment • Learn how to use the ones available to you
Pillows	• Keep small and large pillows handy to support the person in side-lying positions • The pillows remain with the person throughout their hospitalisation and, if used only for positioning, the pillowslips should be changed weekly or when soiled
Felt-tip pen and measuring tape	If contralateral muscles look unequal, they will need measurement. Use the pen to mark the point of measurement on each muscle mass from a nearby joint. Measure with the tape

ASSESS THE MUSCULOSKELETAL SYSTEM

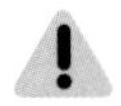

Safety

Musculoskeletal assessment begins with observation and continues on to palpation of muscle, bones and joints in a consistent pattern.

Hand hygiene

Hand hygiene (see **Clinical Skill 5**) removes microorganisms from your hands. It is the most effective preventative measure for cross-contamination, reducing incidences of nosocomial (i.e. hospital- or treatment-acquired) infection.

Obtain a musculoskeletal health history

The past health history of the musculoskeletal system is important in assisting you to focus your assessment. The following should be included (as identified by Estes et al., 2020):

- *Age* – may point to specific disorders, such as rheumatoid arthritis in younger adults, osteoporosis in postmenopausal women or osteoarthritis in older adults.
- *Sex* – may hint at the cause of the problem; for example, females may be prone to developing scoliosis, osteoporosis or multiple sclerosis, and males may be prone to developing gout, muscular dystrophy, amyotrophic lateral sclerosis.
- *Reason for attendance* – this is often due to pain; ask about the seven dimensions: location, radiation, setting, timing, quality, quantity, aggravating and alleviating factors.
- *Change in motor function* – such as a decrease in ability to move a joint or weakness or pain in a limb or muscle group.
- *Limited movement* – in a joint or diffusely in a limb; ask about onset, location, effect on activities of daily living.
- *Deformity* – congenital or acquired, degree of dysfunction caused.
- *Stiffness or inflexibility* – ask about time of day or if it is affected by exercise.
- *Alteration in sensation* – such as tingling in an extremity, numbness or other paraesthesia.
- *Past medical history* – both specific to the musculoskeletal system (e.g. low back pain, poliomyelitis, osteoarthritis and medications such as anti-inflammatory agents or steroids) and general (e.g. malnutrition, diabetes mellitus, obesity, menopause and medications like narcotic analgesics or muscle relaxants).
- *Relevant surgical history* – include such things as joint arthroscopy, repair of meniscus, fractures, injuries like dislocation of a joint and sprains.
- *Social history* – involvement in sports, some hobbies (injury from overuse of muscles); use of tobacco (increases risk of osteoporosis) or alcohol (increases risk of injury, osteoporosis), type of work (manual labour increases incidence of injuries) and use of safety measures like lifting equipment.
- *Family history* – familial linking may indicate conditions like gout or rheumatoid arthritis.

Musculoskeletal assessment

The musculoskeletal assessment should begin when you initially greet the person and assist them into a comfortable position (support painful areas with pillows if necessary). Observe for posture, gait, head position, shoulder and hip symmetry, ability to sit down, stand up, remove their clothing, move their head and move their hands and facial muscles as they talk. Note any unusual joint or muscle movements or stillness. Continue to inspect as you obtain a musculoskeletal history (see 'Obtain a musculoskeletal health history' earlier). Closely attend to the movement or guarding of any part that is reported as a problem or injury and remember to ask about these specifically. Muscles and joints should be symmetrical.

Discussion of the possible abnormalities is beyond the scope of this competency.

> If something about the person's posture, gait, symmetry or movements does not 'look right', make a note of it, ask the person about it and then discuss it with a more senior healthcare professional.

Continue to inspect movement, muscle mass and tone as you begin to palpate the joints. Compare joints and muscles with the contralateral side. Begin with non-affected parts. Inspect each joint as you palpate it – small joints with your thumb and finger pads, and larger joints with the palmar surface of your hand. Inspect and palpate both anterior and posterior surfaces of the joints. Assess the person's ability to move each joint. Identify the anatomical landmarks to aid in documentation. Be systematic and adopt a routine for assessing each joint. Moving from top to toe is an easy routine to remember and makes sense to the person as well. Pain, immobility or limited ROM (i.e. the person can move their left elbow through 45 degrees only) must be documented. Do not move or palpate painful joints or muscles. Additionally, attend to the following:

- Look for colour changes, skin marks, scars, contour changes, bulges or masses, ecchymosis, oedema and muscle atrophy/hypertrophy. Ask the person to move each joint through its ROM while you watch both the joint and their face, and gently palpate the joint.
- Listen to any reports of pain/discomfort or involuntary noises (e.g. moans, grunts) as joints are moved.
- Feel for temperature, masses, tenderness, crepitus (you can also hear this) and joint or bone deformity.

During assessment of the joints, also inspect and palpate the muscles. Look for:

- *Tone* – a normal resting muscle is slightly contracted and ready for action and helps maintain posture; it is not soft or flaccid (hypotonic) nor hard and stiff (hypertonic). Both hypotonia and hypertonia are not normal.
- *Muscle mass* – *atrophy* is a decrease in size and bulk of a muscle; usually due to injury, disuse or disease. *Hypertrophy* is an excessive increase in size and bulk of a muscle, usually due to exercise or medication. If you notice a difference in muscle size, measure the circumference of the muscle mass with a measuring tape on each side of the body. Measure at a point the same distance from a nearby joint. Compare your findings. A difference of 3 cm or more is significant (Estes et al., 2020). Usually this is an estimation, although an ultrasound examination of the thigh can indicate muscle wasting (Martin, Zepeda & Lescas Méndez, 2017).
- *Muscle strength* – assessed both against gravity (ask the person to raise their limb and watch the effort involved) and against resistance (apply force against the limb to see if the person's muscle strength can overcome the resistance). Moderate the force you apply according to the person's condition. Document muscle movement and strength for both right- and left-side muscle groups on a six-point scale where 0 = no movement and 5 = movement with minimal effort. These should be recorded for the best effort (i.e. if the person is unable to raise their leg against gravity, then assessing against resistance would not be done).

Often, as a time-management strategy, the musculoskeletal assessment is integrated into other assessments, such as the cardiovascular and neurological assessments. In doing this, you only assess the limbs once, looking for joint and muscle problems, pulses, skin temperature, capillary refill, hair distribution, varicose veins, oedema, paralysis and paraesthesia.

TABLE 24.1 outlines the movements the person must undertake to enable a nurse to assess the muscle groups.

PERFORM PASSIVE RANGE OF MOTION EXERCISES

During the exercises, adopt a specific systematic pattern so that no joint is forgotten. Start the exercises gradually and work slowly. Movement should be smooth and rhythmic to increase comfort.

During passive ROM exercises, support each joint to prevent over-extension. Move each joint three times, slowly and smoothly. Do these exercises on a scheduled basis. Passive ROM exercises can be incorporated into daily hygiene routines. Move each

TABLE 24.1 Muscle group movements to enable assessment

MUSCLE GROUP	AGAINST GRAVITY	AGAINST RESISTANCE
Shoulders	Shrug (raise) shoulders	Shrug (raise) shoulders against resistance of your hands
Upper arms	Straight arm raises with palm up, both to the side (when standing/sitting) and with arms in front (one at a time)	Straight arm raises against resistance of your hands placed on their wrists
Forearms	Ask person to bring their hand to their shoulder (either lying or sitting)	Apply resistance against the wrist as the person moves it towards their shoulder
Hands	Not applicable	Ask the person to grip your hands tightly and release
Legs	Straight leg raises (from standing or lying; one at a time)	Ask the person to raise their leg while you hold it down
Feet	Plantar flexion and contraction	Plantar flexion and contraction against resistance of your hand placed behind the toes and in front of the toes

joint to the point of resistance but not pain. Use gentle pressure, not force. Start and finish with each joint in its normal, neutral position. Take care to note the person's facial expressions and other non-verbal expressions for evidence of pain. Encouraging the person to do activities of daily living or engage in exercise regimens such as tai chi increases the ROM of all joints and reduces the need to do passive ROM exercises.

TABLE 24.2 outlines the movements possible in each joint in the positions indicated. For a detailed discussion with drawings of these exercises, a good source is DeLaune et al. (2024) *Fundamentals of nursing: Standards and practice.*

Teach the range of movement exercises

The person needs to be taught how to do the ROM exercises. They will need to know the following:

- *what* – which joint is being exercised
- *why* – to maintain mobility and allow specific activities, especially pleasurable ones, to be done
- *how* – use a show-and-tell technique.

Try to make each session relaxing and, if possible, pleasurable, since the person will benefit by taking a more active part.

DOCUMENTATION

Document any abnormalities discovered. Be specific, noting which joint or muscle group is problematic.
For normal findings, simply note that joint configuration and ROM is normal, and that muscle mass, strength and tone are normal. Documentation on ROM exercises should include an initial notation of the joints to be exercised and daily notes that the exercises have been completed, along with any changes.
To document altered ROM, name any joint with limitations and describe its ability to move through its normal range, with or without pain or crepitus (e.g. no limitations; pain or crepitus in left knee ROM noted; or, R elbow movement limited to 90/180 degrees, no crepitus heard; or, fingers of left hand immobile and painful at rest; or, unable to extend R wrist, able to flex only about 10 degrees without pain).

TABLE 24.2 Movements possible in various joints in the supine and prone positions

JOINT	SUPINE	PRONE
Neck (active)	Flex, extend, lateral flex, rotate	Hyperextend
Shoulder	Flex, extend, adduct, abduct, internal and external rotation	Hyperextend
Scapula	Protract	Retract
Elbow	Flex, extend	
Wrist	Flex, extend, ulnar and radial deviation, pronate and supinate	
Fingers	Flex, extend, adduct and abduct	
Thumbs	Flex, extend, oppose	
Hips	Flex, extend, adduct and abduct	Hyperextend
Knees	Flex, extend	Flex, extend
Ankles	Dorsiflex, plantar flex, invert, evert	Dorsiflex, plantar flex
Toes	Flex, extend, adduct and abduct	

NOTE: ALL UPPER BODY MOVEMENTS CAN BE DONE IN A SITTING POSITION.

CLINICAL SKILLS ASSESSMENT

Focused musculoskeletal health history and physical assessment and range of motion exercises

Demonstrates the ability to effectively assess the musculoskeletal systems and to safely maintain a person's joint mobility or teach the person to do so. Incorporates the *National Safety and Quality Health Service Standards*: 2 Partnering with Consumers, 3 Preventing and Controlling Healthcare-Associated Infection, 5 Comprehensive Care, 6 Communicating for Safety, and 8 Recognising and Responding to Acute Deterioration (ACSQHC, 2021).

Performance criteria	1	2	3	4	5
(Numbers indicate NMBA *Registered Nurse Standards for Practice*)	**(Dependent)**	**(Marginal)**	**(Assisted)**	**(Supervised)**	**(Independent)**
1. Identifies indication (1.1, 3.3, 3.4)	☐	☐	☐	☐	☐
2. Evidence of therapeutic interaction with the person, e.g. gives the person a clear explanation of the procedure (1.4, 1.5, 2.1, 2.2, 3.2)	☐	☐	☐	☐	☐
3. Demonstrates clinical reasoning abilities, e.g. safely positions and moves the person with assistance if required, positions the bed, chooses appropriate type of exercise (1.1, 1.2, 1.3, 4.2, 6.1)	☐	☐	☐	☐	☐
4. Gathers equipment (5.5, 6.1): ■ slide sheet ■ lift or hoist ■ small and large pillows as necessary ■ measuring tape, felt-tip pen	☐	☐	☐	☐	☐
5. Performs hand hygiene (1.1, 3.4, 6.1)	☐	☐	☐	☐	☐
6. Assesses the musculoskeletal system: obtains a musculoskeletal health history, inspects musculoskeletal system, assesses and palpates joints and determines muscular strength (4.1, 4.2, 4.3, 6.1)	☐	☐	☐	☐	☐
7. Assists the person to move each joint through its entire range of motion (3.2, 6.1)	☐	☐	☐	☐	☐
8. Teaches the person to accomplish range of movement exercises with minimal assistance (3.2, 6.1)	☐	☐	☐	☐	☐
9. Documents relevant information (1.4, 1.6, 2.2, 2.7, 3.5, 3.7, 6.2, 6.5, 7.3)	☐	☐	☐	☐	☐
10. Demonstrates the ability to link theory to practice (1.1, 3.3, 3.4, 3.5)	☐	☐	☐	☐	☐

Student:

Clinical facilitator: Date:

REFERENCES

Abbott, S., Shuttlewood, E., Flint, S., Chesworth, P. & Parretti, H. (2023). 'Is it time to throw out the weighing scales?' Implicit weight bias among healthcare professionals working in bariatric surgery services and their attitude towards non-weight focused approaches. *EClinical Medicine, 55*, 101770. https://doi.org/10.1016/j.eclinm.2022.101770

Accu-Chek Inform II (2019). *Whole blood glucose testing.* https://www.stjoesonoma.org/documents/Students-Instructors/PVH-Accu-Chek-Inform-II.pdf

Agarwal, E., Ferguson, M., Banks, M., Vivanti, A., Batterham, M., Bauer, J., Capra, S. & Isenring, E. (2019). Malnutrition, poor food intake, and adverse healthcare outcomes in non-critically ill obese acute care hospital patients. *Clinical Nutrition, 38*(2), 759–66. https://doi.org/10.1016/j.clnu.2018.02.033

Agrawal, P., Girish, M., Ramanathan, A., Sudhakaran, M. & Murali, S. (2023). Compartment syndrome and its validation in skeletal injuries. *International Journal of Recent Medical and Surgical Sciences.* https://www.thieme-connect.com/products/ejournals/pdf/10.1055/s-0043-1761415.pdf

Ahmed, S., Adley, R. & Hassan, S. (2019). Nurses' performance regarding care of children with neurological disorders. *Egyptian Journal of Health Care, 10*(1). https://ejhc.journals.ekb.eg/article_251350_ae52e939b5eeed7af3b65e789e4e6bde.pdf

Alkhaqani, A. & Ali, B. (2023). Holistic nursing care for acute myocardial infarction patients: An evidence-based approach. *American Research Journal of Nursing and Health Sciences, 1*(1). https://zapjournals.com/Journals/index.php/arjnhs

Antwi-Baffour, S., Mensah, B., Armah, D., Ali-Mustapha, S. & Annison, L. (2023). Comparative analysis of glycated haemoglobin, fasting blood glucose and haematological parameters of type-2 diabetes patients. *BMC Research Square.* https://doi.org/10.21203/rs.3.rs-2777663/v1

Australian Commission on Safety and Quality in Health Care (ACSQHC) (2021). *National safety and quality health service standards* (3rd ed.). Sydney, NSW: ACSQHC.

Australian Institute of Health and Welfare (AIHW) (2019). *Overweight and obesity: An interactive insight.* https://www.aihw.gov.au/reports/overweight-obesity/overweight-and-obesity-an-interactive-insight/contents/what-is-overweight-and-obesity

Azimirad, M., Magnusson, C., Wiseman, A., Selander, T., Parviainen, I. & Turunen, H. (2022). A clinical competence approach to examine British and Finnish nurses' attitudes towards the rapid response system model: A study in two acute hospitals. *Australian Critical Care, 35*(1), 72–80. https://doi.org/10.1016/j.aucc.2021.02.011

Baamer, R., Iqbal, A., Lobo, D., Knaggs, R., Levy, N. & Toh, L. (2022). Utility of unidimensional and functional pain assessment tools in adult postoperative patients: A systematic review. *British Journal of Anaesthesia, 128*(5), 874–88. https://doi.org/10.1016/j.bja.2021.11.032

Balasubramanian, P., Kiss, T., Tarantini, S., Nyúl-Tóth, A., Ahire, C., Yabluchanskiy, A., Csipo, T., Lipecz, A., Tabak, A., Institoris, A., Csiszar, A. & Ungari, Z. (2021). Obesity-induced cognitive impairment in older adults: A microvascular perspective. *American Journal of Physiology-Heart and Circulatory Physiology, 320*(2), H740–H761. https://doi.org/10.1152%2Fajpheart.00736.2020

Bao, Y. & Zhu, D. (2022). Clinical application guidelines for blood glucose monitoring in China (2022 ed.). *Diabetes Metabolism Research and Reviews, 38*(8), e3581. https://doi.org/10.1002/dmrr.3581

Barreveld, A., Rosén Klement, M., Cheung, S., Axelsson, U., Basem, J., Reddy, A., Borrebaeck, C. & Mehta, M. (2023). An artificial intelligence-powered, patient-centric digital tool for self-management of chronic pain: A prospective, multicenter clinical trial, *Pain Medicine, 24*(9), 1100–10.

Beck, R., Bergenstal, R., Laffel, L. & Pickup, J. (2019). Advances in technology for management of type 1 diabetes. *The Lancet, 394*(10205), 1265–73. https://doi.org/10.1016/S0140-6736(19)31142-0

Bell, S., Lee, C., Zeeman, J., Kearney, M., Macko, L. & Cartwright, C. (2021). Neurological assessment of the hospitalised adult patient. *American Association of Neuroscience Nurses White Paper.* https://aann.org/uploads/about/AANN21_Neuro_White_Paper_V9.pdf

Berg, K., Johnson, D., Nyberg, G., Claeys, C., Ausmus, A., Wilkinson, E. & Clark, N. (2022). Reducing the frequency of pulse oximetry alarms at a children's hospital. *Pediatrics, 151*(5), e2022057465. https://doi.org/10.1542/peds.2022-057465

Bickerton, M. & Pooler, A. (2019). Misplaced ECG electrodes and the need for continuing training. *British Journal of Cardiac Nursing, 14*(3), 123–32. https://doi.org/10.12968/bjca.2019.14.3.123

Birkelbach, O., Mörgeli, R., Spies, C., Olbert, M., Weiss, B., Brauner, M., Neuner, B., Francis, R., Treskatsch, S. & Balzer, F. (2019). Routine frailty assessment predicts postoperative complications in elderly patients across surgical disciplines: A retrospective observational study. *BMC Anesthesiology, 19*, 204 . https://doi.org/10.1186/s12871-019-0880-x

Blake, S., Fries, K., Higginbotham, L., Lorei, C., McGee, M., Murray, R., Priest, M., Rangel, J., Remick-Erickson, K., Schneider, L., Vodopest, B. & Moore, A. (2019). Evaluation of noninvasive thermometers in an endoscopy setting. *Gastroenterology Nursing, 42*(2), 123–31. https://doi.org/10.1097/SGA.0000000000000367

Breda, J., Springston, M., Mariakakis, A. & Patel, S. (2023). FeverPhone: Accessible core-body temperature sensing for fever monitoring using commodity smartphones. *Proceedings ACM Interactive, Mobile, Wearable Ubiquitous Technology, 7*(1), Article 3. https://doi.org/10.1145/3580850

Brekke, I., Puntervoll, L., Pedersen, P., Kellett, J. & Brabrand, M. (2019). The value of vital sign trends in predicting and monitoring clinical deterioration: A systematic review. *Public Library of Science ONE, 14*(1), e0210875. https://doi.org/10.1371/journal.pone.0210875

Buekers, J., Theunis, J., De Boever, P., Vaes, A., Koopman, M., Janssen, E., Wouters, E., Spruit, M. & Aerts, J. (2019). Wearable finger pulse oximetry for continuous oxygen saturation measurements during daily home routines of patients with chronic obstructive pulmonary disease (COPD) over one week: Observational study. *Journal of Medical Internet Research mHealth and uHealth, 7*(6), e12866. https://doi.org/10.2196/12866

Bunney, G., Sundaram, V., Graber-Naidich, A., Miller, K., Brown, I., McCoy, A., Freeze, B., Berger, D., Wright, A. & Yiadom, M. (2023). Beyond chest pain: Incremental value of other variables to identify patients for an early ECG. *American Journal of Emergency Medicine, 67*, 70–8. https://doi.org/10.1016/j.ajem.2023.01.054

Burdette, E., Bartz, D., Pelletier, A. & Johnson, N. (2023). We must address the antiobesity biases we espouse in our operating rooms. *Journal of Surgical Education, 80*(2), 166–9. https://doi.org/10.1016/j.jsurg.2022.09.004

Burgess, S. (2022). Rhabdomyolysis: An evidence-based approach. *Journal of the Intensive Care Society, 23*(4), 513–17. https://journals.sagepub.com/doi/pdf/10.1177/17511437211050782

Cabanas, A. M., Fuentes-Guajardo, M., Latorre, K., León, D. & Martín-Escudero, P. (2022). Skin pigmentation influence on pulse oximetry accuracy: A systematic review and bibliometric analysis. *Sensors, 22*(9), 3402. https://doi.org/10.3390/s22093402

Campbell, B., Richley, D., Ross, C. & Eggett, C. J. (2017). *Clinical guidelines by consensus: Recording a standard 12-lead electrocardiogram. An approved method by the Society for Cardiological Science and Technology (SCST).* http://www.scst.org.uk/resources/SCST_ECG_Recording_Guidelines_2017am.pdf

Cardoso, M., Pinheira, V. & Carvalho, L. (2023). Relationship between O_2 saturation values, functional mobility, physical activity levels and quality of life in older people. In M. J. A. Guardado Moreira, L. S. Carvalho, P. J. Sequeira Gonçalves & V. M. Barreiros Pinheira (eds), *Longevity and development: New perspectives on ageing communities* . Age.Comm 2021. Lecture Notes in Bioengineering. Springer, Cham. https://doi.org/10.1007/978-3-031-22273-3_7

Caswell, M., Brown, D., Frank, J., Wallace, J. & Pardo, S. (2020). Accuracy and user performance evaluation of a blood glucose monitoring system which wirelessly transmits results to compatible insulin pumps. *Current Medical Research and Opinion, 36*(5), 757–64. https://doi.org/10.1080/03007995.2020.1734919

Chan, H., Lau, T., Ho, S., Leung, D. & Lee, D. (2016). The accuracy and acceptability of performing capillary blood glucose measurements at the earlobe. *Journal of Advanced Nursing, 72*(8), 1766–73.

Chatterjee, S., Thakur, R. S., Yadav, R. N., Gupta, L. & Raghuvanshi, D. K. (2020). Review of noise removal techniques in ECG signals. *IET Signal Process, 14*, 569–90. https://doi.org/10.1049/iet-spr.2020.0104

Cheung, A., Whelton, P., Muntner, P., Schutte, A., Moran, A., Williams, B., Sarafidis, P., Chang, T., Daskalopoulou, S., Flack, J., Jennings, G., Juraschek, S., Kreutz, R., Mancia, G., Nebitt, S., Ordunez, P., Padwal, R., Persu, A., Rabi, D., Schlaich, M., Stergiou, G., Tobe, S., Tomaszewski, M., Williams, K. & Mann, J. (2022). International consensus on standardized clinic blood pressure measurement: A call to action. *American Journal of Medicine, 136*(5), 438–45, e1. https://doi.org/10.1016/j.amjmed.2022.12.015

Cho, S.A., Yoon, S., Lee, S.J., Jee, Y.S., Cho, C.K. & Sung, T.Y. (2022). Clinical efficacy of short-term prewarming in elderly and adult patients: A prospective observational study. *International Journal of Medical Sciences, 19*(10), 15–56. https://doi.org.10.7150/ijms.77578

Chow, E. J., Uyeki, T. M. & Chu, H. Y. (2023). The effects of the COVID-19 pandemic on community respiratory virus activity. *Nature Reviews Microbiology, 21*, 195–210. https://doi.org/10.1038/s41579-022-00807-9

Chua, W., Smith, D., Wee, L., Ting, K., Yeo, M., Mordiffi, S. & Liaw, S. (2022). Development and psychometric evaluation of the Attitudes Towards Recognising Early and Noticeable Deterioration (ATREND) scale. *Journal of Clinical Nursing, 32*(11–12). https://doi.org/10.1111/jocn.16350

Chuang, S. Y., Lin, W. L., Lai, C. H., Chung, R. H. & Hsu, C. C. (2022). Pulse pressure associated with physical function decline and frailty syndrome progression. *Journal of Hypertension, 40*(Supplement 1), e1. https://doi.org/10.1097/01.hjh.0000835300.13173.7b

Cirillo, D., Hart, S., Reich, R. & Mason, T. M. (2018). Height measures. *Clinical Journal of Oncology Nursing, 22*(5), 529–33. https://doi.org/10.1188/18.CJON.529-533

Cornish, L., Hill, A., Horswill, M., Becker, S. & Watson, M. (2019). Eye tracking reveals how observation chart design features affect the detection of patient deterioration: An experimental study. *Applied Ergonomics, 75*, 230–42. https://doi.org/10.1016/j.apergo.2018.10.005

Cousins, M., Lane-Krebs, K., Matthews, J. & Johnston-Devin, C. (2022). Student nurses' pain knowledge and attitudes towards pain management over the last 20 years: A systematic review. *Nurse Education Today, 108*, 105169. https://doi.org/10.1016/j.nedt.2021.105169

Craig, K. (2014). Less ouch blood sugar tests. *Diabetic Living.* http://www.diabeticlivingonline.com/monitoring/blood-sugar/less-ouch-blood-sugar-tests.

Damani, D., Sundaram, D., Damani, S., Kapoor, A., Arruda-Olsen, A. & Arunachalum, A. (2021). Investigation of synchronised acquisition of electrocardiogram and phonocardiogram signals towards electromechanical profiling of the heart. *Biomedical Science Instrumentation, 57*(2). https://doi.org/10.34107/BiomedScilnstrum.57.04304

Dao Le, L. (2016). *Pulse oximetry: Clinician information* [Evidence summary]. Adelaide, SA: Joanna Briggs Institute.

Davies, T. L. (2023). Tailoring the mental health assessment to older adults. *The Nurse Practitioner, 48*(1), 10–18. https://doi.org/10.1097/01.NPR.0000902992.34389.1f

Deep, H. S., Kamaldeep, K., Mahajan, D. S. & Brar, H. S. (2019). Comparative study of pulse oximetry and ankle-brachial index as a screening test for asymptomatic peripheral vascular disease in type 2 diabetes mellitus against color doppler ultrasonography as reference standard. *International Journal of Advances in Medicine, 6*(4), 1151–6.

Deering, S. (2023). Clinical public health, climate change, and aging. *Canadian Family Physician, 69*(5), 233–5. https://www.cfp.ca/content/cfp/69/4/233.full.pdf

DeLaune, S., Ladner, P., McTier, L. & Tollefson, J. (2024). *Fundamentals of nursing: Standards and practice* (Australia and New Zealand 3rd ed.). South Melbourne, VIC: Cengage Learning.

Depta, F., Gentile, M., Kallet, R., Firment, P., Leškanič J., Rybár, D., Török, P. & Zdravkovic, M. (2023). Determining respiratory rate using measured expiratory time constant: A prospective observational study, *Journal of Critical Care, 73*. https://doi.org/10.1016/j.jcrc.2022.154174

Díaz-González, C. dl M., Mateos-López, N., De la Rosa-Hormiga, M. & Carballo-Hernández, G. (2023). Influence of hospital environmental variables on thermometric measurements and level of concordance: A cross-sectional descriptive study. *International Journal of Environmental Research and Public Health, 20*(5), 4665. https://doi.org/10.3390/ijerph20054665

Dobbie, L. J., Coelho, C., Crane, J. & McGowan, B. (2023). Clinical evaluation of patients living with obesity. *Internal and Emergency Medicine*, 1–13. https://link.springer.com/article/10.1007/s11739-023-03263-2

Dougherty, L., Lister, S. & West-Oram, A. (eds) (2015). *The Royal Marsden manual of clinical nursing procedures* (9th ed.). Oxford, UK: Wiley-Blackwell.

Douglas, C., Booker, C., Fox, R., Windsor, C., Osborne, S. & Gardner, G. (2016). Nursing physical assessment for patient safety in general wards: Reaching consensus on core skills. *Journal of Clinical Nursing, 25*(13–14), 1890–900. https://doi.org/10.1111/jocn.13201

Dudhe, A., Salunkhe, A., Salunkhe, J., Mohite, V. & Kakade, S. (2023). Effect of sociodemographicals on the post operative hypothermia. *Journal of Pharmaceutical Negative Results, 14*(2), 2100–5. pnrjournal.com

Duncan, A. L., Bell, A. J., Chu, K. & Greenslade, J. H. (2008). Can a non-contact infrared thermometer be used interchangeably with other thermometers in an adult emergency department? *Australasian Emergency Nursing Journal, 11*, 130–4.

Dunning, T. & Sinclair, A. (2020). *Care of people with diabetes: A manual for healthcare practice* (5th ed.). Oxford, UK: Wiley Blackwell.

Earp, B., Monrad, J., LaFrance, M., Bargh, J., Cohen, L. & Richeson, J. (2019). Gender bias in pediatric pain assessment. *Journal of Pediatric Psychology, 44*(4), 403–14. https://doi.org/10.1093/jpepsy/jsy104

Elbaih, A. H. & Basyouni, F. H. (2020). Teaching approach of primary survey in trauma patients. *SunText Review of Surgery, 1*(1), 101. https://www.researchgate.net/profile/Adel-Hamed-

Eley, V., Christensen, R., Guy, L. & Dodd, B. (2019). Perioperative blood pressure monitoring in patients with obesity. *Anesthesia & Analgesia, 128*(3), 484–91. https://doi.org/10.1213/ANE.0000000000003647

Estes, M. E. Z., Calleja, P., Theobald, K. & Harvey, T. (2020). *Health assessment and physical examination* (Australia & New Zealand 3rd ed.). South Melbourne, VIC: Cengage Learning.

Ewens, B., Kemp, V., Towell-Barnard, A. & Whitehead, L. (2022). The nursing care of people with class III obesity in an acute care setting: A scoping review. *BMC Nursing, 21*, 33. https://doi.org/10.1186/s12912-021-00760-7

Faraz, A., Qureshi, A., Khan, M., Bakht Yawar, B., Malik, M., Saghir, M., Faisal, G. & Tarar, M. (2022). Documentation of neurovascular assessment in fracture patients in a tertiary care hospital: A retrospective review. *Annals of Medicine and Surgery, 79*. https://doi.org/10.1016/j.amsu.2022.103935

Fernando, S. M., Fox-Robichaud, A. E., Rochwerg, B., Cardinal, P., Seely, A., Perry, J., McIsaac, D., Tran, A., Stitch, S., Tam, B., Hickey, M., Reardon, P., Tanuseputro, P. & Kwadwo, K. (2019). Prognostic accuracy of the Hamilton Early Warning Score (HEWS) and the National Early Warning Score 2 (NEWS2) among hospitalized patients assessed by a rapid response team. *Critical Care, 23*, 60. https://doi.org/10.1186/s13054-019-2355-3

Fitzwater, J., Johnstone, C., Schippers, M., Cordoza, M. & Norman, B. (2019). Temperature measuring devices in adult acute care. *Medsurg Nursing, 28*(1), 35–41. https://search.proquest.com/openview/69a18ecc2ef0551fea35d16a034d573a/1?pq-origsite=gscholar&cbl=30764

Flack, J .& Adekola, B. (2020). Blood pressure and the new ACC/AHA hypertension guidelines. *Trends in Cardiovascular Medicine, 30*(3), 160–4. https://doi.org/10.1016/j.tcm.2019.05.003

Freeman, L. & Kelly, M. (2018) Describing the pause: Phenomenologic study of physical examination in family practice. *Canadian Family Physician, 64*(2), S1–S115. https://www.cfp.ca

Freund, D. & Bolick, B. (2019). Assessing a child's pain. *American Journal of Nursing, 119*(5), 34–41. https://doi.org/10.1097/01.NAJ.0000557888.65961.c6

Fulton, S., Décarie-Spain, L., Fioramonti, X., Guiard, B. & Nakajima, S. (2022). The menace of obesity to depression and anxiety prevalence. *Trends in Endocrinology & Metabolism, 33*(1), 18–35. https://doi.org/10.1016/j.tem.2021.10.005

Gabb, G., Mangoni, A., Anderson, C., Cowley, D., Dowden, J., Golledge, J., Hankey, G., Howes, F., Leckie, L., Perkovic, V., Schlaich, M., Zwar, N., Medley, T. & Arnolda, L. (2016). National Heart Foundation's guideline for the diagnosis and management of hypertension in adults 2016. *Medical Journal of Australia, 205*(2), 85–9. https://doi.org/10.5694/mja16.00526

Geethavani, G. & Youtham, P. (2022). Evaluation of staff nurses' knowledge regarding the Glasgow Coma Scale (GCS). *International Journal of Research Publication and Reviews, 3*(12), 2525–6. https://ijrpr.com/uploads/V3ISSUE12/IJRPR8919.pdf

Geneva, I. I. & Javaid, W. (2021). Disruption of the body temperature circadian rhythm in hospitalized patients. *American Journal of the Medical Sciences, 362*(6), 578–85. https://doi.org/10.1016/j.amjms.2021.06.021

Givler, A. & Maani-Fogelman, P. (2019). *The importance of cultural competence in pain and palliative care*. StatPearls. https://www.statpearls.com/sp/ph/197/41271

Gordon, C. (2019). Blood glucose monitoring in diabetes: Rationale and procedure. *British Journal of Nursing, 28*(7), 434–9. http://nrl.northumbria.ac.uk/39038/1/Revision%201%20-%20Blood%20glucose%20monitoring%20at%20a%20Glance%20-%20Edited.pdf

Goudsmit, M., van Campen, J., Schilt, T., Hinnen, C., Franzen, S. & Schmand, B. (2018). Comparative diagnostic accuracy of the Rowland Universal Dementia Assessment Scale and the Mini Mental State Examination in a memory clinic population with very low education. *Dementia and Geriatric Cognitive Disorders, 8*(2). https://www.karger.com/Article/FullText/490174#

Greenfield, A., Alba, B., Giersch, G. & Seeley, A. (2023). Sex differences in thermal sensitivity and perception: Implications for behavioral and autonomic thermoregulation. *Physiology & Behavior, 63*, 14126. https://doi.org/10.1016/j.physbeh.2023.114126

Gregory, P., Kilner, T., Lodge, S. & Paget, S. (2021). Accuracy of ECG chest electrode placements by paramedics: An observational study. *British Paramedic Journal, 6*(1), 8–14. https://doi.org/10.29045/14784726.2021.6.6.1.8

Guo, J., Yin, Y., Jin, L., Zhang, R., Hou, Z. & Zhang, Y. (2019). Acute compartment syndrome: Cause, diagnosis, and new viewpoint. *Medicine* (Baltimore), *27*, e16260. https://doi.org/10.1097/MD.0000000000016260

Hadjiantoni, H. (2020). Is the correct anatomical placement of the electrocardiogram (ECG) electrodes essential to diagnosis in the clinical setting: A systematic review. *Research Square*. https://doi.org/10.26502/fccm.92920135

Hak, D. J. (2019). Acute compartment syndrome in children. In C. Mauffrey, D. Hak & M. Martin III (eds), *Compartment syndrome*. Cham, Switzerland: Springer. https://link.springer.com/chapter/10.1007/978-3-030-22331-1_13

Halford, J. & Foran, P. (2022). Understanding the use of tympanic thermometry in the Post Anaesthetic Care Unit: A discussion paper. *ACORN Journal of Perioperative Nursing, 35*(2). https://search.informit.org/doi/epdf/10.3316/informit.542698253302651UndUerstanding

Haller, M. J., Jones, M. C., Bhavsar, S. & Kaiserman, K. (2023). Time–action profile of technosphere insulin in children with type 1 diabetes. *Diabetes Therapy, 14*, 611–17. https://doi.org/10.1007/s13300-023-01368-7

Health Victoria (2021). *Patient care: Frailty*. https://www.health.vic.gov.au/patient-care/frailty

Heart Foundation (n.d.). *Waist measurement*. https://www.heartfoundation.org.au/your-heart/know-your-risks/healthy-weight/waist-measurement

Held, K. (2023). Continuous pulse oximetry monitoring in hospitalised patients: A Doctor of Nursing Practice Project. Doctor of Nursing Practice Dissertation, South Louisiana University. https://www.proquest.com/openview/71ad93f30161aac7eaf643bee0cacfe6/1?pqorigsite=gscholar&cbl=18750&diss=y

Hercelinskyj, G. & Alexander, J. (2020). *Mental health nursing: Applying theory to practice*. South Melbourne, VIC: Cengage Learning.

Hernandez, J. & Upadhye, S. (2017). Do peripheral thermometers accurately correlate to core body temperature? *Annals of Emergency Medicine, 68*(5), 562–3. https://doi.org/10.1016/j.annemergmed.2016.03.030

Herrera, F., Siaron, K., Stutzman, S., Wilson, J. & Olson, D. (2021). Exploring accuracy and precision of noninvasive and intra-arterial blood pressure measurement in neurocritical care patients. *Sigma Repository*. http://hdl.handle.net/10755/20934

Hlavin, D. & Varty, M. (2022). Improving patient safety by increasing staff knowledge of evidence-based pulse oximetry practices. *Critical Care Nurse, 42*(6), e1–e6. https://doi.org/10.4037/ccn2022998

Hohol, A., Gilbert, J. & Johnston, M. (2019). Chronic obesity. In L. Deravin & J. Anderson (eds), *Chronic care nursing: A framework for practice* (2nd ed.). Port Melbourne, VIC: Cambridge University Press.

Holland, M. & Kellett, J. (2023). The United Kingdom's National Early Warning Score: Should everyone use it? A narrative review. *Internal and Emergency Medicine, 18*, 573–83. https://doi.org/10.1007/s11739-022-03189-1

Hunter, M., Vaddi, S., Krvavac, A., Regunath, H. & Guntur, V. (2019). Inpatient management of bronchial asthma for the hospitalist: A concise review. *American Journal of Hospital Medicine, 3*(4). https://doi.org/10.24150/ajhm/2019.015

Jackson, S., Gillespie, C., Shimbo, D., Rakotz, M. & Wall, H. (2022). Blood pressure cuff sizes for adults in the United States: National health and nutrition examination survey, 2015–2020. *American Journal of Hypertension.* https://10.1093/ajh/hpac104

Jakob, D. A., Benjamin, E. R. & Demetriades, D. (2023). Extremity compartment syndrome. In F. Coccolini & F. Catena (eds), *Textbook of emergency general surgery.* Springer, Cham. https://doi.org/10.1007/978-3-031-22599-4_110

Jenkins, M. & Winterbottom, F. (2019). Gerontological alterations. In L. Urden, K. Stacy & M. Lough (eds), *Priorities in critical care nursing* (8th ed.). Maryland, MO: Elsevier.

João, F., Silva, M., Calhau, R., Bellem, T., Nascimento, P., Sousa, L., Ferreira, R., Ferreira, O., Severing, S. & Baixinho, C. (2023). Nursing interventions in the prevention of pressure ulcers associated with medical devices in intensive care: a scoping review. In E. Moguel, L. G. de Pinho & C. Fonseca (eds), *Gerontechnology. Lecture Notes in Bioengineering.* Springer, Cham. https://doi.org/10.1007/978-3- 031-29067-1_9

Jones, T. N., Wilson, P., Hoy, E., Pherwani, S., Meng, J. & Jethwa, N. (2023). 1151 Improving the measurement of postural blood pressure with ad-hoc mobile teaching sessions for nurses and healthcare assistants. *Age and Ageing*, 52(Supplement 1), afac322-106. https://doi.org/10.1093/ageing/afac322.106

Kallioinen, N., Hill, A., Christofidis, M.J.,Horswill, M.S. & Watson, M.O. (2021). Quantitative systematic review: Sources of inaccuracy in manually measured adult respiratory rate data. *Journal of Advanced Nursing, 77*, 98–124. https://doi.org/10.1111/jan.14584

Kapur, V. K., Wilsdon, A. G., Au, D., Avdalovic, M., Enright, P., Fan, V. S., Hansel, N. N., Heckbert, S. R., Jiang, R., Krishnan, J. A., Mukamal, K., Yende, S. & Barr, R. G. (2013). Obesity is associated with a lower resting oxygen saturation in the ambulatory elderly: Results from the Cardiovascular Health Study. *Respiratory Care, 58*(5), 831–7. https://doi.org/10.4187/respcare.02008. PMID: 23107018

Kardong-Edgren, S., Oermann, M. & Rizzolo, M. (2019). Emerging theories influencing the teaching of clinical nursing skills. *Journal of Continuing Education in Nursing, 50*(6), 257–62. https://doi.org/10.3928/00220124-20190516-05

Karlen, W. (2019). *Automated point-of-care processing and interpretation of pulse oximetry for global health applications.* International Engineering and Biomedical Conference, Berlin, July 2019, ETHZurich Research Collection. https://doi.org/10.3929/ethz-b-000359389

Krans, B. (2016). Blood glucose monitoring. *Healthline.* http://www.healthline.com/health/blood-glucose-monitoring#overview1

Kubota, S., Endo, Y., Kubota, M., Miyazaki, H. & Shigemasa, T. (2022). The pressor response to the drinking of cold water and cold carbonated water in healthy younger and older adults. *Frontiers in Neurology, 12*, 2417. https://doi.org/10.1016/j.archger.2023.104988

Kumar, R. & Deo, K. (2019). A cross sectional study of oxygen saturation (SpO_2) of Amarnath Yatris at the Amarnath Holy Cave with a pulse oximeter. *International Journal of Advance Research, Ideas and Innovations in Technology, 5*(5). https://www.ijariit.com/manuscripts/v5i5/V5I5-1162.pdf

Laine, C. & Wee, C. C. (2023). Overweight and obesity: Current clinical challenges. *Annals of Internal Medicine, 176*(5), 699–700. https://www.acpjournals.org/doi/abs/10.7326/M23-0628

Lee, R. R., Rashid, A., Thomson, W. & Cordingley, L. (2020). 'Reluctant to assess pain': A qualitative study of health care professionals' beliefs about the role of pain in juvenile idiopathic arthritis. *Arthritis Care Research, 72*, 69–77. https://doi.org/10.1002/acr.23827

Lima, J., Mesquita, D., Santos, K., Fernandes, K., Mendoca, R., Quinta, C., Silva, D. & Nobrega, L. (2016). The impact of not washing hands on the result of capillary glycaemia. *Journal of Clinical and Molecular Endocrinology.* http://www.clinical-and-molecular-endocrinology.1medpub.com

Lima, M. F. S. d., Oliveira, L. P. d., Cabral, N. L. d. A., Liberalino, L. C. P., Bagni, U. V., Lima, K. C. d. & Lyra, C. d. O. (2018). Estimating the height of elderly nursing home residents: Which equation to use? *PLOS ONE, 13*(10). https://doi.org/10.1371/journal.pone.0205642

Limbert, E. & Santy-Tomlinson, J. (2017). Acute limb compartment syndrome in the lower leg following trauma: Assessment in the intensive care unit. *Nursing Standard, 31*(34), 61. https://doi.org/10.7748/ns.2017.e10708

Lin, F. & Buckley, T. (2019). Cardiovascular assessment and monitoring. In L. Aitken, A. Marshall & W. Chaboyer (eds), *Critical care nursing* (4th ed.). Chatswood, NSW: Elsevier.

Lin, J., Fu, Y., Lin, Y., Yang, H., Zhang, X. & Zhan, Y. (2023). The value of non-contact infrared thermometer in measuring temperatures of different body surfaces: A clinical diagnostic study. *Journal of Health and Environmental Research, 9*(2), 43–50. https://doi.org/10.11648/j.jher.20230902.11

Lin, W. Q., Wu, H. H., Su, C. S., Yang, J. T., Xiao, J. R., Cai, Y. P., Wu, X. Z. & Chen, G. Z. (2017). Comparison of continuous noninvasive blood pressure monitoring by TL-300 with standard invasive blood pressure measurement in patients undergoing elective neurosurgery. *Journal of Neurosurgical Anesthesiology, 29*(1), 1–7. https://doi.org/10.1097/ANA.0000000000000245

Lins, R. (2023). A randomized n-of-1 study comparing blood pressure measured on a clothed arm and on an arm with a rolled-up sleeve. *Acta Clinica Belgica.* https://doi.org/10.1080/17843286.2023

Liu, C., Griffiths, C., Murray, A. & Zheng, D. (2016). Comparison of stethoscope bell and diaphragm and of stethoscope tube length for clinical blood pressure measurement. *Blood Pressure Monitoring, 21*(3), 178–83.

Loewy, M. (2023).Three 'synergistic' problems when taking blood pressure. *Medscape Nurses.* https://www.medscape.com/viewarticle/992902?ecd=wnl_tp10_daily_230607_MSCPEDIT_etid5505767&uac=264686HZ&impID=55 05767

Ma, C. & Zhou, W. (2022). Effects of unfolding case-based learning on academic achievement, critical thinking, and self-confidence in undergraduate nursing students learning health assessment skills. *Nurse Education in Practice, 60.* https://doi.org/10.1016/j.nepr.2022.103321

Mah, A. J., Ghazi Zadeh, L., Khoshnam Tehrani, M., Askari, S., Gandjbakhche, A. H. & Shadgan, B. (2021). Studying the accuracy and function of different thermometry techniques for measuring body temperature. *Biology, 10*(12), 1327. https://doi.org/10.3390/biology10121327

Majder, K., Więch, P., Wojniak, A. & Bazaliński, D. (2020). Knowledge and skills in chest auscultation among nurses. *Pielegniarstwo XXI wieku/Nursing in the 21st Century, 19*(4), 251–7. https://doi.org/10.2478/pielxxiw-2020-0020

Man, H., Veloo, C., Kaur, G., Nazeri, N., Chandrakasan, V., Wah, Y. & Hua, K. (2023). Comparing the accuracy of temperature measurement between infrared forehead thermometer and tympanic thermometer. *Journal of Survey in Fisheries Science, 10*(4S), special issue 4. https://doi.org/10.17762/sfs.v10i4S.764

Marchand, M. & Gin, K. (2022). The cardiovascular system in heat stroke. *Canadian Journal of Cardiology Open, 4*(2), 158–63. https://doi.org/10.1016/j.cjco.2021.10.002

Marston, H. R., Hadley, R., Banks, D. & Duro, M. D. (2019). Mobile self-monitoring ECG devices to diagnose arrhythmia that coincide with palpitations: A scoping review. *Healthcare, 7*(3), 96. https://doi.org/10.3390/healthcare7030096

Martin, A., Zepeda, E. & Lescas Méndez, O. (2017). Bedside ultrasound measurement of rectus femoris: A tutorial for the nutrition support clinician. *Journal of Nutrition and Metabolism*. https://doi.org/10.1155/2017/2767232

Martin, M., Knazovicka, L., Mcevoy, H., Machin, G., Pusnik, I., Cardenas, D., Sadli, M., Chengdu, B., Li, W., Saunders, P. & Girard, F. (2022). *Best practice guide use of infrared ear thermometers to perform traceable non-contact measurements of human body temperature.* Istituto Nazionale Di Ricerca Metrologica Repository Istituzionale. https://iris.inrim.it/bitstream/11696/75939/1/Best%20Practice%20Guide%20for%20Infrared%20Ear%20Thermometers.pdf

Martos-Cabrera, M., Velando-Soriano, A., Pradas-Hernandez, L., Suleiman-Martos, N., Canadas-De-lad Fuente, G., Albendin-Garcia, L. & Gome-Urquiza, J. (2020). Smartphones and apps to control glycosylated hemoglobin (HbA1c) level in diabetes: A systematic review and meta-analysis. *Journal of Clinical Medicine, 9*(3), 693. https://doi.org/10.3390/jcm9030693

Marui, S., Misawa, A., Tanaka, Y. & Nagashima, K. (2017). Assessment of axillary temperature for the evaluation of normal body temperature of healthy young adults at rest in a thermoneutral environment. *Journal of Physiological Anthropology, 36*(1), 18. https://doi.org/10.1186/s40101-017-0133-y

Mathew, T., Zubair, M. & Tadi, P. (2023). Blood glucose monitoring. In *StatPearls*. Treasure Island (FL): StatPearls Publishing. PMID: 32310436. https://www.ncbi.nlm.nih.gov/books/NBK555976

Mattu, A., Grossman, S., Rossen, P., Anderson, R., Carpenter, C., Chang, A., Hirshon, J., Hwang, U., Kennedy, M., Melady, D., Tolia, V. & Wilber, S. (2016). *Geriatric emergencies: A discussion based review.* Oxford, UK: Wiley-Blackwell.

McClean, K., Cross, M. & Reed, S. (2021). Risks to healthcare organizations and staff who manage obese (bariatric) patients and use of obesity data to mitigate risks: A literature review. *Journal of Multidisciplinary Healthcare, 14*, 577–88. https://doi.org/10.2147/JMDH.S289676

McStay, S. (2019). Recording a 12-lead electrocardiogram (ECG). *British Journal of Nursing, 28*(12), 756–60. https://doi.org/10.12968/bjon.2019.28.12.756

Mechanic, O., Gavin, M., Grossman, S. A. & Ziegler, K. (2022). Acute myocardial infarction (nursing). *Stat Pearls, National Library of Medicine*. https://www.ncbi.nlm.nih.gov/books/NBK568759

Medani, S., Hensey, M., Caples, N. & Owens, P. (2018). Accuracy in precordial ECG lead placement: Improving performance through a peer-led educational intervention. *Journal of Electrocardiology, 51*(1), 50–4. https://doi.org/10.1016/j.jelectrocard.2017.04.018

Mehta, R. & Chinthapalli, K. (2019). Glasgow Coma Scale explained. *BMJ: British Medical Journal (Online), 365*. https://doi.org/10.1136/bmj.l1296

Menzies-Gow, E. (2018). How to record a 12-lead electrocardiogram. *Nursing Standard (2014+), 33*(2), 38. https://doi.org/10.7748/ns.2018.e11066

Meo, S. A., Altuwaym, A. A., Alfallaj, R. M., Alduraibi, K. A., Alhamoudi, A. M., Alghamdi, S. M. & Akram, A. (2019). Effect of obesity on cognitive function among school adolescents: A cross-sectional study. *Obesity Facts, 12*(2), 150–6. https://karger.com/ofa/article/12/2/150/240904/Effect-of-Obesity-on-Cognitive-Function-among

Mikkelsen, M., Still, M., Anderson, B., Bienvenu, O., Brodsky, M., Brummel, N., Butcher, B., Clay, A., Felt, H., Ferrante, L., Haines, K., Harhay, M., Hope, A., Hopkins, R., Hosey, M., Hough, C., Jackson, J., Johnson, A., Khan, B., Lone, N., MacTavish, P., McPeake, J., Montgomery-Yates, A., Needham, D., Netzer, G., Schorr, C., Skidmore, B., Stollings, J., Umberger, R., Andrews, A., Iwashyna, T. & Sevin, C. (2020). Society of critical care medicine's international consensus conference on prediction and identification of long-term impairments after critical illness. *Critical Care Medicine, 49*(11), 1670–9. https://doi.org/10.1097/CCM.0000000000004586

Mirajkar, A., Morales-Cruz, M., Fusco, N., Dub, L. & Ganti, L. (2022). Compartment syndrome secondary to vascular transection from a knee dislocation. *Orthopedic Reviews* (Pavia), *14*(3), 36907. https://doi.org/10.52965/001c.36907

Nadolsky, K., Addison, B., Agarwal, M., Almandoz, J., Bird, M., Chaplin, M., Garvey, W. & Kyle, T. (2023). *American Association of Clinical Endocrinology Consensus Statement: Addressing stigma and bias in the diagnosis and management of patients with obesity/adiposity-based chronic disease and assessing bias and stigmatization as determinants of disease severity.* https://doi.org/10.1016/j.eprac.2023.03.272

Nathan, V., Vatanparvar, K., Rahman, M., Nemati, E. & Kuang, J. (2019). *Assessment of chronic pulmonary disease patients using biomarkers from natural speech recorded by mobile devices.* IEEE 16th International Conference on Wearable and Implantable Body Sensor Networks (BSN), Chicago, IL, USA, 2019, pp. 1–4.

National Center for Chronic Disease Prevention and Health Promotion (2020). *Division of nutrition, physical activity and obesity.* https://www.cdc.gov/nccdphp/dnpao

National Nurses Nutrition Group (2017). *Good practice guideline – for accurate body weight measurement using weighing scales in adults and children.* http://www.nnng.org.uk/wp-content/uploads/2017/02/Accurate-Body-Weight-Measurement-GPG-Final-draft-Feb17.pdf

Nursing and Midwifery Board of Australia (NMBA) (2016). *Registered nurse standards for practice.* Dickson, ACT: Nursing and Midwifery Board of Australia.

Ohns, M., Walsh, E. & Douglas, Z. (2019). Acute compartment syndrome in children: Don't miss this elusive diagnosis. *Journal for Nurse Practitioners, 16*(1), 19–22. https://doi.org/10.1016/j.nurpra.2019.07.012

Olinic, D-M., Stanek, A., Tătaru, D-A., Homorodean, C. & Olinic, M. (2019). Acute limb ischemia: An update on diagnosis and management. *Journal of Clinical Medicine, 8*(8), 1215. https://doi.org/10.3390/jcm8081215

Olshansky, B., Ricci, F. & Fedorowski, A. (2022). Importance of resting heart rate. *Trends in Cardiovascular Medicine, 33*(8), 502–15. https://doi.org/10.1016/j.tcm.2022.05.006

Owida, H., Al-Nabulsi, J., Ma'touq, J., Al-Naami, B. & Alnaimat, F. (2022). Validation of earlobe site as an alternative blood glucose testing approach. *Technology and Health Care, 30*(6), 1535–41. https://doi.org/10.3233/THC-220033

Ozone, S., Shaku, F., Sato, M., Takayashiki, A., Tsutsumi, M. & Maaeno, T. (2016). Comparison of blood pressure measurements on the bare arm, over a sleeve and over a rolled-up sleeve in the elderly. *Family Practice, 33*(5), 517–22. https://doi.org/10.1093/fampra/cmw053

Padwal, R., Campbell, N., Schutte, A., Olsen, M., Delles, C., Etyang, A., Cruickshank, J., Stergiou, G., Rakotz, M., Wozniak, G., Jaffe, M., Benjamin, I., Parati, G. & Sharman, J. (2019). Optimizing observer performance of clinic blood pressure measurement: A position statement from the Lancet Commission on Hypertension Group. *Journal of Hypertension, 37*(9), 1737–45. https://doi.org/10.1097/HJH.0000000000002112

Palese, A., Fabbro, E., Casetta, A. & Mansutti, J. (2016). First or second drop of blood in capillary glucose monitoring: Findings from a qualitative study. *Journal of Emergency Nursing, 42*(5), 420–6.

Palk, L. (2019). Assessing and managing the acute complications of diabetes mellitus. *Nursing Standard (2014+), 34*(1), 59. https://doi.org/10.7748/ns.2018.e11250

Palmer, J. H., James, S., Wadsworth, D., Gordon, C. J. & Craft, J. (2022). How registered nurses are measuring respiratory rates in adult acute care health settings: An integrative review. *Journal of Clinical Nursing, 00*, 1– 13. https://doi.org/10.1111/jocn.16522

Pertzov, B., Brachfeld, E., Unterman, A., Gershman, E., Abdel-Rahman, N., Rosengarten, D. & Kramer, M. (2019). Significant delay in the detection of desaturation between finger transmittance and earlobe reflectance oximetry probes during fiberoptic bronchoscopy: Analysis of 104 cases. *Lung, 197*(67), 67–72. https://doi.org/10.1007/s00408-018-0180-0

Peters, M. (2017). *Pain assessment following stroke.* Adelaide, SA: Joanna Briggs Institute.

Phillips, M., Kuruvilla, V. & Bailey, M. (2019). Implementation of the Critical Care Pain Observation Tool increases the frequency of pain assessment for noncommunicative ICU patients. *Australian Critical Care, 32*(5), 367–72. https://doi.org/10.1016/j.aucc.2018.08.007

Pilcher, J., Ploen, L., McKinstry, S., Bardsley, G., Chien, J., Howard, L., Lee, S., Beckert, L., Swanney, M., Weatherall, M. & Beasley, R. (2020). A multicentre prospective observational study comparing arterial blood gas values to those obtained by pulse oximeters used in adult patients attending Australian and New Zealand hospitals. *BMC Pulmonary Medicine, 20*(7). https://doi.org/10.1186/s12890-019-1007-3

Pratley, R. E., Kanapka, L. G., Rickels, M. R., et al. for the Wireless Innovation for Seniors With Diabetes Mellitus (WISDM) Study Group (2020). Effect of continuous glucose monitoring on hypoglycemia in older adults with type 1 diabetes: A randomized clinical trial. *Journal of the American Medical Association, 323*(23), 2397–406. https://doi.org/doi:10.1001/jama.2020.6928

Premalatha, J. & Prince, P. G. (2019). Analysis of non-invasive methods to diagnose blood glucose level: A survey. *Research Journal of Pharmacy and Technology, 12*(6), 3105–8. https://doi.org/10.5958/0974-360X.2019.00525.0

Pretto, J. J., Roebuck, T., Beckert, L. & Hamilton, G. (2014). Clinical use of pulse oximetry: Official guidelines from Thoracic Society of Australia and New Zealand. *Respirology, 19*, 38–46. https://doi.org/10.1111/resp.12204

Puhl, R. (2016). Health professional: Do you have a hidden weight bias? *Medscape Nurses.* http://www.medscape.com/viewarticle/872071

Rahimi, G., Yousefabadi, H., Niyazi, A., Rahimi, N. & Alikhajeh, Y. (2022). Effects of lifestyle intervention on inflammatory markers and waist circumference in overweight/obese adults with metabolic syndrome: A systematic review and metaanalysis of randomized controlled trials. *Biological Research for Nursing, 24*(1) 94–105. https://doi.org/10.1177/10998004211044754

Ratero, L., Andre, J., dos Santos, E., Castiglioni, L., Aparecide, N., de Almeida, S. & Bertolin, D. (2020). Human anatomy and clinical nursing practice. *Journal of Nursing Education and Practice, 10*(10). http://jnep.sciedupress.com

Reece, R. & Hughes, M. (2022). Are digital oral thermometer readings accurate in adult emergency department patients? *Cureus, 14*(2), e22047. https://doi.org/10.7759/cureus.22047

Reinhorn, M. (2020). *Umbilical hernias.* https://bostonhernia.com

Ricciardi, D., Cavallari, I., Creta, A., Di Giovanni, G., Calabrese, V., Di Belardino, N., Mega, S., Colaiori, I., Ragni, L., Proscia, C., Nenna, A. & Di Sciascio, G. (2016). Impact of the high-frequency cutoff of bandpass filtering on ECG quality and clinical interpretation: A comparison between 40 Hz and 150 Hz cutoff in a surgical preoperative adult outpatient population. *Journal of Electrocardiology, 49*(5), 691–5. https://doi.org/10.1016/j.jelectrocard.2016.07.002

Richter, D., Guasti, L., Lionis, C., Abreu, A., Savelieva, I., Fumagali, S., Bo, M., Rocca, B., Jensen, M., Pierard, L., Sudano, I., Aboyans, V. & Asteggiano, R. (2022). Frailty in cardiology: Definition, assessment and clinical implications for general cardiology. A consensus document of the Council for Cardiology Practice (CCP), Association for Acute Cardio Vascular Care (ACVC), Association of Cardiovascular Nursing and Allied Professions (ACNAP), European Association of Preventive Cardiology (EAPC), European Heart Rhythm Association (EHRA), Council on Valvular Heart Diseases (VHD), Council on Hypertension (CHT), Council of Cardio-Oncology (CCO), Working Group (WG) Aorta and Peripheral Vascular Diseases, WG e-Cardiology, WG Thrombosis, of the European Society of Cardiology, European Primary Care Cardiology Society (EPCCS). *European Journal of Preventive Cardiology, 29*(1), 216–27. https://doi.org/10.1093/eurjpc/zwaa167

Rimbi, M., Dunsmuir, D., Ansermino, J., Nakitende, I., Namujwiga, T. & Kellett, J. on behalf of the Kitovu Hospital Study Group (2019). Respiratory rates observed over 15 and 30s compared with rates measured over 60s: Practice-based evidence from an observational study of acutely ill adult medical patients during hospital admission. *QJM: An International Journal of Medicine, 112*(7), 513–17. https://doi.org/10.1093/qjmed/hcz065

Roberts, H. C., Lim, S., Cox, N. & Ibrahim, K. (2019). The challenge of managing undernutrition in older people with frailty. *Nutrients, 11*, 808. https://doi.org/10.3390/nu11040808

Rong, Y. D., Bian, A. L., Hu, H. Y., Ma, Y. & Zhou, X. Z. (2020). A cross-sectional study of the relationships between different components of sarcopenia and brachial ankle pulse wave velocity in community-dwelling elderly. *BMC Geriatrics, 20*, 1–8. https://link.springer.com/article/10.1186/s12877-020-01525-8

Royal Children's Hospital Melbourne (RCHM) (2019). *Clinical guidelines: Neurovascular observations.* http://www.rch.org.au/rchcpg/hospital_clinical_guideline_index/Neurovascular_observations

Royal Children's Hospital Melbourne (RCHM) (2020). *Clinical guidelines: Cardiac telemetry.* https://www.rch.org.au/rchcpg/hospital_clinical_guideline_index/Cardiac_Telemetry

Samani, S. & Rattani, S. (2023). Recognizing early warning signs (EWS) in patients is critically important. *Open Journal of Nursing, 13*, 53–64. https://doi.org/10.4236/ojn.2023.131004

Sapra, A., Malik, A. & Bhandari, P. (2023). Vital sign assessment. In *StatPearls*, Treasure Island, FL: StatPearls Publishing. https://europepmc.org/article/nbk/nbk553213#free-full-text

Satoh, M., Miura, T. & Shimada, T. (2023). Development and evaluation of a simple predictive model for falls in acute care setting. *Journal of Clinical Nursing, 00*, 1–11. https://doi.org/10.1111/jocn.16680

Schick, D. (2023). The do's and don'ts of sternal rub. *Allnurses.* https://allnurses.com/the-dos-donts-sternal-rubs-t454289

Schreiber, M. L. (2016). Neurovascular assessment: An essential nursing focus. *Medsurg Nursing, 25*(1), 55–7. https://search.proquest.com/docview/1765639194?accountid=88802

Schroeder, C., Hengel, R., Nathan, R., Ritter, T., Obi, E., Lancaster, C. Van Anglen, L. & Garey, K. (2022). Appropriate cleaning reduces potential risk of spore transmission from patients with *Clostridioides difficile* infection treated in outpatient infusion centers. *Anaerobe, 77.* https://doi.org/10.1016/j.anaerobe.2022.102617

Schutte, A. E., Kollias, A. & Stergiou, G. S. (2022). Blood pressure and its variability: Classic and novel measurement techniques. *Nature Reviews Cardiology, 19*, 643–52. https://doi.org/10.1038/s41569-022-00690-0

Scuteri, D., Contrada, M., Loria, T., Tonin, P., Sandrini, G., Tamburin, S., Nicotera, P., Bagetta, G. & Corasaniti, M. T. (2022). Pharmacological treatment of pain and agitation in severe dementia and responsiveness to change of the Italian Mobilization–Observation–Behavior–Intensity–Dementia (I-MOBID2) Pain Scale: Study protocol. *Brain Sciences, 12*(5), 573. https://doi.org/10.3390/brainsci12050573

Seidlerová, J., Tumová, P., Rokyta, R. & Hromadka, M. (2019). Factors influencing the accuracy of non-invasive blood pressure measurements in patients admitted for cardiogenic shock. *BMC Cardiovascular Disorders, 19*(150). https://doi.org/10.1186/s12872-019-1129-9

Shahiri, T. & Gélinas, C. (2023). The validity of vital signs for pain assessment in critically ill adults: A narrative review. *Pain Management Nursing, 24*(3), 318–28. https://doi.org/10.1016/j.pmn.2023.01.004

Sharif Nia, H., Chong, P. P., Yiong Huak, C., Gorgulu, O., Taghipour, B., Sivarajan Froelicher, E., Sharif, S. & Rahmatpour, P. (2022). Clinical accuracy and agreement between tympanic and forehead body temperature measurements for screening of patients with COVID-19. *Journal of Clinical Nursing, 31*(21–22), 3272–85. https://onlinelibrary.wiley.com/doi/abs/10.1111/jocn.16166

Sharma, A. P., Kirpalani, A., Sharma, A., Altamirano-Diaz, L., Filler, G. & Noroz, K. (2023). Impact of the 2022 American Heart Association pediatric ambulatory blood pressure monitoring statement on the diagnosis of hypertension. *Pediatric Nephrology, 38*, 2741–51. https://doi.org/10.1007/s00467-022-05856-z

Sharman, J., Tan, I., Stergiou, G., Lombardi, C., Salsdini, F., Butlin, M., Padwal, R., Asayama, K., Avolio, A., Brady, T., Murray, A. & Parati, G. (2023a). Automated 'oscillometric' blood pressure measuring devices: How they work and what they measure. *Journal of Human Hypertension, 37*, 93–100. https://doi.org/10.1038/s41371-022-00693-x

Sharman, J. E., Ordunez, P., Brady, T., Parati, G., Stergiou, G., Whelton P., Padwal, R., Olsen, M., Delles, C., Schutte, A., Tomaszewskil, M., Iackland, D., Khan, N., McManus, R., Tsuyiki, R., Zhang, X., Murphy, L., Moran, A., Schlaich, M. & Campbell, N. (2023b). The urgency to regulate validation of automated blood pressure measuring devices: A policy statement and call to action from the world hypertension league. *Journal of Human Hypertension, 37*, 155–9. https://doi.org/10.1038/s41371-022-00747-0

Shear, D. (2023). Fatima Cody Stanford: Changing the narrative on obesity. *Lancet Perspectives (Profile), 401*(10389). https://www.thelancet.com/journals/lancet/article/PIIS0140-6736(23)00972-8/fulltext

Sheppard, J., Albasri, A., Franssen, M., Fletcher, B., Pealing, L., Roberts, N., Obeid, A., Pucci, M., McManus, R. & Martin, U. (2020). Measurement of blood pressure in the leg: A statement on behalf of the British and Irish Hypertension Society. *Journal of Human Hypertension, 34*, 418–19. https://doi.org/10.1038/s41371-020-0325-5

Shinozaki, K., Jacobson, L. S., Saeki, K., Hirahara, H., Kobayashi, N., Weisner, S., Falotico, J., Li, T., Kim, J. & Becker, L. (2019). Comparison of point-of-care peripheral perfusion assessment using pulse oximetry sensor with manual capillary refill time: Clinical pilot study in the emergency department. *Journal of Intensive Care, 7*(52). https://doi.org/10.1186/s40560-019-0406-0

Showlag, J., Al-Hejin, A., Bataweel, N. & Abu-Zaid. M. (2021). Microbiota molecular identification in the daycare unit in the hospital. *Journal of Applied Sciences Research, 17*(4), 1–5. https://doi.org/10.22587/jasr.2021.17.4.1

Siedlinski, M., Carnevale, L., Xu, X., Carnevale, D., Evangelou, C., Caulfield, M., Maffia, P., Wardlaw, J., Samani, N., Tomaszewski, M., Lembo, G., Holmes, M. & Guzik, T. (2023). Genetic analyses identify brain structures related to cognitive impairment associated with elevated blood pressure. *European Heart Journal*. https://doi.org/10.1093/eurheartj/ehad101

Sillner, A., Berish, D., Mailhot, T., Sweeder, L., Fick, D. & Kolanowski, A. (2023). Delirium superimposed on dementia in post-acute care: Nurse documentation of symptoms and interventions. *Geriatric Nursing, 49*, 122–6. https://doi.org/10.1016/j.gerinurse.2022.11.015

Silva, F. M. & Figueira, L. (2017). Estimated height from knee height or ulna length and self-reported height are no substitute for actual height in inpatients. *Nutrition, 33*, 52–6. https://doi.org/10.1016/j.nut.2016.08.011

Snaith, J. & Holmes-Walker, D. J. (2021).Technologies in the management of type 1 diabetes. *Medical Journal of Australia Perspectives, 214*(5). https://doi.org/10.5694/ mja2.50946

Sonawane, K., Dhamotharan, P., Dixit, H. & Gurumoorthi, P. (2022). Coping with the fear of compartment syndrome without compromising analgesia: A narrative review. *Cureus Online Open Review*. https://assets.cureus.com/uploads/review_article/pdf/121324/20221127-15920-1lza72p.pdf

Sowan, A., Vera, A., Malshe, A. & Reed, C. (2019). Transcription errors of blood glucose values and insulin errors in an intensive care unit: Secondary data analysis toward electronic medical record-glucometer interoperability. *Journal of Medical Informatics Research, 7*(1). https://doi.org/10.2196/11873

Staines, D., Sheridan, S. & Pickering, G. (2020). Respiratory assessment. In S. Wills & R. Dalrymple (eds), *Fundamentals of paramedic practice: A systems approach*. Chichester, UK: Wiley Blackwell.

Starr, K., McDonald, S., Weidner, J. & Bales, C. (2016). Challenges in the management of geriatric obesity in high risk populations. *Nutrients, 8*(5), 262. https://doi.org/10.3390/nu8050262

Stergiou, G., Mukkamala, R., Avolio, A., Kyriakoulis, K., Mieke, S., Murray, A., Parati, G., Schutte, A., Sharman, J., Asmar, R., McManus, R., Asayama, K., De La Sierra, A., Head, G., Kario, K., Kollias, A., Myers, M., Niiranen, T., Ohkubo, T., Wang, J., Wuerzner, G., O'Brien, E., Kreutz, R. & Palatini, P. (2022). Cuffless blood pressure measuring devices: Review and statement by the European Society of Hypertension Working Group on Blood Pressure Monitoring and Cardiovascular Variability. *Journal of Hypertension, 40*(8), 1449–60. https://doi.org/10.1097/HJH.0000000000003224

Stergiou, G., Palatini, P., Parati, G., O'Brien, E., Januszewicz, A., Lurbe, E., Persu, A., Mancia, G. & Kreutz, R. (2021). European Society of Hypertension practice guidelines for office and out-of-office blood pressure measurement. *Journal of Hypertension, 39*(7), 1293–302, https://doi.org/10.1097/HJH.0000000000002843

Stokes, A., Xie, W., Lundberg, D., Hempstead, K., Zajacova, A., Zimmer, Z., Glei, D., Meara, E. & Preston, S. (2020). Increases in BMI and chronic pain for US adults in midlife, 1992 to 2016. *Population Health, 12*, 100644. https://doi.org/10.1016/j.ssmph.2020.100644

Stonko, D., Etchill, E., Giuliano, K., DiBrito, S., Eisenson, D., Heinrichs, T., Morrison, J. & Haut, E. (2021). Failure to rescue in geriatric trauma: The impact of any complication increases with age and injury severity in elderly trauma patients. *The American Surgeon™, 87*(11), 1760–5. https://doi.org/10.1177/00031348211054072

Sunil, K., Savita, K., Neelam, K., Gireesh, D., Sunita, D. & Ravi, B. (2023). Obesity: An important predictor of metabolic syndrome. *Scripta Medica, 54*(1), 81–5. https://scindeks.ceon.rs/Article.aspx?artid=2490-33292301081K

Takayama, A., Nagamine, T. & Kotani, K. (2019). Aging is independently associated with an increasing normal respiratory rate among an older adult population in a clinical setting: A cross-sectional study. *Geriatrics and Gerontology International, 19*, 1179–83. https://doi.org/10.1111/ggi.13788

Thunyacharoen, S., Mahakkanukrauh, C., Pattayakornkul, N., Meetham, K., Charumporn, T. & Mahakkanukrauh, P. (2022). Anatomical variations of the dorsalis pedis artery in a Thai population. *International Journal of Morphology, 40*(1), 137–42. http://www.intjmorphol.com/wpcontent/uploads/2022/02/art_22_401.pdf

Tochihara, Y., Yamashita, K., Fujii, K., Kaji, Y., Wakabayashi, H. & Kitahara, H. (2021). Thermoregulatory and cardiovascular responses in the elderly towards a broad range of gradual air temperature changes. *Journal of Thermal Biology, 99*, 103007. https://doi.org/10.1016/j.jtherbio.2021.103007

Toney-Butler, T. & Unison-Pace, W. (2019). *Nursing admission assessment and examination. StatPearls.* StatPearls Publishing, Treasure Island (FL). https://europepmc.org/article/NBK/NBK493211

Towell-Barnard, A. (2019). Weight bias and stigma: How do we really feel about the obese patient? *Journal of Stomal Therapy Australia, 39*(3), 8–10. https://doi.org/10.33235/jsta.39.3.8-10

Unsworth, J., Tucker, G. & Hindmarsh, Y. (2015). Man versus machine: The importance of manual blood pressure measurement skills amongst registered nurses. *International Journal of Hospital Administration, 4*(6). https://doi.org/10.5430/jha.v4n6p61

Urden, L., Stacy, K. & Long, M. (2017). *Critical care nursing: Diagnosis and management* (8th ed.). St Louis, MO: Elsevier.

Valenzuela, P. L., Carrera-Bastos, P., Castillo-García, A., Lieberman, D., Santos-L ozano, A. & Lucia, A. (2023). Obesity and the risk of cardiometabolic diseases. *Nature Reviews Cardiology, 20*, 475–94. https://doi.org/10.1038/s41569-023-00847-5

van Steen, Y., Ntarladima, A., Grobbee, R., Karssenberg, D. & Vaartjex, I. (2019). Sex differences in mortality after heat waves: Are elderly women at higher risk? *International Archives of Occupational and Environmental Health, 92*, 37–48. https://doi.org/10.1007/s00420-018-1360-1

van Zundert, A., Intaprasert, T., Wiepking, F. & Eley, V. (2022). Are non-contact thermometers an option in anaesthesia? A narrative review on thermometry for perioperative medicine. *Healthcare, 10*(2), 219. https://www.mdpi.com/2227-9032/10/2/219

Vardasca, R., Magalhaes, C., Marques, D., Moreira, J., Frade, R. A., Seixas, A., Mendes, J. G. & Ring, F. (2019). Bilateral assessment of body core temperature through axillar, tympanic and inner canthi thermometers in a young population. *Physiological Measurement, 40*, 094001. https://pubmed.ncbi.nlm.nih.gov/31216516

Victorian Government (2015). Falls Risk Assessment Tool. https://www.health.vic.gov.au/publications/falls-risk-assessment-tool-frat

Voss, R. & Das, J. (2022). Mental status examination. *Stat Pearls.* https://europepmc.org/article/MED/31536288/NBK546682#free-full-text

Wang, J., Fang, P., Sun, G. & Li, M. (2022). Effect of active forced air warming during the first hour after anesthesia induction and intraoperation avoids hypothermia in elderly patients. *BioMedCentral Anesthesiology, 22*, 40. https://doi.org/10.1186/s12871-022-01577-w

Weinstock, R. (2023). Patent education: Glucose monitoring in diabetes (beyond the basics). *UpToDate.* https://www.uptodate.com/contents/glucose-monitoringin-diabetes-beyond-the-basics

Werner, A. & Gunga, H. C. (2020). Monitoring of core body temperature in humans. In A. Choukèr (ed.), *Stress challenges and immunity in space.* Cham, Switzerland: Springer.

Wharton, S., Lau, D., Vallis, M., Sharma, A., Biertho, I., Campbell-Scherer, D., Adamo, K., Alberga, A., Bell, R., … & Wicklum, S. (2020). Obesity in adults: A clinical practice guideline. *Canadian Medical Association Journal, 192*(31), E875–E891. https://doi.org/10.1503/cmaj.191707

Wideman, T., Edwards, R., Walton, D., Martel, M., Hudon, A. & Seminowicz, D. (2019). The multimodal assessment model of pain: A novel framework for further integrating the subjective pain experience within research and practice. *Clinical Journal of Pain, 35*(3), 212–21. https://doi.org/10.1097/AJP.0000000000000670

Wilson, O., Bopp, C., Papalia, Z. & Bopp, M. (2019). Objective vs self-report assessment of height, weight and body mass index: Relationships with adiposity, aerobic fitness and physical activity. *Clinical Obesity, 9*(5). https://doi.org/10.1111/cob.12331

Wood, C., Chaboyer, W. & Carr, P. (2019). How do nurses use early warning scoring systems to detect and act on patient deterioration to ensure patient safety? A scoping review. *International Journal of Nursing Studies, 94*, 166–78. https://doi.org/10.1016/j.ijnurstu.2019.03.012

World Health Organization: Patient Safety (2011). *Pulse oximetry training manual.* https://cdn.who.int/media/docs/defaultsource/patient-safety/pulse-oximetry/who-ps-pulse-oxymetry-training-manual-en.pdf?sfvrsn=322cb7ae_6

Wright, J. J., Williams, A. J., Friedman, S. B., Weaver, R., Williams, J. M., Hodge, E., Fowler, M. & Bao, S. (2022). Accuracy of continuous glucose monitors for inpatient diabetes management. *Journal of Diabetes Science and Technology, 17*(5). https://doi.org/10.1177/19322968221076562

Xie, T., Qi, X., Xing, Z., Yingmu ,T., Hong, R., Chang, L. & Jingyao, Z. (2022). Construction and validation of a nomogram for predicting survival in elderly patients with cardiac surgery. *Frontiers in Public Health, 10*(Oct.). https://doi.org/10.3389/fpubh.2022.972797

Xiong, Y., Pan, G., Huang, W., Yang, W., Hu, R., Mai, Y., Chen, L. Miao, J. & Peng, X. (2022). Accuracy of oxygen saturation measurements in patients with obesity undergoing bariatric surgery. *Obesity Surgery*, 32, 3581–8. https://doi.org/10.1007/s11695-022-06221-7

Yamaguchi, R., Katayama, O., Lee, S., Makino, K., Harada, K., Morikawa, M., ... & Shimada, H. (2023). Association of sarcopenia and systolic blood pressure with mortality: A 5-year longitudinal study. *Archives of Gerontology and Geriatrics, 110*, 104988. https://www.sciencedirect.com/science/article/abs/pii/S0167494323000675

Yang, S., Huang, H., Yeh, T-F., Shen, C-H., Wu, C-L., Y-J., Wu, C-C. & Hung, C-J. (2023). Differences in pain assessments between inpatients and nurses leads to considerable misestimated pain. *Pain Physician, 26*, 61–8. https://www.painphysicianjournal.com/current/pdf?article=NzYyNQ%3D%3D&journal=150

Yıldırım, D. í., Eryılmaz, M. A. & Aydın, M. (2020). Examination of patients' regular participation at an obesity center to evaluate the effects on mental status and blood parameters. *Journal of Obesity and Metabolic Syndrome, 29*(2), 150–7. https://doi.org/10.7570/jomes20030

Younes, J., Chen, M., Ghali, K., Kosonen, R., Melikov, A. & Ghaddar, N. (2023). A thermal sensation model for elderly under steady and transient uniform conditions. *Building and Environment, 227*, Part 2, 109797. https://doi.org/10.1016/j.buildenv.2022.109797

Youngcharoen, P. & Aree-Ue, S. (2023). A cross-sectional study of factors associated with nurses' postoperative pain management practices for older patients. *Nursing Open, 10*, 90–8. https://doi.org/10.1002/nop2.1281

Yuan, L., Chang, M. & Wang, J. (2021). Abdominal obesity, body mass index and the risk of frailty in community-dwelling older adults: A systematic review and meta-analysis. *Age and Ageing, 50*(4), 1118–28. https://doi.org/10.1093/ageing/afab039

Zoler, M. (2023). BMI is a flawed measure of obesity. What are alternatives? *Medscape Medical News.* https://www.medscape.com/viewarticle/991210

PART 4

PROFESSIONAL COMMUNICATION

25 CLINICAL HANDOVER

26 DOCUMENTATION

27 HEALTHCARE TEACHING

Note: These notes are summaries of the most important points in the assessments/procedures and are not exhaustive on the subject. References of the materials used to compile the information have been supplied. The student is expected to have learnt the material surrounding each skill as presented in the references. No single reference is complete on each subject.

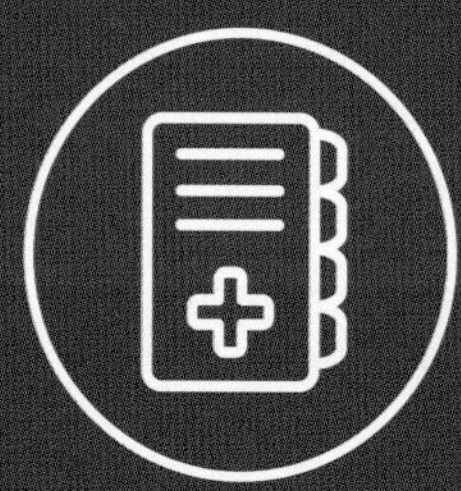

CHAPTER 25

CLINICAL HANDOVER

INDICATIONS

The clinical handover is a verbal report of the condition of a person or group of people. The handover occurs when you are relinquishing care of those people to another healthcare professional. The handover is 'the transfer of professional responsibility and accountability for some or all aspects of care for a patient, or group of patients, to another person or professional group on a temporary or permanent basis' (Australian Medical Association, 2006, p. 3). Handovers occur at change of shift within the care team, when the person is transferred to a different professional group, when the person is moving from one specialty area to another (e.g. from the emergency unit to the medical unit) and when the person is moving from one institution to another (e.g. from acute care to residential care or a community facility) (Australian Commission on Safety and Quality in Health Care [ACSQHC], 2021a).

The handover is vital because it provides safe continuity of care and efficiency by transmitting information (Ghonem & El-Husany, 2023). Handover helps nurses to provide quality care, maintain safety of those in their care and prevent adverse events (Le, Lee & Wilson, 2023). Failures in clinical handover are a major preventable cause of harm to people who use healthcare facilities (ACSQHC, 2012, p. 5). Effective handovers involve two dimensions of communication simultaneously – informational (i.e. content) and interactional (i.e. interpersonal communication styles) (Pun et al., 2020). Problems, errors and misunderstandings can be identified and resolved quickly if the receiving team/individual is encouraged to question, challenge and add information. As well, handovers should have pragmatic recommendations; that is, they should focus on the next shift's required actions as well as what has occurred during the shift just finishing (Awale, Bajracharya & Tviet, 2022).

Clinical handovers also help to update knowledge, build a sense of team, provide support, provide an opportunity for shared critical thinking, permit debriefing, provide informal teaching, and clarify information or point out the need for further action (ACSQHC, 2012). They also reduce stress among staff and increase job satisfaction. The use of a documented form (see the section 'Use a template') or one based on care plans ensures that information is consistent, accurate and timely.

IDENTIFY SAFETY CONSIDERATIONS

Safety

Miscommunication, including incomplete and unstructured clinical handovers, is a major contributing factor to critical incidents, mortality, risk and harm to people in hospitals (Eggins et al., 2019). Accurate knowledge of the person you are handing over is imperative, otherwise the handover is incomplete, which may jeopardise their comfort and safety. Missing, incorrect or 'old' information, or failure in communication, can jeopardise the person's recovery, delay diagnosis, decrease satisfaction with care given, increase the length of the hospital stay and increase the incidence of complications. In order for you and other healthcare professionals to plan and deliver excellent care, you must transfer complete, recent and relevant but concise information in a timely manner. Each person you are caring for should be attended at least hourly (e.g. clinical rounds).

You need to be aware of what information is important and what is superfluous. Use the facility's protocol. Use a consistent order to assist oncoming staff to follow the information (e.g. progressing through people on the unit by room numbers; using a template that is relevant to the unit).

There is another type of handover – a mini-handover, when a nurse is going off the unit (e.g. accompanying someone to X-ray, going on a meal break) for a short while. Another healthcare professional must be informed and becomes responsible for anyone in the 'leaving' nurse's care. Often, this is the team leader. They need to know:

- the identity of the person(s) in care
- any changes in their condition(s) since the start of the shift
- any concerns you have about them or their care
- any imminent care (e.g. intravenous [IV] running down, new bag at bedside, medications due in 20 minutes, pain levels rising with analgesic

ordered for a half-hour from now) to be done while you are off the unit.

Do not leave the unit without handing over an individual's care to another nurse.

ENVIRONMENT

The safety of the vulnerable people in care on the unit is jeopardised by interruptions and distraction creating barriers to effective handover (Vanderzwan et al., 2023). Private information about the person is being transmitted. Turn off mobile phones and pagers to minimise distractions. Interruptions during handover cause loss of concentration and can be minimised by the use of administrative staff and the nurses going off duty (who are not reporting during handover) as gatekeepers to minimise these interruptions (e.g. field telephone calls, answer call bells, see to alarms) (Mayor & Bangerter, 2015). Parallel conversations, superfluous noise and inattention are barriers to communication and thus the individual's safety (de Jesus Amorim et al., 2022). Other healthcare professionals (e.g. doctors, medical students, dietitians) will need education about times of handover and the critical need for uninterrupted reports to minimise mistakes and items being forgotten.

Many, if not most, hospitals in Australia use interactive bedside handovers, where the leaving nurse and the oncoming staff visit each person and, using a protocol, hand over the care of that person. Bedside handovers have proven to be more effective, efficient and safe for the person in care (Kalaf, 2023). The individual is asked for their input. Chien et al. (2022) found that both nurses and the people they care for prefer an interactive bedside handover. Bedside reports are reassuring for the individual. They involve them in their care and promote trust with the nurse, improves safety and a positive health care experience (Street et al., 2022). Healthcare professionals focus more on the person in care in their presence. Small staff numbers are preferred – only the nurse going off duty and the ones coming on makes for a more comfortable handover. Friends and relatives should also be welcome to remain if the person wishes.

With a bedside handover held in a person-centred way, the person in care is usually more positive, engaged and active in their discussion of their medical problems, and more connected to the oncoming nurses. But the handover must be interactional (i.e. actively involve the person). This can be accomplished by using the CARE protocol (Connect, Ask, Respond, Empathise) developed by Eggins and Slade (2016, cited in Chien et al., 2022). The person is introduced to the nurse who will provide care for the shift, and the nurse can 'put a face' to the person in their care. This increases safety. The individual is able to voice their needs and concerns, ask questions, confirm information, provide missing information, correct misconceptions and be kept more up to date with their care planning. A visual inspection of the devices (e.g. IVs, catheters, monitors) is also useful (Paredes-Garza, Lázaro & Vázquez, 2022). Ask the person to participate, ask their opinion, and ask about their condition and care.

If a bedside handover is the unit norm, clinical information may be overheard by other people (patients, visitors, uninvolved staff). In this case, keep voices low and refrain from personal comment other than what is strictly necessary. This will minimise the risk of compromising confidentiality. Johnson, Sanchez and Zheng (2016) suggest a two-step handover: a handover to the whole oncoming team at the nursing station, and then a more detailed one at the bedside for those nurses responsible for an individual's care.

TEAMWORK

Clinical handover is intricately entwined with working with others in a team (Terregino et al., 2023), where each nurse's role for the shift is assigned. Each nurse must work both alone and within a team (solitary teamwork [Nygaard et al., 2023]). Good teamwork is essential for the efficient, safe and effective care of people who are vulnerable, as well as for your engagement and satisfaction with your job and profession (Ruotsalainen et al., 2023). Good teamwork seems to improve the efficacy and efficiency of clinical handovers (Nygaard et al., 2023).

Teamwork can be fostered by:

- assisting others (even if they do not ask for your help, you can offer your abilities and time to lighten their burden if you have completed your work)
- tolerance of diversity
- a positive mindset
- being present and engaged with your work (e.g. paying attention during handovers)
- respecting others
- being fair
- openly communicating
- asking for assistance when you need it.

On the other hand, negativity (e.g. gossip, disrespect, incivility, bullying) can hamper or prevent the development of teamwork. These make the unit/facility a toxic and unpleasant workplace. Avoid negativity.

The team is not limited to nursing staff. Physicians, pharmacists, physiotherapists, dietitians, occupational therapists, chaplains and others become part of your team as the situation demands. Don't forget that the person in your care and their family become part of the team as well. They deserve your attention as part of the team (e.g. ensure open communication, positivity, respecting tolerance, and being present with them and listening to their thoughts and ideas).

USE A TEMPLATE

Handover requires preparation. Assess the person in your care and document the observations. Bring clinical notes up to date (e.g. analgesic administered, laboratory tests completed). It is important to take a few minutes to reflect on your shift and plan what you are going to say (Chan et al., 2023). A handover is a summary of the previous several hours and the current condition of the person. It identifies anticipated problems, imminent tasks and management plans. The content of handovers will be important for future clinical decision making (Samani & Rattani, 2023).

Using a template provides consistency, and using it for every handover assists those who are receiving the report to listen and assimilate the material more easily. Templates plus note taking increase retention of information as well as reducing information omission (Lazzari, 2024). Templates include prompts for basic information and reduce negative clinical management incidents (Awale, Bajracharya & Tviet, 2022). To keep track of information, prepare a table format similar to that shown in TABLE 25.1 or use a template that is used at the healthcare facility. It will have cells to note important information.

The report format ensures content quality and simplifies the communication of complex information. Each unit you work on will have developed a template for information deemed important in that unit. If your current unit does not have a template, use something like the generic one provided in TABLE 25.1. Many units are now providing pre-prepared electronic handover sheets that are up to date and contain all the information necessary to care for the person through the next shift. These are used to support a verbal handover that emphasises relevant aspects of care and allows for questions from oncoming staff and the person in care.

Paterson, Roberts and Bail (2022) suggest that any template should contain the following information (mnemonic is ISBAR):

- *I = Identification of the person* – ensures people are correctly identified; includes three identifiers (e.g. name, date of birth and medical record number).
- *S = Situation and status* – current clinical status (e.g. stable, deteriorating, improving), advanced directives and care requirements, including the prospect of discharge or transfer.
- *B = Background and history* – a summary of background, history (presenting problem, background problems and current issues), evaluation (physical examination and investigation findings, current diagnosis), management to date and effectiveness.
- *A = Assessment and actions* – the latest observations, all tasks to be completed, abnormal or pending results clearly communicated, an established and agreed management and escalation of care plan, a shared understanding of what conditions are being treated, a plan for communication to the senior healthcare professional in charge and clear accountability for actions.
- *R = Responsibility, recommendation, risk management and read back* – face-to-face handover best ensures the transfer of responsibility as staff are leaving the institution, and acceptance of tasks by the incoming team. This ideally includes accepting

TABLE 25.1 Suggested format for a clinical handover

INFORMATION	DESCRIPTION
Demographics	• Identification: name, hospital number, age, location (i.e. room number; if off the ward – where) • Attending doctor's name: often this is added here so that their protocols can be followed
History/complaint, treatment and/or diagnosis, surgery done if applicable	• This might be a combination of all three (e.g. chest pain last night, diagnosed with an MI within two hours and started on …) • Include comorbidities, date, type of surgery and postoperative day
Response to treatment, medications	Includes physical, psychological and emotional response to treatment initiated, alterations in medications or new medications ordered, and the response to medications
Tubes	IVs, nasogastric tubes; include site, fluid, amount, rate, time to change
Wound information	Drains, dressings used, changed; location, type and amount of drainage over the shift; changes due
Physical assessment, vital signs, pain assessment	• Note important information that indicates a change in condition; note normal only if it is a new finding. Ensure recency of information • Risks of harm, worries or concerns about clinical condition • Vital signs are perceived to be indicators of a person's safety and of risk for future adverse events • Each person should have a report on pain levels, even if it is 'none'
Lab work, imaging	What has been done or sent; what needs to be done; any pertinent results
Current treatment plan (keep it simple)	Procedures scheduled, preparation done or needed, education, treatments, consents required, new orders, concerns of staff about the person
Consults (requested or done)	Specialist physicians, physiotherapy, dietitian, occupational therapy, respiratory therapy, psychiatry, chaplain, others
Special needs	Aids (hearing, walking), equipment, family concerns, spiritual or cultural concerns, anything else important not mentioned yet
Future	Discharge planning, healthcare teaching required; community or GP referrals, expected date of discharge

handover sheets or signing of handover sheets. Recommendations are made to the oncoming staff for clinical management, such as increased frequency of observations or when the next pain medication is due (South Australia Health, 2017). Clear communication of risks identified for an individual, and clinical risk management strategies (e.g. alerts for deep vein thrombosis [DVT] prophylaxis) are essential. Read back or check back (i.e. the oncoming staff reading back what they have understood to the reporting nurse) of critical information is helpful to prevent error (Slade et al., 2018).

The acronyms SOAP (Subjective, Objective, Assessment, Planning) or SOAPIE (Subjective, Objective, Assessment, Planning, Implementation, Evaluation) are often used to ensure that the handover (and especially documentation) is clinically complete but concise. SOAP, like ISBAR, ensures the consistency of reporting or documenting. It has mostly been subsumed into the ISBAR format for handover, since it does not include identification or background that impact on the individual's safe care each shift. The ACSQHC recommends the use of ISBAR.

Intra-departmental handovers (e.g. into or out of Theatre, Intensive Care Unit) often incorporate a checklist type of handover (see **Clinical Skill 52** for preoperative care) that prompts reporting of all pertinent information and becomes part of the medical record.

TIMELINESS

Timely reporting means providing up-to-the-minute relevant information about the person. For instance, you might report that 'Mrs Jones' pain levels were stable at around VAS 2 to 3 early this shift, but in the past half-hour she has reported a VAS of 8 along with nausea. Analgesic and anti-emetic were administered at 1445. Please check her during your first round'. This concise summary of what happened on the previous shift prepares the oncoming nurses to assess Mrs Jones within the next half-hour and keep a watch on her pain levels.

Timeliness also means that a handover is time-limited so that this valuable commodity is not wasted. The handover must be well organised, with staff arriving on time and being prepared for their shift (i.e. know who they are caring for on this shift, having their template prepared and knowing the basics for these people). There should be no chatting or gossip.

Clinical handover can be a time-saver as well. Relevant information is not buried in the chart, and is transmitted so the clinical staff can appropriately plan care. The person can be visually assessed (including IV, catheter, monitor readings) during the bedside handover and queried about their comfort (e.g. pain, toilet needs) so an 'extra' trip is eliminated.

USE OF MEDICAL TERMINOLOGY

Using medical terminology when giving a handover permits a report to be complete and concise. It demonstrates your knowledge and acknowledges the professional status of the person you are handing over to. Communication errors are directly associated with the safety of the person in the hospital (Kalaf, 2023), so your knowledge and use of appropriate terminology is important. Be precise in your reporting (e.g. state 'Waiting for lab results on blood drawn for potassium levels', not just 'Waiting for blood results'). This reduces the number of errors that may occur. The oncoming staff must be allowed to question you at handover for clarification and extension of information. You can ask for a read back to ensure that the correct information has been transferred.

RECEIVING HANDOVER

Receiving a handover is every bit as important as providing one. Be prepared. Know which people you will be responsible for (your shift allocation). You should familiarise yourself with the person's diagnosis, surgery and medications (e.g. get your assignment the day before, if possible, and read what you can before arriving at the facility). Prepare your own template (as above), listing the people assigned to you. This will assist you to capture the information presented, organise the work for the day and provide a guide to preparing your handover at the end of the shift. Listen carefully to the handover and ask questions during the read-back time. Often, the nurse providing handover will indicate concern about the person in their care that may alert you to watch for changes in condition. Keep accurate notes on your template (e.g. frequency of vital signs, type of IV fluid and when it is due, when an analgesic is due, trends in vital signs indicating deterioration). Use it as a memory aid and add to it with information gleaned from the individual. Introduce yourself to those in your care (if the leaving nurse has forgotten to do so) and ask them if there is anything they can add to the information given in the bedside handover. Note any information you need to research or ask your clinical educator about. Use the template to organise your workload by prioritising tasks, assessments around the acuity of the person(s) and set time(s) such as meal time, medication rounds or a booked theatre time.

DOCUMENTATION

Facilities will differ in the need for documentation. Currently, documentation may be unnecessary for handovers. However, signing of the handover sheet, and scanning the handover sheet into the person's chart, are being discussed at a national standards level as a safety and accountability measure.

CLINICAL SKILLS ASSESSMENT

Clinical handover

Demonstrates the ability to clearly and concisely report the condition of a person or group of people to another healthcare professional. Incorporates the *National Safety and Quality Health Service Standards*: 2 Partnering with Consumers, 3 Preventing and Controlling Healthcare-Associated Infection, 5 Comprehensive Care, 6 Communicating for Safety, and 8 Recognising and Responding to Acute Deterioration (ACSQHC, 2021b).

Performance criteria	1	2	3	4	5
(Numbers indicate NMBA *Registered Nurse Standards for Practice*)	(Dependent)	(Marginal)	(Assisted)	(Supervised)	(Independent)
1. Identifies indication (1.1, 3.3, 3.4)	☐	☐	☐	☐	☐
2. Conducts or receives the handover in private surroundings or appropriately at the bedside (1.2, 2.1, 2.7, 6.1)	☐	☐	☐	☐	☐
3. Uses a template (1.1, 1.2, 1.6, 3.4, 6.1)	☐	☐	☐	☐	☐
4. Provides information that is accurate, concise and complete (1.1, 1.5, 1.6, 2.7, 3.4, 6.1). Asks questions as appropriate (1.1, 1.5, 1.6, 2.7, 3.4, 6.1)	☐	☐	☐	☐	☐
5. Uses medical terminology appropriately (1.1, 1.4, 2.7, 3.4, 6.1)	☐	☐	☐	☐	☐
6. Delivers information in a timely manner (1.4, 1.6, 2.7, 3.4, 3.6, 3.7, 4.3, 6.1)	☐	☐	☐	☐	☐
7. Demonstrates the ability to link theory to practice (1.1, 3.3, 3.4, 3.5)	☐	☐	☐	☐	☐

Student:

Clinical facilitator: Date:

CHAPTER 26

DOCUMENTATION

INDICATIONS

Documentation is a record of the clinical assessment, the care and its impact, and the professional judgement, critical thinking and decision making used by a healthcare professional in the provision of care for an individual. A critical function of documentation is to enable the healthcare professional to reflect on the effectiveness of the care provided and revise the plan of care if necessary (De Groot et al., 2022). Specific indications for documentation include an admission or baseline notation of assessment and then any changes in the person's condition. People are in hospital because their health condition is relatively unstable and they require around-the-clock care; therefore, any alteration in their condition is significant and needs to be reported.

Professional documentation of an individual's status is both a legal requirement and a professional responsibility. It ensures continuity and timeliness of safe care by providing a mode of communication that is permanent. Hospital accreditation is dependent on sound basic documentation, and nurses are legally protected if their charting demonstrates that a professional standard of care has been delivered. Furthermore, documentation has educational and research applications because students and researchers can use the information for their scientific purposes. All documentation should report accurate and complete facts about a care incident, be current, logically presented and comply with the standards of the profession and the facility.

There are many different types of documentation (or charting), depending on the facility and the circumstances. There are flow sheets, assessment tools, incident forms, risk-assessment tools, discharge-planning forms, nursing-care planning forms and so on. You need to become familiar with the protocols used at the facility where you are attending clinical practice.

This competency addresses only the basic 'in-progress notes' type of documentation. Within in-progress notes, depending on the facility's choice, charting can be narrative, problem-oriented, focused or 'by exception'. As well, many, if not most, facilities will use electronic documentation.

CONTENT

Document facts only – be objective, precise and clinical (i.e. no opinion, no emotion, no guesses, use neutral language). Martin, Bickle and Lok (2022) found that the use of biased language (e.g. 'fat' rather than 'adipose tissue', 'addict' rather than 'person with a substance use disorder', assuming gender rather than asking the person) in communications can influence other clinicians' decisions and judgements about patients, thereby initiating more bias and compromising care provision. Care must be taken to make visible the clinical judgement and care provided by nursing staff. This will ultimately influence the allocation of resources (Rossi et al., 2023). The content of the documentation depends on the person and their condition. For instance, someone who is in hospital for a myocardial infarct will have frequent documentation of their pain levels and sites, their circulation and perfusion, and their anxiety levels, among other parameters. However, someone who has just had a surgical procedure like a knee replacement would have different assessment parameters reported, such as peripheral circulation on the affected leg, pain assessment of the site, drainage from the Hemovac, and circulatory and respiratory status following anaesthetic. Both of these people would have notations about nursing interventions attended (e.g. repositioning, oxygen administration, analgesic administration) and the person's response to these. Document all relevant information, not just in relation to their specific condition (e.g. the person with a myocardial infarct may also report headache or joint pain).

Use medical terminology when documenting because it is accurate and concise, and understood by all healthcare professionals. Often, phrases are abbreviated (e.g. nil by mouth is shortened to NBM); however, this may cause confusion if the abbreviations can refer to different phrases (e.g. 'AC' is listed in one medical lexicon as having four different meanings: abdominal circumference, anterior chamber of the eye, adjuvant chemotherapy and acute). Use only the abbreviations approved by the facility where you are working – there will be a list.

Acronyms and initialisms are formed from the initial letters of the words making the name of a body, such as the Nursing and Midwifery Board of Australia (NMBA). Acronyms and initialisms should also be on an approved list for use in the facility.

Spelling and grammar are important because they make the entry understandable. The entry should be factual, specific (e.g. time of the occurrence; exact findings; the person's, the doctor's and/or your response) and timely (i.e. not completed prior to or long after an event). Do not interpret the facts or use vague or tentative wording (e.g. 'appears' or 'seems'); do not use the words 'mistake' or 'accident'; rather, write exactly what happened. Any change in the person's condition – physical, medical, emotional or psychological – warrants a note in the chart. Assessments must also be specific (e.g. 'slept well' noted at the end of an eight-hour shift is not sufficient; note that the person is asleep at each round or write 'states slept well'). Omissions of scheduled or standardised procedures are also documented (e.g. dressing not attended, Mrs Jones in Theatre from 0800–1200).

STRUCTURE

ISBAR is one frequently used mnemonic that has been adapted for documentation. It is a systematic method of communicating that helps to maintain individual safety (Paterson, Roberts & Bail, 2022). ISBAR (see also **Clinical Skill 25**):

- *Identity* – ensure that you have the correct chart/record. Also, identify yourself at the end of the entry with your printed name, designation and signature.
- *Situation and background* – generally not relevant in contemporaneous charting because the entire nursing note comprises the situation/background; however, outlining these is important during admission and when the person is transferred.
- *Assessment* – upon admission to the unit, a thorough physical assessment and nursing history must be documented as a baseline. Because each nurse takes over the care of the person, their assessment of the person at that time should be noted. After that, alterations in the physical or psychosocial findings are noted. Use the person's own words when possible when reporting subjective data. Generally, changes in medical, physical, emotional or psychological conditions are documented. This alerts other healthcare professionals to potential complications (e.g. unrelieved leg or foot pain in the person with orthopaedic surgery to the leg).
- *Action* – what you did in response to the assessment findings.
- *Response and recommendation* – response to treatment, including analgesia or other prescribed medication. This is important to note so that ineffective treatment can be stopped or effective treatments continued. For example, this might take the following form:

  > 0015 hours – projectile vomiting of murky green fluid commenced three minutes following bolus injection of IV antibiotic. Maxalon IV as per chart given with little effect; 0320 – vomiting lasted from 0010 to 0245 hours, sleeping at present; 0610 – again vomiting of clear green fluid began during bolus injection of antibiotic medication; 0645 – vomiting continues, Dr Jones notified. Will review during morning rounds.

Recommendations may be added, such as health teaching (e.g. name and classification of the antibiotic to be avoided if possible), which would be undertaken at a later time.

Don't report the information charted on flow sheets (e.g. temperature, pulse, respiratory rate or blood pressure) unless that information contributes to pertinent information you are recording (e.g. 0730 – found on the floor, pale, diaphoretic, states 'felt dizzy', BP 100/68, P 58, BGL 2.3). Both observed and measured information give a more complete picture without the need to search the chart. Avoid duplication of information wherever possible.

Interventions and their effect that are not on a flow sheet should be documented. An example for a person with fatigue might be:

> Initial strategy for managing fatigue discussed. Able to explain need to undertake activities early in the day. Stated that 'this makes sense' and will adopt this idea.

Some facilities use a 'systems approach' to charting to organise the content (e.g. St Vincent's Hospital, Melbourne [SVHM, 2017]). You would make a comment on each of the major body systems at least once per shift.

WRITTEN DOCUMENTATION

Types of documentation

Narrative documentation

Narrative documentation is simply a record of what has happened as it happens, listing the observations, the interventions and the person's response to the interventions. Narrative documentation tends to be repetitious and is used only in limited facilities.

Problem-focused documentation

Problem-focused documentation addresses the problems identified during the person's stay, in chronological order. It arises from a physician's notations. Following assessment, you initially generate and number a list of the person's problems. This list is added to as more problems occur. Problems are not prioritised. Written plans are established to deal with each of the problems. Each problem/number is written about separately using a systematic method such as

SOAPIE (Subjective data, Objective data, Assessment, Planning, Intervention, Evaluation) on each shift. As problems are resolved, they are highlighted, and afterwards that problem and its number are no longer addressed in the documentation.

Focus documentation, using something like SOAPIE or DAR (Data [both subjective and objective], Action [or intervention], Response) addresses problems identified during baseline nursing assessment and during care. Problems are named (e.g. pain, nausea, diarrhoea, falls risk). This type of documentation tends to be more nursing-focused and flexible, with specific information easier to find. Foundational and medical-surgical textbooks will provide examples of these types of documentation.

Documentation by exception

Documentation by exception is used by many facilities (especially long-term care facilities) and is appropriate for other situations (e.g. surgical units). Healthcare professionals establish a baseline and accurately document any change from that baseline. Documentation by exception relies on the established flow sheets, graphic records, standard protocols and care plans or pathways to record continuous appropriate care. It assumes that all standards are met unless the event is noted, and requires trust between healthcare professionals that all care was done to an established standard (Ballard, 2018). This mode of documentation focuses on exceptions to the normal or deviations from the usual standards. Documentation of exceptional events continues until there is a return to the previous status or a new level of wellbeing is established for the individual.

LEGAL REQUIREMENTS FOR DOCUMENTATION

This applies to written documentation that is still required in many healthcare facilities. Because the documentation written in the person's chart may become a legal document, there are minimum standards that must be met. Your entry must be:

- legible
- written in black ink
- dated using the dd/mm/yy format and timed using the 24-hour clock; chronology and sequencing may be crucial – i.e. when medications were given, blood pressure (BP) readings taken, transporting to theatre – for medico-legal as well as clinical reasons
- error-free or errors acknowledged with a single line through them and 'error' plus your initials written above; do not erase, scratch out or use correction fluid
- free of blank areas; draw a line through an unused portion of a line
- comprehensible; for example, use only acceptable abbreviations from the facility's list
- signed, acknowledging that it was you who acted or observed, with a printed name and designation after the signature for identification purposes. If you are reporting something seen or heard by another, name this person in the documentation (e.g. Mr Kraft says that his wife [the person in your care] was 'incoherent from about 0930 but until then she had not been confused')
- contemporaneous – made as close to the time of the observation or intervention as is reasonable.

If required, a 'late' entry must follow the last entry (do not squeeze additional information into the notes) and should be noted as such (use either 'addit' or 'late entry' beside the time you actually wrote the notation). Include the time of the occurrence within the notation.

Poor or vague problem-based or narrative documentation is not acceptable because the legal stance is that 'if it was not documented, it was not done'. Therefore, accurate, descriptive and timely documentation is critical, not only for the person's safety and comfort, but also for your security. With documentation by exception, all entries must be supported by the flow sheets. If a legal claim is made, the court would generally take the individual's recall of the incident over that of a healthcare professional. A specific incident is more memorable to the person than to a busy healthcare professional who may encounter similar incidents frequently (Queensland Health, 2013).

ELECTRONIC DOCUMENTATION

As technology advances, evolves and becomes more affordable, electronic health record (EHR) keeping in healthcare facilities is now common. EHRs are computer-based. They are longitudinal; that is, they incorporate previous hospitalisations/healthcare visits and physicians' visits. Thus allergies, previous diagnoses, current medications, treatments and complications are available continuously. Transcriptions are eliminated. Physical examination, laboratory results and pharmaceutical information are all incorporated. The EHR is comprised of electronic forms (e.g. physical assessment forms, doctor's orders, contemporaneous healthcare notes), flow sheets (e.g. vital signs, intake/output) and the electronic medication administration record (eMAR).

EHR keeping affects the work of every nurse (Capriotti, 2019). Ideally, all parts of the system are integrated. The physician's orders, laboratory reports, pharmacy requests, automated entries and nurses' notes use the same system and are cross-referenced, making information available and accessible at the point of care (Lockwood, 2019). Computer terminals may be at point of care (in the person's room), on a mobile computer or at a central nursing area.

There are benefits: records and orders are clear and legible; improved safety in medication administration; reduced time spent in documentation; improved accuracy of documentation; automatic (legible) signatures, dates and times are entered in the system; record tampering is prevented and deletion of information is difficult (Lockwood, 2019). Critical information is more consistently shared with other healthcare professionals. Neither the duration nor the frequency of nursing activities were adversely affected by the introduction of EHR. No significant change in the time spent verbally interacting with the person was noted, as nurses adapted to the new routines (Ang, 2019).

From the nurse's perspective, drawbacks include difficulty in maintaining privacy and security; feeling like the computer is getting more attention than the person; software is often not compiled to enable the healthcare professional to easily track trends and changes in symptoms or vital signs, and automated data entry (e.g. from electronic BP measurement) is often not seen in real time; and data entry is not infallible, and mistakes are easily made. Check boxes and drop-down menus can affect your ability to think critically, since options are given that may or may not fit an individual's condition, and the comment boxes are sometimes insufficient to explain a finding or decision. Many of these disadvantages are being addressed as EHR become more widely used and modified to fit the needs of clinical care (Baniulyte, Rogerson & Bowden, 2023). It may take several weeks or months to become familiar with the system in use at a particular facility, but with practice, EHRs can be efficient.

Much of the material presented in 'Legal requirements for documentation' (above) will be applicable to electronic records. However, there are additional precautions. These include the following:

- Since you cannot 'sign' your note indicating that it was you who saw or did something, you will need a password and PIN unique to you, and you will need to guard it carefully.
- Errors in data entry will still have to be acknowledged and left in the record. You will need to learn how to correct errors.
- Safeguards must be implemented so no unauthorised people can read the notes. These include placing of monitors to prevent inadvertent display of an individual's information and securing the terminal in their room.
- You will have to ensure privacy if voice-activated systems are used.
- Confidentiality will still be a concern and systems will need to be devised to limit access to EHR. Documentation must be secure to remain private and confidential. Healthcare records (both written and electronic) are used only by individuals who are involved in the person's direct care. Leaving charts on the desk or the page open on the computer to be read by non-authorised personnel is a breach of privacy.

Make an effort to track trends, and use your critical thinking skills to think 'outside the box'. Use a standardised nursing language to document care to improve communication within the team and the care given to the individual and create opportunities to demonstrate the effects of nursing skills on improving the health of people in our care (Aleandri, Scalorbi & Pirazzini, 2022).

The individual has a right to see their health record and correct any errors. This right can be overridden by the physician in some cases (e.g. notification of a transmissible disease such as syphilis or dengue fever) (Schnur, 2019). The person in care can follow their own healthcare plans, review the material, absorb information at their own pace, add to it, question it and discuss it with their healthcare professional. Electronic documentation, used without consideration of the individual, arouses feelings that you are focusing on the screen and documenting for the records rather than caring for the person (Kline, 2020). This author suggested the following to personalise your nursing care:

- Tell the person you will be recording information in the computer.
- Place the computer screen where it can be seen by both of you.
- Stop typing while you sit and talk to the person, and use appropriate non-verbal communication skills.
- Make eye contact both before and after typing information into the computer.

Transmitting documentation from one facility to another or from the doctor's office to a facility, laboratory or other external provider requires you to be aware of ensuring security of information, confidentiality and transmissibility of materials. The facility where you are working will have protocols for moving and photocopying material from a person's chart to another setting; these must be followed.

With thanks to Jason Holewa, RN, and Brenda Fleming, RN, for using their experience to validate this information.

CLINICAL SKILLS ASSESSMENT

Documentation

Demonstrates the ability to accurately record information about a person in a timely manner. Incorporates the *National Safety and Quality Health Service Standards*: 2 Partnering with Consumers, 3 Preventing and Controlling Healthcare-Associated Infection, 5 Comprehensive Care, 6 Communicating for Safety, and 8 Recognising and Responding to Acute Deterioration (ACSQHC, 2021b).

Performance criteria	1	2	3	4	5
(Numbers indicate NMBA *Registered Nurse Standards for Practice*)	(Dependent)	(Marginal)	(Assisted)	(Supervised)	(Independent)
1. Identifies indications for documentation in the person's chart/record (1.1, 3.3, 3.4)	☐	☐	☐	☐	☐
2. Uses appropriate medical terminology and approved abbreviations, acronyms and initialisms (1.1, 1.4, 2.7, 3.4, 3.6, 3.7, 6.1)	☐	☐	☐	☐	☐
3. Provides relevant and accurate content in an appropriate structure (1.1, 1.4, 1.6, 2.7, 3.3, 3.4, 3.6, 3.7, 6.1)	☐	☐	☐	☐	☐
4. Adheres to legal requirements (1.4, 1.5)	☐	☐	☐	☐	☐
5. Demonstrates the ability to effectively use the facility's standard forms (1.4, 1.5, 6.5)	☐	☐	☐	☐	☐
6. Demonstrates ability to use the electronic health record system (1.4, 1.5, 6.5)	☐	☐	☐	☐	☐
7. Demonstrates the ability to link theory to practice (1.1, 3.3, 3.4, 3.5)	☐	☐	☐	☐	☐

Student:

Clinical facilitator: Date:

CHAPTER 27

HEALTHCARE TEACHING

INDICATIONS

Teaching is an integral part of the role of a nurse; it is outlined in Standard 3.2 of the *Registered Nurse Standards for Practice* (Nursing and Midwifery Board of Australia [NMBA], 2016).

Early or same-day discharge from hospital, the increasing complexity of healthcare options, financial constraints and increased home healthcare services have combined to make teaching an imperative in quality health care. People need new skills and knowledge to maintain and enhance their health, gain independence and enhance quality of life. Health literacy is an essential foundation to better control of a person's health, helping them to make informed decisions, improve compliance, reduce anxiety levels and actively participate in their treatment (Sak, Rothenfluh & Schulz, 2017). Chronic disease is prevalent, and self-management is important to improve health outcomes.

Formal teaching is a large part of your responsibilities; however, teaching need not all be formal. Use *teaching moments* (Robinson et al., 2020) as well, which are teaching opportunities that occur during the daily routine to influence the person towards more positive health behaviours. People have a right to receive understandable information about their health care in order to make informed decisions about treatment options and lifestyle issues. Offering information relevant to an individual's health supports their efforts to assume responsibility for their own health. You must have the knowledge (know the material), attitude (well prepared), confidence and psychomotor skills to enable you to successfully teach a person (Richard, Evans & Williams, 2016).

People require knowledge (cognitive domain) about numerous things that impact on their health status. These could be medications, pathophysiology and symptoms of complications, various treatments and any number of other sets of information, which help the person to independence in health care. Improving understanding of their disease reduces a person's readmission rate (Prochnow, Meiers & Scheckel, 2019). Multidisciplinary input (e.g. pharmacy, nursing, physiotherapy and physicians reinforcing the material) improves the outcome, and people need different teaching modalities to support their learning preferences (Truccolo et al., 2019).

Individuals must learn to deal with the affective domain – the feelings, attitudes, interests and values motivating us to behave the way we do. Programs to stop smoking, change a diet and keep taking a prescribed medication are based on this internal process that influences the learner's interaction with the environment. This is the most difficult to address.

The psychomotor domain deals with motor and procedural skills: giving oneself an injection, deep-breathing exercises and changing a dressing are skills a person may need to learn. Most teaching should include the individual's support person, so that reinforcement of the information/attitude/skill is available once the person no longer has direct support from the healthcare professional. As well, teaching family members assists them to support the person's recovery.

Teaching and learning is a very complex interaction and process. This Clinical Skill is able to give only a very brief and broad description of the processes involved. Entire textbooks are available on this topic; see for example, Bastable (2017), *Essentials of Patient Education*.

EVIDENCE OF THERAPEUTIC INTERACTION

Good verbal and non-verbal communication skills are imperative. Leahy and Kizilay (1998, p. 245) outline the following characteristics of a good teacher: accurate, reliable, dynamic, supportive, attentive and friendly, with genuine positive regard for the learner. Saxena and Desanghere (2023) add other personal attributes to shape a good teacher. These include interpersonal skills, such as works well with others, available, humble, minimally biased; professional attributes such as compassionate engagement, trustworthiness, uses adaptive reflection, commitment to the profession; a commitment to teach and to learn (i.e. proactively seeks and provides constructive feedback, creates learning opportunities), and work–life balance/integration (e.g. calm demeanour, inspirational). Introduce yourself to the person, use their preferred name, and explain what you will do and the time frame. Decide the depth of knowledge to impart. This is determined by the person's ability and interest, their health literacy and the amount of time available for the teaching. Your own time and other healthcare professionals' scheduling (e.g. theatre schedules) can be the two greatest impediments to good teaching in the healthcare setting.

Planning and organising information is crucial to the success of the teaching session. The following teaching sequence is based on Malcolm Knowles's (1978) principles of adult learning:

- Adults learn best when there is a perceived need. Ensure the person understands the underlying health issue (to be prevented) or illness (to be resolved), prior to teaching. The person has an individual responsibility to learn, so motivation is essential (Herrman, 2020).
- Teaching adults should progress from the known to the unknown. Assess what is known; don't reteach the things they already know.
- Teaching adults should progress from simple to more complex topics.
- Adults learn best using active participation. Use 'teach back' (see 'Teach-back method' below) to encourage learning and to permit clarification.
- Adults require opportunities to practise new skills (e.g. drawing up insulin). (See 'Demonstration coaching' below.) Elaboration is a strategy that asks the person to explain something in their own words and to connect it to previous knowledge (Herrman, 2020). Sammut et al. (2021) found that interactive educational strategies yield better results than didactic (e.g. lecture) approaches, and practical learning strategies (e.g. doing, handling equipment) are preferred over theoretical approaches. Attitudinal change is more easily accomplished with teaching of longer duration.
- Adults need the behaviour reinforced (e.g. allow the person to draw up and give their insulin each time it is due). Read information/handouts with or to the person to individualise it to their situation, to answer questions and to direct attention to specific material. Provide individualised attention over several short sessions. The internet is an important source of health information for many people and should be integrated into the teaching plan as necessary.

Explain the purpose

For each teaching session, link the new knowledge to previous knowledge. Explain the purpose of the new skills to increase interest and motivation. Set learning outcomes with the person for each session. Learning is more effective if directed towards specified and achievable outcomes. Individualising standard material promotes consistency and accuracy. Learners must interact with the material and use effort to incorporate information. Repetition is not enough; making connections and contextualising information help form memory and mental models so the idea becomes embedded (Herrman, 2020). The nurse-teacher is an enabler to vulnerable people's learning of health-associated information and behaviour change (Stănescu-Yadav & Lillekroken, 2023).

DEMONSTRATE CLINICAL REASONING

Assess the person

The ability to learn varies; you need to know the person's level of knowledge. Be aware of your own bias to ascribe health literacy levels to specific groups. Goggins et al. (2016) found that healthcare professionals overestimated health literacy in males and in those with less education. Do not assume a level of previous knowledge. During an assessment, explore the person's knowledge of the phenomena in question. Use previous knowledge to build new knowledge. The ability to learn is based on the person's motivation, their developmental and physical capabilities, the learning environment, their ability to take responsibility for their own learning and the applicability of the information to their situation. Use the inherent strengths and problem-solving capabilities of the individual.

Learning takes energy, concentration and motivation. The person's willingness and ability to learn, and their attitude towards learning, are influenced by: age; gender; level of maturity; level of fear and anxiety; intelligence; educational, cultural and socioeconomic background; lifestyle; language; and support. Assess these factors so you can tailor the teaching to the individual and prioritise their learning needs.

Generally, the person in hospital may have many barriers to effectively learning about their own health management, such as nervousness, emotional response to a new diagnosis, malaise or lack of focus due to the condition, or memory or cognitive difficulties due to medications (e.g. analgesics, sedatives), the condition or a comorbidity (e.g. dementia).

Planning

Check if the healthcare facility has a standardised teaching curriculum for specific groups of people (e.g. people who are post-myocardial infarct, newly diagnosed diabetic, on specific medications such as anticoagulants). These usually include assessments, goals, key steps and information and post-teaching assessments for you to use. If available, use these to co-design an educational plan with the person.

Work with the person to clarify and develop strategies to individualise treatment guidelines, implement continuing education and improve communication skills, in order to assist the person to achieve behavioural change. Careful planning of the teaching session timing reduces physiological barriers (e.g. fatigue and pain). Also, plan teaching to minimise interruptions such as X-ray visits, physician rounds or meals. Physiological problems, such as hearing loss, poor vision, aphasia, organic brain syndrome or loss

GATHER EQUIPMENT

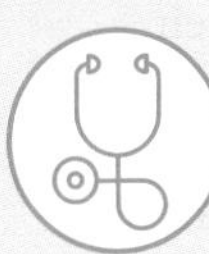

The type of equipment needed depends on what is being taught. The following are general categories rather than a list of items:

EQUIPMENT	EXPLANATION
Audiovisual materials	• These must take into consideration the person's learning ability, vocabulary, reading ability and concentration span. They range from written instructions to videos, DVDs or websites presenting material. Infographics have proved to be as effective as video/YouTube presentations (Ebrahimabadi et al., 2019) • All audiovisual material must be consistent with the information presented by healthcare professionals • Review YouTube presentations for veracity, clarity and suitability before showing/recommending them
Equipment for teaching a psychomotor skill	• Check all items for completeness and working order before teaching begins. Good organisation demonstrates accuracy and reliability • A well-lit room free of distractions makes learning easier
Teaching aids (pamphlet, video, printed information)	• Teaching aids must be assessed for suitability for the learner and consistency with the information being taught • Determine the readability of the written material; for example, print size, complexity of words used, number of concepts/facts presented and suitability for the person

of muscle strength and coordination, require you to use other strategies (e.g. enlarged visual aids, short sessions, primary teaching of the significant other).

Address *psychological barriers to learning*, such as fear, anxiety and perceived loss of control, by first identifying the problem(s) and then discussing the most important concerns and clearly defining the goals (so their priorities motivate their learning). Reduce the negative feelings so that learning can occur. Pace personalised, accurate, consistent and structured information to reduce the perceived threat of new learning. Health promotion programs are especially challenging because lifestyle behavioural change is difficult. Individuals often gain many positive feelings from their past/current behaviour, use the behaviour as a coping strategy (York et al., 2017) and feel negative about making changes. Motivating a person to change a lifestyle behaviour is difficult. Enlist the person's interest and boost their motivation by asking them why the behaviour will improve their life (e.g. a mother who is a smoker may tell you she wants to protect her children and be a better role model to prevent them smoking in the future). Keeping this in mind will be a strong motivating force for her.

Understanding cultural factors is critical in addressing psycho-physical change. All cultures have beliefs about health and illness. These may become barriers to learning because of different perceptions of illness, pain and health care. Locus of control, socioeconomic factors, and beliefs about religion, gender, ageing and ethnicity affect a person's beliefs about maintaining health and preventing and treating illness. Learning approaches are usually culturally based (and biased). You will need to demonstrate respect for the person and their culture. Strive for a culture of self-reflection and self-critique to address unconscious biases within yourself and the health profession. This requires three core values: curiosity, humility and accountability (Yepes-Rios et al., 2023). Healthcare information is important to quality of life, and teaching must be comprehensible to the individual. Provide healthcare information at a level the person can understand. If English is not their primary language, use medical interpreting services to overcome communication problems and to improve the quality of care.

Knowledge of the content is important. The person must perceive you as being competent, trustworthy and supportive. This results from thorough knowledge of self; the procedural, sensory and factual aspects of the subject; the ability to be considerate of the learner's fears and anxieties; and the flexibility to adapt the delivery of the material accordingly.

HEALTHCARE TEACHING

The following is a broad outline of the major points of healthcare teaching. This material, along with the assessment and planning of a teaching session, is adaptable to teaching peers, colleagues, nursing students and the family of the person in your care, as well as the person.

Teaching strategies

Teaching strategies for the *cognitive domain* include lectures (e.g. informing a group about the effects of exercise on diabetes mellitus), audio and video material, discussion, pictures, posters, written instructions, slide presentations and one-to-one teaching. This type of teaching suits sensory, procedural and factual information.

- *Sensory information* – teaching about sensations likely to be encountered during a procedure: sights, sounds, smells, movements and physical and psychological sensations.

- *Procedural information* – what the person is expected to do or have done to them during a procedure: the sequencing, the time involved, medications and what the person can do to facilitate the procedure.
- *Factual information* – provides knowledge about physiology, pathophysiology and treatment, and is usually presented more formally.

Sensory and procedural information are often given only once or twice prior to an event or during an event and do not require much reinforcement. They are often spontaneous, taking place in the context of nursing care rather than as a structured teaching session. This information decreases uncertainty and increases the person's sense of control. By contrast, factual information needs frequent reinforcement if the person uses the information on a regular basis; for example, when teaching about medications, teach back by asking the person to restate the information just taught to them. This is an effective technique to improve retention (Ryan-Madonna, Levin & Lauder, 2019) (see 'Teach-back method').

Affective change is usually facilitated by group discussion and role-playing, with the person as an active participant. One-to-one discussions offer support during change. Changing values and beliefs is not easy and requires time, effort, support and a well-motivated person. Social support from family and healthcare providers is essential to changing behaviour (Dunn, Margaritis & Anderson, 2017).

Teach-back method

The teach-back method is the preferred, comprehensive, standardised best practice that engages people and their caregivers by asking them to explain back, in their own words, what they have learnt. Prochnow, Meiers and Scheckel (2019) found caregivers were able to recall more information about new medications than the person in care was able to, so you should include the family/caregiver when providing health-related education whenever possible. Teach-back health education improves self-management and decreases uncertainty (Ahmadidarrehsima et al., 2020). It is used to increase the person's knowledge of their condition, medications, dietary changes, blood glucose levels, physical restrictions and so on.

The following points outline the use of teach-back:

- Use a caring tone of voice and attitude. Avoid a bored, hurried or disinterested tone. Your non-verbal communication is important.
- Display comfortable body language and make eye contact. Sit down with them if possible. Take into account cultural differences here.
- Use plain language. Explain any medical jargon carefully (e.g. test results, medications).
- Intersperse all teaching with checks for understanding. Don't leave the questions until the end of the teaching session; instead, chunk and check so there are smaller amounts of information for the person to assimilate.
- Ask the person to explain back, using their own words. Take care not to be condescending or derogatory, use non-shaming, open-ended questions; avoid closed questions that can be answered with 'yes' or 'no'.
- Emphasise that the responsibility to explain clearly is on you, the nurse. Do not interrogate. Precede the question with a framing statement to reduce the stigma of possible not understanding so that the focus of the conversation is on the communication between the nurse and the person (Seely, Higgs & Nigh, 2022). An example might be asking: 'Would you put this information in your own words so I can make sure I explained it correctly?', and then asking about the specifics (e.g. 'Can you tell me what this medication is for, how much and how often you should take it and what side effects might arise?'). You may need to ask these as three separate questions, so the person can answer them singly.
- If the person is not able to teach back correctly, explain again and recheck. Try not to simply repeat what you have just taught; use different words or a different approach. For example, 'OK, you are right about the reason you are taking the Frusemide and how it will help you, but you will need to take it twice a day – early in the morning with breakfast and again at about noon, so with lunch. If you take it too late in the day, you will be going to the toilet late into the night.'
- Use reader-friendly print materials to support learning. Review the key material in the handout with the person. Do not assume that they can or will read the information. Circle or highlight the most important points.
- Document use of and the person's response to teach-back.

Adapted from: Agency for Healthcare Research and Quality (AHRQ) (2020). *Use the Teach-Back Method: Tool #5*. Content last reviewed March 2020. Rockville, MD: AHRQ. Retrieved from https://www.ahrq.gov/health-literacy/quality-resources/tools/literacy-toolkit/healthlittoolkit2-tool5.html, accessed 29 March 2020.

Demonstration coaching

The major strategy for teaching psychomotor skills is demonstration coaching. Outline what you are going to do: demonstration, return demonstration, feedback and then performance. For example, you might begin the session by saying, 'Today you will learn to draw up your insulin. I will show you first, then I will repeat it with explanations, then you can talk me through doing it so you remember the steps. Then it will be your turn. You can familiarise yourself with the equipment, practise some of the steps. When you are ready, you will draw up the medication and I will direct you the first time through. After that, you will talk yourself through the procedure and I will help you as needed.'

Demonstration

- Demonstrate the skill to be learnt from beginning to end, with no interruptions. The person can see the skill in its entirety, performed in a seamless and flowing fashion.
- Demonstrate the skill again, breaking it into easy-to-understand steps. Explain each step. Small steps are easier to learn, as the information is assimilated in small amounts at a time. Explanations and rationales for each step increase the ease with which it can be recalled.
- Repeat the demonstration slowly. This time, ask the person to direct your actions and to give explanations for each of the steps. This process helps the person consolidate the progression of the skill without needing to use the motor movements of actually manipulating the equipment.
- Have them handle each piece of equipment and ask questions, try parts of the procedure and practise the steps.

Return demonstration

The person now does the procedure while you coach them through the steps. This gives the person a chance to master the fine motor movements of the skill. A second (or more as needed) return demonstration, with the person coaching themselves through the steps, helps to consolidate and integrate the skill and the rationale. These steps require repetitions before the person masters the skill. Short practice sessions are more effective than one sustained practice period. Finally, the person should demonstrate how to deal with errors and unexpected situational variations (with you coaching as needed). Other strategies often used with demonstration coaching during psychomotor skill development are written instructions, posters, pictures and audiovisual presentations.

Feedback

Feedback is crucial to any type of learning and should be given regularly throughout the teaching session. Feedback provides information about the quality and accuracy of a response or action. It should be positive to increase self-esteem and therefore the self-confidence of the person. Any corrections or negative feedback should follow positive feedback, so budding self-confidence is preserved. It also needs to be timely; that is, it must occur at the time of the error to stop establishing inaccurate mindsets (i.e. bad habits). Negative feedback is more valuable if it clearly specifies what the error was, why the response was wrong and the criteria for correcting it. Feedback must also be honest to preserve the therapeutic relationship.

Feedback is essential in learning psychomotor skills. Frequent feedback is needed during initial sessions, with less and less as the person progresses. Encourage them to give themselves feedback and to compare their performance to a standard. The entire teaching session should be evaluated with the person and the achievement of learning outcomes emphasised, to give the person a feeling of progression towards a goal.

Performance

Encourage the person to perform the new skill or display their new knowledge; this reinforces new learning and increases the likelihood of the knowledge being incorporated into the person's repertoire of skills.

DOCUMENTATION

Documenting the teaching provides for continuity of care and evidence that time was spent teaching the person. What was taught, when it was taught, the method used, the degree of their participation in the teaching activity and whether the learning outcomes were met or not are documented in the person's notes. Note any written material provided. Referral to other healthcare personnel and recommendations for further teaching should be noted both in writing and verbally to ensure appropriate follow-up. If the person has difficulty with a new skill or idea, others can reinforce the information.

PART 4

CLINICAL SKILLS ASSESSMENT

Healthcare teaching

Demonstrates the ability to effectively teach a skill to a person. Incorporates the *National Safety and Quality Health Service Standards*: 2 Partnering with Consumers, 3 Preventing and Controlling Healthcare-Associated Infection, 5 Comprehensive Care, 6 Communicating for Safety, and 8 Recognising and Responding to Acute Deterioration (ACSQHC, 2021b).

Performance criteria	1	2	3	4	5
(Numbers indicate NMBA *Registered Nurse Standards for Practice*)	**(Dependent)**	**(Marginal)**	**(Assisted)**	**(Supervised)**	**(Independent)**
1. Identifies indication (1.1, 3.3, 3.4)	☐	☐	☐	☐	☐
2. Evidence of therapeutic interaction with the person, e.g. gives the person a clear explanation of the procedure (1.4, 1.5, 2.1, 2.2, 3.2)	☐	☐	☐	☐	☐
3. Demonstrates clinical reasoning, e.g. assesses the person, prepares the environment, understands barriers to learning, gathers equipment (1.1, 1.2, 1.3, 1.5, 2.3, 4.1, 4.2, 4.3, 5.1, 6.1)	☐	☐	☐	☐	☐
4. Uses 'teach-back'. Individualises standard material (1.2, 1.3, 2.1, 2.2, 2.3, 2.4, 2.7, 6.1)	☐	☐	☐	☐	☐
5. Provides information at the person's cognitive level (1.2, 1.3, 2.1, 2.5, 2.7)	☐	☐	☐	☐	☐
6. Demonstrates the (psychomotor) skill, and has the person return the demonstration (3.2, 6.1)	☐	☐	☐	☐	☐
7. Facilitates affective learning (3.2, 6.1)	☐	☐	☐	☐	☐
8. Gives feedback (3.2, 6.1)	☐	☐	☐	☐	☐
9. Encourages the person to use the new skill/information (3.2, 6.1)	☐	☐	☐	☐	☐
10. Documents relevant information (1.1, 1.4, 1.6, 2.2, 2.7, 3.5, 3.7, 6.1, 6.2, 6.5, 7.3)	☐	☐	☐	☐	☐
11. Demonstrates the ability to link theory to practice (1.1, 3.3, 3.4, 3.5)	☐	☐	☐	☐	☐

Student:

Clinical facilitator: Date:

REFERENCES

Agency for Healthcare Research and Quality (AHRQ) (2020). *Use the teach-back method: Tool #5.* Rockville, MD: AHRQ. https://www.ahrq.gov/health-literacy/quality-resources/tools/literacy-toolkit/healthlittoolkit2-tool5.html

Ahmadidarrehsima, S., Bidmeshki, E. A., Rahnama, M., Babaei, K., Afshari, M. & Khandani, B. (2020). The effect of self-management education by the teach-back method on uncertainty of patients with breast cancer: A quasi-experimental study. *Journal of Cancer Education, 35*, 366–72. https://doi.org/10.1007/s13187-019-1474-5

Aleandri, M., Scalorbi, S. & Pirazzini, M. (2022). Electronic nursing care plans through the use of NANDA, NOC, and NIC taxonomies in community setting: A descriptive study in northern Italy. *International Journal of Nursing Knowledge, 33*(1), 72–80. https://doi.org/10.1111/2047-3095.12326

Ang, J. (2019). Use of content management systems to address nursing workflow. *International Journal of Nursing Sciences, 6*(4), 454–9. https://doi.org/10.1016/j.ijnss.2019.09.012

Australian Commission on Safety and Quality in Health Care (ACSQHC) (2012). *Safety and Quality Improvement Guide Standard 6: Clinical Handover.* Sydney, NSW: ACSQHC.

Australian Commission on Safety and Quality in Health Care (ACSQHC) (2021a). Communication at clinical handover. *National safety and quality health service standards* (3rd ed.) Sydney, NSW: ACSQHC. https://www.safetyandquality.gov.au/standards/nsqhs-standards/communicating-safety-standard/communication-clinical-handover

Australian Commission on Safety and Quality in Health Care (ACSQHC) (2021b). *National safety and quality health service standards* (3rd ed.) Sydney, NSW: ACSQHC.

Australian Medical Association (2006). *Safe handover: Safe patients. Guidance on clinical handover for clinicians and managers.* https://ama.com.au/article/guidance-clinical-handover. Originates from *Safe handover: Safe patients.* London: British Medical Association, 2006, p. 7.

Awale, S., Bajracharya, S. & Tviet, B. (2022). Chapter 38: ISBAR Communication tool for clinical handover. In A. Nieminen & A. Suikkala, A. (eds), *Tools for Wellbeing and Dignity II – Developing multi-professional collaboration competence among the disciplines of nursing, social work and microbiology.* Diak Publications 3. Diaconia University of Applies Sciences.

Ballard, L. (2018). The nurse and documentation. In L. Ballard & P. Grant (eds), *Law for nurse leaders* (2nd ed.). New York, NY: Springer Publishing Company.

Baniulyte, G., Rogerson, N. & Bowden, J. (2023). Evolution – removing paper and digitising the hospital. *Health and Technology, 13*, 263–71. https://www.semanticscholar.org/paper/Evolution---removing-paper-and-digitising-the-Baniulyte-Rogerson/bf8285491b82dcbf0a655771331393d33ec9a24e

Bastable, S. (2017). *Essentials of patient education* (2nd ed.). Burlington, MA: Jones and Bartlett.

Capriotti, T. (2019). *Document smart: The A-to-Z guide to better nursing documentation* (4th ed.). Philadelphia, PA: Lippincott Williams & Wilkins.

Chan, M. M. K., Chan, C. K. Y., Pang, M. T. H. & Tsang, V. W. Y. (2023). Teaching clinical handover by clinical reasoning. *Nurse Educator, 48*(1), E30. https://journals.lww.com/nurseeducatoronline/Citation/2023/01000/Teaching_Clinical_Handover_by_Clinical_Reasoning.29.aspx

Chien, L., Slade, D., Dahm, M., Brady, B., Roberts, E., Goncharov, L., Taylor, J., Eggins, S. & Thornton, A. (2022). Improving patient-centred care through a tailored intervention addressing nursing clinical handover communication in its organizational and cultural context. *Journal of Advanced Nursing, 78*, 1413–30. https://doi.org/10.1111/jan.15110

De Groot, K., De Veer, A. J. E., Munster, A. M., Francke, A. L. & Paans, W. (2022). Nursing documentation and its relationship with perceived nursing workload: A mixed-methods study among community nurses. *BMC Nursing, 21*(1), 34. https://doi.org/10.1186/s12912-022-00811-7

de Jesus Amorim, E., Silva de Assis, Y., de Carvalho Santos, M., Ferreira da Luz Silva, T., Sant'Ana Souza Santos, R. N., da Silva Cruz, J. & de Lima Fonseca, M. (2022). Procedure for the handover: Nurses' perspective in intensive care units. *Revista Baiana de Enfermagem, 36*, 1–10. https://web.s.ebscohost.com/abstract?direct=true&profle=ehost&scope=site&authtype=crawler&jrnl=01025430&AN=161257061&h=skcBO3jCJKDxnl7Oq9KVzzR8LbaSmywOpKvF5NNqplW4CxLtReNG6V3nz0qJHxpz3BaUUqJPyCRwAhDXrkfh2A%3d%3d&crl=c&resultNs=AdminWebAuth&resultLocal=ErrCrlNotAuth&crlhashurl=login.aspx%3fdirect%3dtrue%26profle%3dehost%26scope%3dsite%26authtype%3dcrawler%26jrnl%3d01025430%26AN%3d161257061

Dunn, P. J., Margaritis, V. & Anderson, C. L. (2017). Understanding health literacy skills in patients with cardiovascular disease and diabetes. *The Qualitative Report, 22*(1), 33–46. https://search.proquest.com/docview/1867930785?accountid=88802.

Ebrahimabadi, M., Rezaei, K., Moini, A., Fournier, A. & Abedi, A. (2019). Infographics or video: Which one is more effective in asthmatic patients' health? A randomized clinical trial. *Journal of Asthma, 56*(12), 1306–13. https://doi.org/10.1080/02770903.2018.1536143

Eggins, S., Pun, J., Slade, D. & Chan, E. A. (2019). *Understanding the complexity of effective nursing handover communication in a bilingual Hong Kong hospital.* 16th International Pragmatics Conference (IPrA 2019), Hong Kong, China. https://scholars.cityu.edu.hk/en/publications/understanding-the-complexity-of-effective-nursing-handover-communication-in-a-bilingual-hong-kong-hospital(3b0697c0-528a-4acc-8ed1-38313bf81d85).html

Ghonem, N. & El-Husany, W. (2023). SBAR shift report training program and its effect on nurses' knowledge and practice and their perception of shift handoff communication. *SAGE Open Nursing, 9.* https://doi.org/10.1177/23779608231159340

Goggins, K., Wallston, K. A., Mion, L., Cawthon, C. & Kripalani, S. (2016). What patient characteristics influence nurses' assessment of health literacy? *Journal of Health Communication, 21*, 105–8. https://doi.org/10.1080/10810730.2016.1193919

Herrman, J. (2020). *Creative teaching strategies for the nurse educator* (3rd ed.). Philadelphia, PA: F. A. Davis.

Johnson, M., Sanchez, P. & Zheng, C. (2016). Reducing patient clinical management errors using structured content and electronic nursing handover. *Journal of Nursing Care Quality, 31*(3), 245–53. https://doi.org/10.1097/NCQ.0000000000000167

Kalaf, Z. (2023). Improving patient handover: A narrative review. *African Journal of Paediatric Surgery* (Jan). https://doi.org/10.4103/ajps.ajps_82_22

Kline, L. (2020). How electronic health records correlate with patient-centered care. *Nursing 2020, 50*(1), 61–3. https://doi.org/10.1097/01.NURSE.0000615140.23834.06

Knowles, M. S. (1978). Andragogy: Adult learning theory in perspective. *Community College Review, 5*(3), 9–20. https://doi.org/10.1177/009155217800500302

Lazzari, C. (2024). Implementing the verbal and electronic handover in general and psychiatric nursing using the Introduction, Situation, Background, Assessment, and Recommendation Framework: A systematic review. *Iranian Journal of Nursing and Midwifery Research, 29*(1), 23–32. https://doi.org/10.4103/ijnmr.ijnmr_24_23

Le, A., Lee, M. & Wilson, J. (2023). Nursing handoff education: An integrative literature review. *Nurse Education in Practice, 68.* https://doi.org/10.1016/j.nepr.2023.103570

Leahy, J. & Kizilay, P. (1998). *Foundations of nursing practice: A nursing process approach*. Philadelphia, PA: Saunders.

Lockwood, W. (2019). Documentation: Accurate and legal. *2019 RN.ORG*. http://www.medceu.co/courses/coursematerial-66.pdf

Martin, K., Bickle, K. & Lok, J. (2022). Investigating the impact of cognitive bias in nursing documentation on decision-making and judgement. *International Journal of Mental Health Nursing, 4*, 897–907. https://doi.org/10.1111/inm.12997

Mayor, E. & Bangerter, A. (2015). Managing perturbations during handover meetings: A joint activity framework. *Nursing Open, 2*(3), 130–40. https://doi.org/10.1002/nop2.29

Nursing and Midwifery Board of Australia (NMBA) (2016). *Registered nurse standards for practice*. Dickson, ACT: Nursing and Midwifery Board of Australia.

Nygaard, A., Haugdahl, H., Brinchmann, B. & Lind, R. (2023). Interprofessional care for the ICU patient's family: Solitary teamwork. *Journal of Interprofessional Care, 37*(1), 11–20. https://doi.org/10.1080/13561820.2022.2038548

Paredes-Garza, F., Lázaro, E. & Vázquez, N. (2022). Nursing bedside handover in an intensive care unit with a mixed structure: Nursing professionals' perception. *Journal of Nursing Management, 30*(8), 4314–21. https://doi.org/10.1111/jonm.13834

Paterson, C., Roberts, C. & Bail, K. (2022). 'Paper care not patient care': Nurse and patient experiences of comprehensive risk assessment and care plan documentation in hospital. *Journal of Clinical Nursing, 32*(3–4), 523–38. https://doi.org/10.1111/jocn.16291

Prochnow, J., Meiers, S. & Scheckel, M. (2019). Improving patient and caregiver new medication education using an innovative teach-back toolkit. *Journal of Nursing Care Quality, 34*(2) 101–6. https://doi.org/10.1097/NCQ.0000000000000342

Pun, J., Chan, A., Eggins, S. & Slade, D. (2020). Training in communication and interaction during shift-to-shift nursing handovers in a bilingual hospital: A case study. *Journal of Nurse Education, 84*, 104212. https://doi.org/10.1016/j.nedt.2019.104212

Queensland Health (2013). *Fact sheet: Good clinical documentation – its importance from a legal perspective.* http://woundcareresource.com/downloads/good_clinical_documentation_QH.pdf

Richard, E., Evans, T. & Williams, B. (2016). Nursing students' perceptions of preparation to engage in patient education. *Nurse Education in Practice, 28*(1), 1–6. https://doi.org/10.1016/j.nepr.2017.09.008

Robinson, A., Slight, R., Husband, A. & Slight, S. (2020). The value of teachable moments in surgical patient care and the supportive role of digital technologies. *Perioperative Medicine, 9*(2). https://doi.org/10.1186/s13741-019-0133-z

Rossi, L., Butler, S., Coakley, A. & Flanagan, J. (2023). Nursing knowledge captured in electronic health records. *International Journal of Nursing Knowledge, 34*, 72–84. https://doi.org/10.1111/2047-3095.12365

Ruotsalainen, S., Elovainio, M., Jantunen, S. & Sinervo, T. (2023). The mediating effect of psychosocial factors in the relationship between self-organizing teams and employee wellbeing: A cross-sectional observational study. *International Journal of Nursing Studies,138*. https://doi.org/10.1016/j.ijnurstu.2022.104415

Ryan-Madonna, M., Levin, R. & Lauder, B. (2019). Effectiveness of the teach-back method for improving caregivers' confidence in caring for hospice patients and decreasing hospitalizations. *Journal of Hospice & Palliative Nursing, 21*(9), 61–70. https://doi.org/10.1097/NJH.0000000000000492

Sak, G., Rothenfluh, F. & Schulz, P. J. (2017). Assessing the predictive power of psychological empowerment and health literacy for older patients' participation in health care: A cross-sectional population-based study. *Bio Med Central Geriatrics, 17*(1), 59. https://doi.org/10.1186/s12877-017-0448-x

Samani, S. & Rattani, S. (2023). Recognizing early warning signs (EWS) in patients is critically important. *Open Journal of Nursing, 13*, 53–64. https://doi.org/10.4236/ojn.2023.131004

Sammut, D., Kuruppu, J., Hegarty, K. & Bradbury-Jones, C. (2021). Which violence against women educational strategies are effective for prequalifying health-care students?: A systematic review. *Trauma, Violence, & Abuse, 22*(2), 339–58. https://doi.org/10.1177/1524838019843198

Saxena, A. & Desanghere, L. (2023). A framework for residents' pursuit of excellence based upon non-cognitive and cognitive attributes. *Postgraduate Medical Journal, 99*(1167), 17–24. https://doi.org/10.1093/postmj/qgac001

Schnur, M. (2019). *Guide to privacy and security of electronic health information*. The Office of the National Coordinator for Health Information Technology. Washington, DC, USA. March, 2019.

Seely, K., Higgs, J. & Nigh, A. (2022). Utilizing the 'teach-back' method to improve surgical informed consent and shared decision-making: A review. *Patient Safety in Surgery, 16*(1), 12. https://doi.org/10.1186/s13037-022-00322-z

Slade, D., Murray, K., Pun, J. & Eggins, S. (2018). Nurses' perceptions of mandatory bedside clinical handovers: An Australian hospital study. *Journal of Nursing Management, 27*(1), 161–71. https://doi.org/10.1111/jonm.12661

South Australia Health (2017). *Clinical handover guidelines. Policy developed by: Safety and Quality, Public Health and Clinical Systems*. http://www.sahealth.sa.gov.au/wps/wcm

St Vincent's Hospital, Melbourne (SVHM) (2017). *Documentation guidelines*. Melbourne, VIC: SVHM. https://svhm.org.au/home/education/nursing-education/undergraduate-nurse/during-placement/documentation-guidelines

Stănescu-Yadav, D-N. & Lillekroken, D. (2023). Nurse preceptors' perceptions of the fundamentals of nursing knowledge gained by students in clinical rotations at nursing homes: A qualitative study. *Journal of Professional Nursing, 44*, 17–25. https://doi.org/10.1016/j.profnurs.2022.11.005

Street, M., Dempster, J., Berry, D., Gray, E., Mapes, J., Liskaser, R., Papageorgiou, S. & Considine, J. (2022). Enhancing active patient participation in nursing handover: A mixed methods study. *Journal of Clinical Nursing, 31*, 1016–1029. https://doi.org/10.1111/jocn.15961

Terregino, C., Jagpal, S., Parikh, P., Pradhan, A., Weber, P., Michaels, L., Nicastro, O., Escobar, J. & Rashid, H. (2023). Critical care teamwork in the future: The role of team STEPPS® in the COVID-19 pandemic and implications for the future. *Healthcare, 11*(4), 599. https://doi.org/10.3390/healthcare11040599

Truccolo, I., Mazzocut, M., Mis, C., Bidoli, E., Zotti, P., Flora, S., Mei, L., Apostolico, M., Drace, C., Ravaioli, V., Conficconi, A., Cocchi, S., Cervi, E., Gangeri, L. & DePaoli, P. (2019). Patients and caregivers' unmet information needs in the field of patient education: Results from an Italian multicenter exploratory survey. *Support Care Cancer, 27*, 2023–30. https://doi.org/10.1007/s00520-018-4439-z

Vanderzwan, K., Kilroy, S., Daniels, A. & O'Rourke, J. (2023). Nurse-to-nurse handoff with distractors and interruptions: An integrative review. *Nurse Education in Practice, 67*. https://doi.org/10.1016/j.nepr.2023.103550

Yepes-Rios, M., Chavan, M., Moncaliano, M. C., Wilson-Delfosse, A. L., Mauer, Y., Croniger, C., Lambrese, J. & Logio, L. (2023). Curiosity, humility, and accountability: Key elements to advance a culture of diversity, equity, and inclusion in health professions education. In *Cases on diversity, equity, and inclusion for the health professions educator* (pp. 289–304). IGI Global. https://www.igi-global.com/chapter/curiosity-humility-and-accountability/317249

York, N. L., Kane, C., Beaton, K., Keown, B. & McMahan, S. (2017). Identifying barriers to hospitalized patients' participation in a free smoking cessation support program. *Medsurg Nursing, 26*(1), 25–32.

PART 5

ASSISTING WITH FLUID AND NUTRITIONAL STATUS

28 ASSISTING WITH MEALS

29 NASOGASTRIC TUBE INSERTION

30 ADMINISTERING ENTERAL NUTRITION

31 INTRAVENOUS THERAPY – ASSISTING WITH ESTABLISHMENT

32 INTRAVENOUS THERAPY – MANAGEMENT

Note: These notes are summaries of the most important points in the assessments/procedures and are not exhaustive on the subject. References of the materials used to compile the information have been supplied. The student is expected to have learnt the material surrounding each skill as presented in the references. No single reference is complete on each subject.

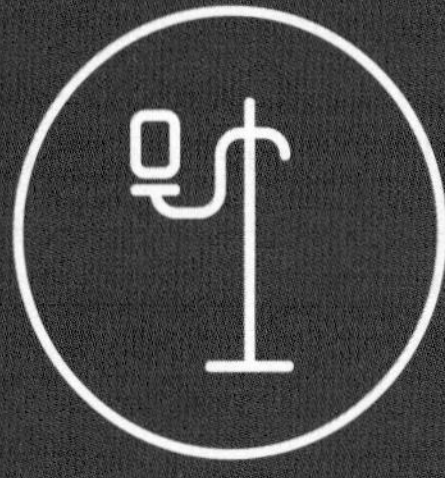

CHAPTER 28

ASSISTING WITH MEALS

INDICATIONS

Assisting with meals is fundamental nursing care. Fundamental nursing care is not common sense – high-quality fundamental care is complex and requires considerable knowledge and skill to provide a consistently high standard of relationship-centred and integrated personal care (Feo et al., 2019).

Disease-related malnutrition occurs in nearly 30 per cent of hospitalised individuals (Stumpf et al., 2023), due to both inadequate intake and the effects of inflammation and other complex pathophysiologies. It contributes to poor outcomes, including death (Sauer et al., 2019). Providing nutritional support (such as supplements, nutritional advice and assistance, and extra snacks) reduces length of stay, readmission and mortality rates in medical inpatients (Gomes, Baumgartner & Bounoure, 2019), as well as the incidence of pressure injuries (Peladic et al., 2019). Nutritional support can be tailored to the individual, the disease and the stage of the disease (Stumpf et al., 2023).

Assisting a person to maintain their nutrition is a care measure that encompasses a range of activities, from preparing food in a manner that permits the person to eat the meal independently to actually putting food into the person's mouth. It is necessary in a range of situations and incapacities.

Dysphagia (i.e. difficulty swallowing) is a functional impairment that can significantly affect a person's chewing, safe swallowing, nutrition and medication dose (Wright, Smithard & Griffith, 2020) as well as their oral health status (Furuya et al., 2020). People with neurological conditions (e.g. those caused by cerebrovascular accidents, advanced dementia, multiple sclerosis) need to have their gag and cough reflexes or dysphagia assessed (usually by a speech therapist, if available). Clinical manifestations of dysphagia include drooling, coughing during meals, hoarse voice following meals, gurgling sounds in the throat, upper respiratory tract infection, wet lung sounds or packing food in the cheeks (Klinedinst, Cohen & Dahlen, 2020). In addition to neurological conditions, the absence of teeth, decreased saliva production, poorly fitting dentures, decreased level of consciousness, certain medications (e.g. anaesthetics, sedatives, psychotropics) increase the risk of dysphagia.

Other people will have physical frailty (e.g. extremes in age), injuries (e.g. wounds of the hands or arms), medical incapacities (e.g. casts or immobilisation) or mental health conditions (e.g. dementia, severe depression) that affect their ability to feed themselves. Malnutrition also arises from disease processes, protein catabolism or decreased appetite, or may have been established prior to hospitalisation.

Irrespective of the cause of the person's eating difficulties, the primary principle is maintaining the person's nutrition and hydration as well as their dignity. Assisting a person to maintain their nutrition as palatably and independently as possible can be achieved by incorporating nursing strategies such as modifying crockery and cutlery, opening food or drink packages, pouring fluids into cups, preparing or cutting food into bite-size pieces, altering the consistency of diet and fluids, providing finger foods where appropriate or positioning the person to reduce aspiration risks.

EVIDENCE OF THERAPEUTIC INTERACTION

Introduce yourself and explain the type of assistance you will provide and your expectations of the person. This will assist with their cooperation. Talking with the person about their interests normalises mealtimes and helps the person relax. Maintaining a positive attitude and making encouraging comments assists the person to eat and drink the necessary amounts. Avoid discussing treatments or medical procedures, unless the person wishes to discuss them.

Cultural and spiritual diversity also require consideration (Sheikh, 2023). For instance, special foods are prepared and consumed for celebrations such as the Jewish Passover or the Hindu Holi. The family will probably provide these foods. Fasting is also part of the spiritual life of many people, and this needs special consideration. Christians may observe Lent (40 days prior to Easter), during which fasting and avoidance of some foods (e.g. meat) is practised. If the person's condition permits, intermittent fasting is possible (e.g. during the month-long Ramadan observed by Muslims, food and fluids can be given before dawn and after sunset). The person who is very ill and cannot fast may have a dispensation from their spiritual leader to eat and drink, and receive IV fluids when necessary.

DEMONSTRATE CLINICAL REASONING

Prepare the environment

Provide privacy to minimise embarrassment. Clean the over-bed table so the food tray can be placed conveniently and hygienically. Note that over-bed tables should be reserved for food, drink and personal items only. Do not place elimination items, linen (clean or soiled) dressing materials or other healthcare items on them. It is not pleasant to see your personal space filled with these items. In some cases, use of the table for anything other than food or drink is culturally repugnant. Remove any distressing material from the room (e.g. dressing materials, bedpans, or anything with a noxious or overpowering odour, including some flowers) and open any windows to air the room if appropriate. Noxious odours and sights diminish the appetite.

Assess the person

Consult the written plan of care for the person to maintain consistency of care provision. Usually, the level of assistance required is available on a care plan. If not, ask the person what help they would like.

Safety

The following three-step nursing swallowing assessment assists to identify dysphagia and reduce the person's risk of aspiration (note to New Zealand student nurses – the nursing swallowing assessment is not within your competencies):

1. Examine the person's level of consciousness, posture, voluntary cough, voice quality and saliva control.
2. Have the person drink one teaspoon of water.
3. If the teaspoon of water clears safely, have the person drink small sips from a glass of water.

Assist the person

Reduce the person's discomfort by assessing their pain and nausea levels 20 to 30 minutes prior to mealtime. If required, administer analgesia or anti-emetic as ordered, ensuring the person is comfortable. This assists relaxation.

If the person needs assistance with elimination, ask them if they would like to use the toilet, urinal or bedpan prior to eating. This improves comfort levels and reduces risks of interruption to the meal. Provide required materials for the person to wash their hands in order to reduce contamination.

Provide oral care prior to mealtime. If they wear dentures, ask if they would like to clean and replace them. If glasses or a hearing aid are required, help the person to put them on.

ELDER CARE

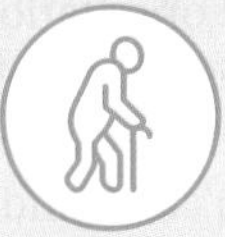

Malnutrition is highly prevalent in older adults, often due to age-related physiological decline, reduced access to nutritious food (cost, difficulty in shopping or preparing food), comorbidities (Dent et al., 2023) and disinterest in eating (e.g. isolation, diminished taste). Malnutrition increases the morbidity and mortality of hospitalised elders (Wu et al., 2023). Nutritional support may be required. This may include individualised nutritional assessment, guidance and counselling, oral nutritional supplements, fortified foods, assistance with preparing and consuming meals and enteral or parenteral nutrition as required (Dent et al., 2023).

Social isolation contributes to poor nutritional intake and inadequate hydration. Poor social connections increase the risk of cardiovascular disease, hypertension, diabetes, infectious diseases, impaired cognitive function, depression and anxiety (*The Lancet*, 2023). Many elderly people are socially isolated, although not every elderly person is lonely or isolated, and loneliness and social isolation are not limited to the elderly, and, indeed, they can manifest at any age. Feelings of social isolation can reduce nutritional intake. Inviting relatives or friends to sit with the person during their meal promotes interaction. Shune and Linville (2019) found individualisation of care and socialisation improved nutritional intake. A television or music may provide some simulated social interaction. However, if the person has dysphagia, distractions should be minimised (Hunter, 2013). Digital technology in the form of Skyping with a loved one or tele-dining supports more interactivity while eating (Spence, Mancini & Huisman, 2019).

THE PERSON LIVING WITH SEVERE OBESITY

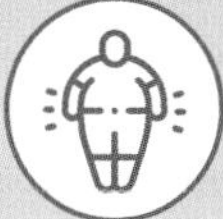

People living with severe obesity are at risk of malnutrition, due to long-term dietary restriction, comorbidities, polypharmacy, lack of nutritional assessment tools and appropriate nutritional guidelines for people living with severe obesity, staff bias (Dickerson et al., 2022) and sarcopenia from, especially, protein lack. Individualised nutritional care, involving the dietician, physician, pharmacist and nursing staff, can help. Elliott et al. (2023) identified that 70.4 per cent of hospitalised people living with obesity were not seen by a dietician.

PART 5

GATHER EQUIPMENT

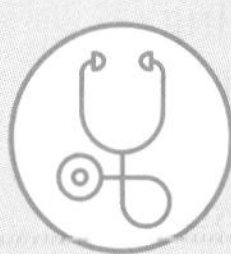

Gather and prepare all the equipment required to assist the person before proceeding to the bedside to minimise disruption for the person during their meal. Various types of equipment are available to increase independence and can be individualised to the person's needs and their dietary requirements; these include but are not limited to the following:

EQUIPMENT	EXPLANATION
Large serviette or hand towel	• Used to protect the person's clothing • Do not call it a 'bib' to preserve self-esteem
Cups with specialised spouts	For a person who has weakened muscles around their mouth, the specialised spouts introduce liquids deep enough into the person's mouth to reduce fluids escaping
Non-slip place mat	Keeps dishes in place, so cutlery can be used more effectively
Large-handled cutlery	• For a person with a weakened grip or reduced fine-motor hand functions, large-handled cutlery allows a person to use a spoon or fork • These often have hand clips to reduce the amount of work needed to grip them
Rimmed plates	Designed to provide an edge against which a spoon or fork can be pushed so the food is piled up on the utensil. They are generally heavier than usual, so they sit still
Weighted utensils	The extra weight and bulk of the cutlery assists those with tremors to hold cutlery
Plastic-covered spoons	Help you to safely introduce food into the person's mouth without fear of chipping teeth or cutting the lip
A plastic apron	Protects your uniform from soiling

When assisting the person to reposition, consider the time required in that position, and your own comfort when assisting them, to prevent self-injury from assuming an awkward position. If the person would like to sit out of bed and it is appropriate, assist them to do so. Sitting upright assists in normalising the meal, reduces risk of aspiration and aids digestion. Alternatively, help the person to sit as upright as their condition permits (see **Clinical Skill 57**).

?

If the person's appetite is poor (i.e. they eat less than half of the food provided), and if permitted, then food brought from home is usually more palatable and more readily eaten than the institutional food. Remember, people eat food, not nutrition (Holst et al., 2017). Family may feel more useful if they are providing some of their loved one's food.

ASSIST A PERSON WITH MEALS

Video

Assisting a person with meals can range from choosing the correct type of food preparation (e.g. toast would be painful to eat with mouth ulcers) to physically feeding them.

Hand hygiene

Hand hygiene (see **Clinical Skill 5**) removes microorganisms from your hands. It is the most effective preventative measure for cross-contamination, reducing incidences of nosocomial (i.e. hospital- or treatment-acquired) infection. In this procedure, it is necessary to prevent food contamination. For this skill, hand washing applies to the person in care as well as you, and is an aesthetic necessity besides being a hygiene one.

Assist a person to maintain nutrition

Minimal assistance required

Some people only need assistance with opening food containers (e.g. the foil seals on juice cups or yoghurt containers, or caps on bottles). You may need to help with their serviette, remove plastic wrap or pour tea, unwrap and butter bread, spread jam, put sauce onto the food (ask first!) or cut meat and vegetables into bite-size pieces.

A person with reduced vision may need orientation to the tray and the location of food on their plate. Tell them exactly what is on their tray and where each item is. Use the clock face (e.g. the meat is at 9 o'clock and the potatoes are at 2 o'clock) to describe their plate. Ask what assistance they require (e.g. to rearrange their tray). Open packets and containers, remove plastic wrap and tell the person where you have put the condiments and extras. Help the person with their serviette or other protection for their clothing.

Assist the person to maintain their hydration by helping them to drink water and their preferred beverages (within the limits of their medical condition) throughout the day. Provide drinks at the preferred temperature.

Total assistance required

Put on a plastic apron to protect your uniform, if necessary. Determine the type of diet the person needs, as recommended by the dietitian or speech therapist. The food may be vitamised in the kitchen and placed in a thermos to keep it at the correct temperature, or it may consist of liquids, soft foods, or a 'normal' diet that you will need to prepare as for someone requiring minimal assistance. Place a large serviette or hand towel over the person's chest to protect their clothing.

Transfer liquids to a feeding cup. Ask the person in which order they would like their meal and if they would like condiments added to their food. If they are unable to advise you, offer the food in the following order: the soup, the main meal and then dessert, followed by tea or coffee. Tell the person what food you are offering and its temperature (e.g. this is warm tomato soup). Place small amounts of liquid in their mouth and watch that this is swallowed before giving more.

For the vitamised food, take about a teaspoonful onto the plasticised spoon, and again tell the person what the food is. Do not mix the food together unless the person specifically asks.

For someone who needs assistance to eat a normal diet, cut the meat and vegetables into bite-sized pieces and use a plastic-covered spoon to convey small amounts to their mouth. Wait until these are chewed and swallowed and the person is ready for more before offering another spoonful.

A person generally requires 20 minutes to eat a meal. However, some people are tired by the simple act of eating and require longer intervals between mouthfuls. You may need to reheat the food to ensure it remains appetising. Rushing a person to eat their meal causes distress, limits their enjoyment, can reduce digestion and reduce nutritional intake. Enjoyment of the tastes and textures of food is an incentive to eat.

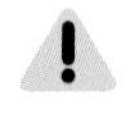
Safety

For people with dysphagia, the following nursing interventions reduce the risk of aspiration:

- rest for 30 minutes before eating
- sit in an upright, chin-down position, head turned to one side
- place food in one side of mouth
- alternate small amounts of solid and liquid foods
- thicken food to a honey consistency (if recommended by the speech therapist)
- avoid rushing or forced feeding: people with dysphagia require approximately 30 minutes for eating/assisted feeding
- minimise distractions (Klinedinst, Cohen & Dahlen, 2020).

Any food the person refuses because of dislike should be noted within their health history and reported to the dietitian so that it is not served again.

Post-procedure

Remove the tray and tidy other debris (wrappers, serviette into the general rubbish). Use or offer a warm washcloth or wipes to clean hands and face. Offer dental care and/or mouthwash. Leave the person sitting in their chair or supported in a semi-Fowler's position (as permitted) for 30 to 45 minutes post-meal to reduce the incidence of regurgitation or aspiration. Leave the person comfortable and with their possessions and the call bell within their reach.

CLEAN, REPLACE AND DISPOSE OF EQUIPMENT

Usually, specialised feeding equipment is cleaned using dishwashing detergent, dried and returned to a storage cupboard. In some facilities, these utensils go to the kitchen for cleaning, and come back with the person's tray for their next meal.

DOCUMENTATION

Relevant information, including date and time, amount and type of food and fluids offered and consumed, is noted, generally on a food chart. Evaluation of the person's responses (until impaired gag and cough reflexes resolve) is documented.

CLINICAL SKILLS ASSESSMENT

Assisting with meals

Demonstrates the ability to effectively and safely assist a person to maintain their nutrition. Incorporates the *National Safety and Quality Health Service Standards*: 2 Partnering with Consumers, 3 Preventing and Controlling Healthcare-Associated Infection, 5 Comprehensive Care, 6 Communicating for Safety, and 8 Recognising and Responding to Acute Deterioration (ACSQHC, 2021b).

Performance criteria	1	2	3	4	5
(Numbers indicate NMBA *Registered Nurse Standards for Practice*)	(Dependent)	(Marginal)	(Assisted)	(Supervised)	(Independent)
1. Identifies indication (1.1, 3.3, 3.4)	☐	☐	☐	☐	☐
2. Evidence of therapeutic interaction with the person, e.g. gives an explanation, converses with the person (1.4, 1.5, 2.1, 2.2, 2.3)	☐	☐	☐	☐	☐
3. Demonstrates clinical reasoning abilities, e.g. prepares the person, administers medications if required, prepares room or bed space (1.1, 1.2, 1.3, 4.2, 6.1)	☐	☐	☐	☐	☐
4. Gathers equipment as needed (5.5, 6.1): ■ protection for clothing ■ feeder cup ■ large-handled utensils ■ rimmed plate ■ plastic-covered spoon ■ apron	☐	☐	☐	☐	☐
5. Adheres to hand hygiene (1.1, 3.4, 6.1)	☐	☐	☐	☐	☐
6. Puts on appropriate personal protective equipment (1.1, 3.4, 6.1)	☐	☐	☐	☐	☐
7. Assists the person to eat (1.1, 1.2, 4.2, 5.1, 6.1)	☐	☐	☐	☐	☐
8. Cleans, replaces and disposes of equipment appropriately (3.6, 6.1)	☐	☐	☐	☐	☐
9. Documents relevant information (1.4, 1.6, 2.2, 3.5, 3.7, 6.2, 6.5, 7.3)	☐	☐	☐	☐	☐
10. Demonstrates the ability to link theory to practice (1.1, 3.3, 3.5)	☐	☐	☐	☐	☐

Student:

Clinical facilitator: Date:

CHAPTER 29

NASOGASTRIC TUBE INSERTION

INDICATIONS

Nasogastric tubes (NGTs) are inserted to:

- decompress the stomach and upper bowel
- empty the stomach of accumulated gas and fluid
- lavage the stomach of toxic fluid
- gain access to stomach contents for gastric analysis
- gain access to the upper gastrointestinal tract for medical intervention (e.g. treatment of oesophageal varices – the procedure is done by physicians for this intervention)
- provide enteral feedings (and medications) when the person is unable to take adequate nutrition orally.

People who are unable to take adequate nutrition orally include those who:

- have difficulty swallowing
- are unresponsive
- have had oral or neck surgery or trauma
- are anorexic
- are seriously ill.

The gastrointestinal tract below the oesophagus must be functional.

A written physician's order is necessary to initiate NGT insertion for enteral feedings. Usually, a dietitian will indicate the type and amount of enteral feedings required.

After the initial insertion, the frequency of NGT replacement is determined by the individual facility.

There are many contraindications to insertion of an NGT, including:

- basal skull fractures
- maxillofacial disorders/surgeries or injuries
- unstable cervical spinal injuries
- nasal/pharyngeal /oesophageal obstruction or ulceration
- oesophageal stricture (e.g. trauma caused by ingestion of a caustic substance causing burns) or other abnormalities of the oesophagus
- post laryngectomy
- actively bleeding oesophageal or gastric varices
- intestinal obstruction (Sigmon & An, 2022).

Verify the written medication order

Verification is a legal requirement. The written medication order usually alerts you to the reason for the NGT, may indicate the size that is needed and state any time limit for leaving the tube in place. The order may indicate the use of lidocaine and a nasal vasoconstrictor to significantly decrease the person's discomfort (Sigmon & An, 2022).

This skill focuses on the insertion of the small bore NGT for supplying nutrition and administering medications.

EVIDENCE OF THERAPEUTIC INTERACTION

The person, whether responsive or not, requires a clear explanation for why an NGT is needed. Inserting it is an uncomfortable procedure. If the person understands the need, what to expect and how to help, they will be more willing to consent, and you will be able to complete the procedure with a minimum of discomfort for the person. Assess the person's mental status and ability to cooperate, as another nurse may be required to assist. A combination of interactive styles that blend the technical or directive style with an affective or comforting style has proved to be both effective and efficient (Penrod, Morse & Wilson, 1999).

DEMONSTRATE CLINICAL REASONING

Safety of the person, their privacy and dignity, and easing the insertion of the NGT are all important aspects of the individual's care.

Safety considerations

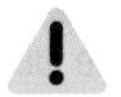

Safety

Several complications, including kinking, coiling, misplacement, aspiration, nasopharyngeal trauma, severe epistaxis and ulceration, are associated with the insertion of NGTs (Vadivelu et al., 2023). Longer-term use for external feeding adds gastrointestinal complications such as nausea, vomiting, diarrhoea or constipation, and metabolic complications such as dehydration and electrolyte disturbances. Be aware of these and watch for signs and symptoms.

X-ray verification of the placement of the NGT is best practice, especially if a guide wire has been used. The placement of the tube must be assessed prior to any fluid (water, enteral feeds or medication) being introduced.

Provision of privacy

Privacy preserves the person's dignity. This procedure can often be distressing. Family members are frequently requested to leave the bedside of the person to minimise their own distress. The person should have the freedom of being in private so that distress can be expressed without embarrassment. Providing comfort measures and pain relief increases the trust the person has in you; they may also increase the person's ability to relax, which will facilitate the insertion of the NGT.

Position the person

Position in a semi- to high Fowler's position if the person's condition permits. This position facilitates insertion because of the force of gravity and the anatomical structure of the nasopharynx and oesophagus. Place a pillow behind the person's shoulders to maintain their position. Assess the pharyngeal (gag) and swallowing reflexes to determine the possibility of aspiration. Touch the back of the palate with a sterile tongue blade to elicit a pharyngeal reflex; ask the person to swallow a sip of water, watch and listen for changes in voice, or coughing, to assess the swallowing reflex. Also assess their abdomen for distension, pain, tenderness and bowel sounds for later comparison if required.

Give the person a glass of cool, fresh water and a straw, if allowed.

ELDER CARE

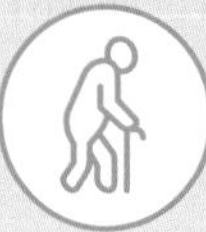

Use a fine-bore, flexible tube for elders (over 65 years) to reduce irritation and erosion of oesophageal and nasal tissue (Vadivelu et al., 2023). Stomach content pH increases with advanced age (Taskiran & Sari, 2022), so aspiration of stomach content is less reliable and X-ray placement verification is extremely important. Rabaut et al. (2022) found that within individuals with severe stroke, the older the age, a diagnosis of pneumonia and number of nasogastric tube insertions were associated with higher mortality.

THE PERSON LIVING WITH SEVERE OBESITY

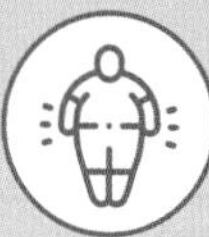

For people living with severe obesity, a guide wire within the NGT aids insertion and increases the 'first attempt' success with fewer complications (kinking, coiling or bleeding) associated with insertion (Vadivelu et al., 2023). The initial feeding tube placement should be assessed by X-ray – again, the guide wire type of tube will be important.

PERFORM NASOGASTRIC TUBE INSERTION

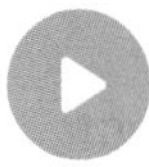

Video

Inserting the NGT is comprised of a number of sequential steps that combine to keep the person safe and help to accomplish the task, as outlined in the following sections.

GATHER EQUIPMENT

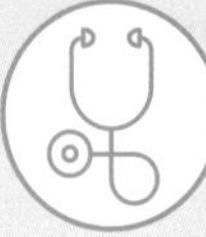

Gathering equipment is an organisational step that helps to create a positive environment for a successful interaction. It ensures that you have all needed material, boosts the person's confidence and trust in you, and increases your self-confidence. While gathering the equipment, you can mentally rehearse the procedure. Equipment required includes:

EQUIPMENT	EXPLANATION
Nasogastric tube NB – the NGT used for enteral feeding/medication administration is colour coded (the colour depends on the size and the manufacturer) If it is used for drainage, the tube will be clear	• A small-calibre, flexible tube with a radio-opaque tip • Its size is determined by the size of the person and the intended use and duration of the tube placement • Small-bore tubes (less than Fr9) are less traumatic to insert and are better tolerated. Large-bore NGTs are used for stomach decompression and emptying, and to administer medication • Immersing the (rubber/silastic) tube in ice may be required to reduce its pliability and aid ease of insertion. A warm-water bath may be required for heavier or stiff plastic tubes to increase their flexibility • The tube will have an attached cap for use with intermittent feedings or medication administration • A guide wire/stylet may be incorporated in the NGT to ease insertion of softer plastic tubes. The guide wire may or may not need to be removed (once removed, it is never reinserted)

EQUIPMENT	EXPLANATION
Emesis basin	• This is precautionary, in case insertion of the NGT causes vomiting
Lubricant or normal saline (NS)	• Reduces friction so the tube is more easily inserted • Follow the facility's protocol
Fresh water and a straw	• For the person to sip and swallow during insertion. This reduces the gag reflex and speeds the insertion • Water can only be given to someone who is able to swallow, can follow instructions and has no contraindications
Clean gloves and an apron	• Worn for your protection (standard precautions)
pH indicator strips (with a range of pH 1–6) in a kidney dish	• Measure the acidity of the stomach contents to verify correct placement of the NGT • The kidney dish is used to minimise mess during testing
Waterproof pen	• To mark the tube and denote the time and date on the tape
50 mL syringe (oral)	• Used to remove a small amount of gastric content to test for pH using the pH indicator strips in the kidney dish
Tongue blade and penlight	• Used initially to check the patency of the nostril and then visually determine the position of the tube in the oropharynx during insertion • An extra tongue blade may be used to check the gag reflex prior to starting the procedure
Low-suction apparatus	• The low-suction apparatus is used to apply suction to decompress the stomach and remove excess fluids and gas without damaging the intestinal mucosa • A doctor's order is needed to apply suction to an NGT
Drainage bag (may be needed)	• Used if gravity drainage is to be used
Feeding apparatus (kangaroo pump, gravity feed, IV stand) and ordered nutritional fluid	• Deliver the appropriate enteral feeding to the tube
Adaptor	• Used to connect the NGT to either the suction tubing or the enteral feeding tubing
Elastic band and safety pin	• Used to secure the tubing to the person's clothing to minimise 'pull' when moving
Hypo-allergenic adhesive tape	• Used to mark the position of the tube (an indelible pen may also be used) and secure the NGT in position • Prepare tape to secure the NGT before starting the procedure. Cut a 10 cm length of tape and split it lengthwise to 5 cm. This will produce a 5 cm length of tape with 2 × 5 cm 'tails'. Cut another small piece of tape to use as a marker. Stick both onto the over-bed table or another easily reached place
Paper (disposable) tape measure	• Used to measure the length of the tube from the nares to the hub following insertion. It is left coiled at the bedside for ongoing use • This is a safeguard in case of dislodgement
Absorbent pad	• Keeps the person and the bedclothes clean and dry
Clamp or plug	• Needed to occlude the tube between feedings (for bolus feedings)
Tissues	• Given to the person because lachrymation (tearing) often occurs during passage of the tube
Oral hygiene equipment	• Mouth care is important following NGT insertion for refreshment and cleansing • See **Clinical Skill 56** for more on oral hygiene

Hand hygiene

This is a clean procedure (as opposed to a medically aseptic procedure). Hand hygiene (see **Clinical Skill 5**) removes microbes and reduces their transmission to the person. Clean gloves are used to comply with standard precautions.

Insert the nasogastric tube

Determine the length of insertion

The length of tube to insert must be decided before you start the procedure, to ensure that the distal tip is long enough to rest in the stomach or duodenum. Estimate the length required by measuring from the person's nares to their earlobe and then to their xiphoid process. This length approximates the distance from the nose to the stomach; however, the tube may need to be inserted further (up to 10 cm) to reach the body of the stomach (Vadivelu et al., 2023). The required length is marked on the tube with a waterproof pen or small piece of tape, or its distance is noted from the measuring marks on the tube so the length is obvious.

Check nostrils for obstruction

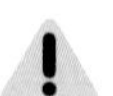
Safety

Ask the person if they have any difficulty in breathing through one nostril or the other, or if they have had nasal surgery or a deviated septum. Ask them to tip their head back (if able) so you can look up each nostril. Use your penlight to assist you. Occlude each nostril and ask the person to breathe through their nose. Listen for breathing difficulties. If there are no obstructions, give the person the choice of which nostril will be used.

Place the absorbent pad on their chest. Ask them to blow their nose to clear any mucus from the nasal passages. Use lidocaine or nasal vasoconstrictor medication as ordered. Wait the recommended time until the medication is effective.

Introduce the nasogastric tube

Wrap the initial 10 cm of the tube around your gloved fingers and release to increase its flexibility. Lubricate the NGT for the first 6 to 10 cm with a water-soluble lubricant or NS to decrease friction and ease insertion. Ask the person to keep their head in a neutral position, if able, so the nares are parallel to the floor (Vadivelu et al., 2023), to straighten the curvature of the nasopharyngeal junction. Insert the tube along the floor of the chosen nostril, with the natural curve of the tube towards the person and towards the ear to avoid the turbinates in the nostril. When the tube is in the nasopharynx, ask the person to flex their neck ('chin tuck') so the NGT will more easily follow the posterior wall of the nasopharynx and enter the oesophagus rather than the trachea.

The NGT should be introduced slowly but steadily. When the NGT reaches the back of the oropharynx, the person may begin to gag. Stop advancing the tube momentarily and ask the person to sip and swallow some water (if not contraindicated). Advance the tube quickly (5 to 10 cm) when the person swallows. The muscular movements of swallowing help to advance the NGT. If the person begins to choke, cough or become dyspnoeic or cyanotic, pull the tube back but do not remove it. Resume advancing the tube with each swallow.

If resistance is met, withdraw the tube, relubricate it and reinsert it through the other nostril. Watch the person closely while inserting the NGT. Observation of coughing, choking or cyanosis indicates that the tube has tracked into the trachea and bronchi. If this occurs, remove the tube and attempt the procedure again when the person has regained their breath. Continuous gagging may indicate that the tube has not continued down the oesophagus and is instead coiled at the back of the throat. Check by looking through the mouth. If the tube is coiled there, remove it to the point where it is straight and continue advancing it. Remember that if the person's level of consciousness is impaired, the cough and gag reflexes will be absent. Do not rely on this indicator. Clean any lubricant or mucus from the person's nose.

Anchor the tube using the prepared tape when the NGT has been inserted to the marked length. Place the non-split half of the tape on the bridge of the nose and wrap one of the tails around the tube. The mark of the tube is observed four-hourly and prior to introduction of any fluid into the tube to check for migration. If this happens, an X-ray is needed for confirmation.

Check the nasogastric tube position

Determine the position of the distal tip of the nasogastric tube. An X-ray is the surest and safest method to determine the placement of the tube and is recommended practice. A 50 mL syringe can also be used to establish position, although aspiration of stomach contents is not an infallible indicator (Taskiran & Sari, 2022). Aspirate a small amount of the gastric contents. Observe the aspirate for colour. Although not an independent indicator of correct placement, a clear, colourless to grassy green to brown liquid can be a helpful clue. Drip it on fresh pH indicator strips (litmus paper is not accurate enough). A reading of 1.5 to 5 indicates that the tip of the NGT is in the stomach (stomach contents usually have a pH below 5). However, Judd (2020) warns that the person cannot have had medications or food for at least an hour prior to testing the stomach contents for the pH to be below 5. Point of care ultrasound is a more reliable method of placement determination but requires the appropriate equipment (at this time, usually in the Intensive Care Unit). It is a convenient and effective tool for monitoring NGT positioning (Wang et al., 2022). Leave the syringe attached to the tube so it does not leak until you are ready to connect it to suction or feeding.

> ?
> **If no aspirate returns, advance the NGT a further 7 to 10 cm and attempt to recover aspirate again for testing. The person may need to be repositioned to place the tip in a pool of stomach contents.**

Secure the nasogastric tube to the person

Once the position of the tube is confirmed to be in the stomach, mark the place where the tube emerges from the nares (so that any migration of the tube can be seen) with either an indelible pen or a strip of tape marked as such. You can also measure the length of tubing from the nares to the hub (with the paper measuring tape) and document this measurement in the nursing notes or care plan. This provides a base measurement to compare in case of dislodgement.

Wrap the remaining tape 'tail' around the tube to reduce the chance of dislodging the tube. Tape the tube to the person's cheek out of their line of vision to reduce annoyance and stabilise the tube. Ensure that there is no traction placed on the nares, to prevent pressure and eventual breakdown of the skin, as well as discomfort. Note the date and time on the tape with a waterproof pen. Tuck the other end of the tube behind the ear or secure it to the person's gown with an elastic band and safety pin to reduce its movement.

Connect the free end of the nasogastric tube

Use the connector to connect the free end of the tube to the low-suction apparatus, a collection bag (gravity drainage) or the enteral feeding tube as appropriate. The tube may also be clamped or plugged for later use. Connections are often taped to prevent disconnection. Suction is commenced as ordered. Monitor and document the amount and character of the drainage. If feeding is ordered, the initial instillation should be a *slow* (gravity-fed) instillation of a small amount of water. This is a precaution taken in case the tube tip has inadvertently been placed into the trachea. A minimal amount of water in the lung causes fewer problems than does an enteral feeding preparation.

If changes in respiratory status occur, withdraw the tube immediately.

Post-procedure

Assist the person to a position of comfort. They may wish to stay in Fowler's position. Clean their nares and offer oral hygiene both for their comfort and to reduce the incidence of hospital-acquired infection. Ensure their personal belongings and the call bell are available. Perform hand hygiene.

Removing the nasogastric tube

When the nasogastric medication administration or nutrition is no longer required (e.g. recovery from post-stroke dysphagia), the person requires a long-term solution (e.g. a percutaneous endoscopic gastrostomy [PEG] formation) or the NGT is on a routine change schedule (e.g. q2 weeks to maintain patency), removal of the NGT is ordered.

You will need:

EQUIPMENT	EXPLANATION
Alcohol-based hand rub (ABHR)	To remove microorganisms from your hands before and after the procedure
PPE, including safety goggles/shield, clean gloves	For protection against splashes of body fluids either contaminating your eyes, or your clothing. This is a clean procedure
Tissues	To assist the person to clean their nares following NGT removal
Emesis basin/bag	In case the person vomits during removal of the tube
Underpad (bluey)	Protection of the person's clothing from mucous or gastric content
Clinical waste bin	To contain used and soiled items
Oral care equipment	To freshen the person's mouth following NGT removal

Procedure

Hand hygiene is completed before touching the person/bed area (hand washing, using ABHR). Provide privacy to maintain dignity. This procedure may be distressing to the person, triggering the gag reflex and vomiting. The procedure is as follows:

- Identify the person by asking their name and verifying with their identification bracelet.
- Explain the reason for removal and the procedure and ask their permission to proceed (i.e. consent). Ask them to 'teach-back' so you know they understand.
- Ask the person to practise taking a breath and exhaling slowly. Again, use the ABHR or wash your hands.
- Turn off suction (if used) and disconnect the NGT from the suction machine or feeding pump. Use ABHR and put on personal protective equipment (PPE).
- Place the underpad on the person's chest to protect their clothing and unpin the NGT from the gown.
- Remove adhesive tape from the nose. Take care, as facial skin is tender.
- Grasp the NGT close to the person's nose and crimp it (fold over on itself and pinch it tightly) to reduce any leakage of remaining fluid.
- Ask the person to take a deep breath and exhale slowly as you remove the NGT tube in a steady, continuous movement. Check the tip of the NGT for intactness, place it onto the underpad and discard both into the clinical waste bin.
- Offer tissues to the person (mucous is expected and the person will need to clean their nares).
- Use ABHR.
- Provide oral care to freshen their mouth.
- Document: In the medical record time, date, skin integrity (nares) and response to removal. In the fluid balance chart record time, date of removal, and cessation of feeding/aspirate monitoring.

SOURCE: ADAPTED FROM NSW HEALTH (2023). *GUIDELINE: INSERTION AND MANAGEMENT OF NASOGASTRIC AND OROGASTRIC TUBES IN ADULTS*. HTTPS://WWW1.HEALTH.NSW.GOV.AU/PDS/ACTIVEPDSDOCUMENTS/GL2023_001.PDF

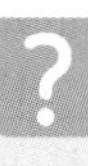

If the tip of the NGT is not intact, contact the senior registered nurse (RN) or medical officer as soon as possible.

CLEAN, REPLACE AND DISPOSE OF EQUIPMENT

Replace equipment to ensure that the next person to use it is not inconvenienced. It is important that pH graded indicator strips are stored as per manufacturer's instructions (usually tightly covered in a dark place). Dispose of used material to reduce clutter at the bedside, to increase the person's psychological comfort and to reduce material on which microorganisms can flourish. Perform hand hygiene.

DOCUMENTATION

The reason for the NGT insertion is documented. Record:

- the person's consent
- the type and size of NGT used
- ease of insertion
- confirmation of placement, and length of the tube from nares to hub
- amount of aspirate and its nature, including pH
- type of apparatus connected (e.g. suction and the pressure setting, kangaroo pump, gravity drain)
- the person's response to the procedure.

This will increase communication between healthcare professionals and comply with legal requirements for reporting changes.

CLINICAL SKILLS ASSESSMENT

Nasogastric tube insertion

Demonstrates the ability to safely and efficiently insert a nasogastric tube (NGT). Incorporates the *National Safety and Quality Health Service Standards*: 2 Partnering with Consumers, 3 Preventing and Controlling Healthcare-Associated Infection, 5 Comprehensive Care, 6 Communicating for Safety, and 8 Recognising and Responding to Acute Deterioration (ACSQHC, 2021b).

Performance criteria	1	2	3	4	5
(Numbers indicate NMBA *Registered Nurse Standards for Practice*)	(Dependent)	(Marginal)	(Assisted)	(Supervised)	(Independent)
1. Identifies indication (1.1, 3.3, 3.4)	☐	☐	☐	☐	☐
2. Verifies the written medication order (1.4, 3.4, 6.1, 6.2, 6.5)	☐	☐	☐	☐	☐
3. Evidence of therapeutic interaction with the person, e.g. gives a clear explanation of the procedure (1.4, 1.5, 2.1, 2.2, 3.2)	☐	☐	☐	☐	☐
4. Demonstrates clinical reasoning abilities, e.g. provides privacy, comfort measures, pain relief, positions the person (1.1, 1.2, 1.3, 4.2, 6.1)	☐	☐	☐	☐	☐
5. Gathers appropriate equipment (5.5, 6.1):	☐	☐	☐	☐	☐
6. Performs hand hygiene and dons gloves (1.1, 3.4, 6.1)	☐	☐	☐	☐	☐
7. Ascertains the length of nasogastric tube to be inserted (1.1, 6.1)	☐	☐	☐	☐	☐
8. Checks nostrils for obstruction (1.1, 4.2, 6.1)	☐	☐	☐	☐	☐
9. Inserts nasogastric tube to the appropriate length (1.1, 1.4, 6.1)	☐	☐	☐	☐	☐
10. Ascertains the placement of the nasogastric tube (1.1, 1.4, 6.1)	☐	☐	☐	☐	☐
11. Tapes the nasogastric tube to the person (1.1, 6.1)	☐	☐	☐	☐	☐
12. Connects the nasogastric tube to appropriate apparatus (1.1, 6.1)	☐	☐	☐	☐	☐
13. Cleans, replaces and disposes of equipment appropriately (3.6, 6.1)	☐	☐	☐	☐	☐
14. Removes NGT efficiently	☐	☐	☐	☐	☐
15. Documents relevant information (1.4, 1.6, 2.2, 2.7, 3.5, 3.7, 6.2, 6.5, 7.3)	☐	☐	☐	☐	☐
16. Demonstrates the ability to link theory to practice (1.1, 3.3, 3.4, 3.5)	☐	☐	☐	☐	☐

Student:

Clinical facilitator: Date:

CHAPTER 30

ADMINISTERING ENTERAL NUTRITION

INDICATIONS

Enteral feeding supplies nutrients to the person who is unable to safely consume adequate nutrition orally. The person must have a functional gastrointestinal tract but be unable to eat. This may be due to trauma or disease of the mouth, neck or throat. Enteral nutrition has positive effects on the gastrointestinal mucosa, nourishing the enterocytes and thereby maintaining the absorptive and immunologic structures of the bowel minimising inflammation and preventing mucosal atrophy (Lai et al., 2022).

Selection of the enteral access route depends on the type and anticipated duration of supplemental requirements, gastric emptying and aspiration risk. Enteral nutrition can be delivered through orogastric, nasogastric (NG), transpyloric gastrostomy and jejunostomy tubes.

Orogastric tube feeding is used almost exclusively for newborns. Orogastric tubes can also be inserted for gastric lavage in adults.

Nasogastric feeding is the most commonly used enteral feed and is suitable for short-term feeding (approximately two to four weeks) (Vadivelu et al., 2023). Fine-bore feeding tubes should be used whenever possible because these are more comfortable for the person than wide-bore tubes. They are also less likely to cause complications such as rhinitis, oesophageal irritation and gastritis (Dietitians Association of Australia [DAA], 2018).

Gastrostomy tubes pass through the abdominal wall directly into the stomach. They are commonly inserted endoscopically (percutaneous endoscopic gastrostomy [PEG]) and can also be placed surgically. Gastrostomy tubes are usually used for those who require medium (six to 12 weeks) to long-term feeding, or where NG access is difficult. Following placement and healing, the insertion site is cared for as part of normal hygiene, using soap and water on the skin around the tube.

Jejunostomy tubes are placed surgically through the abdominal wall into the jejunum. Some are placed via the nasogastric route, but the tube is longer and extended into the duodenum or jejunum. They are generally used when there is a high risk of pulmonary aspiration or in people with delayed gastric emptying, gastroparesis associated with people who are uraemic, or in those who have diabetes. They can also be inserted via a gastric puncture with the assistance of either an endoscope or radiography to guide an extension through the pylorus into the duodenum or jejunum (percutaneous endoscopic gastrostomy – jejunum [PEGJ]). Gastrostomy feeding does reduce the risks associated with reflux and aspiration, but does not entirely eliminate them (DAA, 2018). Jejunostomy feeds must be sterile because the acidic, anti-infective stomach has been bypassed.

Verify the written medication order

Before enteral tube feedings are administered, a nutrition plan is developed by the multidisciplinary team. The person's past medical history, current condition, laboratory results (e.g. urea and electrolytes, renal function, liver function test and blood sugar levels) and current medications are reviewed. Calculation of the person's caloric and protein requirements are made and their hydration is considered.

Verifying the order is a legal requirement. The written medication order also alerts you to the type of formula, and the amount and the method of delivery (either as a bolus or a continuous infusion).

Most enteral feeds come as ready-to-use nutritionally completed preparations, which contain energy, protein, vitamins, minerals, trace elements and fluid, and may include fibre. A ready-to-use standard feed such as Nutrison or Ensure usually contains 15 per cent protein, 30 per cent fat and 55 per cent carbohydrate (DAA, 2018).

The choice of feeding solutions and method of administration (bolus, intermittent or continuous 16 to 24 hours per day) is made by the multidisciplinary healthcare team, having considered the pathophysiology of the gastrointestinal tract, the person's condition and preference, and the method of medication administration. A dietitian usually prescribes the enteral feeding fluid.

Safety considerations

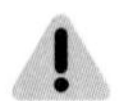
Safety

Know the difference between enteral and parenteral. Fatalities have occurred from mixing up these two forms of nutrition.

Enteral means providing food or fluid through the gastrointestinal tract. It includes feeding oneself or others through the mouth, but, more commonly, it means through a tube that goes into the gastrointestinal tract (nasogastric, orogastric, gastrostomy and jejunostomy tubes). Enteral feeds through a tube are generally commercially prepared formulations with components balanced to provide nutrition.

Parenteral nutrition (also known as total parenteral nutrition) means providing a special sterile pharmaceutical formulation composed of glucose, amino acid, protein, salts, lipids, vitamins and minerals through intravenous access to the cardiovascular system, bypassing ingestion and digestion. The components of parenteral nutrition are in molecular formulation so they can pass into cells from the bloodstream.

EVIDENCE OF THERAPEUTIC INTERACTION

The person, whether responsive or not, requires a clear explanation. This ensures that they understand the purpose of the feed and can provide consent. Discuss the common adverse effects for enteral feeding and ask the person to alert the nursing staff to any changes they note during the administration of the feed. By explaining to the person what to expect and how to help, they will be willing, if able, to assist in the procedure. Assess all of their concerns and complaints.

DEMONSTRATE CLINICAL REASONING

Assessment, elder care, care of the person living with severe obesity, safety considerations, privacy and positioning the person contribute to successful enteral feedings, as outlined in the following sections.

Assessment

Obtain the person's baseline weight; their weight is then monitored daily (see **Clinical Skill 23**). Also assess for any signs of oedema (pedal, sacral, generalised) or jugular venous distension, and auscultate for breath sounds. Commence a fluid balance chart to record intake and output to assess hydration status. Assess for protein calorie malnutrition, including a history of recent weight loss, muscle atrophy, oedema, weakness or lethargy. These physical signs and symptoms indicate the severity of malnutrition and establish a baseline for evaluation of the person's response to nutritional support (DAA, 2018). You should also perform an abdominal assessment (to determine the presence of bowel sounds, any abdominal distension, if the person is passing flatus and bowel motions) prior to each feeding to ascertain the functioning of the gastrointestinal tract (see **Clinical Skill 22**). Assess for respiratory distress, which may indicate migration of the nasogastric tube (NGT) into the airways (cough, choking or dyspnoea) (Bering & DiBaise, 2022).

Safety considerations

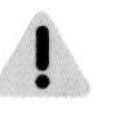
Safety

Be aware that enteral feeding is associated with a number of complications, including aspiration, nasopharyngeal trauma and ulceration. Longer-term use for external feeding can cause gastrointestinal complications such as nausea, vomiting, diarrhoea or constipation, and metabolic complications such as dehydration and electrolyte disturbances (Bering & DiBaise, 2022). Nursing management aims to prevent complications and monitor the person's tolerance of feeding. It is important that you understand the insertion and flushing and can confirm the placement of the feeding tube (see **Clinical Skill 29**).

Other, equally important safety considerations surround the preparation and storage of the feeding

ELDER CARE

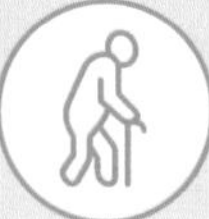

Up to 50 per cent of elderly Australians (both community dwelling and those in residential aged care facilities) are either malnourished or at risk of malnourishment (DAA, 2019). Both malnutrition and under-hydration increase with advancing age, chronic illness (e.g. cancers, neurological diseases [de Oliveira et al., 2023]) and hospitalisation, making enteral nutrition increasingly important (Volkert et al., 2022). These authors suggest identifying risk early and implementing support through preferably oral, then enteral, feeding measures. Fine-bore NGTs are recommended for the elderly and frail person to minimise trauma during introduction and irritation of the tissues from continuous use.

THE PERSON LIVING WITH SEVERE OBESITY

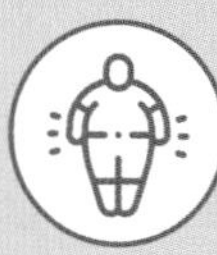

Enteral feeds for the severely obese are often hypocaloric (low carbohydrate, moderate fat and high protein levels) to induce weight loss while preserving muscle mass (Formisano et al., 2023).

fluids. Contamination occurs in more than 30 per cent of hospital and home feeds and can cause serious infections. The following is adapted from DAA (2018), Boullata et al. (2017) and Bischoff et al. (2022):

- Identify the person and verify the order against the solution.
- Use pre-packaged, ready-to-use enteral feeds whenever possible.
- Use minimal handling and Aseptic Non Touch Technique (ANTT) to assemble the feeding and enteral tubes.
- Maintain effective hand decontamination.
- Use a clean work area dedicated to preparation of enteral feeds.
- Reconstitute feeds using sterile or cooled, boiled water and ANTT.
- Store enteral feeding solutions according to the manufacturer's direction.
- Store reconstituted feeds in a refrigerator for up to 24 hours; discard if left at room temperature for four hours or more.

Ready-to-use feeds can be given over 24 hours; reconstituted feeds should be given over four hours. Administration sets and feed containers are single-use only and must be discarded after each session.

The skin around the NGT should be cleaned at least daily, and the tape around the tube changed whenever it is loose or soiled. Check that the taping on the tube is secure to prevent the tube from moving, which may irritate the nares or oral mucosa or cause accidental dislodgement of the tube.

Clean the peristomal skin of gastrostomies daily. Initially, change dressings used around gastrostomy insertion sites daily using an aseptic technique to minimise the risk of infection (see **Clinical Skill 67**). The peristomal skin and stoma are observed for signs of infection, irritation or excoriation. To prevent discomfort and 'buried bumper syndrome' (where a gastrostomy disc is forced under the skin), ensure that the gastrostomy disc or bumper is not pulled tight against the abdominal wall. Tug the tube gently for 1 to 2 mm and rotate between your thumb and forefinger daily to release any sticking and to promote tract formation (DAA, 2018). If the person has a gastrostomy tube retained by a balloon, check the water volume weekly to prevent the tube from falling out.

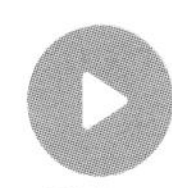
Video

Type of feeding solution

Check the order for the type of solution to be given. There are many types of feeds. Some are specifically formulated for people with requirements for specific disease states, such as those with concentrated kilojoules or those providing low sodium and potassium, or altered mineral content like magnesium or phosphorus, or with added vitamins such as A and D. Low-protein formulae for renal insufficiency and higher-protein formulae are available for people on dialysis (e.g. Nepro). A formula low in carbohydrates, high in fat and concentrated in calories (e.g. Pulmocare) can be used for people with pulmonary dysfunction.

Use of blenderised tube feeding (blended food mixed with liquid into the enteral feeding tube) is increasing, although it has drawbacks, such as more frequent clogging of the tube, greater chances

GATHER EQUIPMENT

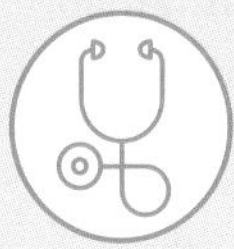

Gathering equipment is an organisational step that helps to create a positive environment for a successful interaction. It ensures that you have all needed material, boosts the person's confidence and trust in you, and increases your self-confidence. While gathering the equipment, you can mentally rehearse the procedure. If a feeding pump is in use, it will be at the bedside. Equipment required includes:

EQUIPMENT	EXPLANATION
Clean gloves	• Worn for personal protection (standard precautions)
pH-test strip in a kidney dish	• To determine if the NGT is in the stomach
50 mL syringe	• Used to remove a small amount of gastric content to test for pH using a pH-test strip in a kidney dish
Tongue blade and penlight	• Used to visually determine the position of the tube in the oropharynx
Feeding apparatus (kangaroo pump, gravity feed, IV stand plus administration set/container)	• Used to deliver the appropriate enteral feeding to the tube • Administration sets are single-use only and must be discarded after each session
Ordered nutritional fluid	• This can be either pre-packaged or reconstituted (as per manufacturer's directions), and should be warmed to ambient temperature and labelled
Adaptor	• Used to connect the feeding apparatus to the enteral feeding tubing
Elastic band and safety pin	• Used to secure the tubing to the person's clothing to minimise 'pull' when moving
Tape	• Used to secure the enteral tube in position
Waterproof, absorbent pad	• Keeps the person and their bedclothes clean and dry

of contamination and increased effort required (Dietitians Australia, 2023). Chandrasekar et al. (2022) found less gastrointestinal tract inflammation and increased microbiome diversity, leading to fewer symptoms, such as constipation, diarrhoea and reflux, in children fed with blenderised food.

Provision of privacy

Privacy preserves the person's dignity. Providing comfort measures and pain relief increases the trust the person has in you. These may also increase the person's ability to relax and participate and assist with the process, as much as they are able.

Position the person

A semi- to high Fowler's position is used if the person's condition permits (Tatsumi, 2019). The head of the bed should be positioned at least 30 to 45 degrees during the infusion of enteral feeds and should remain elevated for one to two hours after the feed is completed. This reduces the risk of aspiration of gastric contents. Some people may prefer to sit on the side of the bed or in a chair. Those who must lie flat (e.g. a person with an unstable neck fracture) need to be monitored closely for aspiration during infusion of enteral feeds.

ENTERAL TUBE FEEDING

An enteral tube feeding includes preparing the formula, verifying the placement of the NGT (or other tube), measuring the residual volume if ordered, flushing the enteral tube, administering the formula and extra water and monitoring the person following the feeding.

Hand hygiene

This is a clean procedure. Hand hygiene (see **Clinical Skill 5**) removes microbes and reduces their transmission to the person. The acid levels in the stomach destroy most microbes that are transmitted in the solution. Clean gloves are used to comply with standard precautions and protect you from bodily fluids.

Prepare the formula

Check the expiration date of the formula. Ensure it is at room temperature, as cold feeds may cause discomfort, abdominal cramps and diarrhoea. When using an open system, clean the top of the container before opening it to minimise the risk of contaminants entering the feeding syringe or feeding bag.

For continuous administration, first close the clamp on the enteral feeding bag and pour up to four hours' measure of formula (or as per facility policy) into the bag or hang the pre-packaged closed-system container of the prescribed formula. There are a number of closed systems available – familiarise yourself with those used in the facility (Boullata et al., 2017).

For intermittent feeding, pour the required amount of formula into an administration bag. Bacterial growth can occur quickly in formulas with high carbohydrate concentration. This can lead to gastritis, nausea, vomiting and diarrhoea. To prevent contamination:

- use scrupulous hand hygiene and aseptic technique
- change the administration sets and syringes used for flushing daily
- do not add new formula to any remaining from the previous administration
- flush the bag with tap water before refilling, swab ports with antiseptic swabs before and after handling.

If using an open system, cover, label and refrigerate unused formula and discard the formula 24 hours after opening. It is best to use a closed system, if possible, to prevent contamination (Boullata et al., 2017).

Labelling

All containers and syringes used in syringe pumps are labelled with the following information: the person's demographics (name, UR number, doctor or nutritionist's name), formula name, type of enteral access (NGT, PEG), the volume to be administered and the rate, duration of the hang time, date and time plus your name/initials as the one preparing and hanging the product, and the expiration date. Compare the prepared label to the order to confirm the correct formula is being administered. Most labels will have 'NOT FOR INTRAVENOUS USE'; if they don't, these words should be added to the label.

Verify correct feeding tube placement

Four-hourly, or before initiating a feeding, providing water or administering medication, you must ensure that the tube is in the correct position (Judd, 2020). Assessing the exit point marked on the (nasogastric) tube helps to determine if the tube has maintained the same position. Observe the PEG exit site for any problems (refer back to the section 'Safety considerations').

A 50 mL syringe is used to aspirate a small amount (1 to 2 mL) of the gastric contents, and this is dripped onto pH-graded test strips. Greater accuracy is possible with the use of a pH-test strip rather than litmus paper. A pH less than 5 is consistent with gastric placement and the contents are unlikely to be pulmonary aspirate. With this reading, it is considered appropriate to proceed with the feed.

If no aspirate returns, or the pH is greater than 5, feeding should not be commenced. Leave the NGT in place and reposition the person if possible. This may assist to place the tip in a pool of stomach contents. Attempt to recover aspirate again for testing. Wait at least one hour after a feed or medication has been administered (either orally or via the tube) to enable it to be absorbed, which will prevent inaccurate pH results (Judd, 2020). Medication and enteral formulas may interact, reducing the effectiveness of the medication or causing enteral feeding adverse effects as well as clogging the tube (Alhashemi, Ghorbani & Vazin, 2019) (see **Clinical Skill 38**).

If a pH of 6 or above is obtained or there is doubt about the result in the range pH 5 to 6, feeding should not be commenced until the person is reviewed and the tube placement is verified because there is an increased risk of the nasogastric tube being incorrectly positioned. Follow the facility's policy if pH is 6 or greater.

The pH method of determining tube placement may not be useful during continuous enteral feeding because the formula raises the gastric pH and lowers intestinal pH (DAA, 2018). Mak and Tan (2020) demonstrated the efficacy of bedside ultrasonography as a supporting method to pH determination. The use of litmus paper or the absence of respiratory distress are unreliable signs of tube dislodgement. They have been shown to give false positive results and should not be used.

The position of a jejunostomy tube is confirmed by noting the position of external markers to determine if movement has occurred. Assessment of bilirubin content of aspirate has also been used as a method to differentiate between respiratory, gastric and intestinal tube placement. Bilirubin levels in the lungs should be almost zero, while levels in the stomach will be approximately 1.5 mg/dL, and in the intestines over 10 mg/dL. Reliable bedside analysis tests have not been developed. In the absence of an X-ray, more than one method should be used to establish tube position.

Evaluate residual volume

Measuring gastric residual volume is controversial (Mutrie & Hill, 2018). If it is the facility's policy, the amount of feed remaining in the stomach is measured regularly until the tolerance for feeds is established. Yasuda et al. (2021) found the effect of measuring gastric residual volume to be uncertain in clinical outcomes including mortality, pneumonia, vomiting, and length of hospital stay. Mutrie and Hill (2018) found that the frequency of gastric tube aspirations could be reduced (that is, longer intervals between aspirations) with no increase in risk to the person, resulting in saved nursing time, decreased risk of contamination of the feeding circuit, and minimised risk of body fluid exposure. As well, aspirating gastric contents can contribute to tube occlusion (Ernstmeyer & Christman, 2021).

If a gastric residual volume is ordered, attach the 60 mL syringe (or appropriate syringe) to the feeding tube. Since fine-bore NGTs differ, refer to the manufacturer's instructions for recommendations on aspiration of the specific tube and for the best method of aspiration.

For nasogastric, nasoenteric or gastrostomy tubes, aspirate contents; if greater than 60 mL, place the return in a clean cup. An increased residual may indicate delayed gastric emptying or that a gastrostomy tube's internal stabiliser (a weighted end) has migrated and could be obstructing the pyloric outlet. If the gastrostomy tube residual cannot be aspirated, the tube may be displaced between the person's stomach and abdominal wall. Peritonitis may develop if a feed is administered. Report an inability to aspirate residual from the gastrostomy tube to the shift coordinator.

If the residual gastric aspirate is above 200 mL with continuous feeding, or greater than 50 per cent of the previous bolus volume, assess the person for other signs and symptoms of possible feed intolerance (abdominal distension, complaints of nausea and/or vomiting, absence of bowel sounds or bowel movement), to avoid contributing to hypocaloric feeding (DAA, 2018). Report the findings to the shift coordinator and follow the facility's policy regarding withholding feeds and do not administer the scheduled formula.

If the tube is in the small intestine, residuals cannot be aspirated.

Return gastric aspirate

Return up to 150 mL of gastric aspirate (or as per facility policy), which contains enzymes and secretions essential for digesting nutrients. Returning more than 150 mL of gastric aspirate may overfill the stomach when the enteral feed is commenced. Some facilities may require the aspirate to be tested for blood, and if positive the aspirate is not returned. Follow the facility's guidelines for testing aspirates for blood.

Flush the feeding tube

Tube occlusion, or clogging, has an incidence as frequent as 23 to 35 per cent, and results in delayed administration of medication and nutrition. Instil 30 to 60 mL of water to prevent the tube clogging. The DAA (2018) recommends using warm tap water unless the person is immunocompromised, in which case, sterile water is used. These flushes should precede and follow each intermittent feeding and each medication administration, including between medications if more than one is ordered (Nielsen et al., 2022). If the person is on continuous feeding, flushes are done at least once every eight hours. This also provides additional free water to the person to improve hydration. Anyone on fluid restrictions (e.g. those with renal failure or heart failure) should have a 15 to 20 mL flush to clean the tube.

Flush the tube with 30 to 60 mL of water before and after feeds and medication to reduce sedimentation from formula or medications and prevent blockages (see **Clinical Skill 38**).

> ?
>
> The most effective way to manage clogged feeding tubes is to prevent them by flushing sufficiently and paying attention to your medication administration techniques. If the feeding tube is blocked, the DAA (2018) recommends the following actions:
>
> - Use the smallest syringe available (usually a 5 mL Luer Lock) that will fit onto the feeding tube.

- Fill it with very warm water (drinkable tea/coffee temperature). Flush into the tube using moderate pressure.
- Clamp tube, wait 10 minutes then withdraw as much of the tube content as possible.
- Repeat.

There is no evidence that other substances (e.g. fizzy soft drinks [Coke or similar] or urinary alkaliniser) are more effective than warm water. Alsamet (2022) adds that acidic juices (e.g. cranberry juice) can cause the precipitation of protein and cause the tube to clog.

If warm water does not work, pancreatic enzyme can be tried; however, this is expensive and should be used only if tube replacement is not a realistic option. Check the facility's policy and confirm with a pharmacist or senior nurse.

- Crush the enteric-coated pancreatic enzyme supplement (2 to 3 capsules or granule scoops of pancreatic enzyme supplement [will differ according to brand and format]) in a mortar and pestle very well.
- Mix very thoroughly with 10 mL very warm tap water with sodium bicarbonate (check with protocol or pharmacist). An alkaline solution is required to activate the enzymes.
- Flush the well-mixed solution into the tube, clamp the tube, wait 10 to 30 minutes, then attempt to flush the tube.

If these measures are not effective, report your findings to a senior nurse. The NGT will probably be removed and replaced. Alternatively, commercial mechanical declogging devices are available. Check the facility's policy and follow the manufacturer's instructions to use such a device. The PEG and PEGJ will need further declogging efforts.

Hang the labelled bag on the IV pole

The bag should be approximately 30 cm above the insertion point into the person. Prime the tubing by squeezing the drip chamber to approximately half its capacity, allow the formula to run down the tubing, then reclamp the tube. This purges the system of air. For continuous enteral feeding, load the administration set into an enteral feeding pump. There are a number of pumps available, and feeding pumps differ from one manufacturer to another. Familiarise yourself with the feeding pumps used in the facility. Follow the tube from connector to origin (nares, PEG) to ensure it is a gastric feeding tube. Connect the distal end of the administration tubing to the feeding tube and ensure it is secure.

Begin the infusion

Unclamp the tubing:

- *For pump feeding* – set the feeding pump to the prescribed flow rate and begin the infusion via the pump.
- *For gravity feeding* – adjust the roller clamp to infuse the formula via gravity over 30 to 60 minutes for intermittent feeds. Feeds that are administered too rapidly can cause flatulence, cramps and/or vomiting and increase the risk of aspiration.
- *For the syringe method* – remove the plunger from a 60 mL syringe. Pour the formula to be administered into a jug. Pinch or clamp the enteric tube to prevent air entering the person's stomach, which can cause distension. Attach the syringe to the feeding tube and position it approximately 20 cm above the person's stomach. Pour the formula carefully and slowly into the syringe barrel and release the enteric tube, trying not to introduce air into the person's gastrointestinal system. Allow the formula to flow in at the prescribed rate by gravity. You can regulate the flow by either raising or lowering the syringe. If the person experiences discomfort during the feed, pinch or clamp the tubing to stop the flow for a couple of minutes.

Administer a water bolus as prescribed

Administer water boluses or flush the feeding tube with 20 to 60 mL of water before and at the completion of each feed to help maintain the patency of the tube.

Pinch or clamp the tubing

Clamp the tubing. Remove the syringe or administration set from the feeding tube and secure the tube. Remove your gloves and perform hand hygiene.

Post-procedure

Offer oral hygiene (see **Clinical Skill 56**) regularly to help clear the palate of unpleasant flavours, and clean the teeth, remove plaque, clean the tongue and oral mucous membranes, simulate salivation and reduce xerostoma. Frequent oral hygiene helps reduce the incidence of nosocomial infections (e.g. pneumonia, oral infections). The risk for respiratory infection (pneumonia) from aspiration of respiratory pathogens is significantly reduced in people receiving regular and frequent oral hygiene (Terech-Skóra et al., 2023). Regular dental care is also a preventative measure to remove calculus and decrease the bacterial load.

Keep the head of the bed elevated for one to two hours following intermittent bolus feeds. If the person is receiving continuous feeds, maintain elevation at 30 to 45 degrees. They may need support from extra pillows. If the person needs to be repositioned at less than 30 degrees, turn the feed off for one hour before repositioning them. Return personal belongings and put the call bell within reach.

CLEAN, REPLACE AND DISPOSE OF EQUIPMENT

Clean and replace equipment to ensure that the next nurse to use it is not inconvenienced. Wash, rinse and allow equipment to dry after each feeding. Return the equipment to the person's bedside. Disposing of used material reduces clutter at the bedside, increases the person's psychological comfort and reduces the presence of material that can grow bacteria. Perform hand hygiene.

DOCUMENTATION

Documentation increases communication between healthcare professionals and complies with legal requirements for reporting changes. For enteral feeding, you should document the following:

- date and time of the procedure
- abdominal assessment findings
- bowel elimination pattern and characteristics
- daily weight
- methods used to determine tube placement
- amount and description of residual gastric fluid (if measured)
- amount, rate and type of formula administered
- fluid balance status
- person's response to the procedure (e.g. nausea, bloating, diarrhoea).

CLINICAL SKILLS ASSESSMENT

Administering enteral nutrition

Demonstrates the ability to safely administer nutrition and care for a person requiring enteral nutrition. Incorporates the *National Safety and Quality Health Service Standards*: 2 Partnering with Consumers, 3 Preventing and Controlling Healthcare-Associated Infection, 5 Comprehensive Care, 6 Communicating for Safety, and 8 Recognising and Responding to Acute Deterioration (ACSQHC, 2021b).

Performance criteria	1	2	3	4	5
(Numbers indicate NMBA *Registered Nurse Standards for Practice*)	(Dependent)	(Marginal)	(Assisted)	(Supervised)	(Independent)
1. Identifies indication (1.1, 3.3, 3.4)	☐	☐	☐	☐	☐
2. Verifies the written medication order (1.4, 3.4, 6.1, 6.2, 6.5)	☐	☐	☐	☐	☐
3. Evidence of therapeutic interaction with the person, e.g. gives the person a clear explanation of the procedure (1.4, 1.5, 2.1, 2.2, 3.2)	☐	☐	☐	☐	☐
4. Demonstrates clinical reasoning abilities, e.g. provides privacy, comfort measures and pain relief; positions the person (1.1, 1.2, 1.3, 4.2, 6.1)	☐	☐	☐	☐	☐
5. Gathers equipment (5.5, 6.1): ■ clean gloves ■ pH-graded paper ■ 50 mL syringe ■ tongue blade and penlight ■ feeding apparatus, administration set ■ ordered nutritional fluid ■ adaptor ■ absorbent pad ■ elastic band and safety pin ■ tape ■ waterproof, absorbent pad	☐	☐	☐	☐	☐
6. Performs hand hygiene and dons gloves (1.1, 3.4, 6.1)	☐	☐	☐	☐	☐
7. Prepares the formula to be administered (open/closed system; intermittent/continuous infusion) (1.1, 6.1)	☐	☐	☐	☐	☐
8. Determines correct placement of the enteral tube; withdraws gastric residual; and returns gastric content if required (1.1, 1.2, 1.3, 4.2, 6.1)	☐	☐	☐	☐	☐
9. Flushes the enteral tube with water prior to commencing feeding (1.1, 6.1)	☐	☐	☐	☐	☐
10. Administers the feed appropriately (via a feed pump, a feeding bag or a syringe) (1.1, 6.1)	☐	☐	☐	☐	☐
11. Administers a water bolus as prescribed or flushes the tube after the feed is completed (1.1, 1.4, 6.1)	☐	☐	☐	☐	☐
12. Disconnects the feed appropriately (1.1, 6.1)	☐	☐	☐	☐	☐
13. Offers the person oral hygiene post-feed (1.1, 6.1)	☐	☐	☐	☐	☐
14. Cleans, replaces and disposes of equipment appropriately (3.6, 6.1)	☐	☐	☐	☐	☐
15. Documents relevant information (1.4, 1.6, 2.2, 2.7, 3.5, 3.7, 6.2, 6.5, 7.3)	☐	☐	☐	☐	☐
16. Demonstrates the ability to link theory to practice (1.1, 3.3, 3.4, 3.5)	☐	☐	☐	☐	☐

Student:

Clinical facilitator: Date:

CHAPTER 31

INTRAVENOUS THERAPY – ASSISTING WITH ESTABLISHMENT

INDICATIONS

Peripheral intravenous cannulas (PIVCs) are inserted to access the venous system. In Australian hospitals, PIVC is one of the most commonly performed procedures, with approximately 7.7 million PIVCs inserted each year (Australian Commission on Safety and Quality in Health Care [ACSQHC], 2021a). It is administered to most hospitalised people (e.g. pre- or postoperatively, during trauma recovery or to administer intravenous [IV] medication and fluids). Intravenous therapy (IVT):

- restores and maintains fluid and electrolyte balance
- permits transfusion of blood and blood products
- supplies kilojoules and nutritional fluids (parenteral nutrition)
- permits rapid administration of medications.

IV infusions introduce sterile fluids into a person's circulation when the use of enteral fluids is not possible, sufficient or appropriate. There are numerous IV fluids available, and each is used for a different purpose. It is the responsibility of every nurse to know the various IV fluid uses and to understand the rationale for their use (Nasa et al., 2022). Fluids are generally divided into crystalloids (fluids that cross from the vessel into the tissues – e.g. normal saline, 5% dextrose in water) and colloids (solutions that pull interstitial fluids into the vessel – e.g. albumin and dextran) (Malina, 2022). Pharmacology texts will provide a detailed explanation of osmolality on which fluid administration is based.

The insertion of the IV cannula is the responsibility of either the medical staff or nurses who have accredited competency in cannulation. Most facilities permit only two cannulation attempts before a more experienced healthcare practitioner is sought (DeLaune et al., 2024).

EVIDENCE OF THERAPEUTIC INTERACTION

Give the person a clear explanation of the procedure. Take time to listen to their concerns so your explanation is effective (Plohal, 2019). They must consent to the procedure (usually tacit). Many people will be apprehensive about receiving fluids via an IV. Determine if they have experienced IVT before and what that experience was like. Some facilities use local anaesthetic gels or patches to minimise the pain during insertion and so reduce the associated anxiety. These patches take time to be effective, so plan ahead. If possible, give the person a choice of IV sites, then assist them to a position of comfort. Reassure the person that the metal 'needle' will be removed, leaving only a plastic 'tube' into their arm.

Warn the person that they may experience some discomfort during insertion or vein irritation during infusion and offer assistance if this occurs (e.g. warm compresses, mild analgesia). Assess all concerns or complaints voiced by the person; this develops trust in the nursing staff. Engage the person in their own care.

Discuss common adverse effects of IVT and ask the person to alert you to any changes that they note following insertion of the IV line or change of an IV bag. Although an adverse reaction is unusual or unexpected, do not ignore the possibility; it needs exploration. Teach the following to the person about IVT:

- its importance
- how they can help protect the site
- what to watch for (regarding infiltration, leaking or infection)
- what to report (pain when a medication is injected, pain along the vein)
- to speak up if they see poor practice (e.g. no hand hygiene prior to touching the ports) (Cooke et al., 2018; Gorski, 2022).

DEMONSTRATE CLINICAL REASONING

Assessing the person (and the probable IV sites) prior to insertion reduces the risk of complications and the need for resiting. The person inserting the cannula will do this; however, for your own knowledge development, please do the following assessment.

LOOK at their baseline vital signs, dominant side, medical diagnosis (especially heart failure, renal failure or bleeding disorders), skin at the proposed site (for rashes, oedema, bruises or abrasions), planned interventions and general condition.

LISTEN to their report of any allergies (e.g. medications, adhesive tape). Shellfish allergies may indicate iodine sensitivity; banana sensitivity may indicate a latex allergy.

FEEL their skin – is it well hydrated? Moist? Dry, thin and fragile? Skin condition will dictate the type of securement of the IV. Also feel the veins – are they stable, mobile, prominent or deep?

The professional who cannulates will assess possible IV sites for suitability. They will take into account:

- *the person's dominant hand* – is left free if possible to allow self-care
- *areas of flexion* – are avoided; for example, antecubital fossa or wrist
- *previous injury* – for example, mastectomy side, affected side of a person following a stroke, arteriovenous shunt
- *inconvenience* – for example, if surgery is proposed for the left shoulder, the left arm/hand is avoided for IV insertion
- *areas of localised oedema, cellulitis, thrombosis, dermatitis or skin grafts* – are avoided
- *the person's choice of sites, if possible.*

Both Rodriguez-Calero et al. (2020) and Marsh et al. (2020) found that situating the catheter in the forearm rather than wrist, antecubital fossa or upper arm, using the smallest diameter catheter possible and insertion by a specialised IV team, improved the ease of insertion and survival of the IV catheter. The size and condition of the veins (the elderly or those with chronic diseases often have fragile skin/delicate veins) and frequency of access are determined. Veins with visible bifurcations and bumps are avoided because these indicate valves. Insertion through a valve increases the risk of thrombosis. Damage to the vein by probing during insertion increases the rate of complication and failure (Major & Huey, 2016). Children have their IV access sited away from joints. Usually, initial IV access is at the most peripheral suitable site, allowing the more proximal sites to be left for subsequent access. Local anaesthetic or vapocoolant spray or anaesthetic patches reduce the pain and stress of IV insertion.

Determine how long the IV access device will be needed. If it is more than a week, many facilities are now using central lines rather than peripheral lines. Peripheral IV catheters remain in place for 72 to 96 hours or until they show signs of complications before they are resited (follow the policy of the facility).

ELDER CARE

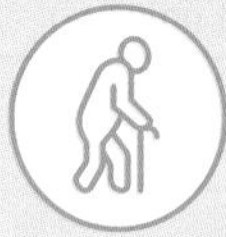

Elders frequently have tortuous, thin veins that tend to roll away from the insertion needle (due to loss of subcutaneous tissue and thinner skin), making insertion more difficult. They also may have comorbidities that affect their veins (e.g. diabetes mellitus, chemotherapy medications for cancer), making them more difficult to find, or more susceptible to damage (phlebitis) or puncturing the other side (infiltration and extravasation). Once the PIVC is established, the thin, frail skin makes securement more difficult. The use of a tubular net bandage over the primary transparent dressing may reduce the need for additional tape and increase security.

THE PERSON LIVING WITH SEVERE OBESITY

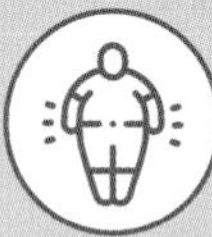

Often there is difficulty in locating appropriate veins in people living with severe obesity because of adipose tissue 'burying' the vessels and obscuring the landmarks. Ultrasound may be necessary to locate the vein and help the medical officer or RN to visualise the insertion path.

GATHER EQUIPMENT

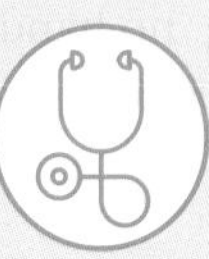

Gathering equipment is an organisational step that helps to create a positive environment for a successful interaction. While gathering the equipment, you can mentally rehearse the procedure. Equipment required includes:

EQUIPMENT	EXPLANATION
Fluid order sheet	• The written order is used to determine the fluid and the amount required per 24 hours • The person's name, hospital number, date of birth and doctor are used to identify the person so the correct fluid and amount are given to the correct person

EQUIPMENT	EXPLANATION
Prescribed fluid (one bag)	• Check for intact outer bag, expiry date, type and strength of fluid • Discard the outer bag/packaging; the inner bag may be damp from condensation • Check sterile contents of the inner bag for colour and clarity of fluid by holding against a dark and a light background • Gently squeeze the bag to check for leaks • Determine if additives are required (see **Clinical Skill 47**) • Generally, two registered healthcare professionals (registered nurse, medical officer or enrolled nurse) are required to check and sign the fluid against the fluid order • Attach a graduated timeline (IV safe label with the time, date, your initials) to the bag • Place the label so it can be read when the bag is hanging, and does not obscure information on the front of the bag
Required cannula and giving set	*Cannulae* • Come in a variety of gauges and types. The advanced practice nurse, unit protocols or physician will determine type • Flexible polyurethane catheters are less damaging and decrease the incidence of phlebitis and thrombosis • Generally, the smallest size that can deliver the volume of fluid needed is used to allow maximum blood flow around the cannula (Zingg et al., 2023) • Most often, an angiocath (i.e. over-the-needle cannula) (Broyles et al., 2017) *Giving sets (administration sets)* • Includes the tubing used to deliver the fluid and an inline drip chamber • Choice depends on the fluid being infused (e.g. crystalloids, colloids, blood, blood products), the person's size and condition and whether an infusion pump is needed (most pumps require specific tubing/drip chambers) • Frail elderly people, children and infants generally require a giving set with a microdrip – 60 drops per mL • Adults usually have a macrodrip – 15 or 20 drops per mL • Note which one is used in the facility where you are practising • There are also 'add-on' devices, such as filter chambers, extension sets and adaptors
Extension set	• These help to secure the catheter in the vein by minimising movement of the PIVC and by securing the line in a different direction (Zingg et al., 2023)
Vascular visualisation device (ACSQHC, 2021a)	• Transilluminator – a light used under the IV site to visualise the veins (especially for newborn and infants) • Infrared, near infrared light – analyses the skin and shows veins as black lines to increase accuracy of first-attempt insertion • Ultrasound – permits visualisation of vessel size, depth and structure to increase accuracy
Clippers as required	• To remove excess hair from the proposed site
Alcowipes, chlorhexidine or Betadine wipes	• Used to scrub clean and disinfect the skin prior to cannula insertion – use sterile gauze if not supplied in a one-time packet • Good skin preparation destroys most resident and all transient bacteria on the skin • ACSQHC (2021a) and Zingg et al. (2023) recommend chlorhexidine 2% in 70% alcohol • Use according to the policy of the facility
Clean gloves	Standard precaution to protect the person inserting the IV cannula or connecting it to the line, from body fluids
Tourniquet	• Apply above the intended IV site to reduce the flow of venous blood back to the heart to distend the veins, making insertion easier • A single-use tourniquet is an effective infection-control measure (Santos-Costa et al., 2022)
Tape	• Type selected is dependent on both the dressing chosen and on the person • Paper tape is gentlest on the skin for the frail person. Adhesive tape is more robust, but also can cause sensitivity and be more difficult to remove • Micropore tape is used frequently because it provides good adhesion and is not difficult to remove • Tape is not applied to the insertion site
Dressing	• Usually a transparent polyurethane, ideally with an adhesive cloth border. ACSQHC standards specify sterile, transparent, semipermeable dressing for IV sites. Check the facility's policy and familiarise yourself with what is available • Transparent dressings permit direct visualisation of the IV insertion site and the adhesive border seals it more securely • Gauze dressings may sometimes be used together with a transparent one
Armboard	• Used to stabilise the wrist or elbow to maintain a regular flow of fluid if the IV site is nearby, because flexion of the joint might restrict infusion rates • Armboards are not comfortable and the IV site should be chosen to avoid any areas of flexion if possible
Securement device	A variety of commercial devices that decrease dislodgement, decrease complications (e.g. infiltration) and prolong the usefulness of the site (Corley et al., 2022)
IV stand	• The IV stand or pole is an extendable support for the fluid bag • Wheeled poles assist the person with mobilisation • Many beds have an integrated IV stand to reduce bedside clutter. In this case, a wheeled stand will be required when the person gets out of bed
Injection tray	To transport the cannula and antiseptic wipes to and from the bedside
Sharps container	Taken to the bedside so that the used inner cannula can be immediately disposed of; reducing the chance of needle-stick injuries
Watch with a second hand	Used to time the infusion rate if there is no infusion pump
Infusion pump	May be required for children, the elderly or anyone who requires exact amounts of fluid

POSITION THE PERSON

Yamagami and Inoue (2020) found the supine position (rather than a seated position) increased vein distension following tourniquet application to increase the success of the first attempt at cannulation. The arm should be supported in a comfortable position to reduce muscle strain and assist to relax the person.

GENERAL CONCEPTS OF MEDICATION ADMINISTRATION AND THE SIX RIGHTS

IV fluids are therapeutic prescriptions and are therefore treated as medications. The general concepts of medication administration and the six rights apply (see **Clinical Skill 37**).

ASSIST TO ESTABLISH INTRAVENOUS THERAPY

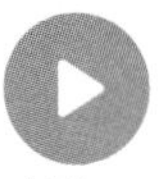
Video

Assisting with the establishment of an IV is a multifaceted skill that takes practice. You will need to assemble the materials, anticipate the physician's needs, support the person, prepare the fluid bag and giving set, insert the line into the cannula and dress the site.

Hand hygiene

Hand hygiene (see **Clinical Skill 5**) is a vital infection-control measure. The fluid being prepared will go directly into a vein, so care needs to be taken to maintain asepsis. Clean gloves should be used to comply with standard precautions.

Assist the physician or advanced nurse to establish an IV access

Assemble and prepare the equipment using aseptic technique. Crucially, support the person. If analgesic patches are ordered, place them on likely sites and cover with transparent dressings at least an hour before cannulation. Other forms of analgesia or anaesthesia may be used (e.g. vapocoolant on the skin). Warm small flat veins with a warm, damp face washer and keep the arm dependent for a few minutes to help distend the vein and make insertion faster and easier.

Prepare the giving set

Safety

Remove the giving set from its packaging and move the roller clamp to about 5 cm below the drip chamber. Tighten the roller clamp to prevent fluid flow until you are ready to prime the line and adjust the flow. The roller clamp should be moved every six hours during the infusion to prevent the tube from denting, which would alter the flow rate. Remove the protective cap over the spike on the top end of the drip chamber. Take care to maintain the sterility of the spike. The needleless connector that connects the line to the hub of the cannula must also remain sterile.

Spike the fluid bag

Pull off the protective sheath to expose the port on the fluid bag. Rest the fluid bag on a table, hang it on the IV pole or hold it firmly under your non-dominant arm to ensure that the port is straight and the spike does not go through the sides of the port. Gently squeeze the drip chamber of the giving set while inserting the spike to prevent air entering the fluid. Take care not to touch the outer edges of the port with the spike while firmly pushing all of its length into the port.

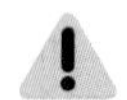
Safety

Prime the line with fluid

Hang the bag of fluid on the IV pole and gently release the drip chamber. Fill until it is half-full. Open the roller clamp and allow fluid to fill the IV line. You may need to remove the protective cap at the distal end of the IV line (some caps permit priming while still in place). Hold the distal end over the kidney dish and higher than its dependent loops so that air is expelled and fluid is not spilled. When the line is full and there are no air bubbles, close the roller clamp, reapply the protective cap and hang the line over the IV pole until it is needed. Make sure the dependent loop is clear of the floor and the end is easily reached. Raise the IV pole to a height not more than 1 m above the person. Tag the line with the time, date and your initials to indicate when tubing change is needed – do not write on the IV bag with a felt-tip pen, as it may leach into the fluid (DeLaune et al., 2024).

> ?
>
> If there are air bubbles in the line, keep the line between the bubbles and the drip chamber straight and slightly taut. Gently tap the line at the level of the air bubbles – a pen can be used, or you can 'flick' the line with your middle finger. If there are bubbles trapped in a port, invert the port and let the air rise into the line, and tap or flick them up. The bubbles will dislodge from the line and ascend into the drip chamber. Keep at it. It may take some work to get them all floating up. Air in the line can be carried into the vein and cause blockage of the vessel. More dire consequences include specific organ failure. Ruiz-Avila, García-Araque and Acosta-Gutiérrez (2022) report that a venous gas embolism occurs when air in the venous system eventually causes an obstruction in the pulmonary circulation.

Prepare the dressing material at this time. Maintain sterility of all dressing material and place cut tape in an easily accessible place (e.g. on an IV pole or the edge of the over-bed table).

Insert the line into an existing cannula hub

Stabilising the cannula in the vein and securing the line to the skin before dressing the IV cannula is important. Insecure peripheral vascular devices may fall out, lead to phlebitis (i.e. irritation or inflammation to the vein wall), infiltration (i.e. fluid leaking into surrounding tissues) or occlusion (i.e. blockage). They increase the risk of catheter-related blood infection because movement of the catheter in the vein allows migration of organisms along the catheter and into the bloodstream (Czajka, Frey & Shears, 2018). This is especially crucial when placing an infusion line in anatomic areas of greater movement (e.g. antecubital veins and saphenous veins in the foot), and for anyone at greater risk of unintentional dislodgement (e.g. those who are confused, combative or developmentally challenged, have changes in mental status, or are toddlers or infants).

Perform hand hygiene and put on clean gloves. Stabilise the cannula in the vein with your non-dominant hand. Carefully remove the protective cap from the primed line and quickly but firmly insert the sterile needleless connector into the cannula hub (venipuncture catheter). Slowly release the roller clamp on the line to allow sufficient fluid through to maintain patency of the cannula. Stabilise the cannula with your non-dominant hand until the first pieces of tape safely hold the cannula in place and the line in position, or while applying the transparent dressing.

Apply the dressing

Use aseptic technique and sterile supplies to apply the dressing. Corley et al. (2022) state that there are significantly more adverse events (dislodgement, infiltration, phlebitis, infection and pain) in those who had poorly secured PIVCs. The dressing type will depend on the facility's protocols and the use of the engineered securement devices (ESDs) or medical cyanoacrylate tissue adhesives. A multi-product (e.g. transparent dressing with additional support [tubular net, transparent tape]) can assist in stabilising the PIVC. Stabilise the cannula by looping about 10 cm of the line back around towards the insertion site and beyond (i.e. a J-loop). Tape securely over the line both above and below the insertion site, taking care to leave the junction itself clear of tape. This reduces the pull on the insertion site. Sterile tape may be applied over the PIVC hub and the catheter wings for additional stability (Corley et al., 2022). Note that the use of adhesive tapes has potential problems, causing some people to develop blisters, bruises, erythema and contact dermatitis, so monitor their use closely.

To apply transparent dressing, carefully remove the adherent backing from one edge of the dressing. Apply the dressing from that edge, smoothing it onto the skin as you remove the backing. It should cover the insertion site and most of the hub of the cannula but not the adaptor, leaving the junction clear of dressing material. Write the date and time of PIVC insertion on the dressing's adhesive border.

Establish the ordered flow

Time with a watch

Determine the flow rate by calculating an hourly rate. To do this, divide the volume to be infused by the number of hours over which the volume is to infuse. For example, 1 L of fluid in an eight-hour period is calculated by dividing 1000 mL by 8 = 125 mL/hr.

This hourly rate is then converted to a 'drops per minute' rate by using one of the following formulae:

- *Microdrop giving set* – hourly volume × 60 drops per mL/60 minutes = drops per minute.
- *Macrodrop giving set* – hourly volume × 20 (or 15; be careful to take note of this information on the giving set packaging) drops per mL/60 minutes = drops per minute.

Time the flow by counting the drops as they fall into the drip chamber for a one-minute period. Adjust the rate of flow by tightening or loosening the roller clamp. Again, time the flow until the rate is as ordered.

The infusion pump

Infusion pumps differ from one manufacturer to another. Familiarise yourself with the infusion pump in use in the facility and ensure that the giving set is the one required for that pump. The following is applicable to most infusion pumps:

1. Slow the IV fluid rate to very slow using the roller clamp.
2. Place the electronic sensor on the drip chamber, above the level of the fluid.
3. Open the door on the face of the pump.
4. Thread the IV tubing through the pump in the direction of flow – tubing nearest the IV bag goes into the top of the pump and the tubing nearest the person comes out the bottom of the pump.
5. Close the door.
6. Turn the power on.
7. Set the pump to volume per hour as appropriate to the pump.
8. Open the roller clamp so that it does not impede the flow of fluid.
9. Press the start button on the infusion pump.
10. Time the flow for one minute to ensure that the pump is working effectively.

CLEAN, REPLACE AND DISPOSE OF EQUIPMENT

Whoever inserts the cannula is responsible for the correct disposal of sharps. Dispose of the insertion stylet from the cannula in the sharps container. Discard alcowipes or Betadine wipes into a contaminated waste bin. Discard the tourniquet if disposable; otherwise, wash and dry it and return it to storage for further use. Wash and dry the injection tray and return it to storage, along with the tape. Perform hand hygiene.

DOCUMENTATION

Note the insertion of the IV cannula on the progress sheet or on the electronic medication administration record (eMAR). Include the type and gauge of the cannula, site of insertion, IV fluid type and amount initiated, and rate of flow, time and date, as well as the name of the healthcare professional who cannulated the person. If more than one attempt was required, note this as well. Initiate a fluid balance sheet if there is not one in use. Note the type and amount of solution and the time initiated on the fluid balance sheet. Keep a record of the amount infused and the time that bags were changed. Record in the progress notes any inspection of the insertion site and the findings at least once per shift. Also record here complaints of any sort. As a courtesy to incoming staff, ensure that the medical staff have ordered enough fluids to last till the following day unless the person needs to be reviewed, and at handover verbally report the amount of fluid remaining to be infused and the rate at which it is infusing.

CLINICAL SKILLS ASSESSMENT

Intravenous therapy – assisting with establishment

Demonstrates the ability to effectively and safely assist in the establishment of intravenous therapy. Incorporates the *National Safety and Quality Health Service Standards*: 2 Partnering with Consumers, 3 Preventing and Controlling Healthcare-Associated Infection, 5 Comprehensive Care, 6 Communicating for Safety, and 8 Recognising and Responding to Acute Deterioration (ACSQHC, 2021b).

Performance criteria	1	2	3	4	5
(Numbers indicate NMBA *Registered Nurse Standards for Practice*)	(Dependent)	(Marginal)	(Assisted)	(Supervised)	(Independent)
1. Identifies indication (1.1, 3.3, 3.4)	☐	☐	☐	☐	☐
2. Evidence of therapeutic interaction with the person, e.g. allays person's anxiety by adequately explaining the procedure (1.4, 1.5, 2.1, 2.2, 3.2)	☐	☐	☐	☐	☐
3. Demonstrates clinical reasoning, e.g. assesses the person and intravenous site, determines how long the intravenous access needs to be (1.1, 2.3, 4.1, 4.2, 4.3, 5.1, 6.1)	☐	☐	☐	☐	☐
4. Gathers equipment (5.5, 6.1): ■ fluid order sheet ■ prescribed fluid (one bag) ■ required cannula and giving set ■ visualisation device (if available) ■ alcowipes, chlorhexidine or Betadine wipes ■ clean gloves ■ tourniquet ■ tape and dressing ■ armboard ■ stabilisation/securement device ■ intravenous stand ■ injection tray ■ sharps container ■ watch with a second hand ■ infusion pump (if required)	☐	☐	☐	☐	☐
5. Uses general concepts of medication administration plus the six rights (1.1, 1.2, 1.4, 1.5, 2.1, 2.2, 3.3, 3.4, 4.1, 4.2, 4.3, 6.1, 6.2, 6.5, 6.6)	☐	☐	☐	☐	☐
6. Performs hand hygiene (1.1, 3.4, 6.1)	☐	☐	☐	☐	☐
7. Prepares the giving set (1.1, 6.1, 6.5)	☐	☐	☐	☐	☐
8. Spikes the fluid bag (1.1, 6.1)	☐	☐	☐	☐	☐
9. Primes the line (1.1, 6.1)	☐	☐	☐	☐	☐
10. Assists the physician/specialist RN to establish intravenous access (1.1, 6.1)	☐	☐	☐	☐	☐
11. Inserts the line into the cannula hub, stabilises the line and applies the dressing (1.1, 6.1)	☐	☐	☐	☐	☐
12. Establishes the ordered flow using either the infusion pump or timing with a watch (1.1, 6.1, 6.2)	☐	☐	☐	☐	☐
13. Cleans, replaces and disposes of equipment appropriately (3.6, 6.1)	☐	☐	☐	☐	☐
14. Documents relevant information (1.4, 1.6, 2.2, 2.7, 3.5, 3.7, 6.2, 6.5, 7.3)	☐	☐	☐	☐	☐
15. Demonstrates the ability to link theory to practice (1.1, 3.3, 3.4, 3.5)	☐	☐	☐	☐	☐

Student:

Clinical facilitator: Date:

CHAPTER 32

INTRAVENOUS THERAPY – MANAGEMENT

INDICATIONS

Intravenous (IV) infusion into a peripheral vein is a common intervention for administration of fluids, electrolytes and medications. Intravenous therapy (IVT) is most often required in acute care settings. Because of the frequency of use, management of the IV and site are often thought to be routine. However, inserting an IV line involves an invasive, stressful and painful procedure (Cooke et al., 2018) that breaks the integrity of the skin, leaving a portal for infection. IVT infection is one of the biggest causes of hospital-acquired infection (HAI). The failure of peripherally inserted IV therapy with unscheduled restarts is high (rates of 33 to 66 per cent or more) (Marsh et al., 2024). To prevent the premature removal of an IV line, the destruction or infection of an IV site, and the need for another painful procedure, proper care and management of the established line are imperative.

To manage an IV infusion, you must know the ordered solution, rate of flow and any further solution(s) ordered following the current one. This information is found on either the physician's order sheet or the fluid balance sheet. Be aware of the reason for IVT, the duration of the therapy and any IV medications prescribed. Know the different parenteral fluids and the rationale for the use of specific prescribed fluids and the effects of IV medications systemically and locally.

Management also includes monitoring the site of insertion and the patency of the infusion, planning subsequent insertions, changing solution bags and dressings, and preparing the equipment and the person for these procedures.

EVIDENCE OF THERAPEUTIC INTERACTION

A person with an IV in situ needs to know about their therapy. Discuss the comfort of the site with the person and reassure them that the frequent checks done on the IVT are a normal occurrence. Emphasise the importance of disclosing any pain, burning, swelling or other abnormal sensation associated with the IVT, because these may point to a complication (Parreira et al., 2019). Always explore any reports of pain, try to determine the cause and provide comfort measures. Pain on insertion and at the insertion site is the earliest sign of phlebitis and is often overlooked (Simões, Vendramim & Pedreira, 2022).

DEMONSTRATE CLINICAL REASONING

Assessments during IV maintenance are subdivided into local, systemic and equipment assessment. Assess the person for signs of each of the possible complications on a regular basis. Eight-hourly assessments are a minimum. Anyone who is unstable or who has signs and symptoms of complications would be assessed more frequently (Brooks, 2016). Usually, these are noted during any interaction with the person. Overall assessment of the person's need for peripheral intravenous cannulation (PIVC) is undertaken daily (usually by the medical officer, with nursing input). The PIVC is removed as soon as possible. Check the facility's protocol.

ELDER CARE

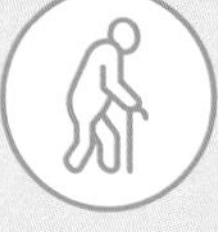

Phlebitis is a concern for older people. The increased administration of medications that damage the intima of the veins (e.g. antibiotics, potassium chloride [KCl]), increased incidences of hypertension and diabetes, and often the administration of hypertonic solutions make phlebitis an important consideration. Also, with the impaired inflammatory response of the elderly, phlebitis may be masked (Salma et al., 2019). Use of a smaller bore catheter produces fewer incidents of phlebitis.

Fluid overload and hyponatraemia are concerns in the elderly due to reduced renal clearance, so keep a close eye on the rate of administration and assess for signs of overload (fluid retention [especially in those with cardiorespiratory or renal dysfunction], weight gain) and electrolyte imbalances (e.g. hyponatraemia manifests as nausea, vomiting confusion, headache and restlessness, among other symptoms). Use an infusion pump, if possible, and check the gravity feed system frequently.

THE PERSON LIVING WITH SEVERE OBESITY

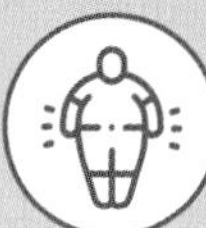

Many people living with severe obesity are diaphoretic, which causes loosening of the securement tape. This must be checked frequently. People living with severe obesity are also relatively immobile, which is a risk factor for the development of phlebitis (Simões, Vendramim & Pedreira, 2022). Take care to monitor closely for complications.

GATHER EQUIPMENT

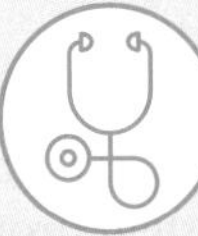

Gathering equipment ensures that you have all needed material, boosts the person's confidence and trust in you, and increases your self-confidence. While gathering the equipment, you can mentally rehearse the procedure. Besides your observation skills, you will need the following items:

EQUIPMENT	EXPLANATION
Fluid order sheet	States the solution and the rate, and is signed by the physician. It may be left at the bedside
Watch with a second hand	Used to time the infusion rate if there is no infusion pump
Clean gloves	Standard precaution to protect against contamination from body fluids
Alcowipes, chlorhexidine in alcohol wipes	• Used to scrub clean and disinfect the skin, hub and lock • The Australian Commission on Safety and Quality in Health (ACSQHC, 2021a) and Zingg et al. (2023) recommend chlorhexidine 2% in 70% alcohol • Use according to the policy of the facility
Sterile intermittent infusion lock device	Caps the IV catheter cannula so that continuous fluid infusion is not necessary, but access to the vein is still available
Syringe with sterile saline (or rarely heparin flush solution)	• The syringe will preferably have a needleless connector, but if a needle is required, use a small gauge • If heparin is used, ensure that the strength is for flushing, not medicating
Sharps container	Use to dispose of sharps directly after use to prevent inadvertent injury to yourself, the person or other staff

Local assessment

Assess the IV insertion site (LOOK, LISTEN, FEEL) for the following:

- *Infiltration* – fluid flowing into the tissue surrounding the vein. Signs are a blanched (pale), cool area with pain/burning at the insertion site, swelling, tightness and a slowed flow rate. It is termed 'extravasation' if the infusing fluid is an irritant or causes severe damage. If infiltration occurs, stop the infusion and remove the catheter, apply a compress – cold for irritating fluid or warm for neutral fluid (depending on the type and amount of infiltrate and the elapsed time), elevate the limb if possible, check the pulses and capillary refill on that limb (compartment syndrome is a possibility [Trinidad, 2022]; see **Clinical Skill 21**), and have the IV restarted in the other arm or well above the site of infiltration.
- *Phlebitis* – inflammation of the vein wall from irritation by the fluid, medications or the cannula. It causes pain, inflammation, heat, swelling and redness at the site, tracks up the vein, possibly causes malaise and an elevated temperature (febrile). The incidence of phlebitis increases with age, catheter size (Fernandes et al., 2020), number of IV medications given, types of medications (Simões, Vendramim & Pedreira, 2022) and length of hospital stay (Rojas-Sánchez, Parra & Camargo-Figuera, 2015). If phlebitis occurs, stop the infusion and remove the catheter, apply a warm pack and have the IV restarted elsewhere.
- *Cellulitis* – an HAI of the tissues surrounding the insertion site. It causes a warm or hot area with swelling. The person could be febrile and report malaise. If cellulitis occurs, stop the infusion and remove the catheter. Culture the tip and any exudate at the site of insertion. Monitor the person's vital signs, call their medical practitioner and anticipate antibiotic administration (Kaur et al., 2019).

Check for leaking fluid and for bleeding. Assess the patency of the IV cannula by compressing the cannulated vein proximal to the insertion site (IV flow should diminish, there should be little discomfort felt).

Systemic assessment

Monitor for signs of circulatory overload, fluid volume deficit, septicaemia, hypersensitivity and pulmonary or air embolism. (Please consult a nursing foundation or surgical text for the signs and symptoms of these conditions.) Remember that pre-existing medical conditions (e.g. cardiorespiratory or renal conditions) will impact on the speed and severity of fluid volume excess or deficit. Zingg et al. (2023) found that bloodstream infections, although uncommon in PIVCs, due to the high frequency of IVT, are significant contributors to morbidity and mortality. Surveillance is essential.

Assessment of fluid and equipment

Assessment of fluid and equipment are completed hourly to:

- determine that the fluid is infusing as ordered
- confirm that the solution is the one prescribed
- determine the rate, and alter it if it is not correct
- calculate the amount absorbed
- note the amount remaining to be infused.

The level remaining in the bag is noted, and a fresh bag (as ordered) is brought to the bedside before the infusing bag is empty.

INTRAVENOUS THERAPY MANAGEMENT

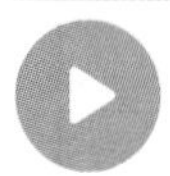

Managing IVT is a frequent task in most nursing units. It should not become a habitual routine. You need to be mindful of the problems and complications to look for and the assistance required by the person with an IV at each encounter (Park et al., 2022). The clinical standard (ACSQHC, 2021b) requires a thorough assessment of the system at least once each shift when assessing the device or if the person has concerns. Patency is checked and the line is flushed (according to the facility's schedule) to minimise PIVC failure.

Hand hygiene

Adequate hand hygiene (see **Clinical Skill 5**) removes transient microorganisms and reduces cross-contamination. It remains the single most effective measure to prevent HAI. Clean gloves should be used to comply with standard precautions.

Monitor or change the flow rate

The flow rate is monitored hourly to ensure correct/safe administration. Check it more frequently if the rate ordered is very fast (i.e. over 120 mL per hour). A flow-rate control device (e.g. burette or volumetric pump) is used for elderly, paediatric and anyone who is critically ill, those with a history of cardiac or renal failure, and for any infusion that has additives (e.g. potassium chloride). Volumetric pumps precisely infuse the fluid in millilitres per hour. Each pump will be subtly different. Familiarise yourself with the model used in the facility. If the flow rate is not as ordered, you will need to change it. See **Clinical Skill 31** for establishing the flow rate. Monitors for IV fluid levels are on the horizon and may soon be available at the clinical facility. These measure the remaining volume and transfer the information to an app carried by the nurse. This aim to improve safety (e.g. by alerting to too rapid infusion, reducing over-/under-infusion) and free up the nurse's time by reducing repeated trips to the person's room to 'check the levels' (Puolitaival et al., 2022).

'Smart pumps' have been developed to reduce medication errors in IV administration. They are interactive and contain pharmaceutical libraries with doses and interactions, programming to prevent medication errors, and connect to the person's electronic health record. If the facility where you are gaining experience is using these, you will need to understand and use this technology for improved care (Hodge et al., 2019).

Alarms on infusion pumps signal when drips cannot be sensed due to an empty IV bag, kinked tubing, an occluded catheter, infiltration of the IV site or a pump malfunction. Assess the entire system (from IV bag to insertion site) if an alarm sounds.

Some IV sites and cannulae are positional; that is, the tip of the cannula may rest against a vein wall in some positions and obstruct the flow. Sometimes the person or a staff member alters the rate of flow, putting the person at risk of under- or over-hydration. The flow rate can also be affected by the patency of the tubing and cannula.

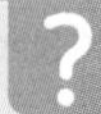

If the infusion is not being delivered at the prescribed rate:

- ensure the height of the infusion is 1 m or slightly more above the IV insertion site
- ensure the drip chamber is half-full of fluid
- check the IV tubing for kinks or for large air bubbles (see **Clinical Skill 31** for clearing air bubbles)
- check that the person is not lying on the IV tubing and thereby reducing or stopping the flow
- look for dependent loops and place excess tubing on the bed (dependent loops of fluid reduce the flow rate)
- check connections for leaks and for security; tighten any loose connections
- if the flow is sluggish or stopped, remove the bag of fluid from the IV stand and lower it below the level of the insertion site. Observe the tubing (blood return indicates patency of the vessel).

If the IV flow has stopped and infiltration is suspected but there are no signs, pinch the tubing just above the cannula hub and watch for blood flowing back into the tubing (it will if the cannula remains in the vein).

Notify the shift coordinator if you are unable to establish flow at the correct rate.

Change clothing for a person with an intravenous line

IV gowns were designed to be put on and removed easily. These have fasteners (buttons, ties, Velcro) along the upper side of each sleeve. However, many people prefer to use their own clothing. To remove a soiled gown (or pyjama top):

1. Provide privacy and prepare the clean gown – unfolded and placed in the proper orientation.
2. Assist the person to remove their unaffected arm and head from the original gown. Move the gown

carefully over the IV insertion site and off the hand so it is lying on the bed with the IV line still running through it.
3. Take the IV bag off the stand and, keeping it above the level of the insertion site, slide the gown off the line and fluid bag. Discard the soiled gown.
4. Thread the clean gown over the IV bag and line, bag first, from the bottom to the armhole to the wrist of the sleeve.
5. Rehang the fluid bag.
6. Carefully slip the gown sleeve over the person's hand and insertion site, and then help them to put the unaffected arm through the other sleeve and their head through the neck of the gown. Adjust the gown for comfort.

If an IV pump is used, the procedure is similar, but the line is clamped (i.e. slowed to keep the vein open) and removed from the pump prior to changing the clothing. Do not forget to replace the line in the machine, unclamp it and restart the pump.

Assist a person with an intravenous line to ambulate

The person will probably require help to get out of and back into the bed. Mind the IV insertion site and lines. Provide a wheeled IV stand when they need to walk. Many prefer to use the IV stand to steady themselves as they walk. Assist from the person's unaffected side and help them to manage the tubing. Keep the IV stand far enough in front or to the side to prevent tripping on the wheels.

Change solutions on an established intravenous line

This process is similar to the initial establishment of IVT except that the line is already fully primed (see **Clinical Skill 31**). Prepare to change the bag when there is still about an hour's worth of fluid remaining in the old bag. Check the IV fluid orders and bring the selected solution to the bedside. Generally, IV fluids need to be checked by two registered healthcare professionals (e.g. registered nurses [RNs], medical officers, enrolled nurses). These people both sign the infusion order. Check the person's identification (use the six rights of medication administration). Inspect the fluid and the container for turbidity, leaks, cracks, particles and the expiry date before you commence.

Do not let the old bag empty entirely, to prevent air entering the drip chamber and line. The manufacturer provides slightly more than 1 L in each bag. When the bag has approximately 50 mL of fluid remaining, wash your hands and, using the roller clamp, stop the flow of solution. Remove the old bag from the IV stand. Remove the spike by firmly pulling it from the old bag, taking care not to contaminate it or spill the remaining fluid. Pull off the protective sheath to expose the port on the new fluid bag. Rest the bag on a table, hang it on the IV pole or hold it firmly under your non-dominant arm to ensure that the port is straight and the spike does not puncture the sides of the port. Firmly push the spike's entire length into the port. Gently squeeze the drip chamber of the giving set while inserting the spike to prevent air entering the fluid. Hang the new bag. Check that the drip chamber is half-full and re-establish the prescribed flow rate.

Change the dressing

IV catheter site dressings anchor the catheter to the skin, reducing movement and microbial migration into the wound, and provide a barrier to reduce microbial entry from the environment (Corley et al., 2022). Assess the IV catheter site dressing at least once per shift and document. When the dressing is soiled, loose or damp, it needs to be changed. A transparent dressing is replaced routinely (72 to 96 hours) (Corley et al., 2022), although many facilities recommend changing the dressing only if it is necessary (e.g. damp, loose or soiled) (Santos-Costa et al., 2022). Discuss the rationale for changing the dressing with the person. Provide privacy. Gather equipment, including a fresh sterile transparent dressing, the antiseptic recommended by the facility, a disposable dressing tray, and sterile tape to secure the hub. Perform hand hygiene and don non-sterile gloves (see **Clinical Skills 5 and 6**).

Establish an aseptic field and prepare all of the equipment (see **Clinical Skill 67**). To remove transparent dressings, loosen opposite edges and pull them apart parallel to the skin – this lifts the material off the skin. Take care that the transparent dressing does not adhere to the catheter and move it.

Inspect the insertion site. If infection is suspected, inform the RN, take a swab of the insertion site with a culture and sensitivity kit and label it (see **Clinical Skill 69**). A requisition for microbiology is required. Remove the gloves, perform hand hygiene and determine if sterile gloves will be required. Continue as for a simple transparent dressing (see **Clinical Skill 67**).

Convert to a saline lock

If no IV fluid is necessary but access to a vein is required for intermittent medication administration, a saline or heparin lock is used. You will need clean gloves; alcowipes or, preferably, chlorhexidine 2% in alcohol 70% wipes (ACSQHC, 2021a) (as per use in the facility); a sterile intermittent infusion lock device; a syringe with the saline solution; and a sharps container. Heparin flushes are no longer recommended and usually not ordered, but if ordered for a peripheral IV lock, be sure to use dilute heparin (10 or 100 units per mL) designated for flushes.

Undertake the following steps:

- Perform hand hygiene.
- Stop the IV infusion by closing the roller clamp or turning off the infusion pump.
- Disinfect (scrub) the catheter hub with alcowipes or chlorhexidine in alcohol for 15 seconds; let it dry for at least 30 seconds.
- Open the sterile saline lock package. Loosen and remove the existing IV tubing from the hub

and insert the saline lock into the hub of the IV cannula using Aseptic Non Touch Technique (ANTT) technique.

- Test the saline lock for patency by first cleansing the lock device with the alcowipe and friction for a minimum of 15 seconds (Corley et al., 2019) and, again, let it dry for 30 seconds.
- Insert the needleless adaptor with the flush solution through the diaphragm of the lock and pull back gently on the syringe; watch for blood return.
- Inject the saline (or dilute heparin) slowly into the lock.
- Remove the syringe/needleless adaptor. Discard the syringe/needleless adaptor into the sharps container. Do not reuse the flush syringe (Arnold et al., 2017).
- Discard the used wipes and your gloves in the contaminated waste bin and perform hand hygiene.
- Assess the person for pain and the site for leakage or infiltration.

Safety

Be rigorous in cleansing the hub and the lock face. The greatest risk for contamination of the IV catheter after insertion is the access hub (33 to 45 per cent are contaminated in normal use). A contaminated hub acts as the immediate portal of entry for intraluminal contaminants (Ryder et al., 2023).

Discontinue intravenous therapy

PIVCs are removed as soon as they are no longer clinically indicated (Zingg et al., 2023). A PIVC is removed if there are signs and symptoms of phlebitis, occlusion, local of systemic infections or the facility has a routine for resiting the PIVC (e.g. every two days). Generally, a doctor's order is needed to discontinue IVT. Use clean gloves and an apron. Bring a dry sterile gauze square and a small sterile dressing and tape (as per the facility's protocol) to the bedside in a kidney basin or on an injection tray. Perform hand hygiene.

Open the gauze square and the dressing aseptically. Cut a 10 cm length of tape and secure it by one edge in a handy place. Perform hand hygiene and put on gloves. Clamp the tubing so fluid cannot flow out onto the person or the bed. Hold the cannula firmly in place and carefully remove the tape securing the line and cannula to prevent damage to the vein. Keep the skin taut to reduce the pull as the transparent dressing is removed. Pull the edges of the transparent dressing outward, parallel to the skin. Remove the dressing and discard it into the kidney basin. Inspect the insertion site for infection or infiltration.

Support the insertion site with the sterile gauze square. Pull the cannula out along the line of the vein to avoid injury to the vein. Be extra gentle with elderly people as their veins and skin are often very fragile. Apply firm pressure to the insertion site with the gauze square for two to three minutes until haemostasis occurs; the person may do this if they are willing. Apply pressure for a bit longer on elderly people as clotting may take extra time (even if they're not taking anticoagulant medications). Check the end of the cannula to make sure it is intact. If it is broken, report it to the shift coordinator or medical staff immediately. Dress the site using the sterile dressing and prepared tape. Place the used dressing, cannula and lines into the kidney basin and carry them and the fluid bag to the utility room for disposal.

The site is monitored for 48 hours for signs of pain, redness or swelling. If the person is being discharged, explain these signs and who they should contact if they arise (ACSQHC, 2021a).

CLEAN, REPLACE AND DISPOSE OF EQUIPMENT

Empty excess solution from the discontinued IV fluid bag down the sink and place the empty bag in the garbage bin. Once removed, dispose of the cannula into the contaminated waste bin or butterfly needle into the sharps container. Dispose of gloves and dressing material into the contaminated waste bin. Wash the kidney basin and return it to storage. Clean the IV pole as per the facility's guidelines and return it to the storage area.

DOCUMENTATION

Document IV interventions on the fluid order sheet and the fluid balance chart and note solution bag changes. Note discontinuation of the IV on the fluid order sheet, the fluid balance sheet and in the progress notes or the eMAR. Record the appearance of the IV site, the amount of fluid infused, the person's response to the procedure and any abnormal or untoward findings (infiltration, prolonged bleeding, broken cannula tip) in the progress notes and also report these to the shift coordinator. Some facilities use specific IV documentation; use the facility's procedure. Clinical handover includes the fluid ordered, the rate and the amount remaining to be infused or the expected time the current bag will take to complete, along with any untoward findings.

CLINICAL SKILLS ASSESSMENT

Intravenous therapy – management

Demonstrates the ability to effectively and safely manage intravenous therapy. Incorporates the *National Safety and Quality Health Service Standards*: 2 Partnering with Consumers, 3 Preventing and Controlling Healthcare-Associated Infection, 5 Comprehensive Care, 6 Communicating for Safety, and 8 Recognising and Responding to Acute Deterioration (ACSQHC, 2021b).

Performance criteria	1	2	3	4	5
(Numbers indicate NMBA *Registered Nurse Standards for Practice*)	(Dependent)	(Marginal)	(Assisted)	(Supervised)	(Independent)
1. Identifies indication (1.1, 3.3, 3.4)	☐	☐	☐	☐	☐
2. Evidence of therapeutic interaction with the person, e.g. allays anxiety by adequately explaining the procedure (1.4, 1.5, 2.1, 2.2, 3.2)	☐	☐	☐	☐	☐
3. Demonstrates clinical reasoning, e.g. assesses the person, the intravenous site, the fluid and the equipment (2.1, 2.2, 2.3, 4.1, 4.2, 4.3, 6.1)	☐	☐	☐	☐	☐
4. Gathers equipment (1.1, 5.5, 6.1): ■ fluid balance sheet ■ watch with a second hand ■ clean gloves ■ alcowipes, chlorhexidine in alcohol wipes ■ sterile intermittent infusion lock device ■ syringe with saline (or heparin) flush solution ■ sharps container	☐	☐	☐	☐	☐
5. Performs hand hygiene (1.1, 3.4, 6.1)	☐	☐	☐	☐	☐
6. Monitors or changes the flow rate (3.4, 4.1, 4.2, 4.3, 6.1, 6.2, 6.5)	☐	☐	☐	☐	☐
7. Changes clothing for the person with an intravenous line (1.1, 6.1)	☐	☐	☐	☐	☐
8. Assists the person with an intravenous line to ambulate (1.1, 6.1)	☐	☐	☐	☐	☐
9. Changes solutions on an established intravenous line (3.4, 4.1, 4.2, 4.3, 6.1, 6.2, 6.5)	☐	☐	☐	☐	☐
10. Changes the intravenous dressing (1.1, 6.1)	☐	☐	☐	☐	☐
11. Converts to a saline lock (3.4, 4.1, 6.1, 6.2, 6.5)	☐	☐	☐	☐	☐
12. Discontinues intravenous therapy (3.4, 4.1, 4.2, 4.3, 6.1, 6.2, 6.5)	☐	☐	☐	☐	☐
13. Cleans, replaces and disposes of equipment appropriately (3.6, 6.1)	☐	☐	☐	☐	☐
14. Documents relevant information (1.4, 1.6, 2.2, 3.5, 3.7, 6.2, 6.5, 7.3)	☐	☐	☐	☐	☐
15. Demonstrates the ability to link theory to practice (1.1, 3.3, 3.4, 3.5)	☐	☐	☐	☐	☐

Student:

Clinical facilitator: Date:

REFERENCES

Alhashemi, S., Ghorbani, R. & Vazin, A. (2019). Improving knowledge, attitudes and practice of nurses in medication administration through enteral feeding tubes by clinical pharmacists: A case-control study. *Advances in Medical Education and Practice, 10,* 493–500. https://doi.org/10.2147/AMEP.S203680

Alsamet, H. (2022). Considerations regarding oral medications delivery to patients on nasoenteral tubes. *Nutrition Clinique et Métabolisme, 36*(1), 21–7. https://doi.org/10.1016/j.nupar.2021.09.002

Arnold, S., Melville, S., Morehead, B., Vaughan, G., Moorman, A. & Crist, M. (2017). Hepatitis C transmission from inappropriate reuse of saline flush syringes for multiple patients in an acute care general hospital. *Morbidity and Mortality Weekly Report, 66*(9), 258–60. http://www.medscape.com/viewarticle/877154?

Australian Commission on Safety and Quality in Health Care (ACSQHC) (2021a). *Clinical standards: Management of peripheral catheters.* https://www.safetyandquality.gov.au/standards/clinical-care-standards/management- peripheral-intravenous-catheters-clinical-care-standard

Australian Commission on Safety and Quality in Health Care (ACSQHC) (2021b). *National safety and quality health service standards* (3rd edn). Sydney, NSW: ACSQHC.

Bering, J. & DiBaise, J. K. (2022). Home parenteral and enteral nutrition. *Nutrients, 14*(13), 2558. https://doi.org/10.3390/nu14132558

Bischoff, S., Austin, P., Boeykens, K., Chourdakis, M., Cuerda, C., Jonkers-Schuitema, C., Lichota, M., Nyulasi, I., Schneider, S., Stanga, Z. & Pironi, L. (2022). ESPEN practical guideline: Home enteral nutrition. *Clinical Nutrition, 41*(2), 468–88. https://doi.org/10.1016/j.clnu.2021.10.018

Boullata, J., Carrera, A., Harvey, L., Escuro, A., Mays, A., McGinnis, C., Wessel, J., Bajpai, S., Beebe, M., Kinn, T., Kiang, M., Lord, L., Martin, K., Pompeii-Wolfe, C., Sullivan, J., Wood, A., Malone, A. & Guenter, P. (2017). ASPEN safe practices for enteral nutrition therapy. *Parenteral and Enteral Nutrition, 41*(3), 520. https://doi.org/10.1177/0148607116673053

Brooks, N. (2016). Intravenous cannula site management. *Nursing Standard (2014+), 30*(52), 53. https://doi.org/10.7748/ns.2016.e10315

Broyles, B., Reiss, B., Evans, M., McKenzie, G., Pleunik, S. & Page, R. (2017). *Pharmacology in nursing* (Australia and New Zealand 2nd ed.). South Melbourne, VIC: Cengage Learning.

Chandrasekar, N., Dehlsen, K., Leach, S. T. & Krishnan, U. (2022). Blenderised tube feeds vs. commercial formula: Which is better for gastrostomy-fed children? *Nutrients, 14*(15), 3139. https://doi.org/10.3390/nu14153139

Cooke, M., Ullman, A., Ray-Barruel, G., Wallis, M., Corley, A. & Rickard, C. (2018). Not 'just' an intravenous line: Consumer perspectives on peripheral intravenous cannulation (PIVC). An international cross-sectional survey of 25 countries. *PLOS ONE, 13*(2), e0193436. https://doi.org/10.1371/journal.pone.0193436

Corley, A., Marsh, N., Ullman, A. J. & Rickard, C. M. (2022). Peripheral intravenous catheter securement: An integrative review of contemporary literature around medical adhesive tapes and supplementary securement products. *Journal of Clinical Nursing, 32,* 1841–57. https://doi.org/10.1111/jocn.16237

Corley, A., Ullman, A. J., Mihala, G., Ray-Barruel, G., Alexandrou, E. & Rickard, C. (2019). Peripheral intravenous catheter dressing and securement practice is associated with site complications and suboptimal dressing integrity: A secondary analysis of 40,637 catheters. *International Journal of Nursing Studies, 100,* 103409. https://doi.org/10.1016/j.ijnurstu.2019.103409

Czajka, C., Frey, A. & Shears, G. (2018). Vascular access device stabilization and line securement. *American Nurse Today, 13*(12), 22–4. https://www.medscape.com/viewarticle/906617_1

de Oliveira, J., de Sales Guilarducci, J., de Moura, L., Carvalho, E., Teixeira, L. & Pimenta, L. (2023). Prevalent clinical conditions in the elderly using home enteral nutrition therapy: A systematic review. *Nutrition Clinique et Métabolisme, 37*(1), 2–9. https://doi.org/10.1016/j.nupar.2022.09.007

DeLaune, S., Ladner, P., McTier, L. & Tollefson, J. (2024). *Fundamentals of nursing* (Australia and New Zealand 3rd ed.). South Melbourne, VIC: Cengage Learning.

Dent, E., Wright, O. R., Woo, J. & Hoogendijk, E. O. (2023). Malnutrition in older adults. *The Lancet, 401*(10380), 951–66. https://www.thelancet.com/journals/lancet/article/PIIS0140-6736(22)02612-5/abstract

Dickerson, R., Andromalos, L., Brown, J., Correia, M., Pritts, W., Ridley, E., Robinson, K., Rosenthal, M. & van Zanten, A. (2022). Obesity and critical care nutrition: Current practice gaps and directions for future research. *Critical Care, 26,* 283. https://doi.org/10.1186/s13054-022-04148-0

Dietitians Association of Australia (DAA) (2018). *Enteral nutrition manual for adults in health care facilities.* https://daa.asn.au/wp-content/uploads/2018/06/Enteral-nutrition-manual-june-2018-website.pdf

Dietitians Association of Australia (DAA) (2019). Malnutrition in older Australians. Royal Commission into Aged Care. https://agedcare.royalcommission.gov.au

Dietitians Australia (2023). *Enteral nutrition.* https://dietitiansaustralia.org.au/health-advice/enteral-nutrition

Elliott, A., Gibson, S., Bauer, J., Cardamis, A. & Davidson, Z. (2023). Exploring overnutrition, overweight, and obesity in the hospital setting: A point prevalence study. *Nutrients, 15*(10), 2315. https://doi.org/10.3390/nu15102315

Ernstmeyer, K. & Christman, E. (eds). (2021). Chapter 17: Enteral tube management. In *Nursing Skills [Internet]. Open Resources for Nursing (Open RN).* Eau Claire (WI): Chippewa Valley Technical College.

Feo, R., Frensham, L., Conroy, T. & Alison, K. (2019). 'It's just common sense': Preconceptions and myths regarding fundamental care. *Nurse Education in Practice, 36,* 82–4. https://doi.org/10.1016/j.nepr.2019.03.006

Fernandes, E., Peres, E., Gomes, H., Pires, B., Leite, D., Péres Júnior, E. & Faria, C. (2020). Occurrence of phlebitis associated with peripheral venous catheterizations in hospitalized patients. *Research, Society and Development, 9*(5), e154953301. https://doi.org/10.33448/rsd-v9i5.3301

Formisano, E., Schiavetti, I., Gradaschi, R., Gardella, P., Romeo, C., Pisciotta, L. & Sukkar, S. G. (2023). The real-life use of a protein-sparing modified fast diet by nasogastric tube (ProMoFast) in adults with obesity: An open-label randomized controlled trial. *Nutrients, 15*(22), 4822. https://doi.org/10.3390/nu15224822

Furuya, J., Suzuki, H., Tamada, Y., Onodera, S., Nomura, R., Hidaka, R., Minakuchi, S. & Kondo, H. (2020). Food intake and oral health status of inpatients with dysphagia in acute care settings. *Journal of Oral Rehabilitation, 47*(6), 736–42. https://doi.org/10.1111/joor.12964

Gomes, F., Baumgartner, A. & Bounoure, L. (2019). Association of nutritional support with clinical outcomes among medical inpatients who are malnourished or at nutritional risk: An updated systemic review and meta-analysis. *Journal of the American Medical Association Network Open, 2*(11), e1915136. https://doi.org/10.1001/jamanetworkopen.2019.15138

Gorski, L. (2022). *Phillips' manual of I.V. therapeutics: Evidence-based practice for infusion therapy.* F.A. Davis Co.

Hodge, L., Walters, W., Sharp, K., King, L. & Smailes, P. (2019). Successful nursing optimization after pump integration with the electronic health record. *Journal of Informatics Nursing, 4*(4), 25–9. https://search.proquest.com/openview/cb7ecdd5cdf7c6efa a17511999bcb050/1?pq-origsite=gscholar&cbl=2044826

Holst, M., Beermann, T., Mortensen, M., Skadhauge, L., Kohler, M., Lindorff-Larsen, K. & Rasmussen, H. (2017). Optimizing protein and energy intake in hospitals by improving individualised meal serving, hosting and the environment. *Nutrition, 34*(Feb), 14–20. https://doi.org/10.1016/j.nut.2016.05.011

Hunter, S. (2013). *Miller's nursing for wellness in older adults* (1st Australian & New Zealand ed.). Philadelphia, PA: Lippincott Williams & Wilkins.

Judd, M. (2020). Confirming nasogastric tube placement in adults. *Nursing 2020, 50*(4), 43–6. https://doi.org/10.1097/01.NURSE.0000654032.78679.f1

Kaur, P., Rickard, C., Domer, G. & Glover, K. (2019). Dangers of peripheral intravenous catheterization: The forgotten tourniquet and other patient safety considerations. *IntechOpen.* https://doi.org/10.5772/intechopen.83854

Klinedinst, R., Cohen, A. & Dahlen, C. (2020). Dysphagia, hiccups and other oral symptoms. In B. Rolling Ferrell & J. Paice (eds), *Oxford textbook of palliative care.* Oxford, UK: Oxford University Press.

Lai, J., Chen, S., Chen, L., Huang, D., Lin, J. & Zheng, Q. (2022). Bedside gastrointestinal ultrasound combined with acute gastrointestinal injury score to guide enteral nutrition therapy in critically patients. *BMC Anesthesiology, 22,* 231. https://doi.org/10.1186/s12871-022-01772-9

Major, M., & Huey, T. (2016). Decreasing IV infiltrates in the pediatric patient: System-based improvement project. *Pediatric Nursing, 42*(1), 14–20. https://search.proquest.com/docview/1765381650/78FABAFFB33240FAPQ/5? accountid=88802

Mak, M. & Tan, G. (2020). Ultrasonography for nasogastric tube placement verification: An additional reference. *British Journal of Community Nursing, 25*(7), 328–34. https://www.magonlinelibrary.com/doi/abs/10.12968/bjcn.2020.25.7.328

Malina, D. (2022). Fluids and electrolytes. In J. Odom-Forren (ed.), *Drain's perianesthesia nursing – ebook: A critical care approach.* Elsevier.

Marsh, N., Larsen, E., Takashima, M., Kleidon, T., Keogh, S., Ullman, A., Mihala, G., Chopra, V. & Rickard, C. (2021). Peripheral intravenous catheter failure: A secondary analysis of risks from 11,830 catheters. *International Journal of Nursing Studies, 124,* 104095. https://doi.org/10.1016/j.ijnurstu.2021.104095

Marsh, N., Larsen, E., Ullman, A., Mihala, G., Cooke, M., Chopra, V., Ray-Barruel, G. & Rickard, C. (2024). Peripheral intravenous catheter infection and failure: A systematic review and meta-analysis. *International Journal of Nursing Studies, 151*(104673). https://doi.org/10.1016/j.ijnurstu.2023.104673

Marsh, N., Webster, J., Ullman, A. J., Gabor, M., Cooke, M., Chopra, V. & Rickard, C. (2020). Peripheral intravenous catheter non-infectious complications in adults: A systematic review and meta-analysis. *Journal of Advanced Nursing, 76,* 33463362. https://doi.org/10.1111/jan.14565

Mutrie, L. & Hill, B. (2018). Providing nutritional support for patients in critical care. *Nursing Standard (2014+), 33*(3). https://doi.org/10.7748/ns.2018.e10804

Nasa, P., Wise, R., Elbers, P., Wong, A., Dabrowski, W., Regenmortel, N., Monnet, X., Myatra, S. & Malbrain, M. (2022). Intravenous fluid therapy in perioperative and critical care setting – knowledge test and practice: An international cross-sectional survey. *Journal of Critical Care, 71,* 154122. https://doi.org/10.1016/j.jcrc.2022.154122

Nielsen, C., Ward, C., Zamora, Z. & Shuck-Conner, C. (2022). A standardized approach to enteral medication administration. *Nursing, 52*(5), 54–7. https://doi.org/10.1097/01.NURSE.0000827136.76706.5f

NSW Health (2023). *Guideline: Insertion and management of nasogastric and orogastric tubes in adults.* https://www1.health.nsw.gov.au/pds/ActivePDSDocuments/GL2023_001.pdf

Park, J., You, S., Kim, H., Park, C., Ryu, G., Kwon, S., Kim, Y., Lee, S. & Lee, K. (2022). Experience of nurses with intravenous fluid monitoring for patient safety: A qualitative descriptive study. *Risk Management and Healthcare Policy, 15,* 1783–93. https://doi.org/10.2147/RMHP.S374563

Parreira, P., Serambeque, B., Costa, P., Mónico, L., Oliveira, V., Sousa, L., Gama, F., Bernardes, R., Adriano, D., Marques, I., Braga, L., Graveto, J., Osorio, N. & Salgueiro-Oliveira, A. (2019). Impact of an innovative securement dressing and tourniquet in peripheral intravenous catheter-related complications and contamination: An interventional study. *International Journal of Environmental Research and Public Health, 16*(18). https://doi.org/10.3390/ijerph16183301

Peladic, N., Orlandoni, P., Dell'Aquila, G., Carrieri, B., Eusebi, P., Landi, F., Volpato, S., Zuliani, G., Lattanzio, F. & Cherubini, A. (2019). Dysphagia in nursing home residents: Management and outcomes. *Journal of the American Medical Directors Association, 20*(2), 147–51. https://doi.org/10.1016/j.jamda.2018.07.023

Penrod, J., Morse, J. & Wilson, S. (1999). Comforting strategies used during nasogastric tube insertion. *Journal of Clinical Nursing, 8*(31), 31–8.

Plohal, A. (2019). Improving communication during I.V. catheter insertion. *Nursing, 49*(9), 60–1. https://doi.org/10.1097/01.NURSE.0000577748.87879.49

Puolitaival, A., Savola, M., Tuomainen, P., Assebug, C., Lundstrom, T. & Soini, E. (2022). Advantages in management and remote monitoring of intravenous therapy: Exploratory survey and economic evaluation of gravity-based infusions in Finland. *Advances in Therapies, 39,* 2096–108. https://doi.org/10.1007/s12325-022-02093-6

Rabaut, J., Thirugnanachandran, T., Singhal, S., Martin, J., Lievliev, S., Ma, H. & Phan, T. (2022). Clinical outcomes and patient safety of nasogastric tube in acute stroke patients. *Dysphagia, 37,* 1732–9. https://doi.org/10.1007/s00455-022-10437-1

Rodriguez-Calero, M., de Pedro-Gomez, J., Molero-Ballester, J., Fernandez-Fernandez, I., Matamalas-Massanet, C., Moreno-Mejias, L., Blanco-Mavillard, I., Moya-Suarez, A., Personat-Labrador, C. & Morales-Asencio, J. (2020). Risk factors for difficult peripheral intravenous cannulation. The PIVV2 multicentre case-control study. *Journal of Clinical Medicine, 9*(3), 799. https://doi.org/10.3390/jcm9030799

Rojas-Sánchez, L. Z., Parra, D. I. & Camargo-Figuera, F. (2015). Incidence and factors associated with the development of phlebitis: Results of a pilot cohort study. *Revista De Enfermagem Referência, 4*(4), 61–7. https://doi.org/10.12707/RIII13141

Ruiz Avila, H., García-Araque, H. & Acosta-Gutiérrez, E. (2022). Paradoxical venous air embolism detected with point-of-care ultrasound: A case report. *Ultrasound Journal, 14*(19). https://doi.org/10.1186/s13089-022-00265-7

Ryder, M., DeLancey-Pulcini, E., Parker, A. & James, G. (2023). Bacterial transfer and biofilm formation in needleless connectors in a clinically simulated in vitro catheter model. *Infection Control & Hospital Epidemiology,* 1–9. https://doi.org/10.1017/ice.2023.60

Salma, U., Sarker, M., Nahida, Z. & Ahamed, K. (2019). Frequency of peripheral intravenous catheter related phlebitis and related risk factors: A prospective study. *Journal of Medicine, 20*(1), 29–33. https://doi.org/10.3329/jom.v20i1.38818

Santos-Costa, P., Paiva-Santos, F., Sousa, L., Bernardes, R., Ventura. F., Fearnley, W., Salgueiro-Oliveira, A., Parreira, P., Vieira, M. & Graveto, J. (2022). Nurses' practices in the peripheral intravenous catheterization of adult oncology patients: A mix-method study. *Journal of Personalized Medicine, 12*(2), 151. https://doi.org/10.3390/jpm12020151

Sauer, A., Goates, S., Malone, A., Gerwirtz, G., Sulz, I., Moick, S., Laviano, A. & Hiesmayr, M. (2019). Prevalence of malnutrition risk and the impact of nutrition risk on hospital outcomes: Results from nutritionDay in the U.S. *Journal of Parenteral and Enteral Nutrition, 43*(7), 918–26. https://doi.org/10.1002/jpen.1499

Sheikh, F. (2023). Celebrating cultural diversity and spirituality in long term care facilities. *Diversity, Equity and Inclusion, 14*(4), 14. https://doi.org/10.1016/j.carage.2023.04.007

Shune, S. & Linville, D. (2019). Understanding the dining experience of individuals with dysphagia living in care facilities: A grounded theory analysis. *International Journal of Nursing Studies, 92,* 144–53. https://doi.org/10.1016/j.ijnurstu.2019.01.017

Sigmon, D. & An, J. (2022). Nasogastric tube. *StatPearls (Internet).* https://www.ncbi.nlm.nih.gov/books/NBK556063

Simões, A. M. N., Vendramim, P. & Pedreira, M. L. G. (2022). Risk factors for peripheral intravenous catheter-related phlebitis in adult patients. *Revista da Escola de Enfermagem da USP, 56,* e20210398. https://www.scielo.br/j/reeusp/a/LccxWRW6JScJZqV3DyFSLTD/?lang=en

Spence, C., Mancini, M. & Huisman, G. (2019). Digital commensality: Eating and drinking in the company of technology. *Frontiers in Psychology, 10.* https://www.frontiersin.org/articles/10.3389/fpsyg.2019.02252

Stumpf, F., Keller, B., Gressies, C. & Schuetz, P. (2023). Inflammation and nutrition: Friend or foe? *Nutrients, 15*(5), 1159. https://doi.org/10.3390/nu15051159

Taskiran, N. & Sari, D. (2022). The effectiveness of auscultatory, colorimetric capnometry and pH measurement methods to confirm placement of nasogastric tubes: A methodological study. *International Journal of Nursing Practice, 28*(2), e13049. https://doi.org/10.1111/ijn.13049

Tatsumi, H. (2019). Enteral tolerance in critically ill patients. *Journal of Intensive Care, 7*(30). https://doi.org/10.1186/s40560-019-0378-0

Terech-Skóra, S., Kasprzyk-Mazur, J., Leyk-Kolańczak, M., Kruk, A., Piotrkowska, R., Mędrzycka-Dąbrowska, W. & Książek, J. (2023). Assessment of oral health in long-term enteral and parenteral nutrition patients: Significant aspects of nursing care. *International Journal of Environmental Research and Public Health, 20*(4), 3381. https://doi.org/10.3390/ijerph20043381

The Lancet (2023). Editorial: Loneliness as a health issue. *The Lancet, 402*(10396), 79. https://doi.org/10.1016/S0140-6736(23)01411-3htt

Trinidad, M. (2022). Peripheral intravenous infiltration and extravasation prevention. *Journal of Nursing Practice Applications & Reviews of Research, 19.* https://mypnaa.org/resources/Documents/JNPARR/Issues/PNAA%20Journal%20Jan%20Volume%2013%20Number%201.pdf#page=21

Vadivelu, N., Kodumudi, G., Leffert, L., Pierson, D., Rein, L., Silverman, M., Cornett, E. & Kaye, A. (2023). Evolving therapeutic roles of nasogastric tubes: Current concepts in clinical practice. *Advances in Therapy, 40,* 828–43. https://doi.org/10.1007/s12325-022-02406-9

Volkert, D., Beck, A., Cederholm, T., Cruz-Jentoft, A., Hooper, L., Kiesswetter, E., Maggio, M., Raynaud-Simon, A., Sieber, C., Sobotka, L., vanAsselt, D., Wirth, R. & Bischoff, S. (2022). ESPEN practical guideline: Clinical nutrition and hydration in geriatrics. *Clinical Nutrition, 41,* 958–89. https://www.espen.org/files/ESPEN-Guidelines/ESPEN_practical_guideline_Clinical_nutrition_and_hydration_in_geriatrics.pdf

Wang, H-Y., Lin, Y-H., Chen, W-T. & Chen, J-B. (2022). Application of point-of- care ultrasound in patients receiving enteral nutrition. *European Review for Medical and Pharmacological Sciences, 26,* 3919–26. https://www.europeanreview.org/wp/wp-content/uploads/3919-3926.pdf

Wright, D., Smithard, D. & Griffith, R. (2020). Optimising medicines administration for patients with dysphagia in hospital: Medical or nursing responsibility? *Geriatrics, 5*(1), 9. https://doi.org/10.3390/geriatrics5010009

Wu, S., Morrison-Koechl, J., McAiney, C., Middleton, L., Lengyel, C., Slaughter, S., Carrier, N., Yoon, M-N. & Keller, H. (2023). Multi-level factors associated with relationship-centred and task-focused mealtime practices in long-term care: A secondary data analysis of the making the most of mealtimes study. *Canadian Journal on Aging/La Revue Canadienne Du Vieillissement,* 1–14. https://doi.org/10.1017/S0714980823000156

Yamagami, Y. & Inoue, T. (2020). Patient position affects venodilation for peripheral intravenous cannulation. *Biological Research for Nursing, 22*(2), 226–33. https://doi.org/10.1177/1099800419893027

Yasuda, H., Kondo, N., Yamamoto, R., Asami, S., Abe, T., Tsujimoto, H., Tsujimoto, Y. & Kataoka, Y. (2021). Monitoring of gastric residual volume during enteral nutrition. *Cochrane Database of Systematic Reviews, 9,* CD013335. https://doi.org/10.1002/14651858.CD013335.pub2

Zingg, W., Barton, A., Bitmead, J., Eggimann, P., Pujol, M., Simon, A. & Tatzel, J. (2023). Best practice in the use of peripheral venous catheters: A scoping review and expert consensus. *Infection Prevention in Practice, 5*(2). https://doi.org/10.1016/j.infpip.2023.100271

PART 6

ASSISTING WITH ELIMINATION

33 ASSISTING WITH ELIMINATION NEEDS

34 ADMINISTERING AN ENEMA

35 SUPRAPUBIC CATHETER CARE – CATHETER IRRIGATION

36 URINARY CATHETERISATION

Note: These notes are summaries of the most important points in the assessments/procedures and are not exhaustive on the subject. References of the materials used to compile the information have been supplied. The student is expected to have learnt the material surrounding each skill as presented in the references. No single reference is complete on each subject.

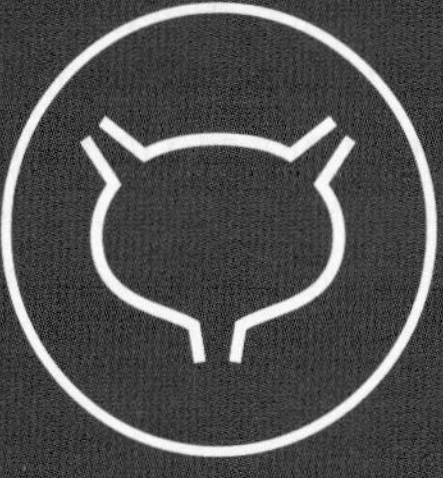

CHAPTER 33

ASSISTING WITH ELIMINATION NEEDS

INDICATIONS

Some people cannot mobilise due to their condition or because of their treatment. They require devices to assist elimination, such as a commode, bedpan or urinal. These provide a receptacle into which the bed-bound person can eliminate wastes, or from which you can obtain a specimen for analysis or accurately measure the person's output.

Physicians may order bed rest 'with toilet privileges', which means the person can use the toilet with as much assistance as necessary. If the order is 'commode', then the person must use a commode or bedpan, whether they are able to physically mobilise or not. 'Bed rest' means using a urinal or bedpan for elimination. Nurses can initiate the use of any of the assistive devices to assist the person.

EVIDENCE OF THERAPEUTIC INTERACTION

This simple nursing measure requires your tact and patience. The basic elimination requirements are intensely private for most people. The cultural mores surrounding elimination are rigid. For example, most of us were very well toilet-trained by the age of two or so and were taught that elimination requires privacy.

Adults are expected to meet their own elimination needs unaided and feel they are regressing when help is needed. Often, people will suppress the urge to defecate and this can lead to constipation (Toney-Butler & Gaston, 2019). Some may restrict their fluids to reduce the number of times toileting assistance is required or bedpan experiences are necessary in the day (Bak, 2018). A bedpan is generally uncomfortable and difficult to move on, and people fear 'missing the pan' and wetting or soiling the bed. Reinforce the reasons for the need for a bedpan or urinal to help reduce the person's feelings of inadequacy. Use tact and consideration to reduce embarrassment about sights, sounds and odours and the dependence on another for accomplishing such a basic function. Attending to the elimination needs of individuals promptly when requested reduces constipation and incontinence, as does prompted voiding (Bak, 2018). Check the chart for orders regarding activity, remember to introduce yourself and explain the necessity of using the bedpan, urinal or commode to increase cooperation.

DEMONSTRATE CLINICAL REASONING

Assess the person's ability to be independent

Refer to the care plan to establish whether manual-handling equipment or assistance from another healthcare professional is required. This determines the choice of assistive devices. If the person can ambulate with assistance, taking them to the toilet is the best option. It is less psychologically unsettling than having to stay in bed to accomplish the most basic of needs. If the person can transfer but is unable to be mobilised, a commode is the next best choice; it is similar to a toilet, out of the bed and less distressing for most people to use. As well, most commodes are wheeled to enable placing them over the toilet bowl. Urinals and bedpans are usually used in the bed, although some males may be able to stand at the bedside to use the urinal. Focus on the person rather than the task.

Management of elimination

Position the person as close to the usual anatomical position for toileting as possible. This promotes maximum comfort. If not contraindicated, raise the back of the bed or support the person with pillows in a high Fowler's position. The person's condition and restrictions will temper this. Ensure privacy and place the call bell within reach. Answering the call bell promptly will decrease falls and increase satisfaction with care (Toney-Butler & Gaston, 2019). Wear clean gloves to protect against body fluids, especially when removing urinals and/or bedpans. Take care that the contents of the bedpan or urinal are not spilled when removing the bedpan/urinal. Toilet paper, air freshener and hand-washing equipment should be in easy reach for the person to assist themselves if they are capable.

ELDER CARE

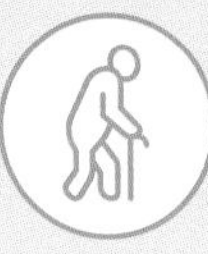

Age-related functional impairments and chronic disease increase the percentage of elderly people who are hospitalised for both acute and ongoing care. Dignity is an important concept when caring for the elimination needs of elders. Providing privacy, treating each elder with respect, promoting their autonomy, improving their health knowledge, safe care, and providing positive, person-centred care contribute to dignified care (Fuseini et al., 2023).

Urinary incontinence is common in the elderly, with significant risk factors of constipation, immobility/wheelchair use, pelvic or spinal damage/surgery (Tai et al., 2021). Elderly women are at increased risk of both stress and urge incontinence (Assis et al., 2023). To assist these people, provide sufficient fluids (30 mL/kg/day in 100 to 300 mL drinks – stop drinking two to three hours before bedtime to avoid nocturia) to dilute the urine, answer the call bell quickly, remind females to do their Kegel (pelvic floor) exercises and to refrain from citrus, alcohol, carbonated drinks or artificially sweetened foods, caffeine (tea, especially, irritates the bladder). Timed toileting can be effective (take the person to the toilet or offer a commode/bedpan q2-3h) or provide with continence undergarments or pads as per the facility's policy. These suggestions are effective for anyone, not just the elderly. Refer to a fundamentals nursing text for further information on urinary incontinence.

Approximately 30 per cent of elderly hospitalised people will suffer constipation (Dowden, 2021). Assessment of the stools (or lack of stools) will alert you to impending constipation. Provide extra fluids of choice (within the treatment regimen), dietary fibre and promote exercise to assist to maintain normal bowel habits for those with short-term (less than three months) constipation. Help establish a 'bowel routine'; that is, a specific time of day, often following a hot drink or a meal to evacuate the bowels. Again, refer to a fundamentals text for more in-depth discussion of bowel elimination.

THE PERSON LIVING WITH SEVERE OBESITY

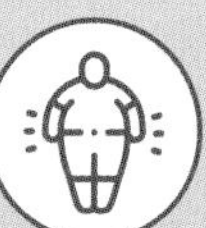

People living with severe obesity can experience elimination difficulties. Bauer, Eglseer and Großschädl (2023) found both urinary and faecal incontinence more common in those with severe obesity. Increased abdominal adiposity, limited mobility, and damage to the pelvic floor vasculature and muscles all contribute. The severely obese person will require increased assistance to toilet and for perineal hygiene (to prevent skin maceration and ulceration). Prompt care is important to preserve dignity and prevent perineal irritation. If they are consistently incontinent, there are large-size containment pads/underwear available.

GATHER EQUIPMENT

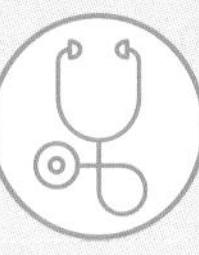

Gathering equipment is an organisational step that helps to create a positive environment for a successful interaction and reduces the person's discomfort and embarrassment. While gathering the equipment, you can mentally rehearse the procedure. Equipment required may include:

EQUIPMENT	EXPLANATION
Commode	• A wheeled armchair with a toilet seat and a receptacle below that collects the urine and faeces • Some have a second plain seat that is closed to transform the commode into a chair • Some can be wheeled over a toilet so there is one transfer only • They have locks on their wheels to prevent the person slipping while being transferred onto the commode • Severely obese people will need a suitably sized commode
Bedpan	• Used for faecal elimination in both males and females and for urinary elimination for most females • Commonly available in two types – regular pan and fracture or slipper pan that is smaller and flatter and is designed for those who have physical limitations or who are unable to lift their buttocks onto the regular bedpan • Disposable bedpans are becoming available and provide an acceptable, less costly and more hygienic alternative to bedpan washers (Meunier et al., 2019) • For hygienic reasons, never place on the floor, bed table or locker • During cold weather, swirl a metal or plastic bedpan with warm water, empty and dry it prior to use to warm it so that the cold metal or plastic against the skin does not reduce the person's urge to void or defecate • Some facilities permit the use of a dusting of talcum powder on the rim of the metal or plastic pan to facilitate repositioning • Bariatric bedpans are available for people up to 544 kg weight (Toney-Butler & Gaston, 2019)

Bedpan liner	These are gel-coated liners used to decrease splashing (e.g. from diarrhoea) and transference of multi-resistant bacteria (Steeves, Vallande & Lonks, 2020)
Urinals	• Deep, narrow receptacles for urine, mostly used by males • Female urinals are available, but are very difficult for most females to use • For hygienic reasons, never place on the floor, bed table or locker • The urinal (empty and clean) is sometimes placed in a bag or wire holder and hung on the bed frame so the person has easy access
Toilet paper or disposable wipes	For cleansing after urinary or faecal elimination
Covers (large flat paper bags or plastic to use if the bedpan does not have an integral cover)	• Used to cover the bedpan and urinal when transporting the used bedpan/urinal to the dirty utility room for disposal • Reduce the dispersal of pathogens during movement through the unit; such pathogens may contribute to the development of multidrug-resistant organisms (van Knippenberg-Gordebeke, 2015). Additionally, it is more aesthetically pleasing to see a covered pan/urinal than an open one
A waterproof sheet or 'bluey'	Used under the bedpan to catch any inadvertent spills so the linen is not soiled
Manual-handling equipment	Lifts and slide sheets are used as appropriate to assist with positioning the person or to move them onto and off a commode
Clean gloves and apron	Worn for personal protection during possible contact with body fluids; standard precautions
Eye goggles	Protect from splashes if emptying the pan/urinal
Hand-washing equipment	A wet, warm washer and a towel and/or alcohol-based hand rub (ABHR) should be available for the person for cleansing hands following elimination
Air freshener	• May be needed to reduce embarrassment from strong faecal odours • Note that people with respiratory difficulties may react adversely to the aerosolised particles, and that perfume in some fresheners is offensive to some people
Perineal care equipment	Includes a basin of warm water, a towel, a washer, pH-neutral cleanser, clean gloves, a bath blanket and ointment if needed to cleanse the perineum and protect against maceration from moisture
Continence promotion aids	Includes pads and pouch pants, uridomes, mattress protectors and are used as needed
Urine-testing equipment	• Require a specimen of fresh urine to test • To obtain the urine, a clean bedpan or urinal will be required, plus the urine-testing reagent strips, paper towel and gloves

ASSIST WITH ELIMINATION

Video

Assisting with elimination includes helping a person onto a commode or a bedpan or providing a urinal, as well as helping the person to complete perineal hygiene if necessary. Disposing of waste appropriately is also part of assisting with elimination. Performing a ward urinalysis and obtaining a stool specimen are also addressed below.

Hand hygiene

Hand hygiene (see **Clinical Skill 5**) removes microorganisms from the hands and prevents cross-contamination. It is the most effective preventative measure against hospital-acquired infection. Hand hygiene should be done before and after assisting with elimination and after handling excreta or the equipment. Assist the person to clean their hands as well.

Assist the person to use a commode

The person is assisted out of bed and onto the commode. A lift may be required. If they are able, leave them in privacy for a few minutes with the call bell in their hands. The person may or may not need assistance to clean the perineal area. If assistance is needed, help the person to stand and lean against the bed. Wrap toilet paper around your gloved hand; for females, wipe the perineal area from the pubic area backwards to the anal area so that faecal material is not brought forward to the urinary or vaginal meatus; for males, wipe from behind the scrotum back towards the anal area. If wiping with dry paper is not sufficient to cleanse the area, assist the person to return to bed and do perineal care (see the section 'Perform perineal care'). Provide them with hand-washing equipment to prevent the spread of microorganisms. Use air freshener to eliminate embarrassing odours if there are no contraindications. Close and remove the commode from the room for cleaning.

Give and receive a urinal

Assist the male to stand at the bedside, if health permits, or to a semi-Fowler's position. Most males are able to position the urinal independently. If not, place the urinal between the male's legs with the handle upward. You may need to pick the penis up using a gloved hand and place it in the urinal neck. Leave the male in privacy and with the call bell in hand. Return when called or in about three to five minutes. Remove the urinal and cover. Wipe the tip of the penis with toilet paper to remove any urine. Make sure the perineum is dry (may require perineal care) then offer hand-washing equipment. Take the covered urinal to the utility room.

Give and receive a bedpan

The person who can assist

Place the warmed/dried (plastic/metal) or a disposable bedpan on the end of the bed or on an adjacent chair. Fold the covers down to expose the hips and adjust the gown so it will not be soiled. Assist the person to raise their buttocks off the bed (you may require the assistance of a second nurse). The supine person should flex their knees and, resting their weight on their heels and back, raise the buttocks. Assist by placing your arm/hand nearest the person's head under the lower back and using your elbow as a fulcrum and your arm as a lever, push upward to give more movement to the person's hips. With your other hand, slip a waterproof sheet and the bedpan, with the open end towards the feet, under their buttocks. Using good body mechanics will reduce injuries from muscle strain in both the person and you. Make sure the smooth, round end of the bedpan is in contact with the buttocks to prevent both skin abrasion and spillage. Check the position of the pan by looking between the person's legs.

A slipper or fracture pan is placed with the flat end under the person's buttocks and the open end towards the feet. Elevate the head of the bed to high or semi-Fowler's position, if not contraindicated by the person's condition, so the person's back is comfortable, and the position is close to normal sitting to help reduce constipation (Toney-Butler & Gaston, 2019). If this position is not possible, and the person is supine, place a small pillow under their back to increase comfort, if permitted by the person's condition. Slip the pan and a waterproof sheet under the buttocks, as above.

Replace the bed linen and side-rails and leave the person in privacy and with the call bell in their hand and the toilet paper within reach.

When the person has finished, fold the covers down and ask the person to raise their buttocks. Remove the bedpan, leaving the waterproof sheet. The person may or may not need assistance to clean the perineal area; if so assist the person as above. Use one stroke per piece of paper; turn the person on their side and spread the buttocks to clean the anal area in the same manner and place soiled toilet paper in the bedpan (unless a specimen is to be taken). Provide perineal care as required. Remove the waterproof sheet. Provide equipment for the person to clean their hands. Use air freshener as indicated. Take the covered bedpan to the treatment room.

The person who is unable to assist

Lock the bed in position, raise it to a comfortable height for you (usually about your hip height) and raise the side-rails on the far side. Lower the head of the bed until the person is supine. Roll the person onto their side with their back towards you – a second person may need to assist. Position a waterproof sheet under the buttock area. Apply powder lightly to the buttocks to prevent the skin from sticking to the pan. The bedpan – usually the fracture pan – is placed against the person's buttocks with the appropriate end towards the feet. Facing the head of the bed, you hold the hip with one hand and the bedpan in place with the other. Smoothly, by transferring weight from front to back leg, roll the person towards you and onto their back with the bedpan in place. Proceed as for the person who is able to assist. Removing the bedpan entails steadying the bedpan in its horizontal position and rolling the person off the pan, towards you for safety. Remove and cover the bedpan, place it on the end of the bed or on a nearby chair. Clean the perineum and proceed as previously described.

Perform perineal care

Cleansing the perineal area is a hygiene and comfort measure. It is done daily and as necessary due to soiling during elimination or incontinent episodes. If left soiled, the perineal area will macerate and skin integrity will be lost, leading to discomfort and possible infection. Perineal care removes normal secretions and odours as well as any traces of excreta. It also prevents infection and promotes comfort. A rinseless skin cleanser with a balanced pH is preferred (Gandhi et al., 2023). Do not use soap or bath gel as these alter the pH, causing dryness and increasing inflammation and infection (Gandhi et al., 2023).

Perform hand hygiene and wear clean gloves. Position the person in a supine position with the bed linen folded down to the foot of the bed. Place a towel under the hips lengthways so that the lower end can be used to dry the anterior area; the upper edge (under the person's buttocks) is used for the anal area. Follow the instructions for either females or males as shown in TABLE 33.1.

PERFORM ROUTINE URINALYSIS

Urine analysis can add to knowledge of a person's health status. Many medical conditions and alterations in fluid volume manifest in the urine, and a simple examination will reveal many abnormalities. Ward urinalysis is undertaken during admission and as indicated by the person's condition. Perform hand hygiene and wear clean gloves. Use a fresh specimen of urine. Use a clean urinal or bedpan to prevent any changes in test results due to contamination.

Observe the amount (use the clear graduated receptacle in the utility room), colour, clarity, visible sediment and odour of the urine. The pH, glucose, ketone bodies, protein, bilirubin, blood, nitrates and others can be determined using reagent strips.

Remove one reagent strip from the bottle and recap the bottle tightly. Immerse the strip to below the last test area in fresh urine and withdraw it. Lightly rest the edge of the strip on the urine container so that excess flows off and does not dribble onto your hand or the test bottle when reading it. Note the time the strip is dipped and, using the guide on the bottle, read the test areas as their reaction time is reached. Do not touch the strip to the test result guide on the

TABLE 33.1 Assisting with perineal care

FEMALES	MALES
1. Ask the woman to flex her legs, then drape her upper body and legs with the bath blanket in a diamond configuration to reduce embarrassing exposure 2. Wrap the tails of the bath blanket around her legs to anchor the blanket and bring the middle up to expose the perineum 3. Wash and dry the upper inner thighs 4. Clean the labia majora and then spread the labia to expose the folds and labia minora. Using the corners of the washer, cleanse from the front towards the anus, using one stroke per corner 5. If she has an indwelling catheter (IDC), or is menstruating, use gauze squares, one for each stroke, to remove the fluids 6. Rinse the area well, if using soap, following the same procedure 7. Inspect for any areas of excoriation, especially between labial folds, and check for odour, excess secretions or any other abnormality	1. Ask the man to flex his legs, then drape the upper body in a bath blanket, bringing the tails down over the legs 2. Expose the genital area 3. Wash and dry the inner upper thighs 4. Wash and dry the penis, using firm strokes, which may prevent an erection 5. If he is uncircumcised, retract the foreskin to expose the glans penis. Clean it with the washcloth, dry it and replace the foreskin 6. Wash and dry the scrotum 7. Scrotal folds in the posterior may need to be washed and dried while he is on his side
BOTH FEMALES AND MALES	
8. Inspect the urinary meatus for people who have an IDC for signs of excoriation of the orifice 9. Dry the perineum well 10. Assist the person to turn onto their side away from you 11. Spread the buttocks and cleanse the anal area 12. Dry well and apply any protective ointment needed 13. Return the person to a position of comfort and readjust the bedclothes	

bottle because you will contaminate the bottle. Some facilities may have an automated urinalysis machine you will need to become familiar with. These devices test the urine and provide a printout of the results.

The usual result is negative, other than the pH and specific gravity (SG), since none of the components should be in the urine of a healthy person. The pH test strip shows the acidity or alkalinity of the urine. The SG is the degree of concentration of the urine compared with that of an equal volume of distilled water (standard). Check the reagent strip used in the facility. The SG may be determined using appropriate reagent strips.

Note on the vital signs sheet the specimen characteristics, SG, pH and any abnormal test results.

STOOL ASSESSMENT

It is important to assess and record the frequency and appearance of the stool. The Bristol Stool Form Scale (Palter & Patel, 2023) aids in accurate and descriptive recording, which ensures consistency between members of the clinical team. The seven types of stool are:

- *Type 1* – Separate hard lumps, nutlike and hard to pass
- *Type 2* – Lumpy but sausage-shaped, hard to pass
- *Type 3* – Sausage-shaped with a cracked surface, easy to pass
- *Type 4* – Sausage-shaped, smooth and soft, easy to pass
- *Type 5* – Soft blobs, clear edges, easily passed
- *Type 6* – Mushy consistency with fluffy ragged edges
- *Type 7* – Liquid with no solids visible.

The first two indicate constipation, the next two are normal because they are easily defecated but without excess liquid, and the last three progress to diarrhoea. The colour, odour and consistency of faeces and alterations in a person's pattern of defecation may indicate a potential health problem (e.g. a melaena stool is an indication of upper gastrointestinal tract bleeding; diarrhoea may indicate a gastrointestinal infection).

> ? If the stool is a Bristol Stool Form Scale 1/2 or a 6/7, then the person will require further assessment (e.g. diet, medications, abdominal examination, pain assessment, vital signs) and perhaps intervention, such as exercise, increased fluid and fibre in the diet for constipation, or an antidiarrhoeal medication.

Obtain a stool sample

A stool sample (using the scoop provided in the stool specimen container) can be taken from the excreta prior to disposing of the contents of the bedpan. Perform hand hygiene and wear gloves to obtain the specimen. Remove gloves after obtaining the sample and cleaning the bedpan, and perform hand hygiene.

CLEAN, REPLACE AND DISPOSE OF EQUIPMENT

Safety

Perform hand hygiene. Wear clean gloves and an apron to protect against body fluids. Cover the commode, urinal or pan during transport to the dirty utility room, as both an infection control and an aesthetic measure. Do not dispose of contents in the person's en suite bathroom, as any contaminants (e.g. bacteria, chemotherapeutic agents) will be aerosolised, putting a vulnerable person at risk (Jardine, 2021).

Observe the bedpan contents, measure liquid contents and do any tests necessary or obtain specimens (stool). If the urine is to be measured, pour carefully into the designated container, note the amount and dispose without splashing into the hopper or sluice.

Most facilities will use a washer/sanitiser machine that only requires you to insert the bedpan/urinal and (separately) the cover into the machine, close the unit and press a start button. The machine automatically flushes, dispenses detergent, washes and then sanitises the bedpan/urinal. This sounds simple, but there are some important considerations. The following material is adapted from the Meiko website (Meiko, n.d.), which produces a washer/sanitiser machine for use in Australian healthcare facilities.

Transporting the bedpan/urinal

After removing the bedpan or urinal from the person, cover it, place it on the floor, tend to the person, wash your hands and put on clean gloves. Designate one hand as 'clean' and one as 'dirty'. Use the clean hand to open doors and the other to carry the utensil.

Placing the utensil in the washer/sanitiser

Use your clean hand to open the door and your dirty hand to position the utensil and cover into the appropriate rack in the machine. Use your clean hand to close the door, select the appropriate cycle and press the start button. Remove gloves and disinfect your hands.

Removing the utensil from the washer/sanitiser

Use clean hands to open the machine and remove the utensil and cover. Place them inverted on the storage rack in a closed cupboard (to reduce contamination by aerosolised microbes [Jardine, 2021]).

When no washer/sanitiser machine is available

If no washer/sanitiser machine is available, dispose of disposable bedpan covers and waterproof sheets in the contaminated waste bin. Empty excreta into the toilet or a hopper in the unit's dirty utility area. Take care not to splash the contents on yourself or the floor. Liquids are measured, tested if necessary, observed for characteristics and flushed. Solids are observed for colour, consistency and amount, a specimen taken if ordered, and then flushed. Residual excreta that stick to the pan must be removed using toilet paper.

Thoroughly scrub the pan using the toilet (or similar) brush designated for the job and soaked in disinfectant between uses. The pan or urinal is washed and disinfected to reduce the growth of potentially multidrug-resistant organisms (Collins, Carson & Riley, 2019), according to the facility's policy, and returned to the person's locker or the rack. Commodes are reassembled and returned to their usual position or the person's bedside (depending on the facility's policy). Some units have pan/urinal flushers, which are designed to do the washing and disinfecting. Their effectiveness is dependent on individual nurses' use (e.g. adding appropriate type and amount of detergent, descaling solution, temperature setting) (Collins, Carson & Riley, 2019). Remove your gloves and perform hand hygiene.

DOCUMENTATION

It is your responsibility to record elimination to assist in the correct diagnosis (Jardine, 2021); for example, hospital acquired *Clostridium difficile* (Palter & Patel, 2023). Note the bowel action on the temperature, pulse and respiration (TPR) and bowel chart (if in use). The documentation of all output is required for some people. In these cases, all urinary and liquid faecal excreta will need to be measured. Knowledge of the individual documentation requirements is necessary. Some people only require a daily note in the progress sheet that indicates that their elimination is sufficient. Any abnormalities in urine or faeces should be reported to the shift coordinator and noted in the progress notes. Urinalysis is documented on the vital signs sheet in most facilities. Specific gravity, pH, colour, clarity and any abnormal findings are to be recorded.

PART 6

CLINICAL SKILLS ASSESSMENT

Assisting with elimination needs

Demonstrates the ability to effectively and safely assist the person with their elimination needs. Incorporates the *National Safety and Quality Health Service Standards*: 2 Partnering with Consumers, 3 Preventing and Controlling Healthcare-Associated Infection, 5 Comprehensive Care, 6 Communicating for Safety, and 8 Recognising and Responding to Acute Deterioration (ACSQHC, 2021).

Performance criteria	1	2	3	4	5
(Numbers indicate NMBA *Registered Nurse Standards for Practice*)	(Dependent)	(Marginal)	(Assisted)	(Supervised)	(Independent)
1. Identifies indication (1.1, 3.3, 3.4)	☐	☐	☐	☐	☐
2. Evidence of therapeutic interaction with the person, e.g. gives the person a clear explanation of the procedure, discusses the rationale for remaining in bed (1.4, 1.5, 2.1, 2.2, 3.2)	☐	☐	☐	☐	☐
3. Demonstrates clinical reasoning abilities, e.g. positions the person appropriately, provides privacy, provides hand-washing equipment (1.1, 1.2, 1.3, 4.2, 6.1)	☐	☐	☐	☐	☐
4. Assesses the person's ability to be independent (1.1, 2.2, 2.3, 4.1, 4.2, 6.1)	☐	☐	☐	☐	☐
5. Gathers equipment (1.1, 5.5, 6.1): ■ commode, bedpan, urinal as required ■ coversheets ■ clean gloves ■ toilet paper ■ waterproof sheet ■ air freshener ■ hand-washing equipment ■ urinalysis equipment ■ perineal care equipment (basin, soap, water, washer, towel) ■ manual-handling equipment as required	☐	☐	☐	☐	☐
6. Performs hand hygiene (1.1, 3.4, 6.1)	☐	☐	☐	☐	☐
7. Assists the person to use the commode (1.1, 6.1, 6.5)	☐	☐	☐	☐	☐
8. Gives and receives a urinal (1.1, 6.1)	☐	☐	☐	☐	☐
9. Gives and receives a bedpan (1.1, 6.1)	☐	☐	☐	☐	☐
10. Performs perineal care (1.1, 6.1)	☐	☐	☐	☐	☐
11. Performs routine urinalysis/obtains a stool sample (1.1, 4.2, 6.1)	☐	☐	☐	☐	☐
12. Disposes of excreta (1.1, 6.1)	☐	☐	☐	☐	☐
13. Cleans, replaces and disposes of equipment appropriately (3.6, 6.1)	☐	☐	☐	☐	☐
14. Documents relevant information (1.4, 1.6, 2.2, 2.7, 3.5, 3.7, 6.2, 6.5, 7.3)	☐	☐	☐	☐	☐
15. Demonstrates the ability to link theory to practice (1.1, 3.3, 3.4, 3.5)	☐	☐	☐	☐	☐

Student:

Clinical facilitator: Date:

CHAPTER 34

ADMINISTERING AN ENEMA

INDICATIONS

Enemas are administered for two reasons:

- to assist bowel evacuation – an evacuant enema
- to administer fluid or medication – a retention enema.

An evacuant enema may be required for constipation or if faecal material is impacted. Extreme frailty, inadequate nutrition and hydration, lack of exercise, use of a bedpan (Mitchell, 2019), opioid or benzodiazepine use (Arco et al., 2022), and some medical conditions contribute to the formation of hard, dry faeces that are difficult to pass. Also, repeated voluntary contraction of the internal and external sphincters prevents expulsion of faeces for some time (e.g. due to fear of pain from haemorrhoids). People who have spinal cord dysfunction resulting in neurogenic bowel dysfunction may require regular enemas to prevent constipation (Rodriguez & Gater, 2022). Before the use of an enema, other measures to encourage faecal elimination should be tried (Wangui-Verry et al., 2019).

An evacuant enema may be indicated if the bowel needs to be cleansed for examination (X-ray, endoscopy or surgery), although oral preparations causing complete evacuation of the bowel are increasingly used instead.

Fluid and medication (e.g. antibiotics, steroids) can be administered rectally by instilling an enema (see **Clinical Skill 43**). Other solutions, such as milk and molasses, may be ordered for constipation (Wangui-Verry et al., 2019). Contrast media, such as barium, can be introduced into the bowel via an enema for radiographic studies. The procedure remains the same except that the fluid or medication is retained rather than expelled.

Verify the medical order

Enemas normally require a medical order; however, some facilities use a protocol. Verify the order before proceeding. Enema administration requires the six rights of medication administration (see **Clinical Skill 37**). Verbal consent is required, as administering an enema is an invasive procedure.

Contraindications

Contraindications for administering an enema include diarrhoea, cardiac arrhythmias, recent myocardial infarction, inflammatory or ulcerative bowel disease, undiagnosed abdominal pain, and recent surgery of the anus, rectum, bowel, vagina or prostate gland. Enemas are also contraindicated in those with rectal or anal pain, latex allergy or a history of abuse (Mitchell, 2019). Use caution when administering an enema, because bowel perforation, especially in those who have repeat or high colonic enemas, is a possibility (Lister, Hofland & Grafton, 2020).

EVIDENCE OF THERAPEUTIC INTERACTION

Give the person a clear explanation of the procedure to reduce their anxiety and gain their consent. Relaxation increases the ease of administering the enema. Tell the person why the procedure is necessary and what it entails. Knowing the purpose will assist them to retain or expel the bowel contents as appropriate. Encourage them to ask questions and voice their concerns so that misconceptions can be corrected and they can participate in their own health care. Ask them not to flush the toilet after expelling the enema, since you must observe the effects of the procedure.

Many people are embarrassed about their elimination and feel very uncomfortable when undergoing this procedure. Tact and consideration are needed. Talk to the person during the insertion of the fluid to distract them from the distension in their bowel. During an evacuant enema, it helps to tell the person approximately how much of the fluid is left to go in (e.g. half-done, three-quarters done, nearly there).

DEMONSTRATE CLINICAL REASONING

Assessment, preparation of the solution, the environment and positioning the person all help to increase the ease and comfort of this procedure.

Assess the person

Determine the amount of assistance that will be needed.

ELDER CARE

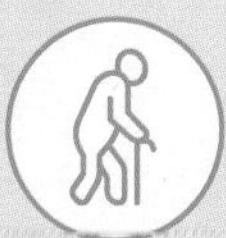

The elderly, and especially females and the frail, have an increased incidence of functional constipation (i.e. constipation with no discernible physiologic causes) that decreases their quality of life (Arco et al., 2022). Management is based on lifestyle, diet and hydration, followed by non-absorbable stool softeners and stimulant laxatives.

Enema use is reserved for people who do not respond to these measures (Cho et al., 2023). Hypertonic enemas (e.g. sodium phosphate solutions) are not recommended for the elderly as they can cause metabolic imbalances in those with comorbidities and renal impairment (Hamilton Smith, Eddleston & Bateman, 2022). Many elderly people will have difficulty with assuming and maintaining the required position (e.g. due to hip or knee arthritis). You may need to modify the position they assume, but ensure that you can clearly see the anus and that there is room to manipulate the enema nozzle. Monitor elderly people closely following an enema as receiving an enema may make them feel weak or even faint. Remember to treat each person with dignity.

THE PERSON LIVING WITH SEVERE OBESITY

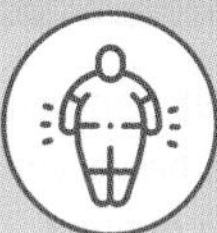

Obesity is one of the causes of the development of haemorrhoids, as is straining at stool (Pullen, 2022). If you are giving an enema to someone who is severely obese, apply an anaesthetic agent (as ordered) prior to administering the enema. Take care to be as gentle as possible and avoid the haemorrhoidal tissue, if possible.

Administering an enema to someone who is severely obese usually requires at least two healthcare workers. Repositioning the person onto their side is often difficult because they have increased difficulty breathing when they are lying down. Buttock and perineal tissue will have to be displaced to enable the nozzle of the enema to be placed in the anus. Mechanical lifts will be needed to help the person onto the commode because their relative immobility precludes mobilisation. Excess weight in the abdomen predisposes the morbidly obese person to faecal incontinence and makes retention of the enema difficult due to weakened pelvic floor muscles (Chilaka, Toozs-Hobson & Chilaka, 2023). Cleansing of the perineum is very important to prevent maceration of the tissues. See **Clinical Skills 15 and 23** for a more comprehensive discussion of issues affecting those living with severe obesity.

LOOK at their mobility – can they move in bed, sit on the side, get out of bed with or without assistance, and walk to the toilet unaided?

LISTEN for comments about being constipated or feeling dizzy or weak (take vital signs); they may need more assistance to get to the toilet. Auscultate and percuss the abdomen if there is no bowel motion for three days or the person is confused or unable to produce a history.

FEEL for a faecal mass in the left lower quadrant.

Prepare the solution

Hospital-prepared solution

Warm the solution (as ordered – oil, normal saline) to the correct temperature. Clamp the outflow tube on the disposable bag. Measure the temperature with the bath thermometer and pour the correct amount of warmed solution into the disposable bag. Prime the tube and clamp it for transport to the bedside, then hang it on the IV pole.

Soapsud enemas are efficacious (Chumpitazi et al., 2016), but infrequently used. They are prepared in the hospital by agitating pure soap in the required amount of warm water until it is cloudy. Pour the solution into a disposable enema bag attached to a clamped tube and a rectal tip, and continue as above.

Commercial solution

If you are using a commercial enema, check it against the order and check its expiry date and intactness. Warm it in a jug of warm water to just above room temperature to help stimulate peristalsis and prevent injury to the bowel mucosa. Take it to the bedside in a kidney basin so there is something to put the used container in after giving the enema.

Prepare the person and the environment

To reduce the person's anxiety, provide privacy and ensure immediate access to a toilet. If access to a toilet is not certain or if the person is less mobile, provide a commode or a bedpan. Ask the person to empty their bladder prior to the procedure to reduce the discomfort and to promote retention of the solution. Help the person to remove their lower garments. Sufficient toilet paper needs to be available.

Position the person

The person's buttocks will need to be exposed. Place a bath blanket or sheet over their upper torso and fold their bed sheets down over the lower body. This provides warmth and preserves some modesty. Position the person in a left lateral position with their upper leg well flexed and their buttocks near the edge of the bed to facilitate inserting the nozzle along the rectal passage.

Place the incontinence pad under the person's hips and buttocks to reduce the chances of soiling the linen and causing an infection risk, and to reduce embarrassment if there is any faecal dribble after inserting the enema. Emphasise the type of enema being given so that the person is better prepared to either retain the solution for a time (oil enema) or expel the bowel contents. Reassurance that the toilet is available helps the person to relax. Place a bedpan on the bed next to the person if there is any question regarding their ability to hold the solution.

GATHER EQUIPMENT

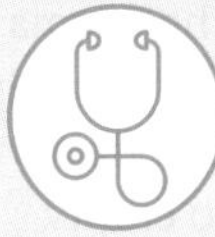

Gathering equipment is an organisational step that helps to create a positive environment for a successful interaction. It ensures that you have all needed material, boosts the person's confidence and trust in you, and increases your self-confidence. While gathering the equipment, you can mentally rehearse the procedure. Equipment required includes:

EQUIPMENT	EXPLANATION
Personal protective equipment	Clean gloves, gown/apron and goggles are required to protect you from body fluids
Incontinence (waterproof) pad	Protects the bed linen from soiling. It is disposable and minimises the risk of exposing ancillary personnel to contaminated linen
Bedpan and cover or commode (if necessary)	Used when the person is non-ambulatory so they can expel the enema. Use the pan cover for the return to the utility room
A bath blanket or sheet	Used for privacy and warmth
Water-soluble lubricant and gauze square	• Helps minimise the trauma to the anal/rectal mucosa during insertion of the tube • Use a gauze square to spread the lubricant up the nozzle
The enema solution as ordered	• The solution is prepared, taken from stock or comes from the pharmacy • Commercial enemas come in premeasured plastic packs that are rolled up from the bottom to force all of the fluid (and no air) into the rectum. They often have a prelubricated tip. You will need a container of hand-hot water to warm the enema pack. Read the manufacturer's directions
Rectal tube and nozzle tip	Needed for the hospital-prepared enema to deliver the prescribed solution into the rectum
A 1 L (or more) container/disposable enema bag	• A container (if the enema is not a commercial one) is used for preparing the solution • A disposable enema bag is needed to hold the solution during administration
Clamp	Placed on the outflow tube to control the flow of the hospital-prepared enema solution
Bath thermometer	• Used to measure the hospital-prepared solution temperature • The ideal temperature is 37 to 40 °C • A cold solution will cause cramping and a hot solution will damage the mucosa
IV pole	Keeps the container of hospital-prepared solution at the correct height of 30 to 60 cm above the level of the anus (Jayasekara, 2013) to ensure that delivery of the fluid is not too fast
Perineal care equipment	• To be used following the procedure • Includes toilet tissue, a washer, a towel, a basin with warm water and a skin cleanser

TABLE 34.1 shows frequently used enema solutions that may be used when administering an enema.

TABLE 34.1 Frequently used enema solutions

SOLUTION	AMOUNT	ACTION	TIME TO RETAIN	ADVERSE EFFECTS
Hypertonic, e.g. Microlax, Fleet – based on sodium phosphate	Under 100 mL	Draws water into the colon to stimulate peristalsis, softens faeces	5 to 10 minutes	Metabolic imbalances: • Sodium retention • Hyperphosphataemia • Mechanical and chemical irritation of the mucosa, leading to injury (Hamilton-Smith, Eddelman & Bateman, 2022)
Hypotonic (e.g. tap water)	500–1000 mL	Provides bulk to distend colon and stimulate peristalsis, softens faeces	Up to 20 minutes	Fluid and electrolyte imbalances, water retention
Isotonic (normal saline)	500–1000 mL	Provides bulk to distend colon and stimulate peristalsis, softens faeces	Up to 20 minutes	Possible sodium retention
Irritant (i.e. soapsuds from pure soap – not often used)	500–1000 mL	Irritates the bowel to stimulate evacuation	10 to 15 minutes	Irritation and possible damage to rectal mucosa
Oil (e.g. arachis, olive, cottonseed, mineral)	90–120 mL	Softens the faecal mass and lubricates it to ease passage	30 minutes to 3 hours (retention)	Arachis oil is a peanut product; take care in case of allergies

SOURCES: ADAPTED FROM DELAUNE ET AL. (2024). *FUNDAMENTALS OF NURSING* (AUSTRALIA AND NEW ZEALAND 2ND ED.). SOUTH MELBOURNE, VIC: CENGAGE LEARNING; LISTER, HOFLAND & GRAFTON (2020). *THE ROYAL MARSDEN MANUAL OF CLINICAL NURSING PROCEDURES*. OXFORD: JOHN WILEY & SONS.

PART 6

ADMINISTER THE ENEMA

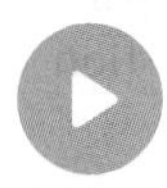

Video

Enema administration consists of steps to promote the person's comfort as well as accomplish the treatment. Lubrication of the nozzle, expelling air from the tube, slow insertion of the nozzle and solution and slow withdrawal of the nozzle help to make this uncomfortable procedure more bearable.

Hand hygiene

Hand hygiene (see **Clinical Skill 5**) removes transient microorganisms and prevents cross-contamination. Don personal protective equipment as necessary – clean gloves and a gown are usually all that is required. Goggles may be required when emptying the bedpan into the hopper. Hand hygiene is completed following the procedure.

Lubricate the enema nozzle

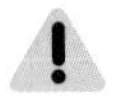

Safety

Liberal lubrication reduces trauma to the rectal mucosa and increases the person's comfort when the enema tube is inserted. Squeeze some lubricant onto the gauze square and use it to ensure the nozzle/tube is covered well for at least 5 cm.

Expel excess air

The enema pack or the rectal tube and tip should be free of air so that only fluid enters the bowel. Air will increase the distension of the bowel and therefore the person's discomfort levels. Clamp the enema tube.

Slowly insert the enema nozzle

Ask the person to take a deep breath and slowly let it out to relax their muscles. Separate the buttocks, and inspect the anal and perineal areas, noting any abnormalities (e.g. haemorrhoids, excoriation). You may need to insert a lubricated finger into the anal canal to determine if there is a faecal mass (for constipation).

Carefully introduce the nozzle into the anus. The entire nozzle is inserted for a commercial enema, or the rectal tube is slowly inserted 10 to 12 cm, past the internal sphincter, to ensure that the solution is in the rectum rather than the anal canal. Direct the nozzle towards the person's umbilicus. Slow insertion reduces stimulation of the anal sphincter and increases comfort. Spasms of the anus, embarrassment, and blockage of the rectum by faeces, haemorrhoids or a tumour can stop the nozzle/tube advancing.

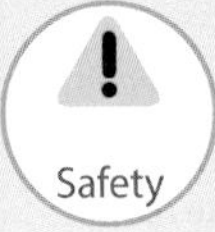

?

If resistance is met, ask the person to take some deep breaths and bear down as if emptying their bowel. If resistance continues, stop inserting, draw the nozzle or tube back a short distance, instil some of the solution and slowly try to insert the nozzle/tube to the correct depth. If resistance is again met, withdraw the nozzle/tube and stop the procedure.

Slowly introduce the fluid

For commercial enemas, slowly roll the container up from the bottom (prevents backflow). For the large-volume enema, regulate the flow by removing the clamp partially or lowering the container as necessary (the higher the container is above the rectum, the faster the inflow). Slow administration reduces the sensation of pressure on the rectal walls. This allows the person to tolerate the entire amount of the enema with less discomfort. Peristalsis will not be immediately stimulated, so more of the solution will be introduced to soften the faeces and provide distension to empty the bowel (evacuant). The slower introduction of the smaller amount of fluid for a retention enema means that it will be easier to retain for the required time. If the person reports pain or inability to hold the enema, stop the flow of fluid and ask them to breathe deeply, then recommence the flow slowly. When nearly all of the solution in the hospital-prepared container is instilled, clamp the tubing to prevent air entering the rectum. If the person cannot retain any more fluid, clamp the tubing before withdrawing to avoid soaking the bed with solution.

Slowly withdraw the nozzle or tube

Slowly withdrawing the nozzle or tube will avoid reflex emptying of the bowel and permit the enema to be retained until the person can reach the toilet, commode or pan, or for the time required for a retention enema. Ask the person to clench their perineal muscles while you gently pinch the cheeks of their buttocks together to assist retention.

Dry the perineal tissue

Use toilet tissue to dry the perineum. This reduces irritation of the perirectal mucosa and increases comfort. It also reduces embarrassment, since there is usually lubricant and some of the solution making the area feel like it is leaking and offensive.

Ask the person to retain the enema

Small evacuant enemas usually are retained for a few minutes. Instruct the person to lie on their left side to assist in retention. Large-volume enemas are more difficult to retain, and the person may need assistance to the toilet, or onto a commode or bedpan. Retention enemas are to be retained for a prescribed amount of time. For these and fluid/nutrient replacement enemas, the foot of the bed can be elevated to reduce the effects of gravity and early expulsion of the solution. Observe the results of the enema (for evacuant enema, note colour, consistency, content and approximate amount of faecal material) and assess the effectiveness of the procedure. Assess the person for any adverse reactions or complications.

Post-procedure

When the enema has been expelled, assist the person to clean their perineal area as needed to minimise irritation from faecal matter and the solution. Help them to wash their hands. Perform hand hygiene. Return them to bed and position them comfortably. Leave a clean, dry waterproof sheet under their buttocks to catch any solution or faeces that may continue to be expelled. Leave the call bell within reach and answer any calls as a priority. The person may urgently need help to the toilet. Assess the person for comfort and ensure that they have water and tissues available.

CLEAN, REPLACE AND DISPOSE OF EQUIPMENT

Wear clean gloves and an apron to protect against body fluids. If a commode or bedpan is used, cover it during transport to the dirty utility room as both an infection control and an aesthetic measure. Dispose of disposable bedpan covers and waterproof sheets in the contaminated waste bin. Observe solids for colour, consistency and amount, and take a specimen, if ordered, before placing in the bedpan washer (see **Clinical Skill 33** for disposal of wastes and cleaning of a bedpan). If the bedpan requires manual cleaning, put on the goggles or eye protection and then empty excreta into the toilet or into a hopper in the unit's dirty utility area, taking care to not splash the contents on yourself or onto the floor. Residual excreta that stick to the pan must be removed using toilet paper. Traces are then removed using the toilet (or similar) brush designated for the job, then the brush is rinsed and soaked in disinfectant between uses.

The disposable enema container, along with the tubing and tip, is placed in the contaminated waste bin. A reusable enema container is washed and sent to central supply for sterilisation. Remove your gloves and apron and dispose of them in the contaminated waste bin. Disinfect the goggles. Perform hand hygiene.

DOCUMENTATION

Documentation assists the healthcare team to monitor the person's bowel function. Administering an enema is a treatment, and it is your responsibility to document the effects of this treatment. For an evacuant enema, note the time, the solution and the amount administered, and the person's response. Note the characteristics of the faeces. Use the Bristol Stool Form Scale (see **Clinical Skill 33**) to ensure consistency between staff observations (Gulati et al., 2018).

CLINICAL SKILLS ASSESSMENT

Administering an enema

Demonstrates the ability to safely administer an enema. Incorporates the *National Safety and Quality Health Service Standards*: 2 Partnering with Consumers, 3 Preventing and Controlling Healthcare-Associated Infection, 5 Comprehensive Care, 6 Communicating for Safety, and 8 Recognising and Responding to Acute Deterioration (ACSQHC, 2021).

Performance criteria	1	2	3	4	5
(Numbers indicate NMBA *Registered Nurse Standards for Practice*)	(Dependent)	(Marginal)	(Assisted)	(Supervised)	(Independent)
1. Identifies indication (1.1, 3.3, 3.4)	☐	☐	☐	☐	☐
2. Verifies there are no contraindications (1.4, 1.5, 2.1, 2.2, 3.2)	☐	☐	☐	☐	☐
3. Verifies the validity of the written medication order (1.4, 3.4, 6.2, 6.5)	☐	☐	☐	☐	☐
4. Evidence of therapeutic interaction with the person, e.g. gives a clear explanation of the procedure (1.4, 1.5, 2.1, 2.2, 3.2)	☐	☐	☐	☐	☐
5. Demonstrates clinical reasoning abilities, such as assessing, preparing the environment, positioning the person (1.1, 1.2, 1.3, 4.2, 6.1)	☐	☐	☐	☐	☐
6. Gathers equipment (1.1, 5.5, 6.1): ■ personal protective equipment ■ incontinence pad ■ bedpan or commode (if necessary) ■ bath blanket or sheet ■ water-soluble lubricant and gauze square ■ enema solution as ordered ■ rectal tube and tip ■ a 1-litre (or more) container/disposable enema bag ■ clamp ■ bath thermometer ■ intravenous pole ■ perineal care equipment	☐	☐	☐	☐	☐
7. Performs hand hygiene (1.1, 3.4, 6.1)	☐	☐	☐	☐	☐
8. Dons personal protective equipment (1.1, 3.4, 6.1)	☐	☐	☐	☐	☐
9. Lubricates the nozzle of the enema or rectal tube (1.1, 6.1)	☐	☐	☐	☐	☐
10. Expels excess air (1.1, 6.1)	☐	☐	☐	☐	☐
11. Slowly inserts the enema nozzle (1.1, 6.1)	☐	☐	☐	☐	☐
12. Slowly introduces the fluid (1.1, 6.1)	☐	☐	☐	☐	☐
13. Slowly withdraws the nozzle or tube (1.1, 6.1)	☐	☐	☐	☐	☐
14. Dries the perineal tissue (1.1, 6.1)	☐	☐	☐	☐	☐
15. Asks the person to retain the enema (as appropriate) (1.1, 6.1)	☐	☐	☐	☐	☐
16. Assists the person to the toilet, commode or bedpan; cares for the person following the procedure (1.1, 6.1)	☐	☐	☐	☐	☐
17. Cleans, replaces and disposes of equipment appropriately (3.6, 6.1)	☐	☐	☐	☐	☐
18. Documents relevant information (1.4, 1.6, 2.2, 2.7, 3.5, 3.7, 6.2, 6.5, 7.3)	☐	☐	☐	☐	☐
19. Demonstrates the ability to link theory to practice (1.1, 3.3, 3.4, 3.5)	☐	☐	☐	☐	☐

Student:

Clinical facilitator: Date:

CHAPTER 35

SUPRAPUBIC CATHETER CARE – CATHETER IRRIGATION

INDICATIONS

Suprapubic catheters are urinary drainage catheters inserted surgically into the bladder through the lower abdomen just above the symphysis pubis. The procedure can be performed at the bedside under local anaesthesia, or it may be performed during surgery. Suprapubic catheterisation is preferable to urethral catheterisation for long-term drainage or where pelvic or urethral trauma, stricture or closure has occurred (Reid et al., 2021). It is well tolerated and commonly used for neurogenic or atonic bladders (Khawaja et al., 2023). Advantages of suprapubic catheterisation over urethral catheterisation include:

- the risk of individuals developing urinary tract infections from bowel microorganisms is reduced (abdominal skin pathologic bacterial count is less than that around the perineal/perianal areas [Lister, Hofland & Grafton, 2020], although Quallich et al. [2023] found bacteriuria was similar in both urethral and suprapubic catheters)
- urethral integrity is retained
- clamping the suprapubic catheter allows for normal voiding to resume postoperatively (it is released if voiding is incomplete)
- pain and discomfort from the urethral catheter are reduced. There is no risk of urethral trauma, necrosis, catheter-induced urethritis or stricture formation
- there is easier access for cleaning and catheter changes, giving greater ability for self-care
- the suprapubic catheter allows for greater freedom of sexuality (fewer impediments to intercourse [Lister, Hofland & Grafton, 2020]).

However, the risks and disadvantages with suprapubic catheterisation include:

- bowel perforation and haemorrhage at the time of insertion
- infection, swelling, encrustation and granulation at the insertion site
- bladder spasm, discomfort or irritation for some people
- bladder stone formation
- altered body image (adapted from Lister, Hofland & Grafton, 2020; Quallich et al., 2023; Reid et al., 2021).

Care of someone with a suprapubic catheter is similar to that of a person with a urethral catheter. Effective catheter management means assessing all aspects of catheter care, activity and mobility (catheter drainage, positioning and kinks). Diet and fluid intake, standards of hygiene and the person's/carer's ability to care for the catheter impact on catheter management. You are responsible for maintaining the catheter while the person is in your care and for teaching the person/caregiver about routine care, so that they can manage their catheter independently once they are able.

Intermittent bladder irrigation

Intermittent bladder irrigation requires a break in the asepsis of a closed drainage system. It should not be undertaken lightly nor done routinely and is used less frequently than in times past as there is little evidence of its efficacy (Werneburg, 2022). Maintaining a closed system is a strategy that minimises infection (Sweeney, 2021). The decision to irrigate the bladder depends on assessment and catheter history. Where possible, time it to coincide with bag changes (five to seven days or as per the facility's policy) so that the catheter system is not disconnected unnecessarily. The greatest risk with bladder lavage or irrigation is introducing infection. Determine the purpose of the irrigation.

Intermittent open catheter irrigation is used to maintain catheter patency. Recurrent catheter blockage is common and may occur because of detrusor spasm, twisted drainage tubing or small clots of blood or mucus. The most common cause is the formation of encrustations on any surface of the catheter, including the tip and the balloon, and within its lumen, with deposits of mineral salts from the urine. These consist of magnesium, ammonium phosphate and calcium phosphate deposits, which precipitate from alkaline urine. Alkaline urine is produced during infection from urease-secreting microorganisms (Lister, Hofland & Grafton, 2020). The most common cause of catheter encrustations is the Proteus species; in particular, the *Proteus mirabilis* hydrolyses urea more rapidly than other urease-producing organisms and moves rapidly over biomaterial surfaces (Wang et al., 2019). Catheters blocked with encrustations may lead to bypassing of the urine, urinary retention, pain and distress for the person, as well as unnecessary catheter changes (Wang et al., 2019). Intermittent bladder irrigation

can also be used to irrigate the bladder with a medication to treat an infection or local bladder irritation.

There are potential risks to the bladder urothelium associated with irrigation. Dilute acid solutions have been shown to remove the surface layer of mucus in the bladder. An increased shedding of urothelial cells has been observed following irrigation with both acidic and neutral pH solutions (Lister, Hofland & Grafton, 2020). Both the chemical irritation and the physical force of the irrigation can be potential risk factors in disrupting the bladder urothelium. There is no consensus and limited research regarding indications for using catheter irrigation nor the method of administration, frequency, duration of administration and the choice of solution (Werneburg, 2022). Comparisons between bladder irrigation with normal saline, chlorhexidine and non-bacteriostatic solutions did not show any difference in infection rate. Sinclair et al. (2017) suggest that currently no recommendations can be made on the effectiveness of catheter irrigations to minimise urinary tract infections and/or encrustations.

Verify the written medication order

Bladder irrigation requires a written medication order in most facilities, although it may be a policy in some. Verify the order before you proceed. The order should indicate the solution required, the amount, the dwell time as well as the purpose of the irrigation – medicinal or preventative.

EVIDENCE OF THERAPEUTIC INTERACTION

Provide a clear explanation of the procedure to the person to ensure understanding and so they can consent, cooperate and assist as able. Gadelkareem et al. (2022) demonstrated the efficacy of using illustrated brochures for teaching about suprapubic catheters to decrease complications. Keep explanations simple and remember to talk about the sensations the person may feel during the procedure. The irrigation can create a sensation similar to voiding or, albeit rarely, pressure. If the person knows what to expect, their anxiety will be diminished and trust increased. This also gives you the opportunity to assess the person.

Demonstrate clinical reasoning

Assess the person:

LOOK at their ability to move in bed and reposition themselves. You may need a helper.

LISTEN to reports of allergies to adhesive, Betadine or chlorhexidine (if these are ordered as a cleansing solution around the catheter site and on the catheter). Ask about bladder comfort (is there any fullness or spasms?). Assess the person's anxiety level and ability to cooperate.

Close the room door, put a 'Do not disturb' sign in a prominent place and close the curtains to provide privacy. Place the bath blanket over the person for privacy and warmth to reduce, to an extent, the discomfort the person must endure. Raise the ambient temperature, if possible, and reduce draughts. Place the container of irrigating solution in a bowl of warm water to warm to 35 to 37 °C to reduce bladder spasm and discomfort.

Clip a plastic rubbish bag to the trolley edge or lower shelf nearest the person and leave the top wide open, enabling you to drop material into it without contaminating your gloves or forceps.

Assist the person into the dorsal recumbent position. Obtain assistance if needed, which indicates forward planning and good assessment skills. Some people will need assistance to maintain the position. Raise the bed to a comfortable working height for you to reduce strain on your muscles. Situate the equipment so that your dominant hand is furthest from the head of the bed and the equipment is in easy reach to facilitate the manipulation of objects. Expose the suprapubic catheter on the abdomen. Place a waterproof sheet under it to prevent soiling of the bottom sheet.

GATHER EQUIPMENT

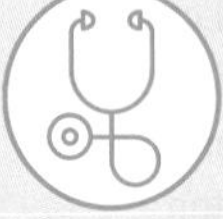

Gathering equipment is an organisational step that helps to create a positive environment for a successful interaction. It ensures that you have all needed material, boosts the person's confidence and trust in you, and increases your self-confidence. While gathering the equipment, you can mentally rehearse the procedure. Equipment varies across facilities. Follow the facility's policy or the medical practitioner's order for the solution and amount to be used for bladder irrigation. Equipment required may include:

EQUIPMENT	EXPLANATION
A bath blanket or similar	Cover the person during the procedure to maintain warmth and dignity
Clean gloves	Non-sterile gloves are needed if the dressing around the suprapubic catheter needs to be removed, and to empty the drainage bag
Waterproof pad	Placed under the catheter to protect the person and the bed linen from being soiled by solutions or urine

EQUIPMENT	EXPLANATION
Clamp	To prevent leakage of urine from the drainage tubing during the procedure
Tray wrapped in a sterile wrapper	• The tray is sterile and provides a barrier to microorganisms. A critical aseptic field is created when the wrapper is opened • May be replaced with a bladder irrigation kit, which eliminates the need to break the system by using a needleless access port just above the drainage bag (only available in some drainage systems) (Holroyd, 2019)
Sterile cap for the drainage tubing	To maintain sterility of the tubing while irrigating the catheter
Plastic bag	Often the tray packaging is clipped (bulldog clip or similar) to the dressing trolley for disposal of used supplies
Personal protective equipment	• Sterile gloves help prevent the introduction of microorganisms into the urinary tract • Goggles and a plastic apron protect you and your uniform from splashes
Drapes	• Used to extend the sterile field and to reduce the transfer of microorganisms • Some facilities use the sterile drape in the basic dressing pack
Small basin	Used to apply solution to the gauze and to act as an initial container for the urine when the catheter is drained
Gauze squares and solution	• The solution is usually normal saline or chlorhexidine in alcohol • Chlorhexidine in alcohol is the preferred cleanser as it offers superior protection due to its rapid and persistent action, a shorter drying time (since it is combined with alcohol) and a longer residual effect at the site of catheter insertion (Nagaraj, 2023) • Used to clean the peristomal area and the catheter
Solution as ordered	• Usually sterile normal saline, although van Veen et al. (2023) demonstrated the safety and efficacy of tap water • Evidence is lacking regarding safety and efficacy of bladder maintenance/irrigation solutions (Dean & Ostaszkiewicz, 2019)
60 mL catheter tip syringe and sterile irrigation fluid	Usually 50 to 100 mL of normal saline (at body temperature to avoid bladder spasm) is used to irrigate the catheter (check the orders or the protocol at the facility)
Specimen container (if required)	• A specimen for microanalysis is collected to reflect the current bacteriology of the urine • A label is also required, as well as a laboratory requisition and a biohazard bag
A new collection bag, tubing and support system	Needed if the drainage bag is due to be replaced
Tape or leg bands	To secure the catheter to the abdomen

IRRIGATE A URINARY CATHETER

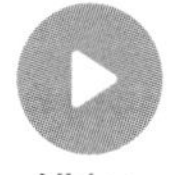
Video

Use Aseptic Non Touch Technique (ANTT) when irrigating a urinary catheter (please review **Clinical Skill 7**) because you will be breaking an aseptic system.

As always, observation and assessment are important components of the skill.

Hand hygiene

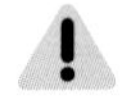
Safety

Perform hand hygiene (see **Clinical Skill 5**) and don clean gloves (see **Clinical Skill 6**) to reduce cross-contamination and to comply with standard precautions. Hand hygiene is the most effective defence against hospital-acquired infections.

Expose the whole length of the catheter

Observe the insertion site for signs of discharge or redness. Position the new urinary drainage bag (as required) on the bed within easy reach. This will not be needed until the end of the procedure. Empty the current drainage bag and note the amount for later calculation of output during the procedure. Discard the drainage bag. If the person has a leg bag, remove the straps and place the bag on the bed. Place an absorbent sheet (bluey) under the catheter junction and clamp the drainage tubing to prevent leakage when the catheter is disconnected.

Remove and discard gloves to reduce cross-contamination and perform hand hygiene. The remainder of the procedure is aseptic.

Establish a critical aseptic field

Use the disposable packaging as a rubbish bag if not already in place. Use a clip to secure it to the dressing trolley in a position between the person and the trolley so that used supplies are not carried over the sterile field. Add any sterile supplies that are not in the dressing tray, such as selected gloves, sterile drape, syringe and sterile bowls. Pour the warmed irrigation solution into the sterile container using aseptic technique.

Don a plastic apron and goggles as a protective measure from accidental spray of body fluids and subsequent contamination. Perform hand hygiene.

Don sterile gloves

Sterile gloves act as a barrier to prevent the transfer of microorganisms from your hands to objects that will contact or enter the bladder, which is sterile (see **Clinical Skill 9**).

Extend the critical aseptic field

Grasp the sterile plain drape by the corners, lift it off the field (protect your sterile gloves by rolling the edge of the sterile drape over your hands) and place it under the junction of the catheter and the tubing of the drainage bag.

Prepare equipment

Arrange equipment for convenience on the sterile field. Draw up irrigating solution into the 60 mL syringe, recap the syringe and return it to the sterile field. Check that the outflow clamp on the drainage bag is closed.

Preparing the field and equipment requires two hands, so it must be completed before you begin cleansing the catheter, which will contaminate the non-dominant hand. Sterile (gloved) hands only touch sterile items.

Clean the peristomal area and the catheter insertion site

Daily care will depend on the facility's policy, but cleaning and dressing the catheter site is similar to that for any surgical drain. Dressings are changed whenever they are damp or soiled (Sweeney, 2021). Haemoserous ooze is expected initially. Use the principles of ANTT.

Use the non-dominant sterile-gloved hand to hold the catheter erect while cleaning. (This hand is no longer sterile – do not touch the critical aseptic field with it.) Use lint-free gauze moistened with cleansing agent to clean the site by swabbing in a circular motion, starting closest to the catheter site and continuing in outward-widening circles for approximately 5 cm. This follows the principles of asepsis, moving from the area of least contamination to the most contaminated, removing microorganisms that could have migrated to the site. Aseptic cleansing of the incision site is not necessary once this area has healed. At this point, the site and catheter can be cleaned during bathing (preferably a shower [Sweeney, 2021]) using soap, water and a clean washcloth (Sharma et al., 2018). Teach the person how to provide hygienic care for the healed site. Use of illustrated brochures proved most effective for this (Gadelkareem et al., 2022).

Next, with a new piece of moistened lint-free gauze, cleanse the catheter at the junction with the drainage bag to remove any microorganisms that may adhere to the tubing. The friction and chemical action reduce the bacterial population at the junction of the catheter and the drainage tubing.

Insert the irrigation fluid

Position a sterile basin on the sterile drape near the person's abdomen. Squeeze (pinch) the end of the catheter just above the connection tubing of the drainage system with the non-dominant hand and hold to stop the urine flow. Using your dominant hand and a dry gauze square, disconnect the catheter from the drainage tubing, and release the catheter tube, allowing urine to flow into the sterile collection basin. Remember, your non-dominant hand is now contaminated. Cover the open end of the drainage tubing with a sterile protective cap (if it is to be reconnected). Use the dominant hand for manoeuvring the cap and position the tubing so that it stays coiled on top of the bed (using the non-dominant hand). This maintains the sterility of the inner aspect of the catheter lumen and drainage tubing, reducing the potential for introducing pathogens into the bladder. Insert the tip of the syringe into the lumen of the catheter, and instil 30 to 50 mL (as ordered/protocol) of the solution slowly and gently to reduce the incidence of bladder spasm. Repeat the procedure, instilling the solution and draining as per the facility's policy (usually twice for catheter maintenance) or until the return is clear. Withdraw the syringe, lower the catheter and allow the solution to flow by gravity into the basin.

?

If strong resistance is noted, do not force the irrigation. If the solution does not return, have the person turn onto their side facing you. Changing the person's position may move the tip of the catheter in the bladder, increasing the likelihood that the instilled fluid will drain. If changing position does not help, reinsert the syringe and gently aspirate the solution.

Calculate the fluid

It is important to calculate the amount of fluid used to irrigate the catheter. Subtract the amount of irrigation solution used from the volume drained to accurately determine urine output.

Attach the drainage collection bag and secure

After the irrigation is complete, attach a new drainage bag to the catheter and hang it on the bed frame, or reattach the old bag, taking care not to contaminate the catheter end. Secure the bag below the level of the bladder, but above the floor (Lister, Hofland & Grafton, 2020). Coil the drainage tubing and secure it to the bottom sheet to facilitate movement of urine. Dependent loops of tubing (i.e. looped lengths of tubing falling over the edge of the bed well below the bladder) encourage pooling of urine in the tube, which may flow back into the bladder (Snyder et al., 2020). Bacteria growing in urine can cause catheter-induced infection, leading to increased formation of encrustations.

Inform the person of the following:

- lying on the tubing impedes the flow of urine
- pulling on the catheter may cause pain and injury
- raising the level of the collection bag above the level of the bladder can cause backflow and is a cause of bladder infections.

Information assists the person to assume responsibility for their own health-related behaviours and to protect themselves from the actions of uninformed care providers.

Secure the catheter

The catheter should be secured at right angles to the abdomen where it emerges from the stoma (Community Infection Prevention and Control Policy for Care Home Settings, 2023; Nagaraj, 2023). Securing the catheter prevents tension on it as the person moves. It may be taped to the abdomen or secured to the upper thigh with a Velcro strap, or both. Nazarko (2020) implicates manipulation and movement of the catheter as a common cause of bladder trauma and, consequently, of bladder infection due to the destruction of the epithelial lining. Observe to ensure that urine is flowing through the catheter tubing.

Remove your gloves, plastic apron and goggles and perform hand hygiene.

Post-procedure

Position the person comfortably and lower the bed to the lowest position and raise the side-rails (as indicated) to promote safety. Leave the call bell within reach. Assess the person's needs and leave items like water, tissues and reading material or similar within reach. Observe the catheter patency and ensure the person's bladder is emptying freely. Observe the person for signs of pain and fever and observe the urine to determine colour, clarity, concentration and odour.

CLEAN, REPLACE AND DISPOSE OF EQUIPMENT

Seal contaminated material in a disposable rubbish bag, then place it in the contaminated waste bin in the dirty utility room. Discard disposable equipment as per facility policy. Make sure you are wearing clean gloves, apron and goggles, then measure the urine amount, empty the basin into the pan washer (or hopper and wipe it down with the recommended disinfectant solution). Wash and dry the basin and any other reusable equipment (e.g. tray, forceps) and send it to central supply for sterilisation. Place soiled linen in the laundry bag on the unit. Perform hand hygiene. Label any solutions that are to be reused with the date and time of opening, and shelve them in front of unopened solutions so that they can be used quickly and to avoid waste.

DOCUMENTATION

Document date and time, amount and characteristics of the urine (colour, viscosity, clarity and presence of clots, solid debris), type and amount of irrigation used, and the person's response to the procedure. This validates the care given and provides a progress report of the person's condition. The date is also used for forward planning if the person requires further bladder irrigation. Establish/maintain a fluid balance sheet as necessary and note on the care plan to monitor intake and output.

CLINICAL SKILLS ASSESSMENT

Suprapubic catheter care – catheter irrigation

Demonstrates the ability to effectively and safely care for a person who requires a catheter irrigation via a suprapubic catheter. Incorporates the *National Safety and Quality Health Service Standards*: 2 Partnering with Consumers, 3 Preventing and Controlling Healthcare-Associated Infection, 5 Comprehensive Care, 6 Communicating for Safety, and 8 Recognising and Responding to Acute Deterioration (ACSQHC, 2021).

Performance criteria	1	2	3	4	5
(Numbers indicate NMBA *Registered Nurse Standards for Practice*)	(Dependent)	(Marginal)	(Assisted)	(Supervised)	(Independent)
1. Identifies indication (1.1, 3.3, 3.4)	☐	☐	☐	☐	☐
2. Verifies the validity of the written medication order (1.4, 3.4, 6.2, 6.5)	☐	☐	☐	☐	☐
3. Evidence of therapeutic interaction with the person, e.g. gives the person a clear explanation of the procedure (1.4, 1.5, 2.1, 2.2, 3.2)	☐	☐	☐	☐	☐
4. Demonstrates clinical reasoning abilities, e.g. provides privacy and warmth, raises bed, positions the person, obtains assistance if needed (1.1, 1.2, 1.3, 3.2, 4.1, 4.2, 6.1)	☐	☐	☐	☐	☐
5. Gathers equipment (1.1, 5.5, 6.1): ■ gloves (clean and sterile) ■ dressing tray and sterile containers ■ sterile drape ■ solutions as per policy ■ absorbent pad or waterproof sheet ('bluey') ■ bath blanket ■ irrigation syringe ■ new urinary drainage system	☐	☐	☐	☐	☐
6. Performs hand hygiene (1.1, 3.4, 6.1)	☐	☐	☐	☐	☐
7. Positions catheter and tubing for ease of access and places an absorbent sheet under the junction of the catheter and the drainage tubing (1.1, 6.1)	☐	☐	☐	☐	☐
8. Establishes a critical aseptic field, dons sterile gloves, prepares equipment (1.1, 3.4, 6.1)	☐	☐	☐	☐	☐
9. Exposes and washes peristomal area if required and cleanses the catheter insertion site (1.1, 6.1)	☐	☐	☐	☐	☐
10. Disconnects the catheter and gently irrigates the catheter (1.1, 6.1)	☐	☐	☐	☐	☐
11. Removes the syringe and allows urine to drain into a sterile container, calculates the irrigant and thus urine output (1.1, 6.1)	☐	☐	☐	☐	☐
12. Attaches a drainage collection bag and secures it after drainage is completed (1.1, 6.1)	☐	☐	☐	☐	☐
13. Secures the catheter (1.1, 6.1)	☐	☐	☐	☐	☐
14. Assists the person to a comfortable position and lowers the bed to its lowest position (1.1, 6.1)	☐	☐	☐	☐	☐
15. Cleans, replaces and disposes of equipment appropriately (3.6, 6.1)	☐	☐	☐	☐	☐
16. Documents relevant information (1.4, 1.6, 2.2, 2.7, 3.5, 3.7, 6.2, 6.5, 7.3)	☐	☐	☐	☐	☐
17. Demonstrates the ability to link theory to practice (1.1, 3.3, 3.4, 3.5)	☐	☐	☐	☐	☐

Student:

Clinical facilitator: Date:

CHAPTER 36

URINARY CATHETERISATION

INDICATIONS

Urinary catheterisation is indicated for:

- *diagnosis* – for example, monitoring urine output, instilling radio-opaque dye and obtaining specimens
- *treatment* – for example, urinary obstruction, or urinary retention following childbirth or anaesthesia, although portable bladder ultrasound devices are often used to determine retention without catheterisation
- *prevention of complications* (preoperative or predelivery insertion) of the urinary tract.

Urinary catheters can be either intermittent; that is, they are inserted, a procedure is done or the bladder is emptied and they are withdrawn; or they may be retained or indwelling (e.g. Foley catheters) so that the urine can drain freely for hours or days at a time.

Catheterisation carries risks and should only be done in the person's best interest. There must be a compelling reason for catheterising an individual. Continence control is not an indication for urinary catheterisation until all other continence measures have been explored and failed. The indication for catheterisation may prepare you for possible difficulties (e.g. prostate enlargement, previous catheterisations).

The complications of catheterisation include urinary tract infection, which accounts for 20 per cent of all hospital-acquired infections in Australia (Gray, Rachakonda & Karnon, 2023), as well as mucosal trauma and hydronephrosis. People describe urinary catheterisation as ranging from very uncomfortable to painful. Many facilities do not allow nurses to catheterise males; consult the policy manual or a senior nurse.

Removal of catheters at the earliest possible time reduces the incidence of catheter-associated urinary tract infections (CAUTIs). Additionally, decreasing catheter use through restricted indications for placement or duration of catheterisation results in lower rates of CAUTI (Holroyd, 2019), as does daily assessment of the need, and the use of strict aseptic technique during insertion and manipulation of the system (Ling et al., 2023).

Self-catheterisation or clean intermittent catheterisation (e.g. people with paraplegia and other conditions) is not addressed in this skill.

Verify the written medication order

Urinary catheterisation usually requires a written medication order, although it is protocol in some situations (e.g. preoperatively for some surgeries). Verify the order before you proceed. The order should indicate the type of catheter (intermittent or indwelling). Usually the size is determined by assessing the person. Indwelling catheters (IDCs) also require an order (or protocol) for removal.

EVIDENCE OF THERAPEUTIC INTERACTION

Catheterising the urinary bladder is an uncomfortable and embarrassing invasion of the body and most people are psychologically affected by it. They may also be anxious about the reason for the procedure, be it diagnostic, treatment or prevention. They may be exceedingly uncomfortable if they need a catheter for urinary retention or obstruction. For these reasons, it is important to provide the person with a clear and full explanation of what will happen, why it is necessary and how the person can help to facilitate the procedure.

Safety: Keep explanations simple. Include a description of the sensations the person may feel during the procedure. Catheterisation creates a sensation similar to voiding or, rarely, pressure and mild burning, and the sensation will cease or diminish when the catheter is in place. Knowledge of what to expect reduces anxiety and increases trust in you. The discussion provides an opportunity to assess the person's anxiety level, their ability to cooperate and their level of mobility, which can all affect the procedure. Verbal consent is needed for urinary catheterisation.

DEMONSTRATE CLINICAL REASONING

Assessment prior to insertion is important.

LOOK at the reason, any contraindications and the choice of equipment; these are factors to consider to provide safe care. Assess the person's mobility and

obtain assistance if needed; this indicates forward planning, good assessment skills and concern for safety. Some people need assistance to maintain the correct position, and someone may be needed to hold a light source.

LISTEN when you ask about a history of strictures, prostate enlargement or other abnormalities that may indicate a healthcare professional with specialised training will need to insert the catheter. Determine allergies to latex (if using), adhesive and lignocaine. Assess anxiety – another nurse may be required to help calm an anxious person.

Close the room door, put a 'Do not disturb' sign in a prominent place and close the curtains to provide privacy. Interruptions are extremely embarrassing for the person. Place the bath blanket over the person for privacy and warmth to reduce, to an extent, the discomfort the person must endure. Raise the ambient temperature, if possible, and reduce draughts. Raise the side-rail opposite you for safety.

Raise the bed to a workable height for you, to reduce fatigue and muscle strain. Position a woman in the dorsal recumbent position with knees bent and abducted to provide access to the urinary meatus. Males should be supine. Place a waterproof sheet under the buttocks to prevent soiling of the linen during the procedure. Clip a plastic rubbish bag to the trolley edge nearest the person and leave the top wide open. Place the equipment so that your dominant hand is furthest from the head of the bed, which helps you manipulate objects comfortably. Place all necessary equipment within easy reach of the dominant hand.

ELDER CARE

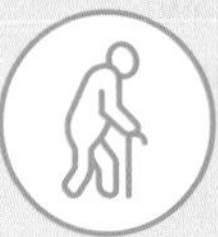

Elderly people, especially those who are frail, are at increased risk of developing a CAUTI (Ling et al., 2023). As well, Giridharan et al. (2023) listed other negative outcomes of IDCs in the elderly, including trauma (from pulling the catheter), restraint, deconditioning, delirium and falls. These consequences indicate the need for serious consideration before inserting an IDC; frequent monitoring of the person/device is required for catheter removal as quickly as practicable.

Use caution with instilling lignocaine in the elderly, those with cardiac dysrhythmias and those with a sensitivity to the medication, because possible injury to the urethral lining during insertion may allow systemic absorption of the medication.

Elderly women usually have very fragile mucous membranes in the perineal area due to loss of oestrogen following menopause. Be very gentle to avoid tearing these membranes.

THE PERSON LIVING WITH SEVERE OBESITY

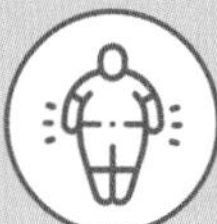

People living with severe obesity are at increased risk for CAUTI (due in part to increased inflammatory mediators and adipokines), so the IDC should be removed as soon as possible. As well, pressure injury/ulcer formation due to lying on the catheter tubing is a consideration. The pressure injury mechanisms specific to this group include increased difficulty repositioning, increased tensile pressure on skin, greater sweat production, increased skin folds, and impaired microcirculation (Anderson & Shashaty, 2021).

You may need a second nurse to assist you if the person is severely obese. The second nurse may be needed to support excess tissue (e.g. mons pubis, labia) or assist a woman to maintain the required position. Women may also need the longer catheter (44 cm) so that the drainage connection is further away from the pendulous folds in the perineum.

GATHER EQUIPMENT

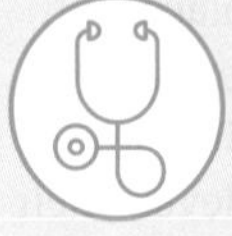

Gathering equipment ensures that you have all needed material, boosts the person's confidence and trust in you, and increases your self-confidence. While gathering the equipment, you can mentally rehearse the procedure.

Equipment varies in each facility. Some facilities supply a catheterisation tray including all of the necessary equipment except the catheter and sterile gloves; others supply a basic tray to which most necessary items need to be added. Prepare the trolley (see **Clinical Skill 7**) and take the supplies to the person's room. You will need the following equipment:

EQUIPMENT	EXPLANATION
Catheter	• The catheter chosen depends on the type of catheterisation and the size of the person's urinary tract • Common types are straight catheters, used for intermittent catheterisation, and IDCs and Foleys • The IDCs have a second lumen with an inflatable balloon near their tip so that when the catheter is in the bladder and the balloon is inflated with sterile water, the catheter stays in place. The balloons come in a variety of sizes, from 5 to 30 mL, with 10 mL or less being preferable • Both straight catheters and IDCs vary in size from French 8 to 10 (children, usually), 10 to 14 (female) and 14 to 18 (male). This is abbreviated to FrXX (e.g. Fr10, Fr16) • Catheter length varies (23 cm for females, 44 cm for males, paediatric lengths are available) • Catheters are made of various materials – PVC, silicone, latex or latex-coated; the latter ease insertion and reduce encrustations. Take care that the person does not have an allergy to latex
10 to 30 mL syringe and sterile water	• Used to inflate the IDC balloon before insertion as a test and again after it has been inserted • Check the size of the balloon on the catheter you have chosen. You will need 3 mL more water to inflate the balloon than the number indicated on the catheter (3 mL of liquid remains in the second lumen)
Cleansing solution/gauze	Usually, normal saline or sterile water are used to cleanse the urinary meatus (Lister, Hofland & Grafton 2020), although Frödin et al. (2022) used chlorhexidine 1% and it decreased the number of CAUTIs
Lubricant	• The type of lubricant incorporating a local anaesthetic agent in a single-use container is used to reduce pain and infection • Ensure it is sterile and water-soluble • Anaesthetic gel is preferred for males and females (Holroyd, 2019)
Catheter drainage valve	• A valve that permits voluntary drainage of the bladder, imitates and maintains bladder tone • Useful for those who do not require continuous drainage, have good cognitive function, manual dexterity and adequate bladder capacity (Lister, Hofland & Grafton, 2020)
Collection bag and tubing and support	• Needed for continued collection of urine as it drains • Various drainage bags are available, ranging from large 2 L capacity bags, commonly used in people who are non-ambulatory and for overnight bags, to leg bags (approximately 750 mL capacity) • Some incorporate urine-measuring burettes used when hourly measurement of urine is required • Some drainage bags and tubing are continuous with the catheter. Do not use a fenestrated drape if this is the case • The bag will require support so it does not drag on the catheter
Specimen container	• To collect a specimen for microanalysis • A label, laboratory requisition and biohazard bag for transporting the specimen to the laboratory are required
Portable light source	Good lighting is needed to provide sufficient light for a female catheterisation
Tray wrapped in a sterile wrapper	Provides the critical sterile field when opened
Clean gloves	Worn during the preliminary cleansing of the perineum
Sterile gloves	Help prevent the introduction of microorganisms into the urinary tract
Forceps	Hold the gauze squares during cleansing of the urinary meatus so that your sterile gloves are not contaminated
Waterproof pad	Placed under the buttocks, protects bed linen from soiling by solutions/urine
Drapes	• Most prepacked catheter trays supply two drapes (one plain, one fenestrated) to extend the sterile field and reduce the transfer of microorganisms • The fenestrated drape has a 10 cm x 10 cm window placed so the opening exposes the labia or the penis; are sometimes omitted because they may slip off a female's pubic area and cause contamination
Bath blanket	Used to cover the person during the procedure
Plastic bag	Often the tray packaging is used for waste disposal; attached with a bulldog clip (or similar) to the dressing trolley
Small basin	• Cleansing solution is poured over the gauze in the basin • Acts as an initial container for urine when the catheter is inserted
Tape or leg bands	Used to secure an IDC to the leg, reducing the trauma potential to the bladder neck and the urethra

URINARY CATHETERISATION

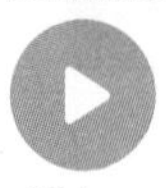

Video

Urinary catheterisation is a complex procedure and requires a great deal of practice to become proficient. Keep in mind the principles of Aseptic Non Touch Technique (ANTT) (see **Clinical Skill 7**) as you manipulate the equipment, clean the perineal area and insert the catheter.

Hand hygiene

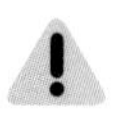

Safety

Perform hand hygiene (see **Clinical Skill 5**) to reduce contamination and minimise hospital-acquired infections, and don non-sterile gloves. The gloves provide a barrier against organisms on the perineum, which may be pathogenic. See **Clinical Skill 6** for gloving and removal of gloves.

Expose and wash the perineal area

For females, place the bath blanket diagonally, with one corner under the chin and the opposite corner draped over the perineal area. The remaining two corners are wrapped around each leg – over the knee, under the calf and over the ankle. The corners are anchored under the heels. This use of the bath blanket reduces the person's feelings of exposure and prevents chilling. For males, place the bath blanket across the torso to reduce exposure.

Expose the person's perineum (for a female, fold up the diagonal piece of the bath blanket; for a male, fold the top sheet down to his mid-thigh). In a male, retract the foreskin prior to washing, then dry and replace. Using the warm washcloth, the solution and the towel, thoroughly wash and dry the perineal area. This reduces the number of microorganisms around the urinary meatus. Sarani et al. (2020) and Mitchell et al. (2021) found that washing with chlorhexidine 2% reduced CAUTIs. The chlorhexidine is bactericidal and bacteriostatic and its effects last for several hours after use. Follow the facility's protocol.

Adjust the light

You will need extra light to catheterise a female. The beam is directed at the perineum, since normal room lights are usually not sufficiently bright to locate the urinary meatus. You may need a helper with a torch if there is no adequate free-standing light source available.

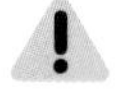

Safety

Perform hand hygiene. Use ANTT for the remainder of the procedure (see **Clinical Skill 7**).

Establish a critical aseptic field

Position yourself at the bedside so your non-dominant hand is closest to the head of the bed to increase the ease of manipulating the sterile items with your dominant hand. Place the wrapped tray between a woman's legs or beside a man's thigh and open it using aseptic technique. Add any sterile supplies that are not in the basic tray or catheterisation tray, such as the selected catheter and gloves or a drape. Pour solutions and add lubricant using aseptic technique. Perform hand hygiene (see **Clinical Skill 5**).

Don sterile gloves

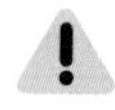

Safety

Sterile gloves prevent the transfer of microorganisms from your hands to objects that will contact or enter the urethra and sterile bladder (see **Clinical Skill 9**).

Prepare equipment

Preparing the field and equipment requires two hands, so it must be completed before you begin cleansing the perineum, which will contaminate the non-dominant hand. Only gloved hands touch sterile items.

Lubricant (preferably with an anaesthetic agent) is spread on the first 5 to 7 cm of the catheter for a female and the first 15 to 20 cm for a male catheterisation. If individual lubricant packages are unavailable and a communal tube (not recommended) must be used, discard approximately 2 cm of lubricant into the plastic rubbish bag to eliminate any contaminated lubricant.

Soak lint-free gauze in solution and wring it out. Open the specimen jar.

Test the catheter balloon (according to the manufacturer's recommendations – some pretest all catheters prior to sterilisation so this step is unnecessary). Fill the syringe with normal saline and attach it to the balloon port. Gently insert the fluid until the capacity of the balloon is reached (indicated on the catheter). Deflate the balloon, but leave the filled syringe attached to the port.

Coil the catheter into the basin with the proximal end within easy reach.

Extend the critical aseptic field

Pick up the folded sterile plain drape on the tray by the corners, move it away from the sterile field and allow it to fall fully open. Follow the instructions for either females or males as shown in TABLE 36.1.

TABLE 36.1 Extending the critical aseptic field before urinary catheterisation

FEMALES	MALES
1. Wrap your gloved hands in each corner of the drape (to prevent their contamination) and ask the woman to lift her buttocks. Slide the drape 5 cm under her buttocks 2. Pick up the fenestrated drape (if using) and place it carefully over the mons pubis area, with the opening exposing the labia	1. The plain drape is slipped under the penis and draped over the man's thighs 2. Pick up the fenestrated drape (if using) and place it so that the tip of the penis is exposed

Clean the urinary meatus

Use the warm normal saline (or prescribed solution) and gauze squares held in forceps in your dominant hand. After this step, your non-dominant hand is contaminated and cannot be used to manipulate anything that is sterile. Follow the instructions for either females or males as shown in TABLE 36.2.

Insert the urinary catheter

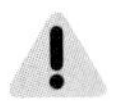
Safety

Place the basin and the catheter near the meatus and tell the person that you are ready to insert the catheter. Ask them to take a deep breath and exhale to relax the sphincter and to minimise irritation. Remind them of the sensations to expect. As they exhale, insert the catheter in the anatomical direction of the urethra. Follow the instructions for either females or males as shown in TABLE 36.3.

If resistance is met at the internal and external sphincters, twist the catheter slightly, then pause and advance carefully. See TABLE 36.4 for solutions to other common problems.

Hold the catheter in place with the non-dominant hand.

Obtain a sterile urine specimen

Allow several millilitres of urine to drain, then pinch or kink the catheter and hold the distal end over the specimen jar (don't rest it on the edge) and release the pinch until sufficient urine has been collected. Again, pinch the catheter and return the distal end to the basin.

If the catheter is a straight one, allow the urine to drain into the basin to completely empty the bladder. Tell the person you are ready to withdraw the catheter and ask them to take a breath and exhale. As they do, pinch the catheter and withdraw it at the same angle it was inserted. Place it in the collection basin.

Inflate the balloon if the catheter is indwelling

Ask the person to immediately report any pain associated with inflating the balloon.

Empty the syringe containing sterile water (already attached to the port of the second lumen) of the requisite amount of fluid. A partially filled balloon irritates the bladder neck and an over-inflated balloon causes discomfort. If there is resistance or pain when you inflate the balloon with sterile water, withdraw the water and advance the catheter further into the

TABLE 36.2 Cleaning the urinary meatus during urinary catheterisation

FEMALES	MALES
1. Spread the labia majora up and outwards by placing the thumb and middle finger of your non-dominant hand about midway down the labia. Gently spread your fingers and pull the tissue upward. This promotes cleansing of the skin folds and meatus, reducing the risk of introducing microorganisms into the urinary meatus 2. Using the forceps and a fresh piece of lint-free gauze for each stroke, cleanse from the labia majora inwards; that is, the first and second strokes are inside the labia majora and downward, the third and fourth are inside the labia minora and downward, and the fifth is around the clitoris and downward over the urinary meatus. Friction reduces the bacterial population around the meatus 3. If the labia are released during cleansing, then repeat the cleansing procedure 4. Insert the nozzle of the lubricant/anaesthetic into the urethra, slowly squeeze the gel in, remove the nozzle and discard the tube. Allow five minutes for the gel's antiseptic and anaesthetic effect to occur 5. The labia must remain open until the catheter is inserted to minimise the chance of recontamination	1. Wrap a sterile gauze around the penis and grasp the shaft just below the glans with the non-dominant hand. You may need to retract the foreskin 2. Using the forceps and lint-free gauze, clean the glans in a circular motion from the meatus outwards. Use three gauze squares to repeat the action three times. Friction reduces the bacterial population of the meatus 3. Insert the nozzle of the lubricant/anaesthetic into the urethra, slowly squeeze the gel in, remove the nozzle and discard the tube 4. Massage the gel along the urethra. Gently squeeze the penis to prevent the anaesthetic gel from escaping and wait approximately five minutes to allow the anaesthetic gel to take effect 5. Hold the penis upright until the catheter has been inserted (straightens the urethra; prevents transfer of microorganisms). If there is an erection, the procedure is abandoned until the erection subsides. If it occurs, treat the situation professionally 6. If the foreskin has been retracted, ensure it is returned over the glans penis

TABLE 36.3 Inserting the urinary catheter

FEMALES	MALES
1. Insert the catheter parallel to the bed, then slightly downwards 5 to 8 cm 2. When urine begins to flow, advance a further 6 to 8 cm to place the balloon deep in the bladder	1. Hold the penis upright, insert the catheter towards the abdomen 25 cm or until it is inserted to the bifurcation of the catheter

TABLE 36.4 Common problems when inserting the urinary catheter

FEMALES	MALES
1. If the labia are touched, the catheter is contaminated and a new sterile catheter will be required (ask another nurse to obtain and open it) 2. If the catheter has been advanced 10 to 12 cm without urine return, it is probably in the vagina (a relatively common occurrence). Leave the catheter in place to mark the vaginal opening, obtain a new catheterisation set-up and begin again	1. If resistance is felt at the external sphincter, increase the traction on the penis slightly and apply steady gentle pressure on the catheter. The resistance may be due to spasms of the external sphincter. Asking the man to strain gently as if he were passing urine can help to relax the external sphincter. Changing the angle of the penis may also help

bladder, and inflate the balloon. Tug *gently* at the catheter to ensure it is snugly seated in the bladder neck (this prevents urine leakage around the catheter). Remove the fenestrated drape so that it does not cause difficulties once the collecting bag is attached.

Attach the drainage collection bag and secure

Attach the sterile drainage bag to the catheter, open the inflow clamp and check that the outflow clamp is closed. Hang the drainage bag on the support on the bed frame above the floor and below the level of the bladder (Anderson & Deamon, 2023; Giridharan et al., 2023).

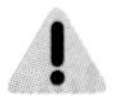
Safety

Coil the drainage tubing on the bed (no dependent loops [i.e. tubing sagging to or below the level of the drainage bag]) and secure it to the bottom sheet to facilitate movement of urine and reduce the incidence of bacteriuria (Anderson & Deamon, 2023). Urine that has pooled in the tubing above an airlock in a dependent loop may flow back into the bladder. Bacteria growing in urine causes catheter-induced infection.

Teach the person that:

- lying on the tubing impedes the flow of urine
- pulling on the catheter may cause pain and injury
- raising the level of the collection bag above the level of the bladder, or resting the bag on the floor can cause infections in the bladder
- they have the right to remind healthcare workers about these precautions.

Information assists the person to assume responsibility for their own health-related behaviours and to protect themselves from the actions of uninformed care providers.

OR

Insert the catheter drainage valve into the catheter lumen. Make sure it is in a closed position. The valve can be attached to a drainage bag for overnight use. Ensure the person knows to open the valve over the toilet at regular intervals.

Secure the catheter

Secure the catheter to prevent tension on the catheter and the bladder neck as the person moves. Tape a female's catheter to the inner thigh and a male's catheter to the anterior thigh or to the abdomen. Some facilities supply leg bands or other support devices that are secured around the thigh and to which the catheter is attached using Velcro tapes. Manipulation and moving the catheter are common causes of bladder trauma and consequently of bladder infection (Nazarko, 2020). Breaking the intact urinary drainage system is a cause of CAUTI (Werneburg, 2022).

Post-procedure

Dry off any solution and wipe off lubricant as a comfort measure, then assist the person to a comfortable position. Lower the bed to suit the person's height and raise the side-rails if appropriate. Leave the call bell within reach and arrange items such as water, tissues and reading material in an accessible position. Assess the person for comfort and provide prescribed analgesia as required.

Establish an intake and output sheet (if not already in use).

REMOVE AN INDWELLING CATHETER

Indwelling catheters are removed as soon as clinically possible to minimise the risk of CAUTIs and to reduce the length of hospital stays (Holroyd, 2020). The need for an indwelling catheter should be assessed daily. Check the care plan for the balloon size and check the medical order sheet to verify the order for removal. Take to the bedside:

- a syringe; must be larger than the amount of liquid in the balloon
- a kidney basin to receive the catheter
- gauze squares or washcloth and solution (usually water)
- a waterproof pad to protect the bed linen from soiling
- two pairs of clean gloves – one to empty the drainage bag and the other to clean the perineum
- an apron to prevent soiling of your uniform and subsequent cross-contamination
- a bag to collect the used tape, gauze squares and any other waste.

Identify the person and tell them that you are going to remove the catheter and what to expect, including possible symptoms that may occur after the catheter is removed (e.g. urinary frequency, urgency or discomfort). Obtain their consent, encourage questions (Bardsley, 2017) and educate them about the importance of removal of the IDC as soon as feasible (Whitaker et al., 2023). Provide for the person's privacy. Perform hand hygiene and put on the clean gloves.

Empty the drainage bag, then expose the catheter and remove the supporting tapes. Use the bedclothes or a towel to cover the person as much as possible for privacy. Place the incontinence pad under the buttocks and the basin between the person's legs. Open the rubbish bag then remove your gloves and dispose of them.

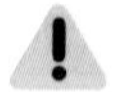
Safety

Wash your hands and put on a fresh pair of gloves. Clean the meatus and the catheter using the gauze squares and water or a washcloth and water. Swab outward/away from the meatus. Attach the syringe to the balloon port and allow all of the fluid to come back into the syringe. Do not pull back on the syringe. Ask the person to breathe deeply and exhale as you *gently* pull to remove the catheter and place it in the basin. Wipe the person's perineum or the tip of the penis dry of urine and mucus.

Remove the equipment. Place the syringe, the pad, the disposable basin and the empty catheter in the rubbish bag and discard it in the contaminated waste bin. Remove the gloves and put them in the contaminated waste bin. Perform hand hygiene.

Make the person comfortable. Record the removal. Document the first voiding post IDC removal, noting amount, colour, clarity and any discomfort or sensation (e.g. need to strain). Monitor for voiding, and intake and output, and assist them to the commode or toilet or provide a urinal or bedpan q2h and measure and record the output (Miranda et al., 2023). If the person is unable to void following removal of the catheter, or if an ultrasound reveals more than 450 mL of residual urine after voiding, inform the physician. The person will likely need to be re-catheterised (Miranda et al., 2023).

?

If the balloon does not deflate:

- leave the syringe attached to the catheter valve and allow the water to seep out slowly. This can take up to 20 minutes
- don't add any more fluid to the balloon in an attempt to burst it or cut the catheter or the inflation arm
- ask about constipation – in a female, this can cause pressure on a urethra/catheter, preventing it from draining
- try a different syringe (the syringe might be faulty)
- check the patency of the inflation channel by inserting 1 to 2 mL of sterile water and drawing back on the syringe. This also indicates if water has been lost from the balloon
- gently squeezing along the catheter tubing may move any blockage and enable the water to drain from the inflation channel
- insert approximately 3 mL of air and draw back using the syringe to create a vacuum, which may aid deflation (Bardsley, 2017).

If all of the above fail, attach a 25-gauge needle to the syringe and pierce the catheter below the valve, inserting the needle into the inflation channel, and draw back using the syringe. This method bypasses a faulty catheter valve (Lister, Hofland & Grafton, 2020).

If the balloon still does not deflate and no water can be withdrawn, seek medical advice.

CLEAN, REPLACE AND DISPOSE OF EQUIPMENT

Seal contaminated material in the disposable plastic bag and place in the contaminated waste bin in the dirty utility room. Measure the urine amount and empty the basin into the hopper. Wipe down the basin with the recommended disinfectant solution, or if it is disposable discard it in the contaminated waste bin. Wash and dry the basin and any other reusable equipment (e.g. tray, forceps) and send it to central supply for sterilisation. Place soiled linen in the laundry bag on the unit. Clean the dressing trolley, including the bulldog clip, and return it to the storage area. Remove your gloves and perform hand hygiene. Label solutions to be reused with the date and time of opening and shelve them in front of unopened solutions so that they can be used quickly and to avoid waste.

DOCUMENTATION

Relevant information to record includes the reason for catheterisation, date and time, amount and characteristics of the urine, type and size of the catheter used, balloon size, type and amount of solution used to inflate the balloon, any problems encountered during the procedure, and the person's response to the procedure. This validates the care given and provides a progress report of the person's condition. The date is also used for forward planning should the person require a catheter for a long period of time. Some catheters are replaced weekly; some (Silastic) need only be replaced monthly. Note the start of a fluid balance sheet if necessary and note on the care plan to monitor intake and output.

CLINICAL SKILLS ASSESSMENT

Urinary catheterisation

Demonstrates the ability to effectively and safely catheterise a person's urinary bladder and remove an indwelling catheter. Incorporates the *National Safety and Quality Health Service Standards*: 2 Partnering with Consumers, 3 Preventing and Controlling Healthcare-Associated Infection, 5 Comprehensive Care, 6 Communicating for Safety, and 8 Recognising and Responding to Acute Deterioration (ACSQHC, 2021).

Performance criteria	1	2	3	4	5
(Numbers indicate NMBA *Registered Nurse Standards for Practice*)	**(Dependent)**	**(Marginal)**	**(Assisted)**	**(Supervised)**	**(Independent)**
1. Identifies indication and verifies order (1.1, 1.4, 3.3, 3.4, 6.2, 6.5)	☐	☐	☐	☐	☐
2. Verifies the validity of the written medical order (1.4, 3.4, 6.2, 6.5)	☐	☐	☐	☐	☐
3. Evidence of therapeutic interaction with the person, e.g. gives the person a clear explanation of the procedure (1.4, 1.5, 2.1, 2.2, 3.2)	☐	☐	☐	☐	☐
4. Demonstrates clinical reasoning abilities, e.g. provides privacy and warmth, raises the bed, positions the person, obtains assistance if needed (1.1, 1.2, 1.3, 3.2, 4.2, 6.1)	☐	☐	☐	☐	☐
5. Gathers equipment (1.1, 5.5, 6.1): ■ catheter ■ 10 to 30 mL syringe and sterile water ■ lubricant ■ collection bag and tubing/catheter valve ■ specimen container ■ portable light source ■ tray wrapped in a sterile wrapper ■ clean gloves and sterile gloves ■ forceps ■ waterproof pad ■ drapes and bath blanket ■ plastic bag ■ gauze squares and solution ■ small basin ■ tape or leg bands	☐	☐	☐	☐	☐
6. Performs hand hygiene (1.1, 3.4, 6.1)	☐	☐	☐	☐	☐
7. Exposes and washes the perineal area (1.1, 6.1)	☐	☐	☐	☐	☐
8. Adjusts the light (1.1, 6.1)	☐	☐	☐	☐	☐
9. Establishes critical aseptic field, dons sterile gloves, prepares equipment (1.1, 6.1)	☐	☐	☐	☐	☐
10. Cleanses the urinary meatus (1.1, 6.1)	☐	☐	☐	☐	☐
11. Inserts the urinary catheter (1.1, 6.1)	☐	☐	☐	☐	☐
12. Obtains a sterile urine specimen (1.2, 5.1, 5.2, 7.1)	☐	☐	☐	☐	☐
13. Inflates the balloon if the catheter is indwelling (1.1, 6.1)	☐	☐	☐	☐	☐
14. Attaches and secures the drainage collection bag (1.1, 6.1)	☐	☐	☐	☐	☐
15. Secures the catheter (1.1, 6.1)	☐	☐	☐	☐	☐
16. Attends to post-procedure care (1.1, 6.1)	☐	☐	☐	☐	☐
17. Removes the indwelling catheter; is able to relate steps if the balloon does not deflate (1.1, 6.1)	☐	☐	☐	☐	☐
18. Cleans, replaces and disposes of equipment appropriately (3.6, 6.1)	☐	☐	☐	☐	☐
19. Documents relevant information (1.4, 1.6, 2.2, 2.7, 3.5, 3.7, 6.2, 6.5, 7.3)	☐	☐	☐	☐	☐
20. Demonstrates the ability to link theory to practice (1.1, 3.3, 3.4, 3.5)	☐	☐	☐	☐	☐

Student:

Clinical facilitator: Date:

REFERENCES

Anderson, J. & Deamon, V. (2023). *Bundle up to improve CAUTI*. Doctor of Nursing Practice Manuscript, South Alabama University. https://jagworks.southalabama.edu/dnp_manuscripts/2

Anderson, M. & Shashaty, M. (2021). Impact of obesity in critical illness. *Chest, 160*(6), 2135–45. https://doi.org/10.1016/j.chest.2021.08.001

Arco, S., Saldaña, E., Serra-Prat, M., Palomera, E., Ribas, Y., Font, S., Clavé, P. & Mundet, L. (2022). Functional constipation in older adults: Prevalence, clinical symptoms and subtypes, association with frailty, and impact on quality of life. *Gerontology, 68*(4), 397–406. https://doi.org/10.1159/000517212

Assis, G., Coelho, M., Rosa, T., Oliveira, F., Silva, C., Brito, M., Oliveira, V., Alves, C., Penha, A., Penha, S. & Sampaio, L. (2023). Proposal for a clinical protocol for the conservative treatment of urge urinary incontinence. *ESTIMA, Brazilian Journal of Enterostomal Therapy, 21*, e0123. https://doi.org/10.30886/estima.v21.1295_IN

Australian Commission on Safety and Quality in Health Care (ACSQHC) (2021). *National safety and quality health service standards* (3rd edn). Sydney, NSW: ACSQHC.

Bak, A. (2018). *Improving hydration of care home residents by addressing institutional barriers to fluid consumption – an improvement project*. PhD thesis, University of West London. http://repository.uwl.ac.uk/id/eprint/6605/1/Bak_Thesis_Final_%28Nov_2018%29_Improving_hydration_of_care_home_residents_by_addressing_institutional_barriers_to_fluid_consumption_an_improvement_project.pdf

Bardsley, A. (2017). How to remove an indwelling urinary catheter in female patients. *Nursing Standard, 31*(19), 42. https://doi.org/10.7748/ns.2017.e10525

Bauer, S., Eglseer, D. & Großschädl, F. (2023). Obesity in nursing home patients: Association with common care problems. *Nutrients, 15*(14), 3188. https://doi.org/10.3390/nu15143188

Chilaka, C., Toozs-Hobson, P. & Chilaka, V. (2023). Pelvic floor dysfunction and obesity. *Journal of Best Practice & Research in Clinical Obstetrics & Gynaecology, 90*, 102389. https://doi.org/10.1016/j.bpobgyn.2023.102389

Cho, Y. S., Lee, Y. J., Shin, J. E., Jung, H. K., Park, S. Y., Kang, S. J., Song, K. H., Kim, J. W., Lim, H. C., Park, H. S., Kim, S. J., Cha, R. R., Bang, K. B., Bang, C. S., Yim, S. K., Ryoo, S. B., Kye, B. H., Ji, W. B., Choi, M., Sung, I. K. & Choi, S.C. … Korean Society of Neurogastroenterology and Motility (2023). 2022 Seoul consensus on clinical practice guidelines for functional constipation. *Journal of Neurogastroenterology and Motility, 29*(3), 271–305. https://doi.org/10.5056/jnm23066

Chumpitazi, C. E., Henke, I. E. B., Valdez, K. L. & Chumpitazi, B. P. (2016). Soap suds enemas are efficacious and safe for treating fecal impaction in children with abdominal pain. *Journal of Pediatric Gastroenterology and Nutrition, 63*(1), 15–18. https://doi.org/10.1097/MPG.0000000000001073

Collins, D., Carson, K., Riley, T. (2019). Microbiological evaluation of the ability of the DEKO-190 washer/disinfector to remove *Clostridium difficile* spores from bedpan surfaces. *Infection, Disease & Health, 24*(4), 208–11. https://doi.org/10.1016/j.idh.2019.07.001

Community Infection Prevention and Control Policy for Care Home Settings (2023). *Urinary catheter care*. Harrogate and District NHS Foundation Trust, Cumberland Council, United Kingdom. https://www.cumbria.gov.uk/elibrary/Content/Internet/327/7041/7047/4408584119.pdf

Dean, J. & Ostaszkiewicz, J. (2019). Current evidence about catheter maintenance solutions for management of catheter blockage in long-term urinary catheterisation. *Australian and New Zealand Continence Journal, 25*(3). https://search.informit.com.au/documentSummary;dn=609061636333370;res=IELNZC

DeLaune, P., Ladner, S., McTier, L. & Tollefson, J. (2024). *Fundamentals of nursing* (Australia and New Zealand 3rd ed.). South Melbourne, VIC: Cengage Learning.

Dowden, A. (2021). The impact of chronic constipation in adults. *Prescriber, 32*, 25–8. https://doi.org/10.1002/psb.1954

Frödin, M., Ahlstrom, L., Gillespie, B. M., Rogmark, C., Nellgard, B., Wikstrom, E. & Andersson, A. (2022). Effectiveness of implementing a preventive urinary catheter care bundle in hip fracture patients. *Journal of Infection Prevention, 23*(2), 41–8. https://doi.org/10.1177/17571774211060417

Fuseini, A-G., Rawson, H., Ley, L. & Kerr, D. (2023). Patient dignity and dignified care: A qualitative description of hospitalised older adults perspectives. *Journal of Clinical Nursing, 32*, 1286–302. https://doi.org/10.1111/jocn.16286

Gadelkareem, R., Abozead, S., Khalaf, R., Mohammed, N. & Khalil, S. (2022). Is reducing the early postoperative complications of percutaneous suprapubic catheterization affected by the method of healthcare education in low-literacy patients? A prospective randomized comparative study. *Current Urology, 16*(3). https://doi.org/10.1097/CU9.0000000000000151

Gandhi, A. B., Madnani, N., Thobbi, V., Vora, P., Seth, S. & Shah, P. (2022). Intimate hygiene for women: Expert practice points. *International Journal of Reproduction, Contraception, Obstetrics and Gynecology, 11*, 2315–9. https://dx.doi.org/10.18203/2320-1770.ijrcog20221962

Giridharan, K., Bradford, D., Lim, S., Feroz, A. & Naeem, O. (2023). 1571 A quality improvement initiative on 'indwelling urinary catheterisations' in hospitalised older adults. *Age and Ageing, 52*(Supplement 2). https://doi.org/10.1093/ageing/afad104.035

Gray, J., Rachakonda, A. & Karnon, J.(2023). Pragmatic review of interventions to prevent catheter-associated urinary tract infections (CAUTIs) in adult inpatients. *Journal of Hospital Infection, 136*, 55–74. https://doi.org/10.1016/j.jhin.2023.03.020

Gulati, R., Komuravelly, A., Leb, S., Mhanna, M. J., Ghori, A., Leon, J. & Needlman, R. (2018). Usefulness of assessment of stool form by the Modified Bristol Stool Form Scale in primary care pediatrics. *Pediatric Gastroenterology & Hepatology Nutrition, 21*(2), 93–100. https://doi.org/10.5223/pghn.2018.21.2.93

Hamilton Smith, R., Eddleston, M. & Bateman, D. N. (2022). Toxicity of phosphate enemas: An updated review. *Clinical Toxicology, 60*(6), 672–80. https://doi.org/10.1080/15563650.2022.2054424

Holroyd, S. (2019). Indwelling urinary catheterisation: Evidence-based practice. *Journal of Community Nursing*. https://www.jcn.co.uk/files/downloads/articles/11---urinary.pdf

Holroyd, S. (2020). Trial without catheter: What is best practice? *Journal of Community Nursing, 34*(2), 60–4, 66–7. https://search.proquest.com/docview/2394932656?accountid=88802

Jardine, X. (2021). Safe handling and disposal of human excreta, protecting the nurse, and the patient. *Professional Nursing Today, 2*, 6–8. https://journals.co.za/doi/abs/10.10520/ejc-mp_pnt_v25_n2_a2

Jayasekara, R. (2013). *Enema: Administration* [Evidence summary]. Adelaide, SA: Joanna Briggs Institute.

Khawaja, F., Flynn, K., Tuong, M., Schlaepfer, C., Metzger, A. & Erickson, B. (2023). MP74-14 Suprapubic catheter drainage for the long-term management of lower urinary tract dysfunction: Longitudinal outcomes and utilization patterns from a tertiary care practice. *Journal of Urology, 209*(4), e1075. https://doi.org/10.1097/JU.0000000000003348.14

Ling, M. L., Ching, P., Apisarnthanarak, A., Jaggi, N., Harrington, G. & Fong, S. (2023). APSIC guide for prevention of catheter associated urinary tract infections (CAUTIs). *Antimicrobial Resistance and Infection Control, 12*(52). https://doi.org/10.1186/s13756-023-01254-8

Lister, S., Hofland, J. & Grafton, H. (eds) (2020). *The Royal Marsden manual of clinical nursing procedures* (10th ed.). Oxford, UK: Wiley-Blackwell.

Meiko (n.d.). Bed pan cleaning. https://www.meiko.com.au/en/meiko-experience/magazine/bedpan-cleaning-instructions?tx_avmeiko_language_selector%5Bcontroller%5D=LanguageSelector&cHash=8744a60d30f5eaf4edddeb150d12fcc9

Meunier, O., Populus, G., Durrheimer, J. M., Duffet, B. & Burger, S. (2019). Single-use: An interesting alternative to bedpan washers. *Hygienes, 27*(4), 205–10. https://hygie.com/wp-content/uploads/2020/02/HY_XXVII_4_Meunier.pdf

Miranda, M., Rosa, M., Castro, M., Fontes, C. & Bocchi, S. (2023). Nursing protocols to reduce urinary tract infection caused by indwelling catheters: An integrative review. *Revista Brasileira de Enfermagen, 76*(2). https://doi.org/10.1590/0034-7167-2022-0067

Mitchell, A. (2019). Administering an enema: Indications, types, equipment and procedure. *British Journal of Nursing, 28*(3), 154–6. https://search.proquest.com/docview/2195371365/415330CB3A654BAEPQ/1?accountid=88802

Mitchell, B., Curryer, C., Holliday, E., Rickard, C. & Fasugba, O. (2021). Effectiveness of meatal cleaning in the prevention of catheter-associated urinary tract infections and bacteriuria: An updated systematic review and meta-analysis. *British Medical Journal Open, 11*, e046817. https://doi.org/10.1136/bmjopen-2020-046817

Nagaraj, C. (2023). Hospital-acquired urinary tract infections. *IntechOpen*. https://doi.org/10.5772/intechopen.110532

Nazarko, L. (2020). *Primum non nocere*: How securement and fixation of indwelling urinary catheters can reduce the risk of harm. *British Journal of Healthcare Assistants, 14*(2), 84–9. https://doi.org/10.12968/bjha.2020.14.2.84

Palter, M. & Patel, R. (2023). Know your poop: How to effectively use stool documentation in the electronic medical record (EMR) to capture *Clostridioides difficile* infections before it's too late! *American Journal of Infection Control, 51*(7), S37–S38. https://doi.org/10.1016/j.ajic.2023.04.069

Pullen, R. (2022). Hemorrhoidal disease: What nurses need to know. *Nursing, 52*(5), 19–24. https://doi.org/10.1097/01.NURSE.0000827128.26047.32

Quallich, S. A., Thompson, T., Jameson, J., Wall, K., Lajiness, M. J., Powley, G., Lutz, A. R., Hemphill, J.: SUNA Suprapubic Catheter Task Force (2023). Management of patients after suprapubic catheter insertion [white paper]. *Urologic Nursing, 43*(2), 61–73, 102. https://doi.org/10.7257/ 2168-4626.2023.43.2.61

Reid, S., Brocksom, J., Hamid, R., Ali, A., Thiruchelvam, N., Sahai, A., Biers, S., Belal, M., Barrett, R., Taylor, J. & Parkinson, R. (2021). British Association of Urological Surgeons (BAUS) and Nurses (BAUN) consensus document: Management of the complications of long-term indwelling catheters. *British Journal of Urology International, 128*, 667–7. https://doi.org/10.1111/bju.15406

Rodriguez, G. M. & Gater, D. R. (2022). Neurogenic bowel and management after spinal cord injury: A narrative review. *Journal of Personalized Medicine, 12*(7), 1141. https://doi.org/10.3390/jpm12071141

Sarani, H., Pishkar Mofrad, Z., Faghihi, H. & Ghabimi, M. (2020). Comparison of the effect of perineal care with normal saline and 2% chlorhexidine solution on the rate of catheter-associated urinary tract infection in women hospitalized in intensive care units: A quasi-experimental study. *Medical-Surgical Nursing Journal, 9*(2), e106739. https://doi.org/10.5812/msnj.106739

Sharma, A., Agarwal, S., Sharma, D. & Veerwal, A. (2018). Spin-top-like encrustation of suprapubic cystostomy catheter: When proper counselling is all that it takes! *British Medical Journal Case Reports*. https://doi.org/10.1136/bcr-2018-226726.

Sinclair, L., Cross, S., Hagen, S. & Niel-Weise, B. S. (2017). Washout policies for the management of long-term indwelling urinary catheterisation in adults (Protocol). *Cochrane Database of Systematic Reviews, 30*(7), 1208–12. https://doi.org/10.1002/14651858.CD004012.pub5

Snyder, M., Priestley, M., Weiss, M., Hoegg, C., Plachter, N., Ardire, S. & Thompson, A. (2020). Preventing catheter-associated urinary tract infections in the pediatric intensive care unit. *Critical Care Nurse, 40*(1), e12–e17. https://doi.org/10.4037/ccn2020438

Steeves, S., Vallande, N. & Lonks, J. (2020). Safety and nosocomial *Clostridioides difficile* infections. *Rhode Island Medical Journal*, March, 21–3. http://www.rimed.org/rimedicaljournal/2020/03/2020-03-21-infection-steeves.pdf

Sweeney, A. (2021). *Best practice guideline: Long-term suprapubic catheter related care at home*. Continence Nurse Society Australia. https://www.consa.org.au/images/files/Best_practice_guideline_-_Long-term_suprapubic_catheter_realted_care_at_home.pdf

Tai, H., Liu, S., Wang, H. & Tan, H. (2021). Determinants of urinary incontinence and subtypes among the elderly in nursing homes. *Frontiers in Public Health, 9*. https://www.frontiersin.org/articles/10.3389/fpubh.2021.788642

Toney-Butler, T. & Gaston, G. (2019). Nursing bedpan management. *StatPearls [Internet]*. Treasure Island (FL): StatPearls Publishing. https://www.ncbi.nlm.nih.gov/books/NBK499978

van Knippenberg-Gordebeke, G. G. (2015). Worldwide improper bedpan-management: Risk for spreading (multi drug) resistant organisms. *Journal of Microbiology, Immunology and Infection, 48*(2), S37. https://doi.org/10.1016/j.jmii.2015.02.055

van Veen, F., Hoedi, S., Coolen, R., Bockhorst, J., Scheepe, J. & Blok, B. (2023). Bladder irrigation with tap water to reduce antibiotic treatment for catheter-associated urinary tract infections: an evaluation of clinical practice. *Frontiers in Urology, 3*. https://doi.org/10.3389/fruro.2023.1172271

Wang, L., Zhang, S., Keatch, R., Corner, G., Nabi, G., Murdoch, S., Davidson, F. & Zhao, Q. (2019). In-vitro antibacterial and anti-encrustation performance of silver-polytetrafluoroethylene nanocomposite coated urinary catheters. *Journal of Hospital Infection, 103*(1), 55–63. https://doi.org/10.1016/j.jhin.2019.02.012

Wangui-Verry, J., Farrington, M., Matthews, G. & Tucker, S. (2019). Are milk and molasses enemas safe for hospitalized adults? A retrospective electronic health record review. *American Journal of Nursing, 119*(9), 24–8. https://doi.org/10.1097/01.NAJ.0000580148.43193.76

Werneburg, G. (2022). Catheter-associated urinary tract infections: Current challenges and future prospects. *Research and Reports in Urology, 14*, 109–33. https://doi.org/10.2147/RRU.S273663

Whitaker, A., Colgrove, G., Scheutzow, M., Ramic, M., Monaco, K. & Hill, J. (2023). Decreasing catheter-associated urinary tract infection (CAUTI) at a community academic medical center using a multidisciplinary team employing a multi-pronged approach during the COVID-19 pandemic. *American Journal of Infection Control, 51*(3), 319–23. https://doi.org/10.1016/j.ajic.2022.08.006

PART 7

MEDICATION ADMINISTRATION

37 ORAL MEDICATION

38 ENTERAL MEDICATION

39 TOPICAL MEDICATION

40 OPTIC MEDICATION

41 OTIC MEDICATION

42 VAGINAL MEDICATION

43 RECTAL MEDICATION

44 INHALED MEDICATION

45 PARENTERAL MEDICATION

46 INTRAVENOUS MEDICATION ADMINISTRATION – VOLUME-CONTROLLED INFUSION SET

47 INTRAVENOUS MEDICATION ADMINISTRATION – INTRAVENOUS CONTAINER

48 INTRAVENOUS MEDICATION ADMINISTRATION – BOLUS

Note: These notes are summaries of the most important points in the assessments/procedures and are not exhaustive on the subject. References of the materials used to compile the information have been supplied. The student is expected to have learnt the material surrounding each skill as presented in the references. No single reference is complete on each subject.

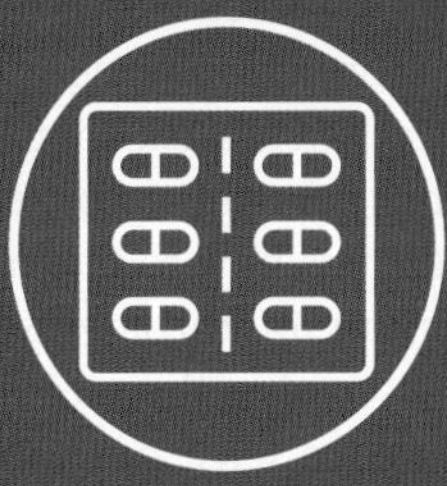

CHAPTER 37

ORAL MEDICATION

INDICATIONS

Oral medications are the most common form of medication. Oral administration is a form of *enteral* administration, and is differentiated here for clarity (see **Clinical Skill 38** for enteral administration via a gastric tube). Enteral medications are absorbed more slowly due to the time required to digest and absorb them.

Oral administration is both the least expensive and least offensive way of administering medications. The main method of oral administration involves swallowing the medication in some form. Two topical medications are included here because they are administered in the oral cavity: *sublingual* administration (e.g. nitroglycerin) causes fast and easy absorption through the mucous membranes under the tongue; and *buccal* administration, where a tablet or lozenge placed in the cheek cavity dissolves and is absorbed over time; neither involves digestion.

'Medication' is the most acceptable term used in health care, but you will also hear the term 'drug' used to indicate prescribed medications as well as illicit substances.

Verify the written medication order

A valid, signed order from a qualified healthcare provider is a requirement for legal administration of a medication. Medical officers, dentists and some nurse practitioners are licensed to prescribe a limited number of medications. A valid order consists of the person's full name, the time, day, month and year the order is written, the medication name (clearly written and correctly spelled), the dose, the strength, the amount or number of tablets, the route of administration and the frequency and/or time of day to take it. Some medications, such as opioid analgesics or antibiotics, also require a finish or stop time. Some over-the-counter (OTC) medications can be given without an order. These are usually listed in the facility's policy manual.

You are responsible and accountable for questioning and clarifying any order that is unclear or incomplete, or that seems inappropriate or unreasonable for the person (e.g. a very high dose, the same medications with two different names). Potentially harmful prescribing errors often go undetected (Kessemeier et al., 2019). Nurses are partly responsible (along with the physician) if an inappropriate order is followed. To question an order, you *must know* the person's diagnosis, the purpose of the medication, its therapeutic effect, any adverse or toxic effects and the usual dose. Your knowledge of pharmacology is crucial to safe medication administration. Anticipate any pertinent nursing implications (e.g. the person's ability to swallow) as well as individual factors that mediate response to medications (e.g. age, weight, psychological factors). Be aware of any drug or food allergies so that potentially harmful substances are not administered. The person must be able to take the medication by mouth (i.e. not be 'nil by mouth', or if so, medications must be allowed), have no trauma to the mouth or throat, have no nausea or vomiting, and be able to swallow.

EVIDENCE OF THERAPEUTIC INTERACTION

Clearly explain the procedure, name the medication and determine the person's knowledge of it. They should be able to state its name, the dose they take, its expected effects and probable adverse effects. This information provides a basis for their decision about treatment. Ask about any drug or food allergies. Once the person has consented to take the medication, discuss how to maximise the intended effects and minimise the adverse effects of the medication. Discussing the medication with the person gives them a sense of control. It also allows you to assess if more teaching is required, and to gauge the person's understanding of their treatment. Ask if they have any questions and answer them.

DEMONSTRATE CLINICAL REASONING

Assess the person

Some medications require assessment of the person prior to administration (e.g. pulse, blood pressure, fluid balance, respiratory assessment). Check with the person and on the medication administration sheet that there are no allergies to the medication, and check on the medication administration sheet that the medication is due and has not been given already. Use LOOK, LISTEN and FEEL to assess individuals for their ability to sit, swallow and follow instructions, to ensure their safety.

Obtain an appropriate form of the medication to facilitate its administration. A person unable to swallow a tablet may find the liquid form of the medication appropriate; however, check with the prescribing practitioner or pharmacy, since liquid medication is absorbed more quickly than solid forms. Many pills may be crushed (exceptions are enteric-coated, slow-release and foul-tasting tablets), so determine the crushability of medication before proceeding, and phone the pharmacy if you are unsure.

Food, health supplements and other medications can interact with many medications to either enhance or reduce their effectiveness. For example:

- grapefruit reduces or even eliminates the effectiveness of some anticoagulants (Mayo Clinic, 2022)
- herbal supplements (e.g. St John's wort) can reduce the amount of circulating digoxin and thus its effect (McAdoo, 2022)
- other medications (e.g. non-steroidal anti-inflammatories) can interfere with antihypertensive drugs (Townsend, 2022).

This needs consideration when you are familiarising yourself with the medication ordered and the individual for whom it is ordered.

Position the person

Position the person to facilitate administering the medication, usually sitting them upright to swallow comfortably. If sitting is impossible, position them for safety and comfort (e.g. lying on their side rather than supine).

Cultural diversity

Cultural traditions related to medication use can usually be accommodated; for example, during Ramadan oral medications can be rescheduled to before dawn or after sunset if this will not interfere with the therapeutic effects (Sheikh, 2023).

General concepts of working with therapeutic substances

Legal responsibilities

Medications must be securely stored and safely administered (Australian Commission on Safety and Quality in Health Care [ACSQHC], 2021; Institute for Safe Medication Practices [ISMP], 2019). If the facility does not have automatic dispensing cabinet technology, controlled substances (schedule medications) are kept in locked cabinets. The keys are passed from one registered nurse (RN) to an oncoming RN at shift change or when leaving the unit. At shift change, all the unit's controlled medications are counted and signed for by both RNs. A precise inventory of all controlled medications is kept as they are used, wasted or added to the unit stock. Many medications require the signature of two licensed healthcare professionals on the inventory sheet as they are administered. These measures (two

ELDER CARE

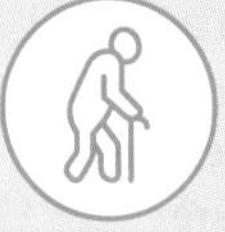

As people age, their gastrointestinal functioning declines. Dysphagia, and especially difficulty in swallowing pills, is relatively common and requires assessment prior to administering an oral medication (especially anyone with a diagnosis of stroke, Parkinson's disease, cancer of the neck/oesophagus, frailty and declining functional status) (Chen et al., 2020). It may indicate the need for a change in oral form from a solid to a liquid. Administering an increased numbers of pills required (polypharmacy) also becomes difficult. Give the person plenty of time to swallow one medication before offering the next. Thirst also diminishes. Offer a glass of water with the medications and urge more fluids (if not contraindicated) to help 'the medicine go down' and assist with preventing dehydration.

THE PERSON LIVING WITH SEVERE OBESITY

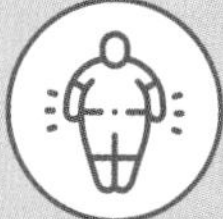

Obese people have, by definition, a greater ratio of fat to lean body tissue. This alters their ability to absorb, use and store various medications. Some medications are highly soluble in fat (e.g. diazepam, opioid analgesics) and stored in fatty tissue, while others (e.g. digoxin, paracetamol) are water-soluble and stored in lean tissue (Appelbaum, Rodriguez-Gonzalvez & Clarke, 2020). Weight-based doses are generally ordered for those living with severe obesity, and are based on the individual's weight and concomitant organ damage (e.g. liver, kidneys) (Erstad & Barletta, 2020), so be prepared for doses that are not within the 'normal' range. Ask either the pharmacist or a senior healthcare professional if you are unsure.

As well, obesity alters physiological responses (electrolyte imbalance, metabolic processes). This means that the pharmacy should be intimately involved in the care planning with the physician and nursing staff, and the person should be carefully monitored for both under-medication and toxicity of any medication prescribed. (See **Clinical Skills 15 and 23** for a brief explanation of bariatric issues.)

Weight loss supplements (OTC or purchased via the internet) have no evidence-based effect on weight loss, but they do have side effects and toxic effects that are unpleasant or worse. Advise any person living with severe obesity to discuss any proposed supplement with their prescribing practitioners. There are several proven weight loss medications available.

professionals witnessing and signing for the schedule medication) may be an added precaution if an automated dispensing cabinet (ADC) is in use.

No medication can be administered without a valid, signed order written by the prescribing physician on the medication administration sheet (there are exceptions for some OTC medications). Verbal and telephone orders are acceptable at some facilities, but there is a protocol for their use. The RN receiving the order has both the order and the transcription verified by a second RN. The physician responsible must sign the order within a specific time frame – usually 24 hours. Any abbreviation used in a written medication order must be approved by the facility.

Accurate dosage calculation

Calculating accurate dosages is a vital skill required to safely administer a medication. Medications are usually supplied in the dosages most commonly used, but an individual may require less or more of the medication. You will need to do a mathematical calculation to determine the dose for a specific person. Calculating paediatric and geriatric dosages is especially critical because of the physiological differences in the young and the very old. Their relative body size and immature or degenerating organ systems make the margin for error smaller, and the response to the medication more unpredictable. Independent double-checking of calculations (each nurse calculates the dose or identifies the medication or person independent of the other) has been demonstrated to reduce medication errors (Brindley, 2020). Check any medication calculations with a senior nurse. Ensure that the environment is distraction-free (Kollstedt, Fowler & Weissman, 2019). Consult your nursing foundations and pharmacology texts for formulae to calculate doses.

Medication names and classifications

Medication or drug names and classifications organise the vast amount of information known about medications. Medications generally have three names:

- *chemical name* – reflects the chemical composition of the drug
- *generic name* – derived from the chemical name, but shorter. Medications are listed in the MIMS under this and are usually ordered by this name (MIMS [2024] is a website/book with independent medicine information for Australian healthcare professionals, known for its high level of editorial integrity. The facility or university will have a subscription to this website to enable you to research medications)
- *trade name* – the manufacturer's name; used for marketing purposes.

For example, acetylsalicylic acid (chemical name) or aspirin (generic name) is sold in pharmacies as Cardiprin (trade name), among others.

Medications are classified according to the following:

- the body systems on which they exert their effects (e.g. cardiac, renal, musculoskeletal)
- the clinical indications (e.g. antihypertensive, diuretic, anti-inflammatory)
- the physiologic properties (e.g. beta-blockers, calcium channel blockers).

It is necessary that you are aware of the name, classification and indication for any medication you administer, as well as the information listed above. Take care to check the name of the medication, as many medication errors are caused by the similarity in names (Musafiri & Daniels, 2020).

Mechanisms of medication administration

Understand the facility's system for administering medications

There are generally two drug-administration systems in use. The first is the stock supply/individual supply, in which stock and labelled individual prescriptions are kept on a trolley or in a locked drawer in the person's bedside locker and dispensed as needed from the bulk supplies and the person's prescriptions.

The second system in common use is the unit dose system (e.g. Webster-paks). In this system, all medications (other than control/schedule medications) that the person will take in a 24-hour period are dispensed by the pharmacy. They are individually packaged for appropriate administration times with the drug name, dose and expiration date, as well as the person's name, their hospital number and the name of the ordering physician.

A third system is becoming available in some facilities. It is an ADC system and works in a similar way to automated bank teller machines. Access the system (password protected), choose the person's name from the list and their medications are displayed. Choose the medication, which is then dispensed from the machine ready to administer. The ADC system has been demonstrated to reduce medication errors by up to 60 per cent (Shitu et al., 2019). These systems are secure, have an optimal inventory and display important information about the person and the medication (ISMP, 2019). Although ADCs are designed to dispense controlled medications (e.g. opioids), Zheng et al. (2021) found that to safeguard against inappropriate use of these medications there need to be processes in place to supplement the technology. Be very cautious if you use the 'override' feature to obtain a medication – this is the biggest source of error (ISMP, 2020). The ADC system uses a scanning technology (e.g. barcoding) to verify five of the six 'rights' of administration (right person, right medication, right dose, right time and right route) and increase efficiency. The scan verifies the person's identity and the medication being administered at the bedside. Barcoding technology has been proven to reduce medication errors (Hutton, Ding & Wellman, 2021). However, Zheng et al. (2021)

urge caution since they found evidence of error due to damaged or inaccurate barcodes and workarounds still occur, and contribute to medication error. Most systems also document (the sixth 'right') the administration of the medication concurrently on the electronic medication administration record (eMAR).

Preparation

Safety

Márquez-Hernández et al. (2019) found that errors (excluding timing errors) occur during 9 per cent of medication administration in hospitals. To reduce errors, administer only medications that you have personally prepared, and undertake the following precautions:

- *Prepare medications in a quiet place without distractions* – avoid interruptions/conversations. Focus your concentration on preparing the medication. Use a 'Do not disturb' sign on the medication trolley and wear a brightly coloured 'attention vest' to reduce distractions and interruptions (Dragon, 2020). As well, visual posters in the medication preparation area and education of the person and their family on medication importance help to minimise medication error (Dall'Oglio et al., 2017).
- *If interrupted by a more urgent task when preparing medications* – return the medications to the storage area, secure them and repeat safety checks when resuming the medication round. This reduces the errors made by losing concentration.
- *Use only medications from containers whose labels are entire and clear* – this helps to avoid mistaking one medication for another.
- *Check the label on the medication container* – for the medication name, strength and cautionary labels.
- *Check the expiration date on each medication* – the potency of out-of-date medications may be affected. Do not give discoloured, sedimented or cloudy liquid medication if they should not be so.
- *Do not touch the medication with your hand* – not only is it unsanitary, but you may pick up minute quantities of the drug on your skin, which may irritate or be absorbed. Wearing gloves is mandatory for some medications (e.g. antibiotics, chemotherapeutic medications). Pour the tablet(s) into the cap of the container and then tip them into a paper cup.
- *Do not leave medications unattended or out of your sight* – they may be taken or removed by unauthorised individuals (including children).
- *Do not return any unused or unlabelled medications to a container* – to prevent the inadvertent mixing of medications or the placement of a medication into the wrong container.
- *Some medications need to be checked by two RNs as a special precaution* – this is normally because of their potency or to prevent accidental errors in dosage. These include, but are not limited to, paediatric doses, narcotic/opioid medications, insulin, intravenous (IV) medications and anticoagulants. Check the policy of the facility for others.
- *Be aware of allergies* – check the medication administration sheet for an allergy caution, look for an allergy armband (red) and ask the person if they are allergic to anything. Ask them if they have taken this medication before and, if so, have they tolerated it.
- *Ask the person to state their name* – don't ask them if their name is 'Mary Smith', for example, they may say 'yes' regardless of who they are (e.g. they may be deaf, confused, non-English-speaking).
- *Observe that the person takes their medication* – do not leave a medication on a bedside locker for them to take at a later time. This ensures that the prescribed drug is correctly administered to the correct person at the correct time.
- *Listen to the person* – many, if not most, people know their medications well, and any query by them as to the dose or appearance of the medication should be taken seriously before administering the dose. Recheck the medication administration sheet and the medication bottle and ask the prescriber about the drug. This validates the person's knowledge and prevents drug-administration errors.
- *Initial the medications sheet/eMAR* – do this as soon as the medication is administered to prevent a potential overdose (e.g. another nurse might administer a second dose of the medication thinking it has not been given). Bar code administration systems do this automatically. Do not sign prior to giving the medication, only after the administration.
- Bar code medication administration systems (where you scan your identification, the person's identification on their wristband and the data on the medication to be administered) reduce transcription and administration error by verifying the six rights (see 'The six rights of administering medication' below) and either alert you to error or approve administration in real time. The ACSQHC (2019) calls these electronic medication management (EMM) systems when they are integrated with the person's electronic diagnostic orders and results, their allergies and adverse drug reactions, other clinical information that influences medication decisions, medication histories on admission and discharge prescriptions and summaries. EMM systems require point-of-care computer access.
- The information is automatically recorded on the eMAR.

Responsibility to the person

Your responsibility involves this generalised assessment (but remember to also use LOOK, LISTEN and FEEL for each individual prior to administering a medication), teaching, advocacy and evaluation of the effect of the medication administered.

Assess the physiological or psychological function that the medication is expected to affect prior to administering medications (e.g. pain assessment before administering analgesia, pulse assessment before administering digoxin). The assessment may indicate that the medication should be withheld and the shift coordinator informed, or it may provide a baseline for evaluating the medication's effectiveness.

Assess the person's medication history (current and past medications: prescribed, OTC, herbal preparations or recreational) and history of allergies or adverse reactions. Some OTC medications (including herbal preparations) may interfere with prescription medications (e.g. ibuprofen, vitamin E and cranberries interact with warfarin [Mayo Clinic, 2020b]). Some medications have a narrow therapeutic range (e.g. digoxin, phenytoin, warfarin, gentamicin), and the person's blood levels are monitored to ensure an effective level and avoid under- or overdosing (Hull, Garcia & Vazquez, 2023). It is especially important in those of extreme age.

Teach the person the name, dose and reason for the drug they are taking, its frequency, adverse effects and how to minimise them. They need to know any implications of taking the medication (e.g. if it should be taken with meals or on an empty stomach or taken at a specific time of day). Discuss maintaining the drug regimen at home, and any adaptations to accommodate the person's home schedule (without compromising the medication's efficacy). Teach the person about the importance of regular monitoring; for example, warfarin will require regular monitoring of international normalised ratio (INR), and the dosage may need adjusting (Hull, Garcia & Vazquez, 2023). Be alert to any cues the person or their family might give about not continuing to use a medication, such as concerns about the cost or inconvenience. Forgetting to take the medication or to fill the prescription, not understanding the instructions, not feeling unwell, having side effects, being reminded of chronic ill health and preference for 'natural remedies' are all reasons people do not adhere to their medication regimen. Discussing these things may improve the person's understanding and commitment to sustaining the prescribed treatment.

Advocacy includes alerting the medical practitioner to adverse effects or any reason the person tells you that would influence their continuation of the medication.

Evaluation is crucial in administering medications. You and the prescribing doctor need to be aware that the drug is doing what it is meant to. Reassess the person following administration of such medications as analgesics, bronchodilators, antihypertensives, anxiolytics, sedatives or diuretics, among others. This should be done within a reasonable time frame from the administration (usually 30 minutes to one hour following) and the effects documented. This evaluation is critical following the initial administration of a medication.

GATHER EQUIPMENT

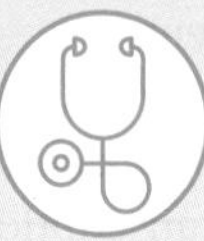

Gathering equipment is an organisational step that helps to create a positive environment for a successful interaction and reduces the risk of errors when preparing medication. Equipment includes the following items:

EQUIPMENT	EXPLANATION
Medication trolley (if there is no ADC system)	• Locked and the key is passed from RN to RN at shift change • Usually stocked with all the necessary equipment for administering a medication as well as a range of alphabetically arranged stock medications or the unit-dose packages • Individual drawers may be used to hold non-stock prescription medications for each person • If the unit-pack system is used, the trolley contains some means of organising the packs • Familiarise yourself with the trolley in the facility
Medication administration sheet (eMAR now in use in many facilities)	• The medication sheet with the signed, valid order is used to identify the person, the medication required, the route, the dose, and the time. It is also the documentation of administering the medication • Usually kept at the person's bedside or may be kept separately with the medications
Paper cups	• In which to place the tablet to give to the person
Graduated plastic cups or oral syringes	• Measures liquid medication and helps administer the medication
Pill cutter or knife	• Used to cut a scored tablet if the dose requires a half tablet
Pill crusher or mortar and pestle	• If a pill cannot be swallowed whole, it can (with some exceptions) be crushed or ground to a powder and given in some soft food
Tongue blade	• Scrapes as much crushed pill out of the mortar as possible. Paper towel (dampened) can remove the rest
Clean gloves	• Used to protect you from contact with the medication
Paper towels	• Paper towels are used for general clean-up – wiping out the mortar (dampened), wiping up spilled medication
Glass of fresh cold water and a straw (if required)	• Used to help the person swallow the medication • Determine the person's preferred fluid to take medication • Cold fluids minimise the bitter aftertaste of some medications and can be swallowed quickly to take the tablets out of the mouth before they dissolve • Provide a straw if the person is unable to sit upright
Soft food like yoghurt, custard or apple sauce	• If a person is unable to swallow liquids, soft food should be added to the trolley to assist them to take oral medication

THE SIX RIGHTS OF ADMINISTERING MEDICATION

Safety

Many *rights* of medication administration are used. Vera (2023) recommends 10 'rights', while Broyles et al. (2017) describe 12; however, Hanson and Haddad (2022) found there is little empirical evidence to support the effectiveness of 'the five (or more) rights' system in reducing medication error, but it is a commonsense practice to improve safe medication administration.

Right time

The *right time* clause in medication administration contributes to the greatest percentage of medication errors (Salami et al., 2019). In most facilities, a scheduled time to administer medications is set (e.g. BD [twice a day], QID [four times per day]) and used as an organisational time-management strategy. If this standard schedule would compromise the written medication order, an individual's needs or the effectiveness of the medication, you have the discretion to accommodate the person's preferences (e.g. giving a QID drug at 0600, 1200, 1800 and 00h rather than 0800, 1400, 2000 and 0200h) or to maximise drug effectiveness. Some medications *must* be given at a specified time, such as insulin being given prior to a meal. Medications given within 30 minutes of the ordered time (with the exception of preoperative medication, insulin and other time-critical medications) are considered to have been given on time.

Right medication

The *right medication* is chosen after verifying the validity of the order. The expiry date is checked. The name of the medication on the container label is checked three times against the written medication order: once when the container is picked up from the trolley, once when the medication is poured and once when the medication container is returned to the trolley. Take care, as many medications have VERY similar names.

Right route

The *right route* is noted from the medication administration sheet. Altering the route (e.g. intramuscular to oral) because of changed conditions requires an order from the physician. Using a different form of the medication within the same route (e.g. oral tablets or a liquid) in consultation with the person, the pharmacy and physician is appropriate. Ensure that the person adheres to the sublingual or buccal routes if they have been ordered and does not swallow the medication.

Check the diet order/restriction of the person prior to administering an oral medication (Scott, 2020). Seek guidance if medications are to be withheld because of fasting/nil by mouth (NBM) orders or protocols (note that these terms are often used interchangeably). Some of these (e.g. fasting prior to surgery) may mean the person could have sips of water with oral medications up to an hour prior to surgery. An NBM order (e.g. on a person following a stroke) means they can have nothing orally as they are at risk of aspiration. Clarify which protocol to use (To, Brien & Story, 2020).

Right dose

The *right dose* is imperative to gain a therapeutic level of the medication. If the dose is anything other than that supplied, calculate the dose to be given and check your calculations with an RN. Check that the units of measurement are the same (e.g. micrograms, millilitres). If not, convert the stock's units into the prescribed dose's units. Take care to ensure the correct formulation when different formulations and/or dosages are available. For example, verapamil is available in 40 mg, 80 mg, 120 mg or 160 mg tablets; and a sustained release (SR) formulation of verapamil is available as 180 mg or 240 mg tablets (National Library of Medicine, 2016). Check the formulation carefully to avoid serious consequences (e.g. substituting three 80 mg tablets of verapamil [will act quickly], when verapamil SR 240 mg is ordered [is formulated to be released over 24 hours] would cause an overdose).

Right person

The *right person* receiving the medication is vital. Ask the person to give you their name and check their name and hospital number (on the identification band) against the label on the medication administration sheet. People may have the same or similar names, so make it a habit to check the identification of any individual any time a medication is administered. If the facility uses the bar code system, adhere to their protocols.

Right documentation

The *right documentation* is completed when the medication has been given. This is noted on the medication administration sheet for most medications. Initial the slot beside the time that the medication was given. This will be beside the individualised written medication order, which describes the medication name, dose, route, time and prescriber's details. Use of the bar code medication administration system means the information is automatically recorded on the eMAR. If the medication was not given or was refused, note this on the medication administration sheet and describe the reason and the actions you took in the progress notes.

Other rights

Other *rights* have been proposed, and their use is encouraged. They include:

- right reason
- right preparation
- right to refuse
- right assessment
- right identification of allergies
- right evaluation
- right education (Broyles et al., 2017).

The additional 'rights' can be found in pharmacology and nursing foundation texts. The university or facility you work in will specify which additional 'rights' are to be used.

Medication administration is not a linear process or routine in nature, as numerous influences, distractions and challenges impact it and cannot be addressed by the 'rights' framework alone (Martyn, Paliadelis & Perry, 2019). It is a framework that is required to learn the process and initiate safe medication administration, and you will learn to combine this framework with clinical judgement to safely and effectively manage the process. Giving a medication within the complexity of modern nursing is not as simple as suggested by the list of 'rights', no matter how long it is. Martyn, Paliadelis and Perry (2019) suggest person-centred care with strategies that respond to individual circumstances will help maintain safety.

ADMINISTER ORAL MEDICATION

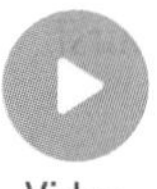

Video

Preparing and administering oral medications is a frequent clinical task. Do not let it become routine or habitual. Think about what you are doing.

Hand hygiene

Hand hygiene (see **Clinical Skill 5**) is an infection-control measure. Administering oral medication is a clean procedure. Ensure the medication never touches your hand by using non-touch pouring techniques to reduce transfer of microorganisms to the alimentary tract of the person and reduce your exposure to the medication.

Hand hygiene – generally using alcohol-based hand rub (ABHR), unless hands are visibly soiled – is to be undertaken prior to and following each individual contact, before beginning a medication round and after it is completed.

Prepare the medication

Pour tablets or capsules from the container into the lid of the container, then transfer them to the medication cup so the medication is not touched. Several different tablets and capsules can be placed in the same cup. Keep the tablets or capsules that require an assessment prior to administration separate in an extra cup so they can be withheld if necessary. Place unit dose medications, still wrapped, in the medicine cup to keep them clean and facilitate identification.

Pre-scored tablets can be broken for a half-dose. Use a gloved hand and a pill cutter, use only if the break is clean to ensure the correct dose in each half (Broyles et al., 2017).

Place tablets to be crushed in a clean mortar and grind to a fine powder with the pestle (some cannot be crushed; check with the pharmacy if in doubt). A clean mortar and pestle prevents contamination of the medication with traces of previous medications. Capsules can be emptied of their powder. Mix the powder with soft food (e.g. yoghurt, custard, apple sauce) for administration. When mixing powders with water or juice, do so at the bedside so there is no time for them to solidify and become difficult to swallow. Give effervescent powders/tablets quickly after they dissolve, as this often improves the palatability.

Shake a suspension to distribute the drug evenly through the liquid. Remove the cap of a liquid and place it upside down on a clean surface to avoid contaminating the inside. Hold the bottle with the label towards the palm of your hand and pour the liquid away from the label to avoid obscuring it with spills. Place the plastic medication cup on a firm surface at eye level and pour the medication to the desired level as measured at the bottom of the meniscus. If using the more accurate oral dosing syringe, remove the syringe from its packaging, place the tip below the top of the liquid and withdraw the plunger slowly until the correct dose is obtained. Wipe the lip of the bottle with a damp paper towel to prevent the cap from sticking.

Take the medication trolley or the wheeled ADC and the original order sheet to the person's bedside.

Administer the medication

In most instances, you need only hand the person the medicine cup and a glass of fresh water or cold beverage of their choice. Help them to use a straw if they must remain supine or side-lying. However, it is your responsibility to see that the medication is swallowed at the time it is prescribed. Do not leave medication at the bedside to be taken 'later'. Some people may not wish to take a medication and will put it in their mouth but not swallow it, then remove the tablet when you have gone. Watch the person swallow the medication. You may need to check under their tongue and in the buccal pouches with a sterile tongue blade for unswallowed medication.

Tablets placed on the back of the tongue stimulate the swallowing reflex and are more easily swallowed. Tipping the head slightly forward facilitates swallowing capsules. If the person cannot hold the medication cup, use the cup to introduce the tablets one at a time into their mouth. Give them plenty of time to swallow each medication before introducing another.

Liquid medications (other than antacids or cough medicine) are diluted with about 15 mL of water or juice to facilitate both emptying the cup and their absorption. If a medication has an objectionable taste, give the person some ice chips to suck just prior to taking the medication and ask them to hold their nose while swallowing, since the cold desensitises the taste buds and the olfactory sensations contribute to taste.

Sublingual tablets are placed under the tongue and left there to dissolve. They are absorbed through the thin mucous membranes into the capillary bed. Their absorption and thus action are quicker than swallowing and digesting before absorption. Remind the person not to swallow the medication, and not to eat, drink or smoke. The tablet dissolves over several minutes. Sublingual medication is not given (except in emergencies) if there are open sores in the mouth.

Buccal tablets (lozenges) are placed between the gums and the cheek to dissolve over several minutes. They are absorbed in the same way as sublingual tablets. Remind the person not to swallow them or suck on them, as this will increase the immediate dose of the medication. Eating, drinking and smoking also alter the absorption of the medication (Brotto, 2020). Again, do not give if there are open sores in the person's mouth.

CLEAN, REPLACE AND DISPOSE OF EQUIPMENT

Discard any disposable items used to administer a medication (e.g. paper medication cups), and clean and replace non-disposable items (e.g. mortar and pestle, knife). Wipe the cart clean of spills or debris, and replace stocks of supplies (e.g. medication cups, paper towel). Wipe any spills from individual bottles or from sticky caps. Order stock medications and individual prescriptions from the pharmacy if they are running low. When they arrive on the unit, place them in the medication trolley with their labels visible to reduce the possibility of errors. (Pharmacy will restock an ADC.) Return the medication administration sheet to its designated place for the next medication round.

DOCUMENTATION

Initial or sign the medication administration sheet or the eMAR in the appropriate timeslot beside the written medication order. If an assessment was done (e.g. pulse, blood pressure), note it in the designated slot. The effects of the medications, expected or unexpected, are assessed 30 minutes to one hour after administration, and are then documented. Adverse effects should be reported to the shift coordinator and the medical staff, and the remaining doses of the medication withheld.

Your laboratory will have medication administration records (MARs) and eMARs to help you become familiar with them. There will also be a list of acceptable medication administration abbreviations that have come from facilities where you will gain experience.

> ?
>
> If a medication has been refused or some other untoward event occurs, document it briefly on the medication administration sheet in the appropriate timeslot (e.g. nauseated, refused), then document it more fully in the progress notes.

CLINICAL SKILLS ASSESSMENT

Oral medication

Demonstrates the ability to effectively and safely administer oral medication. Incorporates the *National Safety and Quality Health Service Standards*: 2 Partnering with Consumers, 3 Preventing and Controlling Healthcare-Associated Infection, 5 Comprehensive Care, 6 Communicating for Safety, and 8 Recognising and Responding to Acute Deterioration (ACSQHC, 2021).

Performance criteria	1	2	3	4	5
(Numbers indicate NMBA *Registered Nurse Standards for Practice*)	(Dependent)	(Marginal)	(Assisted)	(Supervised)	(Independent)
1. Identifies indication (1.1, 3.3, 3.4)	☐	☐	☐	☐	☐
2. Verifies the validity of the written medication order (1.4, 3.4, 6.2, 6.5)	☐	☐	☐	☐	☐
3. Evidence of therapeutic interaction with the person, e.g. gives the person a clear explanation of the medication, discusses adverse effects of the medication (1.4, 1.5, 2.1, 2.2, 3.2)	☐	☐	☐	☐	☐
4. Demonstrates clinical reasoning abilities, e.g. assesses the person if warranted, positions the person, obtains the appropriate form of the medication (1.1, 1.2, 1.3, 4.2, 6.1)	☐	☐	☐	☐	☐
5. Adheres to the general concepts of working with therapeutic substances (1.1, 1.3, 1.5, 3.3, 3.4, 4.1, 4.2, 4.3, 6.2, 6.5, 6.6)	☐	☐	☐	☐	☐
6. Gathers equipment (1.1, 5.5, 6.1): ■ medication trolley ■ medication administration sheet ■ paper cups, graduated plastic cups or oral syringes ■ pill cutter or knife ■ pill crusher or mortar and pestle ■ tongue blade ■ clean gloves ■ paper towels ■ glass of fresh cold water and a straw (if required) ■ soft food like yoghurt, custard or apple sauce	☐	☐	☐	☐	☐
7. Uses the six (or more as designated by the facility/university) rights to administer the medication (1.1, 1.2, 1.3, 1.4, 1.5, 2.2, 3.4, 4.1, 4.2, 4.3, 6.1, 6.2, 6.5, 6.6)	☐	☐	☐	☐	☐
8. Performs hand hygiene (1.1, 3.4, 6.1)	☐	☐	☐	☐	☐
9. Prepares the medication (1.1, 3.4, 6.1)	☐	☐	☐	☐	☐
10. Assists the person to take the medication (1.1, 2.2, 6.1)	☐	☐	☐	☐	☐
11. Cleans, replaces and disposes of equipment appropriately (3.6, 6.1)	☐	☐	☐	☐	☐
12. Documents relevant information (1.4, 1.6, 2.2, 3.5, 3.7, 6.2, 6.5, 7.3)	☐	☐	☐	☐	☐
13. Demonstrates the ability to link theory to practice (1.1, 3.3, 3.4, 3.5)	☐	☐	☐	☐	☐

Student:

Clinical facilitator: Date:

CHAPTER 38

ENTERAL MEDICATION

INDICATIONS

Oral medications are the most common form of medication, and the main method of oral administration involves swallowing a medication in some form. However, this is not possible for some people, such as those who are unconscious or have head injury, mouth or neck trauma and so on. In this case, a nasogastric tube (NGT) is introduced via the nasopharynx into the stomach. Alternatively, a simple surgical procedure is performed to place a percutaneous epigastric tube (PEG) through the abdominal wall into the stomach or into the jejunum (PEGJ). The person is then fed and given medication through the tube. (See **Clinical Skills 29 and 30** for more on NGT insertion and administration of enteral nutrition.)

Verify the written medication order

No medication can be legally administered without a valid, signed order from a qualified healthcare provider (see **Clinical Skill 37** for a description of a valid order). Question any unclear order, or any order that seems incomplete or inappropriate for the person. Be especially aware of pertinent nursing implications, such as the availability of the medication in a liquid form, or its ability (or not) to be crushed or removed from its capsule, as well as individual factors that mediate response to medications such as age, weight and psychological factors. Determine any drug or food allergies that the person may have so that potentially harmful substances are not administered. The person must have a patent NGT, PEG or PEGJ in situ and have no nausea, vomiting or diarrhoea.

EVIDENCE OF THERAPEUTIC INTERACTION

Establish the identity of the person. If they are unconscious, tell them what you are doing. If they are conscious, give them a clear explanation of the procedure, name the medication and determine their knowledge of it. Ensure they are aware of the medication name, the dose they take, its expected effects and probable adverse effects. This gives them information on which to base decisions about treatment.

Once the person has consented to take the medication, talk with them about how they can maximise the intended effects and minimise the adverse effects. Discussing the medication with the person gives them a sense of control. It also allows you to assess if more teaching is required, and to gauge the person's understanding of their treatment. Ask if they have any questions and answer them.

DEMONSTRATE CLINICAL REASONING

Assess the person

LOOK at the person's individual condition before administering a medication (e.g. a respiratory assessment before administering a bronchodilator, fluid balance for a person receiving diuretics, pulse assessment before administering digitalis, or respiratory rate and depth before administering a narcotic).

LISTEN to reports of any medication allergies.

THE PERSON LIVING WITH SEVERE OBESITY

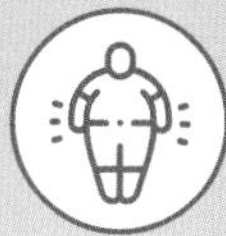

Weight-based doses are generally ordered for those living with severe obesity, and are based on the individual's weight and concomitant organ damage (e.g. liver, kidneys) (Erstad & Barletta, 2020), so be prepared for doses that are not within the 'normal' range.

Assess the medication

Obtain an appropriate form of the medication to facilitate its administration. Consult the pharmacy if in doubt. Liquids are the most suitable for enteral administration; however, not all liquid medications are appropriate for enteral administration. Some are oily, or thick and very viscous, and cannot pass through the narrow lumen of the tube. Some contain large amounts of sorbitol and cause gastrointestinal problems.

Many pills may be crushed or removed from their capsules, with exceptions such as enteric-coated or slow-release tablets (Wright, Smithard & Griffith, 2020), but determine the crushability of medication before proceeding. Some medications are too irritating to be powdered and dispersed in water (e.g. chemotherapy medications) or will combine with the protein in the feeding solution to block the tube (e.g. some antacids and antibiotics) (British Association for Parenteral and Enteral Nutrition and The British Pharmaceutical Nutrition Group, n.d.; Wright, Smithard & Griffith, 2020).

Position the person

Position the person to facilitate administration of the medication; supine is preferable, although prone is well tolerated when necessary (Savio et al., 2020). Supine generally requires the head of the bed to be raised to 30 degrees in order to reduce the possibility of regurgitation and subsequent aspiration into the bronchial tree.

General concepts of working with therapeutic substances

Please review the general concepts and mechanisms of medication administration presented in **Clinical Skill 37**. The following safety concerns are specific to enteral medications:

- Understand the facility's system for administering medications. Generally, for enteral medications, the pharmacy is aware of the person's needs and supplies the medication in a form that can be administered through an enteral tube.
- Use only water to liquify enterally administered medications.
- Flush the tubing prior to and following administration to avoid interaction between the medication and feeds.

GATHER EQUIPMENT

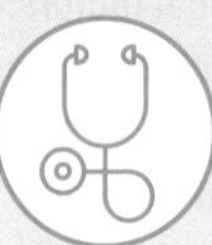

Gathering equipment is an organisational step that helps to create a positive environment for a successful interaction and reduces the risk of errors when preparing medication. Equipment includes the following items:

EQUIPMENT	EXPLANATION
Medication trolley	• Kept locked and the key is passed from registered nurse (RN) to RN at shift change • It is usually stocked with all of the necessary equipment for administering an enteral medication, as well as a range of alphabetically arranged medications • Individual drawers may be used to hold non-stock prescription medications for each person • Check that the trolley contains sufficient stocks of the required items • Familiarise yourself with the trolley or medication dispensing system in the facility (e.g. mobile automated dispensing cabinet [ADC])
Medication administration sheet/eMAR	• The medication sheet/computer file and bar code with the signed, valid order is used to identify the person, the medication required, the route, the dose, and the time. It is also the documentation of administering the medication • Usually kept at the point of care, the eMAR will be on the person's file
Graduated plastic cups or oral syringes	• Used for measuring the liquid medications • Oral syringe tips do not fit into needle hubs, IV needle hubs or Luer Lock devices. Some (e.g. Enfit) are coloured. Come in 10 to 60 mL sizes
Large oral syringe (30 to 60 mL)	The barrel is needed to introduce the medication into the NGT. These are colour coded and incompatible with parenteral equipment (Government of Western Australia: WA Country Health Service, 2019)
Pill cutter or knife	• To cut a scored tablet if the dose requires a half tablet • Use gloves to protect yourself from contact with the medication for hygienic reasons
Pill crusher or mortar and pestle	• To powder tablets so they can be dissolved in water for administration through the NGT, if the medication cannot be obtained in a liquid form • Ensure the equipment is clean to prevent contamination of the medication with traces of previous medications
Large plastic cup	To mix the ground powder with water (White & Bradnam, 2017) if not using the dispersal method
Tongue blade	Scrapes as much crushed pill out of the mortar as possible
Clean gloves	To protect you from contact with the medication
Paper towels	For general clean-up – wiping out the mortar (dampened), wiping up spilled medication

EQUIPMENT	EXPLANATION
Bottle of pH measurement strips, a tongue blade and a penlight	This equipment can be either on the trolley or at the person's bedside and is used to determine the placement of an NGT
Sterile (or fresh tap water – often used at home)	• To flush the tube; check the policy of the facility, as some use tap water • Sterile water contains no contaminants that might interact with the medications (White & Bradnam, 2017) • Check that the person is not on fluid restrictions – if so, the physician will order the amount of flush water to be used

THE SIX RIGHTS OF ADMINISTERING MEDICATION

See **Clinical Skill 37** for a complete description of the rights of medication administration. In summary, they include:

- *right time* – the first consideration
- *right medication* – verify the validity of the order and then choose from the medications on the trolley. Crushing a pill is a last resort if no other formulations are available. Crushing a compressed tablet alters its dosing accuracy (by up to 25 per cent [White & Bradnam, 2017]) and needs a physician's order
- *right route* – confirm this as noted on the medication administration sheet
- *right dose* – is imperative to gain a therapeutic level of the medication
- *right person* – it is vital to verify the correct person is receiving the medication
- *right documentation* – must be adhered to.

ADMINISTER ENTERAL MEDICATION

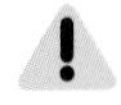
Safety

Take extra care in the early morning (0600 to 0900). This is the time of day that most errors occur due to frequent distractions.

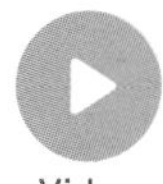
Video

Hand hygiene

Enteral medication administration is a clean procedure. Hand hygiene (see **Clinical Skill 5**) and the use of non-touch pouring reduce the microorganisms that could be transmitted to the alimentary tract of the person. Take the medication trolley/ADC (mobile one) and the original order sheet to the person's bedside. Check that a continuous feeding tube is clamped for medication administration prior to and for 30 minutes following medication administration.

Prepare the medication

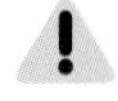
Safety

If in doubt about the suitability of a medication for liquifying for enteral administration, consult the manufacturer's information or the pharmacy.

Crushing

Pour tablets or capsules from the container into the lid of the container (confirm that they are either crushable or suitable to remove from the capsule and the physician has noted to crush the tablet [Alhashemi, Ghorbani & Vazin, 2019]) and then transfer them to the mortar and pestle for crushing, so that hands do not touch the medication and excess tablets are not contaminated. Prescored tablets can be broken to deliver a half-dose; use a gloved hand and a knife or a pill cutter.

To crush tablets, place them in a clean pill crusher, or in a mortar and grind to a fine powder with the pestle. Grind the compressed tablet finely to reduce clogging of the tube (Rosana et al., 2020). Powders are mixed with 10 mL of sterile water and the mortar is rinsed twice with 10 mL of water, which is drawn up into the administering syringe (Government of Western Australia: WA Country Health Service, 2019). This is done at the bedside so there is no time for the mixture to solidify and become difficult to get down the tube. Scrape the mortar clean, rinse and wipe dry with paper towels between tablets. Pull capsules apart and empty into the cup. Discard the gelatin capsule. Mix the crushed pill/powdered medication with tepid water to disperse or dissolve the powder. Each medication is prepared and administered separately.

Dispersal method

Kunieda et al. (2022) have demonstrated the efficacy of a simple suspension method for preparing medication for administration through an enteral tube. They placed a tablet (e.g. furosemide) in a 20 mL syringe with 10 mL of warm water, let the solution sit for 10 minutes, gently agitated it until the tablet was completely dispersed, and then administered it. This method reduced clogging of the finer bore NGTs (8-16Fr) they used with less medication loss than the conventional crushing method. This method of enteral medication administration is being expanded (Institute for Safe Medication Practices [ISMP], 2022b).

Liquid medication

If a liquid medication is a suspension, shake it well (this distributes the drug evenly through the liquid). Remove the cap and place it upside down on a surface to avoid contaminating the inside. Hold the bottle with the label towards the palm of your hand and pour the liquid away from the label to avoid obscuring it with spills. Hold the plastic medication cup at eye level and pour the medication to the desired level as measured at the bottom of the meniscus. Thick medications will require dilution.

Alternatively, use an oral syringe to draw up and measure the liquid. Make sure that the medications are drawn up and dispensed only in oral syringes (not syringes intended to give parenteral injections) in order to avoid the accidental parenteral administration of an oral formulation (Scott, 2020). Wipe the lip of the bottle with a damp paper towel to prevent the cap from sticking. Consider that some liquid medications are based on sorbitol and can cause osmotic diarrhoea.

Assess enteral tube placement

Safety

The nasogastric (or other) tube must be in the stomach to avoid possible complications. Aspiration of the medication into the bronchial tree is the most common complication; however, irritation and erosion of the oesophagus are also considerations. If the person is on continuous feedings, stop the flow of solution 30 minutes prior to medication administration to permit emptying of the stomach contents.

The NGT has an indelible mark or a piece of tape where it emerges from the nares. Check that this mark has not migrated away from the nares.

Perform hand hygiene and put on clean gloves.

Aspirate some of the stomach contents to determine if they are acidic. Pinch the tube and disconnect the NGT from the feeding system. Attach the 50 mL oral syringe to the NGT (not the coloured air tube) and gently aspirate some fluid. Drip the fluid onto a pH test strip (do not use litmus paper, if possible, because it is not as accurate). Determine the pH of the fluid. A reading of 4 to 5.5 indicates that the tip of the NGT is in the stomach (stomach contents usually have a pH below 5). If no aspirate returns, the person may need to be repositioned to place the tip in a pool of stomach contents. Return the aspirate to the stomach. Obtaining aspirate demonstrates tube patency.

Some facilities require that you determine the residual volume of fluid to ensure that the material is moving through the gastrointestinal tract. Check the relevant policy of the facility. If this is the case, withdraw as much fluid as you can, measure the volume and return it to the stomach. If a large amount (greater than 200 mL) is obtained, withhold the medication and consult with a senior RN.

Flush the NGT with 30 mL of tepid water placed in the barrel of the syringe (no plunger), holding the syringe above the level of the stomach to allow gravity to gently move the water down through the tube. It should flow freely. Occlusion of the NGT is most often the result of mixing feeding formula and medication, so it is imperative to flush before and after each medication is introduced.

To prevent build-up of material within the NGT lumen, Abdelhadi, Barakat and Lyman (2022) recommend pulsing the flushes. Use a 50 mL syringe and tap or sterile water, and the plunger reinserted (so more pressure can be applied than the gravity feed without the plunger), to gently pulse the water in with short pushes on the plunger. Adhere to the facility's policy.

?

If there is an occlusion, and the attempt to flush fails, pinch the tube and remove the syringe. Return the plunger to the barrel and try to aspirate the solution above the blockage, then attempt to flush again. If the occlusion remains, use the hospital's protocol for unblocking the NGT (often a solution of bicarbonate of soda and a pancreatic enzyme in water is used to liquify the obstruction). The facility may have another protocol to unblock the tube (e.g. a declogger). If this is unsuccessful, the tube will need to be replaced.

PEGs and PEGJs are usually anchored into the stomach and there is no need to determine their placement before administering medication. Flushing the tube with water will demonstrate patency.

Administer the medication

To administer the medication, remove the plunger of the syringe (now containing about 30 mL of medication/water mixture), pinch the tubing and attach the barrel to the NGT. Unkink the tube. Hold the barrel of the syringe about 30 cm above the person's head (or above the entry point of the tube for PEG or PEGJ) and permit the fluid to flow under gravity only. Raise or lower the syringe to speed or slow the flow of fluid. Administer only one medication at a time. Flush the tube with 10 to 15 mL of sterile water (Bischoff et al., 2022; Rosana et al., 2020) between medications to prevent possible interactions or altered viscosity of medications because of differences in solution bases. Flush the tube with water when the medication has been completely administered. Pinch the tubing every time you detach the plunger to prevent air entry into the tubing. Cap the NGT for 30 minutes to improve the absorption of the medication(s). Reattach the feeding tube.

CLEAN, REPLACE AND DISPOSE OF EQUIPMENT

Discard any disposable items used to administer a medication, and clean and replace non-disposables in the trolley. Thoroughly clean the mortar and pestle. Replace stocks of supplies (e.g. plastic medication cups, large oral syringes, paper towels) as applicable, and order medications from the pharmacy if they are running low. When the medication arrives on the unit, place it so the label is visible to reduce the possibility of error. Finally, return the medication administration sheet to its designated place for the next medication round.

DOCUMENTATION

Document on the medication administration sheet (or electronic medication administration record [eMAR], which is automatic if using the bar code medication administration system), using an initial or signature in the appropriate timeslot beside the written medication order. Record the amount of liquid given on the intake sheet. If an assessment was done (e.g. pulse or blood pressure), also note it in the designated slot on the medication administration sheet. The effects of the medications, expected or unexpected, are assessed 30 minutes to one hour after administration, and are then documented. Adverse effects should be reported to the shift coordinator and the medical staff, and the remaining doses of the medication withheld.

PART 7

CLINICAL SKILLS ASSESSMENT

Enteral medication

Demonstrates the ability to effectively and safely administer medication enterally via nasogastric tube, percutaneous endoscopic gastrostomy tube or percutaneous endoscopic gastrojejunostomy tube. Incorporates the *National Safety and Quality Health Service Standards*: 2 Partnering with Consumers, 3 Preventing and Controlling Healthcare-Associated Infection, 5 Comprehensive Care, 6 Communicating for Safety, and 8 Recognising and Responding to Acute Deterioration (ACSQHC, 2021).

Performance criteria	1	2	3	4	5
(Numbers indicate NMBA *Registered Nurse Standards for Practice*)	**(Dependent)**	**(Marginal)**	**(Assisted)**	**(Supervised)**	**(Independent)**
1. Identifies indication (1.1, 3.3, 3.4)	☐	☐	☐	☐	☐
2. Verifies the validity of the written medication order (1.4, 3.4, 6.2, 6.5)	☐	☐	☐	☐	☐
3. Evidence of therapeutic interaction with the person, e.g. gives the person a clear explanation of the procedure, discusses adverse effects of the medication (1.4, 1.5, 2.1, 2.2, 3.2)	☐	☐	☐	☐	☐
4. Demonstrates clinical reasoning abilities, e.g. positions the person, obtains the appropriate form of the medication, assesses the person if warranted (1.1, 1.2, 1.3, 4.1, 4.2, 4.3, 6.1)	☐	☐	☐	☐	☐
5. Adheres to the general concepts of working with therapeutic substances (1.1, 1.3, 1.5, 3.3, 3.4, 4.1, 4.2, 4.3, 6.2, 6.5, 6.6)	☐	☐	☐	☐	☐
6. Gathers equipment (1.1, 5.5, 6.1): ■ medication trolley ■ medication administration sheet ■ graduated plastic cups or oral syringes ■ large oral syringe (30 to 50 mL) ■ pill cutter or knife ■ pill crusher or mortar and pestle ■ large plastic cup ■ tongue blade ■ clean gloves ■ paper towels ■ bottle of pH measurement strips, a tongue blade and a penlight ■ sterile or fresh tap water	☐	☐	☐	☐	☐
7. Uses the six (or more) rights to administer the medication (1.1, 1.2, 1.3, 1.4, 1.5, 2.2, 3.4, 4.1, 4.2, 4.3, 6.1, 6.2, 6.5, 6.6)	☐	☐	☐	☐	☐
8. Performs hand hygiene (1.1, 3.4, 6.1)	☐	☐	☐	☐	☐
9. Prepares the medication (1.1, 3.4, 6.1)	☐	☐	☐	☐	☐
10. Ascertains the placement of the nasogastric tube, disconnects the tube from the feeding line (1.1, 4.1, 4.2, 4.3, 6.1)	☐	☐	☐	☐	☐
11. Flushes the tube, administers the medication, flushes the tube (1.1, 6.1, 6.2, 6.5)	☐	☐	☐	☐	☐
12. Reconnects and re-establishes the feeding flow (1.1, 4.1, 6.1, 6.2)	☐	☐	☐	☐	☐
13. Cleans, replaces and disposes of equipment appropriately (3.6, 6.1)	☐	☐	☐	☐	☐
14. Documents relevant information (1.4, 1.6, 2.2, 3.5, 3.7, 6.2, 6.5, 7.3)	☐	☐	☐	☐	☐
15. Demonstrates the ability to link theory to practice (1.1, 3.3, 3.4, 3.5)	☐	☐	☐	☐	☐

Student:

Clinical facilitator: Date:

CHAPTER 39

TOPICAL MEDICATION

INDICATIONS

The skin is the largest organ in the body. It plays an active role in immunity by providing a protective barrier to most pathogens, it prevents water loss and it has a low permeability to most foreign substances (e.g. toxins) because they cannot penetrate through the layers and diffuse into the tissues and systemic circulation. Intact skin also insulates, maintains temperature, transmits sensation, synthesises vitamins, and absorbs oxygen and some medicines. The development of techniques and substances to increase the permeability of skin has permitted more medications to be successfully absorbed.

Topical medications are lotions, pastes, creams, foams, gels, ointments, films or patches that have active medication properties and are placed on the skin to be absorbed. These medications are absorbed locally (i.e. epicutaneously) for action at the point of application or just below the surface, but some may act systemically after being absorbed by the tissues (e.g. transdermal application and transdermal patches) and thus into the circulation. The vascularity of the skin influences the rate of absorption and thus the dose and effectiveness of the medication. Many of the types of medication administration – optic, otic, rectal, vaginal and inhalation – are actually topical applications (DeLaune et al., 2024); these are each addressed in separate skills, see **Clinical Skills 40 (optic), 41 (otic), 42 (vaginal), 43 (rectal) and 44 (inhaled)**. Buccal and sublingual medication are also topical; they are covered in **Clinical Skill 37 (oral)**.

Topical medications are applied to intact skin to:

- provide slow, even delivery of the medication to maintain a therapeutic dose over a long period of time (e.g. hormonal creams, glyceryl trinitrate, nicotine patches)
- bypass the gastrointestinal tract (e.g. if the medication causes gastrointestinal symptoms like nausea, diarrhoea; or if it is metabolised in the liver and rendered less effective)
- affect a local area, such as a topical anaesthetic or analgesic cream (e.g. Voltaren cream)
- protect skin in excoriation-prone areas (e.g. zinc cream for the perineal area during nappy changes)
- sooth damaged, inflamed skin (e.g. oatmeal, calamine lotion, corticosteroids)
- protect the skin by moisturising or blocking damaging rays (e.g. sunscreen).

Topical medications such as antiseptics and antimicrobials are also applied to open wounds to prevent or treat infection. Some topical medications are used for protection of an open wound, such as antiseptic sprays and liquid bandage, which seals the cut or abrasion and protects it from microbes.

Transdermal administration is a type of topical administration that occurs when a dose of a medication (a cream or ointment or gel) is applied to the skin and left for a period of time. Dose variations occur due to inconsistency in measuring, loss of medication due to removal by clothing, or increased dose by rubbing in the medication. The person must also deal with a potentially messy or perhaps staining product. Some of these problems are dealt with by covering the dose with a non-absorbent, impermeable strip that is taped in place.

Verify the written medication order

No medication can be legally administered without a valid, signed order from a qualified healthcare provider (see **Clinical Skill 37** for a description of a valid order). Some topical medications, such as antibiotics or steroid medications, require a finish or stop time. Most over-the-counter (OTC) topical medications (e.g. calamine lotion) can be given without an order. These are usually listed in the facility's policy manuals.

Nurses are responsible and accountable for questioning and clarifying any order that is unclear, incomplete or that seems inappropriate or unreasonable for the person (e.g. very high dose, contraindicated for their diagnosis, same medication with two different names). They are partly responsible (along with the physician) if an inappropriate order is followed. To question an order, you *must know* the person's diagnosis, the purpose of the medication, its therapeutic effect, any adverse and toxic effects, and the usual dose. Anticipate any pertinent nursing implications, such as the need to cover the area after application, as well as any personal factors that mediate response to medications, such as age, weight and psychological factors. Know any drug or food allergies that the person may have so that potentially harmful substances are not applied. The person's skin must be intact; that is, not have a traumatic injury, scarring or rashes to the area that would prevent the topical medication's absorption, unless the topical medication has been prescribed for the treatment of the bruise, rash, open area or scar.

PART 7

ELDER CARE

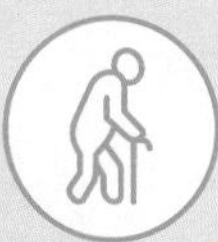

If elderly people are able to use them, topicals can be very effective and decrease drug–drug interactions and side effects by bypassing the gastrointestinal system (e.g. topical non-steroidal anti-inflammatory drugs [NSAIDs] for pain relief) or other systemic difficulties (e.g. decreased renal excretion). Elderly people often have comorbidities that reduce the effectiveness of topical medications (e.g. peripheral vascular disease). Elderly people need more astute assessment because their skin is generally thinner and more fragile, so tape or patches may tear the skin (Qiao, 2023). Although the absorption rate between younger and older skin is similar, due to other age-related changes, such as diminished renal and hepatic function, the medication dose may need to be adjusted to gain the desired effect, as with oral medications (Qiao, 2023). Adjustments of doses or frequency of application become necessary.

THE PERSON LIVING WITH SEVERE OBESITY

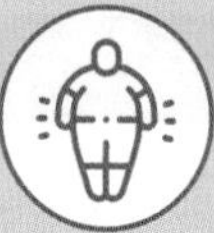

Diaphoresis often plagues people living with severe obesity. Take care that the skin where you intend to apply a topical medication is dry, both to assist in absorption and to help the adhesive covering (e.g. transdermal patches, tape from calibrated strips) to adhere.

EVIDENCE OF THERAPEUTIC INTERACTION

Help the person to better understand their medication regimen. This assists in reducing apprehension, anxiety and fear, increases their ability to relax and increases trust in healthcare personnel. The person may provide information vital to their care, such as sensitivities or allergies to the medication. Good communication will help gain their consent (verbal or tacit). Professional communication improves their comfort and safety, their trust in nurses and ultimately their health and wellbeing.

DEMONSTRATE CLINICAL REASONING

Topical medications require the same vigilance in their administration/application as do any other forms of medication. Be mindful that you are working with an active substance.

Position the person

Position the person to facilitate administering the topical medication. Expose just the area to be covered with the medication; do not expose the person unnecessarily, because it is important to preserve dignity and self-esteem. Make sure the area to be treated is easily accessible so you do not injure yourself while applying the medication. For application to intact skin (transdermal medications), choose areas that are relatively hairless and central to the body, such as the upper arms, chest or upper back (Cohrs & Kerns, 2020).

Assess and prepare the person

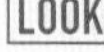 at the site chosen for medication administration. If the topical medication is transdermal, assess the site for irritation or skin breakdown. Broken skin will absorb medication at a faster rate than required and may cause systemic effects or increased irritation.

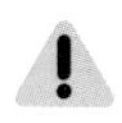

Safety

Changing the site frequently will prevent irritation and skin breakdown. If the previous medication was covered or a transdermal patch was used, carefully remove the patch or dressing, folding the medicated side inward and sealing it closed with the remaining adhesive. Dispose of this package into the clinical waste receptacle. Do not touch the medicated adhesive with bare fingers, because the medication is meant to be transcutaneous.

Take care that the patch or dressing is properly disposed of because contact could be injurious or even deadly to children or pets (e.g. fentanyl) (Cohrs & Kerns, 2020). Wash the area (intact skin) with a mild soap and water to cleanse the area of previous medication and debris and prevent overdose (or to remove oils, sweat and microorganisms from a fresh site). Encrustations can harbour microorganisms and increase the possibility of infections, and previously applied medication can prevent the absorption of the fresh medication and reduce its beneficial effects. Conversely, previously applied transdermal medications can still remain active and contribute to a dose of the medication that is greater than the therapeutic range. Old topical medication is removed generally by irrigation (see **Clinical Skill 69**).

LISTEN to any comments about pain or itchiness at the previous site. The medication or the adhesive may need to be altered.

FEEL the skin at the site chosen for moisture and dry the skin thoroughly before applying a topical medication. If the skin is dry and flakey, gently clean and leave it damp to apply a topical medication to retain the moisture.

General concepts of working with therapeutic substances

Legal responsibilities

Medications must be securely stored and safely administered. Topical medications will usually be stored in the medication trolley, either as a general medication or in the individual's drawer. Consent is required (usually tacit).

Calculating accurate dosages

Topical medications are no different than other methods of administration in the need for accuracy of dosing. Tubes of topical medications are often accompanied by a calibrated measuring strip onto which the medication is squeezed to the desired dose, and the strip is inverted onto the skin and taped in place to allow the medication to be absorbed over a specified period of time. Sometimes an order will specify the amount (e.g. 1 pump, 2 cm or a fingertip unit). A *fingertip unit* is the amount of medication expressed from a tube with a 5 mm opening onto the nurse's index finger from the skin crease of the first joint to the tip of the finger. Some orders will ask for the cream to be applied to an area 'thickly' or 'sparingly' (this may be used for an open wound like a burn). Other dosage instruments include foam or cream actuators that extrude a measured dose when the top is pushed, graduated syringe-type extruders, measuring scoops and tongue depressors. Many topical medications come with their own dosage system. You must become familiar with what is available and the dosage applicator for the medication that has been ordered.

Medication names and classifications You must be aware of the name, classification and indication of any medication you administer. See **Clinical Skill 37** for a discussion of medication names.

The formulations of topical medication include the following:

- *Solutions* – non-viscous mixtures containing the active medication dissolved in water or alcohol (e.g. the surgical scrub solution Betadine, a non-irritating antiseptic [check for iodine allergy]).
- *Lotions* – similar to solutions, but thicker. They often have oil in the mixture and tend to separate. Shake lotions well before use to re-suspend or emulsify all the ingredients (e.g. calamine lotion).
- *Creams* – emulsions of equal amounts of oil and water with the active ingredient homogenised into the mixture. They are thick and maintain their shape when removed from the container but loosen with body heat. They often provide moisturisation for the skin as well as the effect of the medication (e.g. nitroglycerin cream).
- *Ointments* – semi-solid, generally greasy (80% oil, 20% water) concoctions that may or may not be medicated. Non-medicated ointments are used to moisturise the skin and protect it. They provide a semi-occlusive cover (e.g. barrier ointments such as zinc oxide). Medication is added to an ointment base (e.g. beeswax, paraffin or almond oil) and is released to penetrate the skin for absorption into the tissue or to the bloodstream (e.g. Bacitracin ointment).
- *Gels* – semisolid emulsions in an alcohol base. Many melt at body temperature and are drying because of the alcohol (e.g. Picato gel used for removal of solar keratosis).
- *Foams and aerosol sprays* – aerated emulsions often medicated with steroids or antibiotics; (e.g. BenzEFoam used to treat acne).
- *Powders* – finely ground medication mixed with a carrier such as cornflour (e.g. antifungal Micatin powder).
- *Pastes* – ointment in which a powdered medication is suspended (e.g. Kenalog in Orabase, a corticosteroid used inside the mouth).
- *Tinctures* – alcohol-based solutions; are very drying (e.g. tincture of Benzoin).
- *Transdermal patches* – available in three basic types: adhesive (a medication-containing adhesive on a backing material); a layered or matrix (medication is in a matrix, with an adhesive layer and a backing material); and a reservoir (a reservoir of medication enclosed in a membrane layer, an adhesive layer and a backing material). Transdermal delivery uses percutaneous absorption to reach systemic therapeutic levels. It can be delivered distally from the site of action (e.g. patch on arm, action on heart). This type of delivery system can provide a precise dosage over a specified time, although delay in reaching therapeutic levels may be 18 to 48 hours (Tverdohleb, Candido & Knezevic, 2019). Cutting the patch affects the dose delivered and may reduce the dose due to drying of the base medication. A nicotine patch is an example.

Transdermal patches have several advantages over oral medications:

- They bypass the first pass metabolism in the liver faced by oral medications (Qiao, 2023).
- The level of medication can be maintained within a therapeutic range longer than with oral medications.
- There are fewer adverse effects; particularly gastrointestinal, such as nausea, vomiting and other gastrointestinal symptoms (Shukla, Shukla & Srivastava, 2023).
- Their effect can be stopped immediately by removing the patch.
- There may be fewer medication interactions if the person is taking more than one medication (Shukla, Shukla & Srivastava, 2023).
- Antibacterial topical medication is preferred over systemic administration for skin infections due to the higher concentration of medication to the site of infection and reduced toxicity and bacterial resistance (Amirthalingam et al., 2015), although some medications require a 12-hour break to prevent irritation (Leppert et al., 2018).

However, not all medications are suitable for administering via a patch; medications that irritate the skin and those that are not potent enough to cross the dermal barrier and remain effective cannot be given this way.

Mechanisms of medication administration

Preparation

To reduce errors, administer only medications that you have personally prepared, and undertake the following:

- *Be aware of allergies* – check the medication administration sheet for an allergy caution, look for an allergy armband (red) and ask the person if they are allergic to anything. Ask them if they have taken this medication before and, if so, have they tolerated it.
- *Ask the person to state their name* – don't ask them if their name is 'Mary Smith', for example; they may say 'yes', regardless of who they are (e.g. they may be deaf, confused, non-English speaking or mischievous).
- *Listen to the person* – many, if not most, people know their medications well, and any query by them as to the amount or appearance of the topical medication should be taken seriously before administering the dose. Recheck the medication administration sheet and the medication container and ask the prescriber about the medication. This validates the person's knowledge and prevents medication-administration errors.
- *Sign or initial the medications sheet/electronic medication administration record (eMAR)* – do this as soon as a dose of medication is applied. This prevents a potential overdose (i.e. another nurse might administer a second dose of the medication thinking it has not been given). Most facilities do not allow you to sign prior to giving the medication, only after the dose has been given. Bar code medication administration systems automatically record the administration when the person's ID, your ID and the medication bar code are read.

Responsibility to the person

Your responsibility involves assessment, teaching, advocacy and evaluation of the effect of the medication administered.

Assess the physiological or psychological function that the medication is expected to affect prior to applying a topical medication. Examples would be pain assessment prior to administering an analgesic cream (e.g. Voltaren), pulse assessment prior to administering a nitroglycerin patch and a local inflammation assessment prior to administering a corticosteroid. The assessment may indicate that the medication should be withheld and the shift coordinator informed, or it may provide a baseline for evaluating the medication's effectiveness.

Also assess the person's medication history (i.e. a review of the person's current and past drugs – prescribed, OTC, herbal preparations or recreational) and history of allergies or adverse reactions.

Teach the person the name and dose of the medication they are taking, its frequency, adverse effects and how to minimise these. Measuring and applying the correct dose is an important aspect of teaching people to care for themselves. They need to know any implications of taking the medication (e.g. if the area should be covered or remain open to the air, or the medication rubbed in or not). They need to know if the medication will stain their clothing and should be covered. They must know not to use heat (heating pads, hot water bottles) over the area treated with a topical medication as heat increases circulation and therefore speeds absorption rate of the medication, increasing the risk of toxicity or overdose (Cohrs & Kerns, 2020). Discuss maintaining the medication regimen at home and adapt the regimen to accommodate the person's home schedule (without compromising the efficacy of the medication). They need to be aware of the importance of regular monitoring required for some medications (e.g. nitroglycerin patches). Be alert to any cues the person or their family might give about not continuing to use a medication, such as concerns about the cost, inconvenience, adverse effects, or a negative self-concept. Discuss disposing of used material (tongue depressors, cling wrap, bandages) safely, as ingestion of some medications by a child or pet may be fatal, or at least cause severe symptoms (Asad, Boothe & Tarbox, 2019). Discussing these things may improve the person's commitment to sustaining the prescribed treatment.

Advocacy includes alerting the medical practitioner of adverse effects, or any reason the person tells you that would influence their continuation of topical medication use.

Evaluation is a very important aspect of your responsibility in administering medications. You (and the prescribing doctor) need to be aware that the medication is doing what it is meant to. Reassess the person following administration of medications such as anti-inflammatories, antibiotics, anaesthetics, analgesics, corticosteroids, among others. This should be done within a reasonable time frame from the administration (usually 30 minutes to one hour following) and effects noted. Watch out for unexpected effects such as rashes due to reactions to carrier ingredients in the topical medication. This evaluation is crucial following the initial administration of a topical medication.

GATHER EQUIPMENT

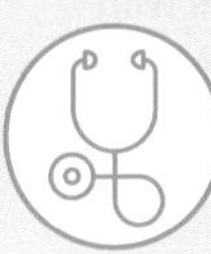

Gathering equipment is an organisational step that helps to create a positive environment for a successful interaction. The medication trolley is usually stocked with all of the necessary equipment for administering a topical medication along with the prescribed topical medication. Drawers with individual names may be used to hold non-stock prescription medications for each person. Familiarise yourself with the trolley used in the facility. The trolley should contain:

EQUIPMENT	EXPLANATION
Calibrated measuring strips	Are marked in millimetres and used to measure the dose of ointments and creams. Come in booklets and torn out as needed
Sterile tongue depressors	To scoop medicated cream out of a large jar and to spread it on an area of skin. Clean depressor required for each 'scoop' into the jar.
Medication swabs (giant cotton buds)	To spread softer creams and lotions over an area of skin
Clean gloves	• To apply topical medication to intact skin • Protect you from absorbing the medication
Sterile gloves	For open wounds (e.g. burns) so there is less chance of contaminating the wound
Cling wrap and net gauze (or similar)	To cover the medicated area to both keep the medication in place and in contact with the skin and to prevent staining of clothing

THE SIX RIGHTS OF ADMINISTERING MEDICATION

See **Clinical Skill 37** for a complete description of the rights of medication administration. In summary, they include:

- *right time* – the first consideration
- *right medication* – verify the validity of the order and then choose from the medications on the trolley
- *right route* – confirm this as noted on the medication administration sheet
- *right dose* – it is imperative to gain a therapeutic level of the medication. Many topical medications come in a range of strengths – be sure you have the right one
- *right person* – it is vital to verify the correct person is receiving the medication
- *right documentation* – must be adhered to.

ADMINISTER TOPICAL MEDICATION

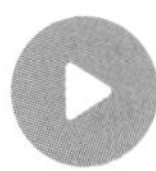

Video

The process of topical medication administration includes preparing the person and the medication (measuring an accurate dose), positioning the person, administering the medication to the appropriate site and then covering the site if required.

Hand hygiene

Prior to and following each individual contact, before beginning a medication round, and after it is completed, hand hygiene is undertaken. Usually this is alcohol-based hand rub (ABHR), unless your hands are visibly soiled. Hand hygiene (see **Clinical Skill 5**) is especially important following topical medication administration in case of inadvertent contamination of your skin with the medication.

Applying medications to open wounds, such as burns, is treated as an aseptic procedure and requires surgical asepsis (see **Clinical Skills 7, 8 and 9**).

Prepare the medication

Topical medications generally require little preparation. Lotions and emulsions are shaken. The lips of tubes or jars of cream, gel or ointment are wiped to remove old residue. Transdermal patches are removed from their packaging and handled by the edges of the patch, leaving the protective plastic covering over the adhesive until you are ready to apply it.

Administer the medication

Hand hygiene is imperative. Clean gloves are used to apply most topical medications to unbroken skin. Sterile gloves are used for broken skin to reduce the spread of infection. Both clean and sterile gloves prevent your contact with the medication (you can absorb it, too). The following suggestions increase absorption and comfort.

Creams, ointments, gels

- Use a measuring scoop or tongue depressor to take the required dose of topical medication from the container and transfer it to your gloved fingers or a medication applicator swab.
- If an ointment is 'stiff', warm it by rubbing between your gloved hands to soften it.
- Centre and firmly tape a calibrated strip over the area to be treated.
- Spread the medication over the affected area with long, sweeping strokes, working in the direction of the growth of hair to reduce the amount of medication forced into the hair follicles. If using for a rash or scaly skin, apply to the edges of the affected area, or as prescribed.

- Depending on the medication, you may need to gently massage the medication into the area or just leave it spread over the area. Do not rub vigorously unless the order directs it to be rubbed in – take care to be gentle.
- Many medicated areas will need to be covered (as ordered) to contain the cream/gel/ointment, increase absorption and prevent its removal by bed clothing or the person's clothing, to prevent staining and to provide a reminder to the person not to rub it in. Check with the pharmacy, as wrapping the area increases heat and moisture and alters the absorption of the medication. Clear plastic wrap (e.g. cling wrap) is often used for this because it is non-absorbent and remains in place reasonably well without adhesive tape. It may be wrapped with an elastic net bandage or a gauze bandage for extra security.

Medicinal powders

- Powders must not be applied to damp skin (they will cake and fall off).
- Powders can irritate the respiratory tract, so ask the person to turn their head away.
- Cover the site (if ordered) to prevent soiling of clothing and increase absorption.

Transdermal patches

- Transdermal patches are applied as soon as they are removed from their packaging to prevent any deterioration in the potency of the medication. Remove the protective plastic covering from the adhesive (like a Band-Aid) without touching the adhesive/medication so the dose will not be affected.
- Apply to a clean, dry hairless area (clip hair if necessary to avoid irritation from shaving) to provide a consistent surface for absorption.
- Hold the patch by the edges only to place the patch, then hold it in place with your palm for approximately 10 seconds, and smooth out the adhesive edges to increase adherence. The heat of your hand and the pressure assist the patch to adhere. Take care that the patch is well adhered around the edges to prevent premature or accidental removal and thus an altered dose.
- Write a date and time along with your initials on the edge of the patch so that other staff know when the medication must be reapplied. Many patches are removed overnight to prevent tolerance to the medication – check orders.

?

If the medication is transdermal but not a patch, you will probably need to cover it. Covering the dose with a non-absorbent, impermeable strip that is taped in place prevents its removal and ensures that the entire dose is available for absorption. Often, the calibrated measuring strip is used for this.

Post-procedure

Ask the person to inform you if the area becomes itchy, tender or inflamed. This could indicate a sensitivity to the medication or worsening of any skin lesions that are being treated. Any such occurrences should be reported to the physician. Check back with the person to determine if there is any irritation of the area, especially for the first several doses.

CLEAN, REPLACE AND DISPOSE OF EQUIPMENT

Discard any disposable items used to administer a topical medication (e.g. gloves, tongue depressor), and clean and replace non-disposable items in the trolley (e.g. measuring scoop). Replace stocks of supplies. Wipe the cart clean of spills or debris and wipe any spills from individual bottles, or from sticky tubes and around the caps. Order stock medications and individual prescriptions from the pharmacy if they are running low. When they arrive on the unit, place them in the medication trolley with their labels visible to reduce the possibility of errors. Return the medication administration sheet to its designated place for the next medication round.

DOCUMENTATION

Initial or sign the medication administration sheet in the appropriate timeslot beside the written medication order and note if an assessment was done (e.g. skin condition, pain). Use the bar code medication administration system and the eMAR in the facility as provided. Also document briefly on the medication administration sheet in the appropriate timeslot if an individual has refused to take the medication or some other untoward event occurs, then document it more fully in the progress notes. The effects of the medications, expected or unexpected, are assessed 30 minutes to one hour after administration, and are then documented. Adverse effects should be reported to the shift coordinator and the medical staff, and the remaining doses of the medication withheld.

CLINICAL SKILLS ASSESSMENT

Topical medication

Demonstrates the ability to effectively administer topical medication. Incorporates the *National Safety and Quality Health Service Standards*: 2 Partnering with Consumers, 3 Preventing and Controlling Healthcare-Associated Infection, 5 Comprehensive Care, 6 Communicating for Safety, and 8 Recognising and Responding to Acute Deterioration (ACSQHC, 2021).

Performance criteria	**1**	**2**	**3**	**4**	**5**
(Numbers indicate NMBA *Registered Nurse Standards for Practice*)	**(Dependent)**	**(Marginal)**	**(Assisted)**	**(Supervised)**	**(Independent)**
1. Identifies indication (1.1, 3.3, 3.4)	☐	☐	☐	☐	☐
2. Verifies the validity of the written medication order (1.4, 3.4, 6.2, 6.5)	☐	☐	☐	☐	☐
3. Evidence of therapeutic interaction with the person, e.g. gives the person a clear explanation of the procedure (1.4, 1.5, 2.1, 2.2, 3.2)	☐	☐	☐	☐	☐
4. Demonstrates clinical reasoning, e.g. positions the person, exposes the site, assesses and cleans the site (1.1, 1.2, 1.3, 4.2, 6.1)	☐	☐	☐	☐	☐
5. Adheres to the general concepts of working with therapeutic substances (1.1, 1.3, 1.5, 3.3, 3.4, 4.1, 4.2, 4.3, 6.2, 6.5, 6.6)	☐	☐	☐	☐	☐
6. Gathers equipment (1.1, 5.5, 6.1): ■ calibrated measuring strips ■ sterile tongue depressors ■ medication swabs (giant cotton buds) ■ clean gloves ■ sterile gloves ■ cling wrap and net gauze (or similar)	☐	☐	☐	☐	☐
7. Uses the six (or more, according to facility/university requirements) rights to administer the medication (1.1, 1.2, 1.3, 1.4, 1.5, 2.2, 3.4, 4.1, 4.2, 4.3, 6.1, 6.2, 6.5, 6.6)	☐	☐	☐	☐	☐
8. Performs hand hygiene (1.1, 3.4, 6.1)	☐	☐	☐	☐	☐
9. Measures the topical medication (1.1, 6.1)	☐	☐	☐	☐	☐
10. Applies the medication appropriately (1.1, 6.1)	☐	☐	☐	☐	☐
11. Covers the medicated site as appropriate (1.1, 6.1)	☐	☐	☐	☐	☐
12. Cleans, replaces and disposes of equipment appropriately (3.6, 6.1)	☐	☐	☐	☐	☐
13. Documents relevant information (1.4, 1.6, 2.2, 3.5, 3.7, 6.2, 6.5, 7.3)	☐	☐	☐	☐	☐
14. Demonstrates the ability to link theory to practice (1.1, 3.3, 3.4, 3.5)	☐	☐	☐	☐	☐

Student:

Clinical facilitator: Date:

CHAPTER 40

OPTIC MEDICATION

INDICATIONS

Optic (or ophthalmic) medications are medicated drops or ointment that are administered into the eye. They:

- keep the eye moist
- prevent corneal damage if the person is unconscious, has reduced production of lacrimal fluid or has ectropion
- reduce inflammation
- fight bacterial, viral or fungal infections
- control glaucoma
- constrict or dilate the pupil
- vasoconstrict (e.g. Visine) or treat allergy symptoms (e.g. antihistamines).

Verify the written medication order

A valid, signed order from a qualified healthcare provider (see **Clinical Skill 37** for a description of a valid order) is required. Follow the written medication order to ensure the person receives the right medication and dosage (i.e. number of drops) at the right time and in the correct eye.

Instilling eye medication is the same as any medication procedure. Two nurses check the medication 'rights' at the bedside. Follow the policy at the facility you are attending.

Medication-loaded contact lenses are being developed and used. They demonstrate improved bioavailability of the medication, improved safety, good biocompatability and reduced side effects (Zhao et al., 2023). This skill addresses instillation of optic drops and ointments only.

EVIDENCE OF THERAPEUTIC INTERACTION

The person will be more willing and able to cooperate if they are aware of what to expect during the procedure. Explanation also reduces apprehension and promotes relaxation. People need to know the expected sensations and effects of the medication. Warn the person of the expected temporary effect of the medication on their vision, to wear sunglasses and avoid driving following instillation of drops (Broyles et al., 2017). Instruction in instilling eye drops is essential to ongoing care (The Eye Practice, 2020).

DEMONSTRATE CLINICAL REASONING

Clinical reasoning when administering medications involves assessment, consideration of the person's safety and comfort, knowledge of the medication, the person's condition, the general concepts and the mechanisms of medication administration.

Privacy, safety and comfort

Provide privacy, comfort measures and pain relief as necessary. Privacy reduces anxiety and feelings of embarrassment. Comfort measures such as toileting, positioning, fluids or pain relief increase comfort and minimise disruptions to the procedure.

Adequate lighting enables maximum observation to reduce harm or discomfort. Remove soft or gas-permeable contact lenses before instillation and reinsert after an interval of at least 15 minutes after the eye drops (Glaucoma Australia, 2023).

ELDER CARE

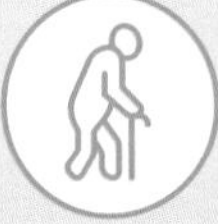

Dry eyes from either underproduction of tears or increased tear evaporation plagues about half of all elderly adults, and is more prevalent in females (due to altered hormones). This causes blurred vision, pain, 'foreign object' sensation, photosensitivity and excess tearing. People will be ordered (among other things) a prescription ointment and artificial tears (Erdinest et al., 2021). Elderly people often have problems instilling the drops/ointment (due to arthritic fingers or tremor, for example) reducing the efficiency of the medication and often leading to contamination of the bottle/tube (Zhao et al., 2023). Assistive devices are available that help 'place' the dropper in the correct position and reduce the force required to squeeze the bottle.

THE PERSON LIVING WITH SEVERE OBESITY

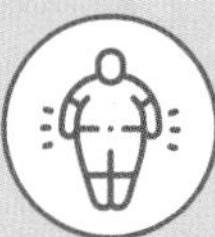

Bayat et al. (2023) demonstrated tear abnormalities (amount, viscosity, tear breakup time) in children who are obese, causing 'dry eye'. These abnormalities were exacerbated by insulin resistance and metabolic syndrome. Ismail, El-Azeim and Saif (2023) found similar changes in older people living with severe obesity due to low level inflammation affecting tear production. As well, people living with severe obesity may be unable to administer their own eye medication due to dexterity (reaching both hands to the eye area or extending the neck) and may need a helper for this procedure.

Position the person

Ask the person to sit or lie down. Have them tilt their head back (unless there is cervical spine trauma), turn it towards the side to be treated and open their eyes (Glaucoma Australia, 2023). This position provides an area furthest away from the tear duct in which to place the medication. Any excess will flow away from the tear duct and minimise systemic absorption of the solution. Ask the person to roll their eyes upwards and away from you, to reduce the blink reflex, to move the cornea away from the lower lid and reduce the risk of corneal damage from inadvertently touching the medication dropper to the cornea, or from dropping solution onto it (The Eye Practice, 2020).

Assess and prepare the person

LOOK at the external eye structures.

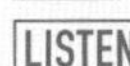

LISTEN to any comments about pain or itchiness in the eye, or about altered vision. Document these.

General concepts of working with therapeutic substances

The concepts of working with medications have been explained in **Clinical Skills 37 and 38**. Please review these if necessary.

Mechanisms of medication administration

Single-dose containers are often used to prevent contamination of the solution. Yilmaz et al. (2023) demonstrated bacterial contamination of ophthalmic drops and ointments in 12.9 per cent of people tested over 23 countries. They suggest not using the same container for both eyes, especially in those with infections (e.g. conjunctivitis, keratitis) or after intraocular surgeries (e.g. cataracts).

However, Palmer et al. (2022) argue for the use of multidose containers for multiple people undergoing ophthalmologic surgery, demonstrating the safety of this practice if stringent clinical guidelines are followed, and reducing waste and cost. Follow the policies of the facility where you are practising.

Different medications or different dosages may be ordered for each eye. If more than one medication is ordered for each eye, the timing of each should be staggered to promote maximum absorption. If two different drops are required at the same time, allow a minimum interval of five minutes before instilling the second preparation to allow maximum absorption and to prevent dilution or overflow (American Academy of Ophthalmology, 2023). However, when separate solutions of miotic drops and adrenaline are needed, wait two to 10 minutes after the miotic drops before instilling the adrenaline. If both eye drops and ointment are ordered for the same eye, instil the drops first to promote better absorption.

Responsibility to the person

Your responsibility involves assessment, teaching, advocacy and evaluation of the effect of the medication administered.

Medication cannot work if it is not taken. Adherence to the medication regimen is often problematic due to arthritis, tremors, forgetfulness, unpleasant side effects (e.g. blurred vision) and 'invisibility' of the condition (e.g. glaucoma where symptoms are insidious) (Biran et al., 2023). Individual instruction increases adherence and persistence to the medication regimen (Talha, 2023). Teaching includes:

- the name of and reason for taking the drops or ointment (this is especially important in a disease like glaucoma – symptoms are very slow to appear but result in loss of sight).
- frequency and dose – you will need to stress the interval between the doses if there are two or more medications
- good instruction on instilling the drops/ ointment (see **Clinical Skill 27** for information on healthcare teaching)
- use of reminder devices such as phone apps (Glaucoma Australia supplies an app that organises medications at the pharmacy and reminds the person of each dose) or tying the administration to meals or bedtime (Javidi et al., 2020).

Safety

Eye administration of non-ocular medications is under-recognised. Conversely, accidental eye administration of 'superglue' (cyanoacrylates) mistaken for eye drops is well documented. Teach the person the following to minimise the possibility of accidental administration of non-ophthalmic medication into the eye:

- Keep optic medications in a separate place from all other drops and ointments.
- Read the name of the medication each time you administer it.
- Keep the optic medication in its original box (so you read the name twice).

Refer to previous chapters for more information on this aspect of administering medications.

GATHER EQUIPMENT

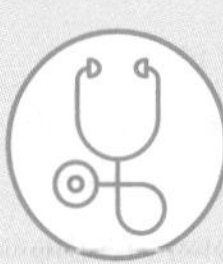

Gathering equipment is an organisational step that ensures that you have all needed material, boosts the person's confidence and trust in you, and increases your self-confidence. The following materials are brought to the bedside and placed on a clean surface:

EQUIPMENT	EXPLANATION
Written medication order	To check the five rights and to complete the sixth one (see **Clinical Skill 37** for a further explanation of the 'six rights' of medication administration)
Ophthalmic drops or ointment	• Check it is marked 'For Ophthalmic Use' • Check the prescribed medication's name and strength, the expiry date, any discolouration, precipitation or cloudiness (if not meant to be) • Clearly mark a new bottle of drops with the person's name and expiry date – usually 28 days after opening (Rull, 2016) • Often kept at the person's bedside and are not used for anyone else
Eye patch and tape	May be required for children, those with diminished consciousness, following local anaesthesia that reduces the blink reflex, anyone who has a large amount of drainage or is photosensitive
Clean gloves	For your protection and that of the person
Gauze pads and sterile water	To cleanse the eye (follow the policies of the facility you are practising in)
Tissues or sterile gauze squares	To blot excess drops or secretions that run out of the conjunctival sac

THE SIX RIGHTS OF ADMINISTERING MEDICATION

See **Clinical Skill 37** for a complete description of the rights of medication administration. In summary, they include:

- *right time* – the first consideration
- *right medication* – verify the validity of the order and then choose from the medications on the trolley. Check that it is designated 'For OPTIC use'
- *right route* – as noted on the medication administration sheet. Check again that it is for optic administration
- *right dose* – it is imperative to gain a therapeutic level of the medication
- *right person* – it is vital to verify the correct person is receiving the medication
- *right documentation* – must be adhered to.

For optic medication, ensure that the correct eye is being treated.

ADMINISTER OPTIC MEDICATION

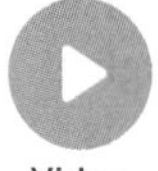

Video

The process of optic medication administration includes assessing and preparing the person and the medication (measuring an accurate dose), positioning the person, and administering the medication to the appropriate eye, either by instilling drops or applying ointment.

Hand hygiene

Hand hygiene (see **Clinical Skill 5**) reduces the spread of microorganisms. Gloves (see **Clinical Skill 6**) protect you from the person's secretions and reduce the spread of microorganisms.

Cleanse the eye

Remove secretions, old medication and any debris from the lids as necessary, using sterile water, normal saline (NS) and a fresh, sterile, low-lint gauze square (or warm tap water and a clean area of the washcloth). Bathe the eyes with the lids closed to prevent damaging the cornea when removing any crusted discharge (Gwenhure & Shepherd, 2019). Cleanse the lower lid first, then the upper lid. Start each stroke at the medial canthus and sweep towards the outer canthus to prevent material being introduced into the lacrimal ducts. If there is a large amount of matter at the medial canthus, remove it first, using a dabbing stroke so that the matter is not moved back across the eye. If matter is crusted on the lids, soak low-lint gauze squares in sterile water or NS (or use a warm, damp washcloth) and rest it on the closed lids for several minutes to soften the crusting and make removal easier.

Prepare the ophthalmic drops

Check the expiration date; once opened, optic drops are considered 'expired' at 30 days (Reed, 2022). Gently roll the bottle between your palms to mix the solution. Open the bottle and place the lid securely on a clean surface, either on its side or with the open portion uppermost. This reduces the chance of contaminating the lid and then the solution. If using an eye-dropper rather than a direct-dispenser container, open it at this point, fill it to the required level and rest it in the open bottle until it is needed.

Instil ophthalmic drops

Always treat the uninfected or uninflamed eye first to reduce the risk of cross-infection, Wear clean gloves.

Steady the dominant hand

Put the heel of your dominant hand on the person's forehead. It will move with the person's head to reduce the chance of inadvertently touching or damaging the eye with the container/dropper. Cover the fingers of your non-dominant hand with a gauze square and gently pull the lower lid downwards, forming a sac in the conjunctival fold to place the medication. This also reduces the ability to squint or blink. The fingers pulling the lower lid gently downwards should rest on the bony orbit to minimise the risk of touching the cornea and to prevent any pressure being put on the eyeball. Approach the eye from the side to reduce the blink reflex. Keep the tip of the container away from the lashes, eyeball or conjunctiva.

A new administration device is becoming available that has a silicone sleeve on the side of the dropper bottle. This balances on the bridge of the nose to steady the dropper, position it over the correct location, and prevents contaminating the dropper (Sanchez et al., 2020).

Administer ophthalmic drops

Hold the medication dropper/container tip vertically 1 to 2 cm above the conjunctival sac to minimise the chance of accidental contact and causing injury to the eye or contamination of the medication. Bacterial colonisation of the medication following contamination occurs quickly if the tip is touched to the eye or by the fingers. If the tip touches anything, the medication is contaminated and must be discarded. Place the drop in the outer third of the conjunctival sac to reduce discomfort (i.e. from stimulation of the cornea) and avoid immediate loss of the drops into the nasolacrimal drainage system (Glaucoma Australia [n.d.]).

Occlude the punctum by applying gentle pressure near the bridge of the nose below the eye for one to two minutes to increase the contact of the medication with the eyeball and decrease the chance of systemic absorption. The person may do this using a moistened, sterile, lint-free gauze square or clean tissue. Ask them to blink to distribute the medication over the entire eyeball. Blot excess medication, increasing comfort and reducing the possibility of skin irritation. If required, a sterile eye pad is taped securely over the closed affected eye. See FIGURE 40.1.

> ?
>
> If the person cannot keep their eyelid open so you can place the drop into the lower conjunctival sac, ask the person to lie down, and administer the drops into the medial canthus. Comparable concentrations of most optic medications were found when drops were applied either way (Great Ormond Street Hospital for Children, 2020).

Administer ointment

Squeeze out a small amount of ointment and discard it to remove any that has been contaminated by the lid or during use. Next, holding the tip of the tube 1 cm above the conjunctival sac, squeeze a ribbon of ointment into and along the conjunctival sac (as above) from the inner to the outer canthus. Do not touch the tip to the conjunctiva. To prevent pulling the ribbon of ointment out of the conjunctival sac, when you lift the tube up and away, turn your hand. Ask the person to gently close their eye, keep it closed for one minute and roll their eye. Rolling their eyes behind closed lids melts the ointment with body heat and distributes the medication over the eyeball. Warn the person that their vision may be blurred for a short while following ointment administration. If two ointments are ordered, wait 30 minutes after the first ointment before administering the second (see FIGURE 40.1).

Post-procedure

Assist the person into a comfortable position. Help them to remove excess ointment from their lids, as it can cause irritation and possibly contact dermatitis. Assess the effect of the medication.

CLEAN, REPLACE AND DISPOSE OF EQUIPMENT

Remove gloves and discard along with any soiled tissues into a waste bin. If no contamination has occurred, return medication to appropriate storage (generally, below 25 °C and protected from the light, or as stated on the manufacturer's information sheet). Some ointments and drops require refrigeration.

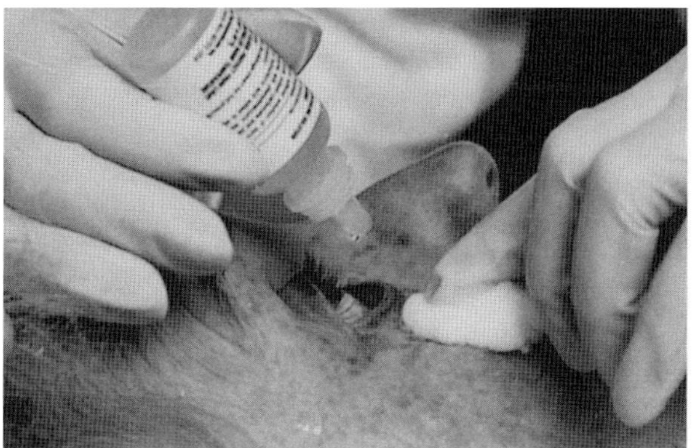

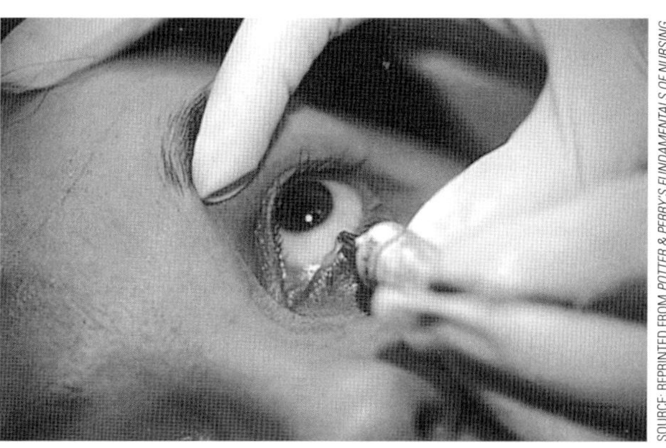

FIGURE 40.1 Administering eye medication: drops and ointment

DOCUMENTATION

Initial or sign the medication administration sheet in the appropriate spot beside the written medication order. Include which eye the medication was instilled into, and the time it was given. Or use the electronic medication administration record (eMAR) and the bar code medication administration system as appropriate. Note the appearance of the eye in the progress notes. If the medication was refused or you were unable to administer it for some other reason, document this on the medication sheet briefly and explain it in the progress notes. Report any adverse effects of the medication so a decision can be made whether to continue with it or change the prescription.

CLINICAL SKILLS ASSESSMENT

Optic medication

Demonstrates the ability to effectively administer optic medication. Incorporates the *National Safety and Quality Health Service Standards*: 2 Partnering with Consumers, 3 Preventing and Controlling Healthcare-Associated Infection, 5 Comprehensive Care, 6 Communicating for Safety, and 8 Recognising and Responding to Acute Deterioration (ACSQHC, 2021).

Performance criteria	**1**	**2**	**3**	**4**	**5**
(Numbers indicate NMBA *Registered Nurse Standards for Practice*)	**(Dependent)**	**(Marginal)**	**(Assisted)**	**(Supervised)**	**(Independent)**
1. Identifies indication (1.1, 3.3, 3.4)	☐	☐	☐	☐	☐
2. Verifies the written medication order, identifies the eye to be treated (1.4, 3.4, 6.2, 6.5)	☐	☐	☐	☐	☐
3. Evidence of therapeutic interaction with the person, e.g. gives the person a clear explanation of the procedure, positions the person (1.4, 1.5, 2.1, 2.2, 3.2)	☐	☐	☐	☐	☐
4. Demonstrates clinical reasoning abilities, e.g. provides privacy, comfort measures and pain relief as necessary (1.1, 1.2, 1.3, 4.2, 6.1)	☐	☐	☐	☐	☐
5. Adheres to the general concepts of working with therapeutic substances and understands the mechanisms of medication administration (1.1, 1.3, 1.5, 3.3, 3.4, 4.1, 4.2, 4.3, 6.2, 6.5, 6.6)	☐	☐	☐	☐	☐
6. Gathers equipment (1.1, 5.5, 6.1): ■ written medication order ■ ophthalmic drops or ointment ■ eye patch and tape ■ clean gloves ■ gauze pads and sterile water ■ tissues or sterile gauze squares	☐	☐	☐	☐	☐
7. Uses the six (or more) rights to administer the medication (1.1, 1.2, 1.3, 1.4, 1.5, 2.2, 3.4, 4.1, 4.2, 4.3, 6.1, 6.2, 6.5, 6.6)	☐	☐	☐	☐	☐
8. Performs hand hygiene (1.1, 3.4, 6.1)	☐	☐	☐	☐	☐
9. Assesses and prepares the person (1.1, 4.2, 6.1)	☐	☐	☐	☐	☐
10. Steadies the dominant hand on the person's forehead (1.1, 6.1)	☐	☐	☐	☐	☐
11. Pulls the lower lid down with the non-dominant hand (1.1, 6.1)	☐	☐	☐	☐	☐
12a. Instils drops into the conjunctival sac (1.1, 6.1)	☐	☐	☐	☐	☐
12b. Asks the person to blink (1.1, 6.1)	☐	☐	☐	☐	☐
12c. Uses a tissue to blot excess medication off lid/cheek (1.1, 6.1)	☐	☐	☐	☐	☐
13a. Squeezes a little ointment out and discards it (1.1, 3.4, 6.1)	☐	☐	☐	☐	☐
13b. Squeezes a ribbon of ointment into the lower conjunctival sac (1.1, 6.1)	☐	☐	☐	☐	☐
13c. Asks the person to roll their eyes behind closed lids (1.1, 6.1)	☐	☐	☐	☐	☐
14. Cleans, replaces and disposes of equipment appropriately (3.6, 6.1)	☐	☐	☐	☐	☐
15. Documents relevant information (1.4, 1.6, 2.2, 3.5, 3.7, 6.2, 6.5, 7.3)	☐	☐	☐	☐	☐
16. Demonstrates the ability to link theory to practice (1.1, 3.3, 3.4, 3.5)	☐	☐	☐	☐	☐

Student:

Clinical facilitator: Date:

CHAPTER 41

OTIC MEDICATION

INDICATIONS

Otic medications are those administered into the ear. Ear drops and ointment are used to treat pain, inflammation, bacterial or fungal infection or to remove cerumen (wax). Medications are often combined (e.g. corticosteroids plus antimicrobials) and administered as drops, solutions, ointments or creams (Australian Commission on Safety and Quality Health Care [ACSQHC]/NPS Medicinewise, 2022). They may be used to treat local conditions (e.g. otitis externa) or be meant to cross the tympanic membrane (trans-tympanic to treat otitis media). Local medication delivery into the ear canal or trans-tympanic delivers a high local therapeutic dose with minimal systemic effects (Takahashi et al., 2023).

While the structures of the outer ear are not sterile, it is important to use sterile drops or solutions in case the eardrum is perforated. Contaminated solutions entering into the middle ear can cause serious infections.

Avoid forcing any solutions into the ear. It is important not to occlude the ear canal with the dropper, as this can increase pressure within the canal during instillation and cause injury to the skin or the tympanic membrane. The World Health Organization (WHO, 2023) notes that ear drops containing alcohol-based antiseptics such as chlorhexidine should not be administered if the tympanic membrane is perforated.

Verify the written medication order

The written medication order ensures that the person receives the medication and dosage (i.e. concentration and number of drops) at the right time and in the correct ear. Words and abbreviations used can easily be misinterpreted (e.g. 'otic' and 'optic', or 'QID' and 'QD'), and caution is needed during administration to guard against medication errors. Similar dropper bottles can contribute to the confusion (Boyd, 2019; Institute for Safe Medication Practices [ISMP], 2022a).

Different medications or different dosages may be ordered for each ear. If more than one medication is ordered for each ear, stagger the timing to promote maximum absorption. Fifteen minutes between different drops is suggested by Fullington et al. (2017). If ear drops and ointment are both ordered for the same ear, instil the drops first to promote better absorption.

EVIDENCE OF THERAPEUTIC INTERACTION

Establish the person's level of understanding regarding the medication. Determine their motivation to self-administer drops. This influences the teaching required and guides the teaching approach you should use. The person will be more willing and able to cooperate if they are aware of the techniques of the procedure. Explanation reduces apprehension and promotes relaxation. People need to know the expected sensations and effects of the medication.

DEMONSTRATE CLINICAL REASONING

Providing privacy and comfort, positioning, assessing the person's ear and using the general concepts of medication administration demonstrate clinical reasoning.

Privacy and comfort

The internal ear structures are sensitive to temperature extremes. Warm medications in your hand or a warm bath to reduce discomfort and to prevent vertigo and/or nausea (these may incapacitate the person for several minutes, putting them at risk of falls) (Cleveland Clinic, 2023). Comfort measures, such as toileting, positioning, fluids or pain relief (analgesia, warm compresses), will increase the person's comfort and minimise disruptions to the procedure.

ELDER CARE

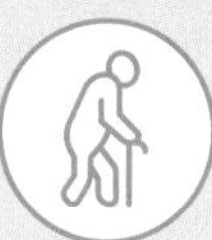

Impacted cerumen (ear wax) can affect up to 30 per cent of elderly people (due to long ear hairs, altered composition of cerumen [Cheng, 2019], hearing aid use, in-ear speakers [Kacker, Fraser & Pierce-Smith, 2022]), causing hearing loss, itchiness and pain. Assessing the ear canals for cerumen, removing it promptly using softening oils/drops and/or irrigating the ears prevents the problems.

THE PERSON LIVING WITH SEVERE OBESITY

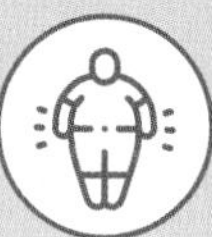

Obesity and increased waist circumference have been demonstrated as risk factors for hearing loss (Yang et al., 2020); however, the mechanism is still uncertain (e.g. central adiposity causing pro-inflammatory adipokines that damage the cochlea; comorbidities of cardiovascular diseases).

Assess the person

Disorders of the ear canal tend to be very painful. Occlusion of the external ear canal by oedema, discharge or cerumen can also reduce hearing. These conditions alter after medication administration.

LOOK at the condition of the external ear structure (pinna, tragus) and canal to provide a baseline to evaluate local response to medication, and to determine if the person's condition is improving or if it is necessary to clean the external ear before administering drops.

LISTEN to reports of pain and use a whisper test to assess hearing.

FEEL the pinna for heat indicating inflammation.

Clean the external ear

Perform an irrigation to remove debris and accumulated wax prior to administration of otic medication if necessary. Use an otoscope to assess the ear canal, if possible, as an oedematous ear canal is extremely painful and will preclude use of the otoscope. Look for an intact tympanic membrane, the condition of the skin of the ear canal, and any obstructions or debris such as crusting, cerumen and discharge. Cerumen and discharge harbour microorganisms and can decrease the distribution and absorption of medication as well as impair hearing.

Cleansing the external ear canal consists of gently syringing the ear canal with warm sterile water or saline. Follow this procedure:

- Explain the steps to the person and ask their permission to continue.
- Gather a 20 mL syringe, a large ampoule of sterile water/saline warmed in a small basin of warm water, a waterproof pad and cotton balls.
- Perform hand hygiene.
- Assist the person to sit or lie with their head tilted towards the affected ear.
- Place the waterproof pad under the ear on their shoulder. Ask them to hold the (now empty) small basin below their ear.
- Cleanse the pinna and the meatus of the ear canal as necessary (use some of the irrigating solution and a cotton ball).
- Fill a 20 mL syringe with the warmed water/normal saline.
- Straighten the ear canal by pulling the pinna up and back for an adult.
- The syringe tip is inserted to about the first third of the ear canal (approximately 8 mm), and the water is aimed at the top/roof of the ear canal (not the tympanic membrane) in a slow and steady stream.
- Allow the solution to flow out.
- When the irrigation is complete, place a cotton ball loosely at the meatus of the ear canal.
- Ask the person to lie on their side (affected ear down) to assist in removing the last of the solution.

?

If cerumen and discharge occlude the outermost portion of the ear canal, wipe the meatus and behind the tragus gently with a cotton-tip applicator using a rotating motion. Replace it if it becomes soiled. Do not force wax or debris inwards, because it might block or occlude the canal.

Position the person

Have the person lie on their side (unless contraindicated) or turn their head so the ear to be treated is upward. Alternatively, they may prefer to sit in a chair or on the bedside with their head tilted to the side to provide easy access for instillation of the medication. Stabilise their head with your hand, which promotes safety during instillation of the medication. For adults and children over three, gently pull the pinna up and back. Developmental differences in children aged three or less require the pinna to be gently pulled down and back to straighten the ear canal. Straightening the ear canal allows gravity to pull the medication more deeply into the ear canal (Cleveland Clinic, 2023).

General concepts of working with therapeutic substances

The concepts of working with medications have been explained in **Clinical Skills 37 and 38**. Please review these if necessary.

PART 7

GATHER EQUIPMENT

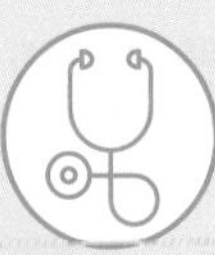

Gathering equipment ensures that you have all needed material, boosts the person's confidence and trust in you, and increases your self-confidence. The following materials are brought to the bedside and placed on a clean surface:

EQUIPMENT	EXPLANATION
Written medication order	For confirming the six rights
Otic medication	• Check it is an otic medication, the expiration date and look for any discolouration, precipitation and cloudiness (if not meant to be) • Clearly mark a newly opened bottle with the person's name and the date • Each person has an individual bottle of their prescribed medication, or it may be supplied in a minim • If the tip is inadvertently touched to anything, the medication is contaminated and must be discarded
Clean gloves	To protect both you and the person
Cotton-tipped applicator and sterile water or normal saline (NS)	May be needed to cleanse the pinna and auditory meatus of the ear
Gauze squares or tissues	• To blot the ear dry after cleansing
Small bowl of warm water	• Warm water (37 to 40 °C) is used to warm the solution • Make sure the label is waterproof (Broyles et al., 2017)

THE SIX RIGHTS OF ADMINISTERING MEDICATION

See **Clinical Skill 37** for a complete description of the rights of medication administration. In summary, they include:

- *right time* – the first consideration
- *right medication* – verify the validity of the order and then choose from the medications on the trolley. Make sure the medication is for OTIC administration
- *right route* – confirm OTIC administration as noted on the medication administration sheet
- *right dose* – it is imperative to gain a therapeutic level of the medication
- *right person* – it is vital to verify the correct person is receiving the medication
- *right documentation* – must be adhered to.

For otic medication, ensure that the correct ear is being treated.

ADMINISTER OTIC MEDICATION

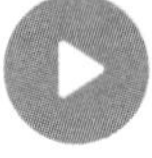

Video

Otic medication administration includes preparing the medication and instilling the drops or ointment.

Hand hygiene

Hand hygiene (see **Clinical Skill 5**) reduces the spread of microorganisms. Gloves protect you from the person's secretions and reduce the spread of microorganisms, and should be used.

Prepare the medication

Warm the medication in either a bowl of warm water or in your hand. This reduces discomfort and vertigo (Cleveland Clinic, 2023). If the medication is a solution, shake the bottle to distribute the contents evenly. Open the bottle and place the lid securely on a clean surface, either on its side or with the open portion uppermost. If a minim is being used, twist the top off and rest the body of the minim on the 'top' that you just removed to keep the opening as clean as possible. If using an ear ointment via cannula (rather than administering from a direct-dispenser container), open and fill it to the required level and rest it in the open bottle until it is needed.

Instil the prescribed drops

Straighten the ear canal (as above). Holding the dropper/minim or individual dispenser bottle vertically 1 cm above the canal, allow the prescribed number of drops to fall into the meatus of the ear; this prevents the tip from becoming contaminated (Nanno et al., 2020). Forceful instillation of drops into an occluded canal can injure the skin and the tympanic membrane (Lister, Hofland & Grafton, 2020). Ask the person to remain in a side-lying position for 15 minutes (Safer Care Victoria, 2019).

Once the drop or ointment is instilled, apply gentle pressure to the tragus with your finger to improve distribution of the medication. Pressure and massage moves the medication inward along the canal. If medication is ordered for both ears, ask the person to stay in the side-lying position for 15 minutes after the first dose before turning onto the other side for the additional medication.

A small piece of a cotton ball may be inserted loosely into the outermost part of the canal. This prevents the medication from draining out of the ear when the person stands or sits (Nanno et al., 2020). Do not force the cotton into the canal. The cotton should not block the canal to impair hearing or prevent absorption of the medication and should be removed after five to 15 minutes. This time period promotes medication distribution and absorption.

Insert otic ointment

Ask the person to sit or lay comfortably with the affected ear upwards. Squeeze the ointment into the syringe barrel after the plunger has been removed. Replace the plunger and attach a special wide-bore, blunt cannula to the syringe. Alternatively, apply ointment directly from the supply tube using the cannula tip provided. Follow the manufacturer's advice for preparing the ointment for instillation. Pull the pinna gently (as above) to straighten the auditory canal. Introduce the cannula just inside the canal and fill the canal until the ointment appears at the meatus.

A foam applicator is a pump device that delivers a measured amount of medication into the ear canal via a delivery tube. Medication must be formulated for this application. It is gentle, and the medication stays in contact with the ear canal skin/tympanic membrane for longer (Martin, 2019).

Ear wicks/otowicks

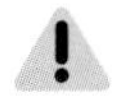

Safety

Wicks are used for severely swollen ear canals. They are sponge or gauze strips placed in the ear canal (by the physician) and saturated with medication several times a day. They transport the drops to the ear canal surface and, when soaked, expand to maintain medication contact with the skin and apply pressure to decrease oedema. Drops are applied to the wick several times a day. They may be used for the first 24 to 48 hours of otitis externa, and replaced every 48 hours if needed for longer. However, the ear wick normally extrudes spontaneously in 12 to 36 hours, after the oedema has subsided.

Healthcare teaching

It is important the person is aware of the correct way to cleanse their ears. To evaluate learning (see **Clinical Skill 27**), ask them to explain or demonstrate the method for cleaning the ears, instilling ear drops and the reasons for the medication. Depending on their response, they may need to be reminded/taught not to put objects into their ears (e.g. bobby pins or cotton-tipped applicators, as these could traumatise skin, foster infection, cause cerumen impaction and puncture the tympanic membrane [Rodríguez et al., 2022]).

Children must be taught not to put any objects into their ears. It is imperative that parents of children with chronic otitis media be taught signs of hearing loss, about the need for follow-up appointments and ways to reduce ear infections.

Post-procedure

Assist the person to a comfortable position

Help the person to sit or lie comfortably. Ask them to keep their head on the side for 15 minutes to aid absorption of the medication.

Assess the effect

After drops or ointment have been absorbed, ask the person if they felt any discomfort when the drops or ointment were administered. This determines if the procedure was performed correctly and can establish the severity of symptoms. Evaluate the condition of the external ear between instillations of drops to determine the person's response to the medication. The person's hearing acuity should be evaluated as hearing may be changed after medication administration.

CLEAN, REPLACE AND DISPOSE OF EQUIPMENT

Discard soiled tissues into the waste bin. Remove gloves and wash hands. Return medication to appropriate storage.

DOCUMENTATION

Record your initials on the medication chart/electronic medication administration record (eMAR) immediately after administering medication. If using the bar code medication administration, it will automatically record the time, dose and your identification. Document the condition of the ear canal and any sudden deterioration in the person's hearing and report it to the shift coordinator and medical staff. Note also any adverse effects or responses to medication and report these to the shift coordinator.

If the medication was withheld, the facility's policy for noting withheld doses should be used to record this on the medication chart. Document the reasons in the person's notes and inform the shift coordinator and the medical officer.

CLINICAL SKILLS ASSESSMENT

Otic medication

Demonstrates the ability to effectively administer otic medication. Incorporates the *National Safety and Quality Health Service Standards*: 2 Partnering with Consumers, 3 Preventing and Controlling Healthcare-Associated Infection, 5 Comprehensive Care, 6 Communicating for Safety, and 8 Recognising and Responding to Acute Deterioration (ACSQHC, 2021).

Performance criteria	1	2	3	4	5
(Numbers indicate NMBA *Registered Nurse Standards for Practice*)	**(Dependent)**	**(Marginal)**	**(Assisted)**	**(Supervised)**	**(Independent)**
1. Identifies indication (1.1, 3.3, 3.4)	☐	☐	☐	☐	☐
2. Verifies the written medication order; identifies the ear to be treated (1.4, 3.4, 6.2, 6.5)	☐	☐	☐	☐	☐
3. Evidence of therapeutic interaction with person, e.g. gives a clear explanation of the procedure, obtains consent (1.4, 1.5, 2.1, 2.2, 3.2)	☐	☐	☐	☐	☐
4. Demonstrates clinical reasoning abilities, e.g. provides privacy, comfort measures and pain relief as necessary, positions the person (1.1, 1.2, 1.3, 4.2, 6.1)	☐	☐	☐	☐	☐
5. Adheres to the general concepts of working with therapeutic substances (1.1, 1.3, 1.5, 3.3, 3.4, 4.1, 4.2, 4.3, 6.2, 6.5, 6.6)	☐	☐	☐	☐	☐
6. Gathers equipment (1.1, 5.5, 6.1): ■ written medication order ■ otic medication ■ clean gloves ■ cotton-tipped applicator and sterile water/normal saline ■ gauze squares or tissues ■ small bowl of warm water	☐	☐	☐	☐	☐
7. Uses the six (or more) rights to administer the medication (1.1, 1.2, 1.3, 1.4, 1.5, 2.2, 3.4, 4.1, 4.2, 4.3, 6.1, 6.2, 6.5, 6.6)	☐	☐	☐	☐	☐
8. Performs hand hygiene (1.1, 3.4, 6.1)	☐	☐	☐	☐	☐
9. Warms the drops to body temperature (6.1)	☐	☐	☐	☐	☐
10. Pulls the pinna appropriately (1.1, 6.1)	☐	☐	☐	☐	☐
11. Instils the prescribed drops or ointment (1.1, 6.1)	☐	☐	☐	☐	☐
12. Asks the person to remain in a side-lying position and applies gentle pressure to the tragus of the ear with a finger (1.1, 6.1)	☐	☐	☐	☐	☐
13. Applies and removes the cotton ball appropriately (1.1, 6.1)	☐	☐	☐	☐	☐
14. Assists the person to a comfortable position after the drops are absorbed (6.1)	☐	☐	☐	☐	☐
15. Cleans, replaces and disposes of equipment appropriately (3.6, 6.1)	☐	☐	☐	☐	☐
16. Documents relevant information (1.4, 1.6, 2.2, 3.5, 3.7, 6.2, 6.5, 7.3)	☐	☐	☐	☐	☐
17. Demonstrates the ability to link theory to practice (1.1, 3.3, 3.4, 3.5)	☐	☐	☐	☐	☐

Student:

Clinical facilitator: Date:

CHAPTER 42

VAGINAL MEDICATION

INDICATIONS

The vagina is a highly effective site for administration of both local and systemic medications. The mucosal lining (as all mucosa) is rich in blood vessels, has a large surface area and is moist, making it ideal for absorbing many medications. Vaginal medications come as solid tablets, suppositories, creams, gels, foams and pastes with active properties. Pharmaceutical pessaries or rings are medicated devices that deliver a controlled dose of a medication over time (e.g. contraceptives) and are inserted by a physician or nurse practitioner. Douches are a type of liquid vaginal medication that flows in a stream over the vaginal mucosa, usually to reduce inflammation or infection.

Vaginally delivered medications are absorbed locally but can act systemically after being absorbed by the vaginal mucosa.

Vaginal medications are applied to intact vaginal mucosa for many reasons:

- to provide rapid delivery of a medication (creams or some suppositories) for immediate effect (e.g. hormones during labour)
- to provide slow, even delivery of the medication to maintain a therapeutic dose over a long period of time (e.g. anti-yeast medications)
- to bypass the gastrointestinal tract (e.g. if the medication causes gastrointestinal symptoms like nausea and diarrhoea, or if it is metabolised in the liver and rendered less effective). This means lower or less frequent doses than oral medications to maintain a therapeutic range
- to affect the local area (e.g. anti-fungal vaginal cream) or to stimulate contractions of the uterus during labour.

Vaginal delivery of medications does have some disadvantages:

- The vagina may be easily irritated by either the medication or the insertion of it.
- Inserted medicated devices such as rings or pessaries must be sterile.
- Only medications that are easily absorbed (i.e. with small molecules) can be used.
- Absorption can be affected by a female's hormonal cycle, pregnancy, vaginal discharge or postmenopausal status.
- The medication can leak, causing stains and discomfort.

You must understand the anatomy and physiology of the perineal and vaginal areas to safely administer a vaginal medication.

Verify the written medication order

No medication can be legally administered without a valid, signed order from a qualified healthcare provider (see **Clinical Skill 37** for a description of a valid order). Some vaginal medications such as antibiotics or steroid creams require a finish or stop time. Question and clarify any order that is unclear, incomplete or that seems inappropriate or unreasonable for the woman (e.g. very high dose, contraindicated for the diagnosis, same medication with two different names or routes – oral and vaginal, for example). The nurse along with the physician is responsible if an inappropriate order is followed. To question an order, you *must know* the woman's diagnosis, the purpose, therapeutic effect, any adverse and toxic effects and the usual dose of the medication.

You must anticipate any pertinent nursing implications, such as individual factors that mediate response to medications (e.g. age, weight and psychological factors). You must also know any drug or food allergies that the woman may have so that potentially harmful substances are not administered. Their vaginal mucosa must be intact; that is, not have had recent surgery to the area that would endanger the vaginal wall by the administration procedure.

EVIDENCE OF THERAPEUTIC INTERACTION

Help the woman to better understand her medication regimen and discuss the reason for this form of administration. Some females find the idea of vaginal insertion of a medication distasteful. Discussion assists in reducing apprehension, anxiety and fear, and increases the person's ability to relax, making insertion less uncomfortable. The woman may provide information vital to her care. She may prefer to administer the medication to herself if she is able. Professional communication improves the woman's comfort and safety, her trust in nurses and ultimately her health and wellbeing.

ELDER CARE

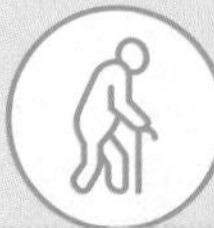

Ageing and oestrogen deficiency (post menopause) cause changes in the vulvovaginal skin and mucous membranes, making them thinner, drier and more fragile. This increases the occurrence of inflammation, infection, pruritis and subsequent damage to the tissues. Take care to assess the perineal area for redness, swelling, evidence of scratching and maceration from urine contact. Liberal use of water soluble lubricant on vaginal medication/insertion devices will minimise further damage. As well, take care during positioning as painful joints and underused muscles may make attaining and maintaining either position slow, difficult and very uncomfortable.

THE PERSON LIVING WITH SEVERE OBESITY

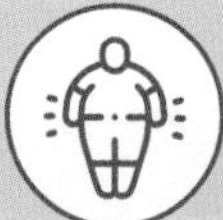

Repositioning of the woman who is severely obese will require at least one extra nurse. Perineal care (see **Clinical Skill 33**) is important because of excess perspiration, difficulty in cleaning the area and often faecal and urinary incontinence (Wang, Lodhia & Chen, 2021). The excess tissue of the thighs, buttocks and perineum will need to be moved aside by the other nurse so that the vagina is visible, the area can be assessed (excoriation of the perineal skin is common) and the vagina can be accessed to insert the medication. (See **Clinical Skills 15 and 23** for a brief explanation of issues for people living with severe obesity.)

DEMONSTRATE CLINICAL REASONING

Clinical reasoning incorporates the concepts of working with medications, including your legal responsibilities, your ability to accurately calculate the dose required and a solid understanding of the medications to be given. You must be aware of elder care and of people living with severe obesity, and issues of privacy and comfort.

Provide privacy

Close doors and curtains. Expose just the area to be accessed – the perineal area – and drape the rest of the woman to preserve dignity and self-esteem. Do not expose her unnecessarily.

Position the woman

Ask regarding toileting requirements. Sometimes, inserting a vaginal medication stimulates voiding. Position the woman to facilitate administering the vaginal medication – usually on her left side with the right leg drawn up to visualise the vaginal opening and ease discomfort of insertion. Alternatively, ask her to lie on her back, feet drawn up and knees abducted. This position is uncomfortable for any length of time, but is quick and easy for vaginal medication administration. Expose just the perineal area; drape the rest of the woman to preserve dignity and self-esteem. Place an incontinence pad under her buttocks in case of accidental discharge.

For a douche, you will need to position the woman on a bedpan (dorsal recumbent position) with her legs spread. Douches can also be used while she is lying in a bath tub, or sitting on the toilet; although if sitting, the labia will need to be held closed for a few minutes to allow the liquid to bathe the vaginal walls and the medication to be absorbed. You may need a torch to visualise the vaginal canal or a helper to assist with maintaining the position if there are conditions (e.g. arthritis) that make it painful or tiring to do so.

General concepts of working with therapeutic substances

Legal responsibilities

Medications must be securely stored and safely administered. Vaginal suppositories will usually be kept in the refrigerator, and vaginal tablets, creams, gels and pastes will usually be stored in the medication trolley or at the woman's bedside. A valid consent (verbal or implied) is required to administer a vaginal medication.

Calculate accurate dosages

Vaginal medications are no different to other methods of administration in the need for accuracy of dosing. Suppositories have fixed doses and should not be cut because the active ingredient may not be homogenous within the base gel. Creams and gels generally come with a calibrated applicator. You must become familiar with what is available and the dosage available for the medication that has been ordered.

The formulations of vaginal medication include:

- suppositories
- vaginal tablets
- creams, pastes and gels
- liquids to be diluted for douches.

Medication names and classifications

It is necessary that you are aware of the name, classification and indication of any medication you administer. See **Clinical Skill 37** for a discussion of medication names.

Mechanisms of medication administration

Preparation

To reduce errors, administer only medications that you have personally prepared, and undertake the following:

- *Be aware of allergies* – check the medication administration sheet for an allergy caution, look for an allergy armband (red) and ask the woman if she is allergic to anything. Ask her if she has had this medication inserted before and, if so, has she tolerated it. For administration of a douche, check if the woman is allergic to iodine or Betadine because these may be the base antiseptic for the douche.
- *Ask the woman to state her name* – don't ask if her name is 'Mary Smith', for example, as she may just agree regardless of who she is (e.g. she may be deaf, confused or non-English speaking).
- *Listen to the woman* – many, if not most, people know their medications well, and any query by them as to the dose or appearance of the vaginal medication should be taken seriously before administering. Recheck the medication administration sheet and the tube of cream or suppository/tablet wrapper, and ask the prescriber about the medication. This validates the woman's knowledge and prevents medication administration errors.
- *Sign or initial the medications sheet* – do this as soon as the cream, suppository or tablet is inserted. (The bar code medication administration system automatically records the medication dose and your identification on the electronic medication administration record [eMAR].) This prevents a potential overdose (i.e. another nurse might administer a second dose of the medication thinking it has not been given). Most facilities do not allow you to sign prior to giving the medication, only after the dose has been given.

Responsibility to the woman

Your responsibility involves assessment, teaching, advocacy and evaluation of the effect of the medication administered.

Assess the physiological function that the vaginal medication is expected to affect prior to applying it (e.g. degree of pruritus prior to administration of an antifungal) to provide a baseline for use in evaluating the effectiveness of the medication. Assess the perineum prior to administering the medication.

LOOK for drainage (Perry, Potter & Ostendorf, 2019), redness or discolouration of the labia. Assess her medication history (i.e. a review of current and past drugs – prescribed, over-the-counter, herbal preparations or recreational) and medical history (e.g. vaginal surgery, recent childbirth, allergies, any vaginal bleeding or discharge). These assessments may indicate that the medication should be withheld and the shift coordinator informed, or a different route ordered.

LISTEN when you ask about pruritus, burning or discomfort, if she is menstruating (as appropriate). Ask her about any vaginal bleeding or discharge, recent childbirth or vaginal surgery or trauma.

Safety

Teach the woman the name and dose of the medication she is taking, its expected effect, its frequency, adverse effects, how to minimise these and how to insert the medication. She may feel more comfortable inserting the medication herself. She needs to know any implications of taking the medication (e.g. if it will drain out and she will need to wear a perineal pad, but avoid a tampon). Discuss maintaining the medication regimen at home and adapt the regimen to accommodate her home schedule (without compromising the efficacy of the medication). Be alert to any cues the woman or family might give about not continuing to use a medication (e.g. cost, difficulty in inserting the medication, negative self-concept). Discussing these things may improve the woman's commitment to sustaining the prescribed treatment. Take the opportunity to discuss perineal hygiene and prevention of vaginal infections. Emphasise (Felix et al., 2020):

- wearing cotton underwear (increases the aeration of the labia, vaginal opening to help maintain temperature/humidity to prevent changes in the vaginal microbiota)
- not wearing tight pants or jeans (reduces heat, pressure and irritation on labia and perineum)
- perineal hygiene (cleansing with toilet paper after each elimination in an anterior posterior direction, washing perineum once to three times daily with a pH-balanced soap, depending on the climate).

Advocacy includes alerting the medical practitioner of adverse effects, or any reason the woman tells you that would influence her continuation of the vaginal medication.

Evaluation is a very important aspect of your responsibility in administering medications. You (and the prescribing doctor) need to be aware that the medication is doing what it is meant to. Reassess the woman following administration of a medication (e.g. antibiotics). This should be done within a reasonable time frame from the administration (usually 30 minutes to one hour following) and effects noted. Watch out for unexpected effects such as pruritus due to reactions to carrier ingredients in the vaginal medication. This evaluation is crucial following the initial administration of any medication.

GATHER EQUIPMENT

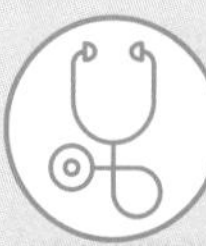

Gathering equipment is an organisational step that ensures that you have all needed material, boosts the woman's confidence and trust in you, and increases your self-confidence. Equipment includes the following items:

EQUIPMENT	EXPLANATION
Medication administration sheet	To identify the woman, the medication required, the route, the dose and the time. It is also the documentation of administering the medication
Tray or trolley	Use to assemble and take the equipment to the woman's bedside
Vaginal medication	*Suppositories* • Thin, bullet-shaped masses composed of water-soluble gels that melt at body temperature, releasing the medication to be absorbed • Often stored in the refrigerator to prevent melting • Do not carry in your hand or pocket; inserting a soft suppository is difficult • If soft, hold it, still in its wrap, under cold running water until it hardens • Check expiration date *Tablets* • Powdered medication pressed into an oval form to be inserted into the vagina • An applicator is often used • Use a water-soluble lubricant prior to insertion and ensure the woman is well hydrated to absorb the medication
	Creams, pastes, gels and foams • Are contained in various densities of carriers • Are administered using an applicator that is well lubricated with a water-soluble lubricant *Medicated douche* • An aqueous base infused with medication • Come pre-packaged and in a container that is designed to deliver the medication into the vagina (with an integrated nozzle or tube) • May need to add warm water to a designated level prior to use • Check expiration date
Waterproof pad	Protects bed linen in case of accidental drainage or spillage and reassures the woman that she will not soil the bed
Bedpan	To catch the outflow of liquid when administering a douche
Water-soluble lubricant	• Reduces friction between the vaginal mucosa and the medication or applicator to ease insertion • A gauze square is used to apply the lubricant to the suppository or douche nozzle
Clean gloves	• For personal protection and to prevent spread of microorganisms • Also worn to protect you from absorbing the medication
Tissues	To clean the perineal area of excess lubricant following insertion of the medication and withdrawal of the inserting finger or applicator
Large drape	Provide cover for maintaining modesty and dignity
Perineal pad	Protects underclothes from wetting/staining with discharge following medication insertion

THE SIX RIGHTS OF ADMINISTERING MEDICATION

See **Clinical Skill 37** for a complete description of the rights of medication administration. In summary, they include:

- *right time* – the first consideration
- *right medication* – verify the validity of the order and then choose from the medications on the trolley/in the refrigerator
- *right route* – confirm this as noted on the medication administration sheet
- *right dose* – it is imperative to gain a therapeutic level of the medication
- *right person* – it is vital to verify the correct person is receiving the medication
- *right documentation* – must be adhered to.

ADMINISTER VAGINAL MEDICATION

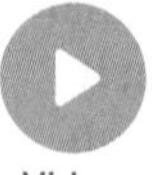
Video

The process of vaginal medication administration includes preparing the medication, positioning the woman (see above) and administering the medication.

Hand hygiene

Hand hygiene (see **Clinical Skill 5**) reduces the spread of microorganisms. Hand hygiene is especially important following vaginal medication administration in case of inadvertent contamination of your skin with the medication. Gloves protect you from secretions, the medication, and reduce the spread of microorganisms.

Prepare the medication

Vaginal medications generally require little preparation. The suppository is contained in a sealed foil package and is usually found in the refrigerator. Take it out a few minutes before administering to warm to room temperature, but do not carry it in your pocket or hand. At the bedside, take the suppository or vaginal tablet with the required dose of medication out of its wrapping. Place it on a gauze square ready for use. There may be a suppository/pill applicator available (this is a long thin cylinder with flexible 'fingers' at the end of the barrel into which the tablet/suppository is inserted and after inserting the applicator into the vagina, the tablet/suppository is ejected by pushing the integrated plunger). Apply a liberal amount of water-soluble lubricating gel to the suppository or tablet with the gauze and to your inserting finger (usually index finger of your dominant hand).

Vaginal creams/gels/pastes are extruded into the applicator to the ordered dose. Lubricate the tip.

Containers of douche medication may need to be diluted. Add warm (approximately 40 °C) water to the indicated level. Lubricate the tip of the nozzle. Use an IV stand to hang the container about 50 cm above the woman's hips.

Administer the medication

Stand with your dominant hand towards her feet (makes manipulating the medication and spreading the labia more comfortable for you). Spread the buttocks to expose the labia using your non-dominant hand. Visually assess the perineal and labial tissue. Tell the woman she will feel a cool sensation and pressure in her vagina so she is prepared. Ask her to take a few deep breaths to relax the perineum. Hold the labia apart with your non-dominant hand.

- *Suppository or vaginal tablet* – use the index finger of your dominant hand to insert the suppository or tablet, with the round end in front (or use the supplied applicator), into the vagina for 8 to 10 cm, to the posterior fornix. Withdraw your finger and wipe it on the tissue. Wipe the perineal area clean of lubricant.
- *Cream, gel or paste* – fill the applicator to the ordered dose indicator (from the tube of gel/cream/paste) and insert the lubricated applicator into the vagina and extend it so the tip of the applicator is in the posterior fornix of the vaginal vault (8 to 10 cm along the posterior vaginal wall). Push the plunger to extrude all of the medication.
- *Foam* – refit the removable nozzle onto the foam container and insert the nozzle of the container into the vagina and extend it so the tip is in the posterior fornix of the vaginal vault (as above). Depress the button to release the foam into the vagina.
- *Douche* – take the cap off the nozzle or the end of the tube of the douche container. Unclamp the tube to permit the tube to fill with solution. Reclamp. Apply a liberal amount of water-soluble lubricating gel to the rounded end. Tell the woman she will feel a warm sensation so she is prepared. Slowly insert the rounded end of the nozzle into the vagina. Unclamp the tube/nozzle and let a small amount of the liquid flow into the vagina so the temperature can be assessed. Rotate the tube/nozzle so the liquid reaches all areas of the vagina. Keep the end of the nozzle against the vaginal wall to improve contact with the medication. Withdraw the tube/nozzle and wrap it in a tissue. Wipe the perineal area clean of lubricant and any of the medicated fluid.

Post-procedure

Remove the bedpan and contents following a douche. Ask the woman to remain in a recumbent position for five to 10 minutes to optimise the absorption of the medication.

Drainage is usual (DeLaune et al., 2024) following vaginal medications. Ask her to inform you if there is vaginal discharge – note amount, odour, colour. Assist her with a perineal pad as needed. Advise her not to use a tampon when she is having a vaginal medication, as the tampon interferes with the delivery of the full dose (Mayo Clinic, 2020a).

CLEAN, REPLACE AND DISPOSE OF EQUIPMENT

Discard any disposable items used to administer a vaginal medication (e.g. gloves, tissues, administration nozzle). Often, the applicator for gel/cream/pastes or nozzle for a foam applicator is reusable; if so, wash it in warm, soapy water, rinse and dry it, replace it in its original container (labelled with the woman's name) and store it in her bedside drawer. If a bedpan was used, cover it, take it to the utility room, sanitise it in the pan washer or empty and clean it, then return it to storage. Wipe the cart or tray clean of spills or debris and replace stocks of supplies. Order stock medications and individual prescriptions from the pharmacy if they are running low. When they arrive on the unit, place them in the refrigerator or medication trolley with their labels visible to reduce the possibility of errors. Return the medication administration sheet to its designated place for the next medication round.

DOCUMENTATION

Initial or sign the medication administration sheet in the appropriate timeslot beside the written medication order and note if an assessment was done (e.g. skin condition, pain). (Or use the bar code medication administration system to record the dose on the eMAR.) Also document briefly on the medication administration sheet in the appropriate timeslot if the woman has refused to take the medication or some other untoward event occurs, then document it more fully in the progress notes. The effects of the medications, expected or unexpected, are assessed 30 minutes to one hour after administration, and these are documented. Adverse effects should be reported to the shift coordinator and the medical staff, and the remaining doses of the medication assessed or withheld.

CLINICAL SKILLS ASSESSMENT

Vaginal medication

Demonstrates the ability to effectively administer vaginal medication. Incorporates the *National Safety and Quality Health Service Standards*: 2 Partnering with Consumers, 3 Preventing and Controlling Healthcare-Associated Infection, 5 Comprehensive Care, 6 Communicating for Safety, and 8 Recognising and Responding to Acute Deterioration (ACSQHC, 2021).

Performance criteria	1	2	3	4	5
(Numbers indicate NMBA *Registered Nurse Standards for Practice*)	**(Dependent)**	**(Marginal)**	**(Assisted)**	**(Supervised)**	**(Independent)**
1. Identifies indication (1.1, 3.3, 3.4)	☐	☐	☐	☐	☐
2. Verifies the written medication order (1.4, 3.4, 6.2, 6.5)	☐	☐	☐	☐	☐
3. Evidence of therapeutic interaction with the woman, e.g. gives a clear explanation of the procedure, obtains consent (1.4, 1.5, 2.1, 2.2, 3.2)	☐	☐	☐	☐	☐
4. Demonstrates clinical reasoning abilities, e.g. provides privacy, assists with positioning (1.1, 1.2, 1.3, 4.2, 6.1)	☐	☐	☐	☐	☐
5. Adheres to the general concepts of working with therapeutic substances (1.1, 1.3, 1.5, 3.3, 3.4, 4.1, 4.2, 4.3, 6.2, 6.5, 6.6)	☐	☐	☐	☐	☐
6. Gathers equipment (1.1, 5.5, 6.1): ■ medication administration sheet ■ tray or trolley ■ vaginal medication ■ waterproof pad ■ bedpan ■ water-soluble lubricant ■ clean gloves ■ tissues ■ large drape ■ perineal pad	☐	☐	☐	☐	☐
7. Uses the six (or more) rights to administer the medication (1.1, 1.2, 1.3, 1.4, 1.5, 2.2, 3.4, 4.1, 4.2, 4.3, 6.1, 6.2, 6.5, 6.6)	☐	☐	☐	☐	☐
8. Performs hand hygiene (1.1, 3.4, 6.1)	☐	☐	☐	☐	☐
9. Prepares the medication, e.g. warms the douche (6.1)	☐	☐	☐	☐	☐
10. Inserts the prescribed medication (1.1, 6.1)	☐	☐	☐	☐	☐
11. Asks the woman to remain in a side-lying position (1.1, 6.1)	☐	☐	☐	☐	☐
12. Assists the woman to a comfortable position after the medication is administered (6.1)	☐	☐	☐	☐	☐
13. Cleans, replaces and disposes of equipment appropriately (3.6, 6.1)	☐	☐	☐	☐	☐
14. Documents relevant information (1.4, 1.6, 2.2, 3.5, 3.7, 6.2, 6.5, 7.3)	☐	☐	☐	☐	☐
15. Demonstrates the ability to link theory to practice (1.1, 3.3, 3.4, 3.5)	☐	☐	☐	☐	☐

Student:

Clinical facilitator: Date:

CHAPTER 43

RECTAL MEDICATION

INDICATIONS

Rectal mucosa absorbs most medication equally as well as the upper part of the gastrointestinal tract and acts faster as no digestive processes are needed. Absorption from aqueous and alcohol-based medications is rapid, leading these solutions to be used as a base for medications for emergent situations, such as convulsions (e.g. diazepam, especially in children). Absorption from oil-based liquids and most suppositories is slower. You must understand the anatomy and physiology of the anal and rectal areas to safely administer a rectal medication.

Rectal medications are used when oral administration is unsuitable (difficulty or inability to swallow, unconscious, severe nausea/vomiting), when the gastrointestinal tract is unavailable (severe irritable bowel disease, gastritis) or often during palliative care. They are also used to soothe the anal areas (external haemorrhoids, anal pruritis), relieve constipation and for both local and systemic effects.

Rectal medication formulations are solid tablets, suppositories, creams or liquids inserted via an enema (see also **Clinical Skill 34**) with active properties. These medications are absorbed locally but can act systemically after being absorbed by the rectal mucosa.

Rectal medications are applied to intact rectal mucosa to:

- provide rapid delivery of a medication for immediate control of specific symptoms (e.g. convulsions, migraine)
- provide slow delivery of the medication that produces and/or maintains a therapeutic dose over a long period of time (e.g. strong analgesics, corticosteroids)
- bypass the gastrointestinal tract (e.g. if the medication causes gastrointestinal symptoms like nausea or diarrhoea; or if it is metabolised in the liver and rendered less effective) or if there are pre-existing upper gastrointestinal upsets like nausea or swallowing difficulties (Hua, 2019)
- affect a local area (e.g. rectal anaesthetic or analgesic cream) or to stimulate defecation (e.g. Microlax).

Rectal administration of medication has a few major drawbacks. It is less acceptable to the person receiving the medication than other forms, and absorption of the medication is interrupted by defecation; it can also be mildly uncomfortable.

There are contraindications: rectal medication should not be given to people who have stomach pain of unknown origin, diarrhoea, recent rectal, bowel or prostate gland surgery, rectal bleeding or prolapse and those who are immunocompromised. Additionally, anyone with an acute coronary condition is at risk of vagal stimulation during insertion of a rectal medication (DeLaune et al., 2024, p. 776).

Verify the written medication order

Generally, medication cannot be legally administered without a valid, signed order from a qualified healthcare provider (see **Clinical Skill 37** for a description of a valid order). Some rectal medications, such as antibiotics or steroid medications, require a finish or stop time. Most over-the-counter (OTC) rectal medications (e.g. glycerine suppositories) can be given without an order. These are usually listed in the facility's policy manuals.

Question and clarify any order that is unclear, incomplete or that seems inappropriate or unreasonable for the person (e.g. very high dose, contraindicated for the diagnosis, same medication with two different names or routes – oral and rectal, for example). The nurse along with the physician is responsible if an inappropriate order is followed. The person's rectal mucosa must be intact; that is, it must not have had recent surgery to the area that would endanger the rectal wall by the administration procedure.

EVIDENCE OF THERAPEUTIC INTERACTION

Help the person to better understand their medication regimen and discuss the reason for this form of administration. Most people find the idea of rectal insertion of a medication repugnant, and some feel panic-stricken at the thought. Discussion assists in reducing apprehension, anxiety and fear, and increases the person's ability to relax, making insertion less uncomfortable. The person may provide information vital to their care. Professional communication improves their comfort and safety, their trust in nurses and ultimately their health and wellbeing.

DEMONSTRATE CLINICAL REASONING

Clinical reasoning includes caring for diverse people and incorporates the concepts of working with medications, including your legal responsibilities, your ability to accurately calculate the dose required, a solid understanding of the medications to be given and assessment of the individual. You must be aware of privacy and comfort.

Provide privacy

Close doors and curtains. Expose just the buttock area, and drape the rest of the person to preserve dignity and self-esteem. Do not expose the person unnecessarily. Embarrassment is a common reaction to rectal medication administration (Brotto, 2020).

Assess the person

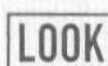

at the perianal tissue for inflammation, haemorrhoids, evidence of bleeding or pruritus (usually just prior to insertion of medication). Assess the person's ability to position themselves and maintain that position (you may need a helper). Assess their medication history (i.e. a review of the person's current and past drugs – prescribed, OTC, herbal preparations or recreational) and medical history (rectal or prostate surgery, allergies, coronary conditions, any rectal bleeding or discharge).

LISTEN to reports of any pruritus, rectal bleeding or discharge. Ask them when their bowels last opened and do not give the medication if there has been bleeding or if the person is due to defecate soon, unless the medication was prescribed for relieving constipation. Check their chart for any contraindications (e.g. cardiac condition).

Position the person

Position the person to facilitate administering the rectal medication, usually on their left side with the right leg drawn up to ease discomfort of insertion. You may need pillows under the upper leg to provide support. Drape appropriately to preserve dignity and self-esteem. Place an incontinence pad under their buttocks in case of accidental faecal discharge.

ELDER CARE

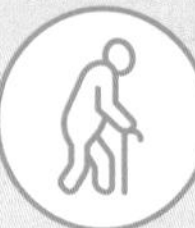

Some elderly people have difficulty positioning themselves with the right leg drawn up and will need help to maintain this position. You may need to alter the position to supine with knees bent and abducted. Again, a second person may be required to help them establish and maintain this position.

If you are administering a stimulant medication, the elderly person may require assistance to the toilet or commode, or onto the bedpan.

THE PERSON LIVING WITH SEVERE OBESITY

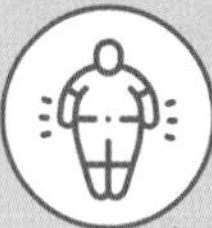

Administering rectal medication to a severely obese person can be challenging. They may be unable to reposition themselves and you will require an assistant and perhaps a lift to help the person move, as well as an assistant to help them to remain on their side. Excess buttock and perineal tissue will need to be moved out of the way so that the rectal area is visible and assessable and you can see well enough to insert the medication. The area will likely need to be cleansed before insertion of the medication since severely obese people frequently experience incontinence due to pressure of the abdominal contents, as well as excess perspiration in the deep skin folds in the groin, buttock and perineal areas. They often have great difficulty in maintaining their perineal hygiene (Earlam & Woods, 2020). You will need a bariatric-sized bedpan and help putting the person on the pan in the case of administering a stimulant medication. (See **Clinical Skills 15 and 23** for a brief explanation of some issues facing people living with severe obesity.)

General concepts of working with therapeutic substances

Legal responsibilities

Medications must be securely stored and safely administered. Rectal suppositories will usually be in the refrigerator because they melt at body temperature and can become difficult to insert at a warm room temperature. Rectal tablets and medicated enemas will usually be stored in the medication trolley, either as a general medication or in the individual's drawer. A valid consent (verbal or implied) is required to administer a rectal medication.

Calculate accurate dosages

Rectal medications are no different than other methods of administration in the need for accuracy of dosing. Suppositories have fixed doses. They should not be cut since the active ingredient may not be homogenous within the base gel. Become familiar with what is available and the dosage available for the medication that has been ordered.

The formulations of rectal medication include: suppositories, rectal tablets, oral medications crushed to a powder and suspended in a solution, and enemas.

Medication names and classifications

It is necessary that you are aware of the name, classification and indication of any medication you administer. See **Clinical Skill 37** for a discussion of medication names.

Mechanisms of medication administration

Preparation

To reduce errors, administer only medications that you have personally prepared, and undertake the following:

- *Be aware of allergies* – check the medication administration sheet for an allergy caution, look for an allergy armband (red) and ask the person if they are allergic to anything. Ask them if they have had this medication inserted before and, if so, have they tolerated it.
- *Ask the person to state their name* – don't ask them if their name is 'Mary Smith', for example, as they may agree, regardless of who they are (e.g. they may be deaf, confused, non-English speaking).
- *Listen to the person* – many, if not most, people know their medications well, and any query by them as to the dose or appearance of the rectal medication should be taken seriously before administering. Recheck the medication administration sheet and the suppository/tablet wrapper and ask the prescriber about the drug. This validates the person's knowledge and prevents medication administration errors.
- *Sign or initial the medications sheet* – do this as soon as the suppository or tablet is inserted to prevent a potential overdose (i.e. another nurse might administer a second dose of the medication thinking it has not been given). Most facilities do not allow you to sign prior to giving the medication, only after the application.

Responsibility to the person

Your responsibility involves assessment, teaching, advocacy and evaluation of the effect of the medication administered.

Assess the physiological or psychological function that the rectal medication is expected to affect prior to applying it (e.g. pain assessment prior to administering an analgesic suppository, such as MS Contin) to provide a baseline for use in evaluating the effectiveness of the medication. Be aware of the possibility of a vagal response to the anal stimulation (bradycardia, hypotension, dizziness, fainting, sweating), especially in anyone with a cardiac condition. These assessments may indicate that the medication should be withheld (and the shift coordinator informed) or an order sought for a different form of the medication (e.g. oral, parenteral).

Teach the name, intended function and dose of the medication to the person, its frequency, adverse effects, how to minimise these and how to insert the medication. They need to know any implications of taking the medication, such as how long they need to retain it. Discuss maintaining the medication regimen at home and adapt the regimen to accommodate the person's home schedule (without compromising the efficacy of the medication). The person needs to be aware of the importance of regular monitoring required for some medications. Be alert to any cues the person or family might give about not continuing to use a medication (e.g. revulsion, difficulty in inserting the suppository, painful haemorrhoids, negative self-concept). Discussing these things may improve the person's commitment to sustaining the prescribed treatment.

Advocacy includes alerting the medical practitioner of adverse effects, or any reason the person tells you that would influence their continuation of the rectal medication.

Evaluation is a very important aspect of your responsibility in administering medications. You (and the prescribing doctor) need to be aware that the medication is doing what it is meant to. Reassess the person following administration of such medications as antibiotics, analgesics, corticosteroids among others. This should be done within a reasonable time frame from the administration (usually 30 minutes to one hour following) and effects noted. Watch out for unexpected effects such as pruritus due to reactions to carrier ingredients in the rectal medication. This evaluation is crucial following the initial administration of a rectal medication.

GATHER EQUIPMENT

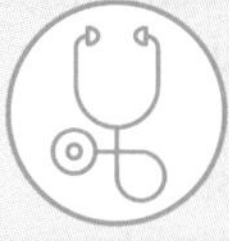

Gathering equipment is an organisational step that helps to create a positive environment for a successful interaction. It ensures that you have all needed material, boosts the person's confidence and trust in you, and increases your self-confidence. Equipment includes the following items:

EQUIPMENT	EXPLANATION
Medication administration sheet	To identify the person, medication, route, dose, time, and to document the successful administration of the medication
Tray or trolley	To organise and transport the equipment

EQUIPMENT	EXPLANATION
Rectal medication	*Suppositories* • Thin, bullet-shaped masses composed of water-soluble gels that melt at body temperature releasing the medication to be absorbed • Often stored in the refrigerator to prevent melting. Do not carry in your hand or pocket – inserting a soft suppository is difficult • Check the expiration date *Rectal tablets* • Powdered medication pressed into an oval form to be inserted into the rectum • Lubricated with water gel prior to insertion • The person must be well hydrated to absorb the medication *Medicated enema* • An aqueous, alcohol or oil base infused with medication prepared by pharmacy or the pharmaceutical company • Are generally less than 15 mL (micro-enema) • Oil-based solutions release their medication more slowly than water- or alcohol-based solutions • Come pre-packaged in a container designed to deliver medication into the rectum (with an integrated nozzle or tube) • Paediatric enemas have shorter nozzles or tubes • Check the expiration date
A (Macy) rectal catheter	• Recently introduced into emergency, critical and palliative care units • Similar to a Foley urinary catheter with two ports (medication administration and balloon inflation), a balloon near the distal end, and multiple holes beyond the balloon for the fluids and medication to be dispersed through • Used for multiple medication administrations over a period of time, and for administration of hypotonic fluids when oral and intravenous routes are inappropriate • Inserted so the balloon is beyond the anal sphincter in the lower third of the rectum and inflated, and the tube is taped to the thigh to keep it in place • A Luer syringe is needed to introduce the medications/fluids through the medication port (personal communication B. Macy, 8 February 2017) • It is safe, easy to use, comfortable, inexpensive and the users report no leakage (Parker, 2020) • This is a clean procedure (Parker, 2020)
Water-soluble lubricant and gauze square	• Reduces friction between the anal skin and the medication to ease insertion • A gauze square is used to apply the lubricant to the suppository, catheter or enema nozzle
Waterproof pad	Protects the bed linen in case of accidental defecation and reassures the person that they will not soil the bed
Bedpan or bedside commode	Needed if the medication is meant to stimulate defecation (see **Clinical Skill 34**)
Clean gloves	For personal protection from body fluids and the medication and to prevent spread of microorganisms
Tissues	To clean the anal area of excess lubricant following insertion of the medication and withdrawal of the inserting finger or nozzle
Drapes	Provides cover for exposed body parts (often bed linen is used)

THE SIX RIGHTS OF ADMINISTERING MEDICATION

See **Clinical Skill 37** for a complete description of the rights of medication administration. In summary, they include:

- *right time* – the first consideration
- *right medication* – verify the validity of the order and then choose from the medications on the trolley or the refrigerator. Check that the formulation is for rectal administration.
- *right route* – confirm this as noted on the medication administration sheet
- *right dose* – it is imperative to gain a therapeutic level of the medication
- *right person* – it is vital to verify the correct person is receiving the medication
- *right documentation* – must be adhered to.

ADMINISTER RECTAL MEDICATION

Video

Rectal administration of medication requires patience and compassion as well as skill. Preparation and administration of the various types of rectal medication are described.

Hand hygiene

Hand hygiene (see **Clinical Skill 5**) reduces the spread of microorganisms. Practise hand hygiene prior to and following each individual contact, before beginning a medication round, and after it is completed. Usually this is alcohol-based hand rub (ABHR), unless your hands are visibly soiled. Hand hygiene is especially important following rectal medication administration in case of inadvertent contamination of your skin with the medication or body fluids.

Administering rectal medication is a clean procedure. Clean gloves are worn to protect you from absorbing the medication as well as a personal protective measure. Ensure the medication never touches your hand.

Prepare the medication

Rectal medications generally require little preparation. The suppository is contained in a sealed package and is usually found in the refrigerator. Take it out a few minutes before administering to warm to room temperature. The micro-enema comes fully prepared from the pharmacy. If you are using a Macy catheter, you may need to powder an oral medication and add it to up to 50 mL of a prescribed solution (check with the pharmacy to ensure the oral formulation is safe to use rectally). Mix it well before drawing it up into an appropriate size of Luer syringe.

> ?
>
> If the suppository is soft (so it does not retain its shape within the wrapper), hold it, still in its wrap, under cold running water until it hardens or return it to the refrigerator to harden.

Administer the medication

Suppository or rectal tablet

Take the suppository or rectal tablet with the required dose of medication out of its wrapping. Place it on a gauze square ready for use. Apply a liberal amount of water-soluble lubricating gel to the suppository with the gauze and to your gloved inserting finger (usually index finger of dominant hand). Spread the buttocks to expose the anus using your non-dominant hand. Tell the person they will feel a cool sensation and pressure in their anus so they are prepared. Ask them to take a few deep breaths to relax the anal sphincter. Holding the buttocks apart, slowly insert your finger into the anus, past the internal sphincter to determine if there is a faecal mass. Withdraw your finger. Remove the glove, keeping the contaminated surface on the inside as you take it off. Perform hand hygiene and put clean gloves on.

If there is a faecal mass, wait until post-defecation to insert the medication (unless the medication is meant to stimulate defecation). If not, slowly insert the end of the suppository or tablet in front of your finger into the anus, about 4 cm, past the internal sphincter. Follow the manufacturer's instruction and the facility's policy about which end of the suppository (tapered or blunt) is to be inserted. The most effective way to insert a suppository remains mostly un-researched. Abd-El-Maeboud et al. (1991), in a very small research project, demonstrated the blunt end first insertion to reduce anal irritation and assist in retention. Other larger research projects have challenged this idea (Mitchell, 2019). If the medication is to treat constipation, slowly insert your finger with the *rounded* end of the suppository or tablet first into the anus, about 4 cm, past the internal sphincter; that is about 7.5 cm in total in an adult (Estes et al., 2020). Keep the suppository/tablet against the rectal wall to improve absorption of the medication. Withdraw your finger and wipe it on the tissue. Wipe the perianal area clean of lubricant. Again, remove the glove as above. Perform hand hygiene.

Medicated enema

Take the cap off the nozzle or the end of the tube of the enema. Apply a liberal amount of water-soluble lubricating gel to the rounded end. Spread the buttocks to expose the anus using your non-dominant hand. Tell the person they will feel a cool sensation and pressure in their anus so they are prepared. Ask them to take a few deep breaths to relax the anal sphincter. Holding the buttocks apart, slowly insert your finger into the anus, past the internal sphincter to determine if there is a faecal mass. Withdraw your finger. Remove the glove as above. Perform hand hygiene and put clean gloves on. If there is a faecal mass, wait until post-defecation to insert the medication. If not, slowly insert the rounded end of the nozzle into the anus, past the internal sphincter. Keep the end of the nozzle against the rectal wall to improve absorption of the medication. Squeeze the container to push the fluid into the rectum. Withdraw the nozzle and wrap the enema container in the tissue. Wipe the perianal area clean of lubricant. Remove the glove as above. Perform hand hygiene.

Ask the person to retain the medication for at least 20 minutes.

Rectal cream

Take the cap off the end of the tube of cream (individual measure) or of the rectal syringe with the cream measured into it from a larger tube. Apply a liberal amount of water-soluble lubricating gel to the rounded end. Spread the buttocks to expose the anus using your non-dominant hand. Tell the person they may feel a cool sensation and pressure in their anus so they are prepared. Ask them to take a few deep breaths to relax the anal sphincter. Holding the buttocks apart, slowly insert the rounded end of the nozzle into the anus, up to or past the internal sphincter, depending on the reason the cream is required. Keep the end of the nozzle against the rectal wall to improve absorption of the medication. Squeeze the container/syringe to push the cream into the anal canal or the rectum. Withdraw the nozzle and wrap the container in the tissue. Wipe the perianal area clean of lubricant. Remove your glove as above. Perform hand hygiene.

Macy catheter administration

Apply a liberal amount of water-soluble lubricating gel to the distal end of the catheter tube. Spread the buttocks to expose the anus using your non-dominant hand. Tell the person they will feel a cool sensation and pressure in their anus so they are prepared. Ask them to take a few deep breaths to relax the anal sphincter. Holding the buttocks apart, slowly insert the catheter to the marks on the tube. Inflate the balloon, and *gently* tug it to make sure it is above the anal sphincter. Tape it in place on the thigh. Draw up the medication into the syringe and attach the Luer syringe to the catheter tube. Slowly push the plunger to place the medication into the rectum. The Macy catheter can be clamped and left in place for further medication administration (Parker, 2020).

Post-procedure

Ask the person retain any systemic medication (e.g. analgesic, anxiolytic, antiemetic) for as long as possible (ideally, at least an hour), but to inform you if they are unable to retain the medication for the required time. Medication for constipation may be expelled more quickly. Remove your gloves and perform hand hygiene. Check back with them to determine the effect of the medication within 30 minutes.

CLEAN, REPLACE AND DISPOSE OF EQUIPMENT

Discard any disposable items used to administer the rectal medication (e.g. gloves, tissues, administration nozzle). Wipe the cart clean of spills or debris and replace stocks of supplies. Order stock medications and individual prescriptions from the pharmacy if they are running low. When they arrive on the unit, place them in the refrigerator or medication trolley with their labels visible to reduce the possibility of errors. Pharmacy will replace any medication in the automated dispensing cabinet (ADC) if one is in use. Return the medication administration sheet to its designated place for the next medication round.

DOCUMENTATION

Initial or sign the medication administration sheet/electronic medication administration record (eMAR) in the appropriate timeslot beside the written medication order and note if an assessment was done (e.g. skin condition, pain). Also document briefly on the medication administration sheet in the appropriate timeslot if an individual has refused to take the medication, or if some other untoward event occurs, document it more fully in the progress notes. The bar code medication administration system will automatically record the medication, dose and time as well as your identification on the eMAR. The effects of the medications, expected or unexpected, are assessed 30 minutes to one hour after administration, and are then documented. Adverse effects should be reported to the shift coordinator and the medical staff, and the remaining doses of the medication withheld.

CLINICAL SKILLS ASSESSMENT

Rectal medication

Demonstrates the ability to effectively and safely administer rectal medication. Incorporates the *National Safety and Quality Health Service Standards:* 2 Partnering with Consumers, 3 Preventing and Controlling Healthcare-Associated Infection, 5 Comprehensive Care, 6 Communicating for Safety, and 8 Recognising and Responding to Acute Deterioration (ACSQHC, 2021).

Performance criteria	1	2	3	4	5
(Numbers indicate NMBA *Registered Nurse Standards for Practice*)	**(Dependent)**	**(Marginal)**	**(Assisted)**	**(Supervised)**	**(Independent)**
1. Identifies indication (1.1, 3.3, 3.4)	☐	☐	☐	☐	☐
2. Verifies the validity of the written medication order (1.4, 3.4, 6.2, 6.5)	☐	☐	☐	☐	☐
3. Evidence of therapeutic interaction with the person, e.g. gives the person a clear explanation of the medication, discusses adverse effects of the medication (1.4, 1.5, 2.1, 2.2, 3.2)	☐	☐	☐	☐	☐
4. Demonstrates clinical reasoning abilities, e.g. positions the person, obtains the appropriate form of the medication, assesses, teaches, advocates for and evaluates the person regarding this medication; provides privacy, comfort measures (1.1, 1.2, 1.3, 4.2, 6.1)	☐	☐	☐	☐	☐
5. Adheres to the general concepts of working with therapeutic substances (1.1, 1.3, 1.5, 3.3, 3.4, 4.1, 4.2, 4.3, 6.2, 6.5, 6.6)	☐	☐	☐	☐	☐
6. Gathers equipment (1.1, 5.5, 6.1): ■ medication administration sheet ■ tray or trolley ■ rectal medication ■ a (Macy) rectal catheter and clamp ■ water-soluble lubricant ■ waterproof pad ■ bedpan or bedside commode ■ clean gloves ■ tissues ■ drapes	☐	☐	☐	☐	☐
7. Uses the six (or more) rights to administer the medication (1.1, 1.2, 1.3, 1.4, 1.5, 2.2, 3.4, 4.1, 4.2, 4.3, 6.1, 6.2, 6.5, 6.6)	☐	☐	☐	☐	☐
8. Performs hand hygiene (1.1, 3.4, 6.1)	☐	☐	☐	☐	☐
9. Prepares the medication (1.1, 3.4, 6.1)	☐	☐	☐	☐	☐
10. Administers the medication (1.1, 2.2, 6.1)	☐	☐	☐	☐	☐
11. Cleans, replaces and disposes of equipment appropriately (3.6, 6.1)	☐	☐	☐	☐	☐
12. Documents relevant information (1.4, 1.6, 2.2, 3.5, 3.7, 6.2, 6.5, 7.3)	☐	☐	☐	☐	☐
13. Demonstrates the ability to link theory to practice (1.1, 3.3, 3.4, 3.5)	☐	☐	☐	☐	☐

Student:

Clinical facilitator: Date:

CHAPTER 44

INHALED MEDICATION

INDICATIONS

Administering inhaled medication involves assisting the person to inhale a measured dose of medication into their respiratory tract, where the medication is immediately absorbed into the bloodstream through the alveolar–capillary interface. The types of inhaled medication are:

- nebulised inhalant – single measured dose of a respiratory medication (e.g. a corticosteroid or bronchodilator), usually diluted in saline. Compressed air or oxygen is passed through the solution, aerosolising the liquid to be inhaled into the lungs via a mouthpiece or a mask
- measured dose inhaler (MDI) – multiple-dose canister of pressurised medication (of various types, e.g. Ventolin puffer) that delivers a small dose of the medication in an inert propellant, ejected directly into the person's mouth for simultaneous inhalation. Careful teaching of the technique is required
- measured dose inhaler with spacer – MDI canister with a spacer (an air-filled chamber) attached to permit the aerosolised medication to be inhaled more slowly, either through a mouthpiece or a mask. This is recommended for all children (Asthma Australia, 2020)
- dry powder inhaler (Spinhaler, turbuhaler) – uses a dry form of medication, tiny particles of which are dispersed by the turbulent air and inhaled directly into the respiratory tract. Single- and multiple-dose varieties are available.

Inhalers of all types have the advantage of achieving high medication concentration in the airway, reducing systemic adverse effects, providing a rapid onset of action, convenience and comfort during use. There are disadvantages – improper technique reduces the dose inhaled, and some people find some of the inhalers difficult to use either due to age or to incapacity (poor vision, grip weakness, arthritis, cognitive disability). The incorrect use of inhaler devices can result in a poorly controlled disease or condition (Caminati et al., 2021). Eighty per cent of people with asthma and 67 per cent of healthcare providers are unable to demonstrate the correct technique for inhaler use (Global Initiative for Asthma, 2019).

As for all medications, the person must be closely monitored for both therapeutic and toxic effects of the inhalation as well as checking their technique for inhaler device use.

Verify the written medication order

Check the medication administration sheet for time, route, dose and medication. The physician also orders the type of inhaler to be used. Question any order that is unclear, incomplete or that seems inappropriate or unreasonable for the person.

To question an order, you *must know* the person's diagnosis, the usual dose, the purpose of the medication, its therapeutic effect, any adverse effects, any pertinent nursing implications, and individual factors that mediate response to medications such as age, weight and psychological factors. Determine any drug allergies that the person may have so that potentially harmful substances are not administered.

EVIDENCE OF THERAPEUTIC INTERACTION

There are generally two situations in which inhalant medication is required, each requiring a different approach. The first is as a therapeutic administration or a prophylactic measure. Seek the person's consent for the treatment. Your greatest job is to teach the person the correct technique for inhaling their medication and to supervise their technique until it is learnt. The second situation is during a respiratory crisis. During an acute attack, you need to control your own anxiety and administer the medication while calmly explaining your actions.

DEMONSTRATE CLINICAL REASONING

ELDER CARE

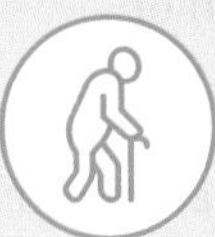

Ageing can cause deterioration of respiratory function, increased susceptibility to infection and malignancy, as well as an increased incidence of chronic obstructive pulmonary disease (COPD) and idiopathic pulmonary fibrosis (Sachi et al., 2023). Inhaling medications is influenced by slower and weaker peak inspiratory flow affecting the dosage. Usami (2022) demonstrated that teaching and reinforcing correct techniques (full exhalation, strongest inhalation and gargling following each administration via an MDI) were effective in reducing errors and improving the elder's condition. Hagmeyer et al. (2023) recommend using a spacer with a one-way valve to improve doses to the lung tissues for elderly people who lack strength and coordination.

THE PERSON LIVING WITH SEVERE OBESITY

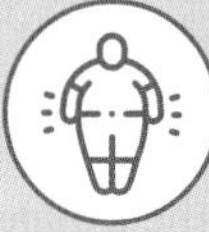

Severe obesity reduces lung function by both mechanical impairment of the lungs/chest wall (e.g. adiposity pressing on diaphragm), the increased production of inflammatory cytokines and alteration in immune cells. These result in both asthma and asthma-like symptoms (e.g. dyspnoea, wheeze and airway hyperresponsiveness) (Dixon & Peters, 2018). Adherence to inhaled medication regimens can assist a severely obese person to undertake weight loss and increase their physical activity (Gibson, McDonald & Thomas, 2023). Again, teaching the correct technique and reinforcing the importance of adhering to the regimen is important.

General concepts of working with therapeutic substances

Please review **Clinical Skill 37** for general concepts of medication administration. The following safety concerns are specific to inhaled medications. You need to know:

- the strength of the medication/solution
- whether the diluent (nebuliser) has been mixed with it
- whether oxygen (and in what dose) or compressed air is to be the propellant (nebuliser)
- the length of time over which the medication is to be given (this is usually the number of 'puffs' or when the mist stops flowing from the nebuliser)
- how to use the device (metered dose inhaler, dry powder inhaler, nebuliser) with the correct technique.

Mechanisms of medication administration

Preparation

To reduce errors, administer only medications that you have personally prepared, and undertake the following:

- *Be aware of allergies* – check the medication administration sheet for an allergy caution, look for an allergy armband (red) and ask the person if they are allergic to anything. Ask them if they have taken this medication before and, if so, have they tolerated it.
- *Ask the person to state their name* – don't ask them if their name is 'Mary Smith', as they may agree, regardless of who they are (e.g. they may be deaf, confused or non-English speaking).
- *Listen to the person* – many, if not most, people know their medications well, and any query by them as to the dose or appearance of the inhaled medication should be taken seriously before administering.
- *Sign or initial the medications sheet* – do this as soon as medication is administered to prevent a potential overdose (i.e. another nurse might administer a second dose of the medication thinking it has not been given). Most facilities do not allow you to sign prior to giving the medication, only after the administration.

Responsibility to the person

Your responsibility involves assessment, teaching, advocacy and evaluation of the effect of the medication administered.

Assess the physiological function that the medication is expected to affect prior to administering an inhaled medication (e.g. respiratory assessment prior to administering an inhaler or nebuliser) to provide a baseline for use in evaluating the effectiveness of the medication. You must also assess the person's medication history (i.e. a review of the person's current and past drugs – prescribed, over-the-counter [OTC], herbal preparations or recreational) and medical history (e.g. respiratory infections, tumours, pneumothorax). These assessments may indicate that the medication should be withheld and the shift coordinator informed.

LOOK at the person's colour, ease of respiration, depth of respiration, use of accessory muscles and flaring of nostrils. This will provide a baseline to determine the effectiveness of the medication.

LISTEN for quiet breathing. If there is distress/difficulty, auscultate the chest and listen for adventitious breath sounds.

FEEL for the respiratory and pulse rates.

If the person is in respiratory crisis, such as worsening asthma, or experiencing an acute attack, you must undertake an immediate and thorough clinical respiratory assessment covering the following:

- their ability to talk
- a brief mental status assessment (especially disorientation and confusion)
- auscultate their chest
- monitor their respiratory rate and effort
- cough
- monitor their pulse
- note their general appearance for anxiety, pallor, cyanosis
- note any sputum production (note amount, colour, viscosity and document).

Stay with the person. Help them to remain calm by slowing their breathing. Ask them to breathe with you and breathe increasingly slower. If you must ask questions, use closed questions wherever possible so answers can be non-verbal.

The medication procedures are the same as below, but you may have to accomplish the steps yourself. A mask would be necessary if nebulisation or a spacer is used. Notify senior staff and the physician for further orders.

Teach the name, intended function and dose of the medication to the person, its frequency, adverse effects, how to minimise these and how to use the medication (see individual types of inhaled medication listed in the 'Gather equipment' box). Discuss maintaining the medication regimen at home and adapt the regimen to accommodate the person's home schedule (without compromising the efficacy of the medication). The person needs to be aware of the importance of regular monitoring required for some medications. Be alert to any cues the person or family might give about not continuing to use a medication (e.g. inability to manipulate equipment due to arthritis). The cost of inhaled medication can reduce adherence to a medication regimen (Tudball et al., 2019). In Australia, the co-payment (out-of-pocket costs) is higher for many of the asthma medications. The person needs to discuss any financial constraints so the physician knows to order generic brands, or use simple medications (e.g. corticosteroids as opposed to combinations) as appropriate. Discussing these things may improve the person's ability or commitment to sustaining the prescribed treatment.

Advocacy includes alerting the medical practitioner of adverse effects, or any reason the person tells you that would influence their continuation of the inhaled medication as required.

Evaluation is a very important aspect of your responsibility in administering medications. You and the prescribing doctor need to be aware that the medication is doing what it is meant to. Reassess the person following administration of such medications as bronchodilators and corticosteroids, among others. This should be done within a reasonable time frame from the administration (usually 30 minutes following inhalation) and effects noted. This evaluation is crucial following the initial administration of an inhaled medication or if the person was having difficulty breathing prior to the medication.

GATHER EQUIPMENT

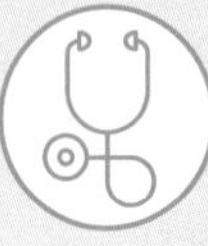

The following list provides a description of the types of equipment you will require to administer inhaled medications. Clean hands and gloves are required while preparing nebulisation so that medication is not contaminated, and you do not contact and absorb the medication. Equipment required includes the following:

EQUIPMENT	EXPLANATION
NEBULISER	
Medication administration sheet	Contains the valid order, the person's name, the medication name, dose, route and time, and provides a place to document its administration
Medication	Prescribed and in a liquid form
Nebule (single dose) or syringe marked with [for inhalant only]	To carefully measure the dose
Sterile saline	To dilute the medication so the dose can be delivered over a prescribed amount of time. The amount will be specified
Sterile nebuliser pack	• Consists of a nebuliser cup that is attached to the compressed air or oxygen by the tubing • The medication and saline are placed in the cup that the air is forced through. It is screwed into the nebuliser body. These can come as a sealed unit with the medication already prepared
Tubing and connector	• Oxygen tubing (green) carries the air or oxygen to the nebuliser cup • A connector is needed to attach the tubing to the outlet • An integral hose carries the medicated aerosol from the nebuliser body to the mask or mouthpiece

EQUIPMENT	EXPLANATION
Oxygen or compressed (wall) air	• Compressed air is needed to create a cloud of droplets the correct size for inhalation/absorption into the bronchial tree • Ultrasonic or vibrating mesh aerosolisation of the medication is increasingly used because it is more effective, quieter and more portable (Vizzoni et al., 2023), although it is more expensive (Hagmeyer et al., 2023)
Mouthpiece or mask	To seal the medication into the person's oropharynx so that none is lost to the atmosphere
Clean disposable gloves	To comply with standard precautions, prevent your absorption of the medication and to protect both you and the person from cross-contamination
METERED DOSE INHALER	
Medication administration sheet	As above
Medication	• A pressurised canister with medication provides a number of doses of the prescribed medication • Devices with dose counters and an add-on phone app to provide feedback on correct inhalation are the most accurate medication therapy (Mahmoud et al., 2023) • Obtained from pharmacy and is not shared with others
Metered dose inhaler device	• A metered dose inhaler device (puffer) accepts the canister, which is pressed to provide the medication for inhalation, consisting of the measured dose and the propellant • This is a personal device
Spacer	• This is a chamber into which the inhaler device fits snugly • The outlet at the other end is put in the person's mouth for them to breathe through • The spacer slows down and contains the aerosolised medication for several seconds while the person inhales it more slowly, reducing the need for coordination between actuation of the MDI and inhalation (Hagmeyer et al., 2023) • All children should use a spacer, and they are recommended for adolescents and adults (Asthma Australia, 2020) • Kept at the bedside
Clean disposable gloves	To comply with standard precautions, prevent your absorption of the medication and to protect both you and the person from cross-contamination
DRY POWDER INHALER	
Medication administration sheet	As above
Medication	Powdered medication (capsules or contained in a multi-dose format) is often used in preference to the MDI because it is effective without the use of chlorofluorocarbon propellants, which damage the ozone layer
Dry powder inhaler (DPI)	• Available in several formats, but generally consists of a small chamber to which the powdered medication (usually in a capsule) is placed • Make yourself aware of the types of devices available where you are gaining experience • The person must continue to use the same device, as a difference in dosage between devices has been noted (Hagmeyer et al., 2023; Salama et al., 2022) • It is important to hold the device according to the manufacturer's instructions (usually horizontally) • To pierce the capsule, activate the device by twisting the halves of the chamber together, so the medication will be released • The person must breathe in long and hard for the air entrainment to produce sufficient turbulence to carry the powder. Power (battery) assisted devices are available to overcome low respiratory flow and increase lung deposition (Kumar et al., 2022). • Not suitable for people experiencing an asthma attack. These people lack sufficient inspiratory flow rates to entrain the medication and then carry it into their lungs • The inhaler must be closed after use (National Asthma Council Australia, 2021)
Clean disposable gloves	To comply with standard precautions, prevent your absorption of the medication and to protect both you and the person from cross-contamination

THE SIX RIGHTS OF ADMINISTERING MEDICATION

The six rights of medication administration are particularly important when administering inhalant medication because of the rapid onset of effects. This leaves little time to intervene if a mistake occurs. See **Clinical Skill 37** for a complete description of the rights of medication administration. In summary, they include:

- *right time* – the first consideration
- *right medication* – verify the validity of the order and then choose from the medications on the trolley
- *right route* – confirm this as noted on the medication administration sheet

- *right dose* – it is imperative to gain a therapeutic level of the medication
- *right person* – it is vital to verify the correct person is receiving the medication
- *right documentation* – must be adhered to.

For inhaled medications, you must also consider the *right device* and adhere to the *right technique*.

ADMINISTER INHALED MEDICATION

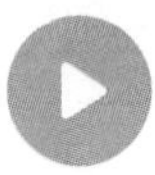
Video

Inhaled medication can be given via metered dose inhaler, nebuliser or dry powder inhaler. Each of these is described in the following sections.

Hand hygiene

Clean hands and gloves are required while preparing nebulisation so that medication is not contaminated, and you do not contact and absorb the medication. Hand hygiene is attended to before and after each contact with the person and at the completion of the treatment (see **Clinical Skill 5**).

Administer the medication

Metered dose inhaler

Medication such as low-dose corticosteroids, and, increasingly, antidepressants, insulin medication and others, are often administered daily or even more often by metered dose inhalation (Fonceca et al., 2019). The person needs to know how to administer the medication, as follows:

1. Seat the canister firmly into the applicator and remove the mouth cap. Check the dose counter (if the MDI has one) to ensure there are doses remaining.
2. Hold the canister upright shake it and applicator vigorously to disperse the medication.
3. Hold the applicator upright with the mouthpiece at the bottom (if using a spacer, place the applicator mouth into the spacer at this point).
4. Breathe out gently away from the mouthpiece.
5. Place the mouthpiece in the mouth between the teeth.
6. Keep the chin up and the applicator upright and breathe out fully.
7. Use the lips to form a seal around the mouthpiece.
8. Press the top of the canister down once (to release the medication and propellant) at the same time as taking a long deep slow breath in.
9. Hold the breath for at least five seconds or longer if comfortable (if using a spacer, breathe normally).
10. Release the pressure from the canister and remove it from the mouth while holding your breath.
11. If multiple doses are ordered, wait a minimum of one minute and repeat the procedure including vigorously shaking the canister.
12. Replace the cap (National Asthma Council Australia, 2021).

After the person has administered the medication, assess the effect of the treatment.

The DPI is administered in a similar way after the medication has been put into the container. The person should be asked to demonstrate their use of an inhaler if you are in doubt about their ability to self-administer an inhaled medication.

Nebulisation

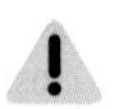
Safety

Nebulised medication is easily deposited on your skin. To reduce your dermal exposure to the medication, stand well back from the person, away from the ventilated outflow port, and ask the person to take deep breaths (Ishau et al., 2020).

This therapy is used effectively for management of long-term respiratory conditions such as chronic bronchitis and other obstructive pulmonary diseases. Nebulisation is used if the person requires oxygen; otherwise, inhaling the medication through a spacer is just as effective (Asthma Australia, 2020). It is administered daily or more often. Seat the person upright if possible and in a supported and relaxed position. Provide diversion, as this treatment can take 10 to 15 minutes to administer. Use the following steps:

1. Place the nebuliser machine on a clean, flat, stable surface and plug it into a power source.
2. Attach the oxygen tubing to the oxygen flow meter or the wall air outlet.
3. Undo the top of the nebuliser unit and add the solution to be nebulised (medication plus diluent that has been carefully measured according to the orders) to the cup.
4. Replace the top of the nebuliser and attach the oxygen tubing to the base of the nebuliser.
5. Connect the mask (if a mask is used, check the facility's policy for providing protective eye wear) or mouthpiece/hose to the top of the nebuliser unit.
6. Turn the oxygen/air flow to 6 to 8 L per minute and check that the mist is issuing from the face mask or mouthpiece.
7. Apply the face mask or give the mouthpiece to the person and check that there is a good seal.
8. Ask the person to breathe through their mouth, slowly and deeply before exhalation, holding their breath. If possible, every 5th breath is held to allow medication to settle into the lung tissue (Cleveland Clinic, 2019).
9. When the mist has stopped (five to 15 minutes), assess the effect of the treatment.

Post-procedure

Many inhaled medications predispose the person to oral health problems, such as dental decay or candidiasis (McCormick et al., 2019). At a minimum, ensure the person rinses their mouth/gargles after using an inhaled medication. Tooth brushing and use of an antimicrobial mouthwash help to reduce the incidence of oral health problems. Chewing sugar-free gum and drinking water help to reduce oral dryness.

CLEAN, REPLACE AND DISPOSE OF EQUIPMENT

Rinse the mask and the nebuliser in warm water after each use and allow to air-dry. The nebuliser should be labelled with the name of the person and the medication, and will be kept at the bedside in a sealed plastic bag. The mask, the tubing and the nebuliser unit are discarded when no longer needed. Perform hand hygiene.

The MDI applicator is a personal-use device. It should be washed and air-dried prior to initial use and after each use. Spacers should be washed in detergent and air-dried and checked for cracks and valve integrity on a monthly basis (Asthma Australia, 2020). The National Asthma Council Australia (2020) further recommends not to rinse or wipe dry, as this causes static build-up inside the spacer to which medication adheres.

DOCUMENTATION

The medication administration is noted on the medication administration sheet or on the electronic medication administration record (eMAR) when using the bar code medication administration system. Assessment information is charted in the progress notes and should include rate and depth of respiration, effort needed, and adventitious breath sounds, both before and following medication administration.

PART 7

CLINICAL SKILLS ASSESSMENT

Inhaled medication

Demonstrates the ability to effectively and safely administer inhaled medication. Incorporates the *National Safety and Quality Health Service Standards*: 2 Partnering with Consumers, 3 Preventing and Controlling Healthcare-Associated Infection, 5 Comprehensive Care, 6 Communicating for Safety, and 8 Recognising and Responding to Acute Deterioration (ACSQHC, 2021).

Performance criteria	1	2	3	4	5
(Numbers indicate NMBA *Registered Nurse Standards for Practice*)	(Dependent)	(Marginal)	(Assisted)	(Supervised)	(Independent)
1. Identifies indication (1.1, 3.3, 3.4)	☐	☐	☐	☐	☐
2. Verifies the validity of the written medication order (1.4, 3.4, 6.2, 6.5)	☐	☐	☐	☐	☐
3. Evidence of therapeutic interaction with the person, e.g. gives the person a clear explanation of the procedure (1.4, 1.5, 2.1, 2.2, 3.2)	☐	☐	☐	☐	☐
4. Demonstrates clinical reasoning (1.1, 1.2, 1.3, 4.2, 6.1)	☐	☐	☐	☐	☐
5. Adheres to the general concepts of working with therapeutic substances (1.1, 1.3, 1.5, 3.3, 3.4, 4.1, 4.2, 4.3, 6.2, 6.5, 6.6)	☐	☐	☐	☐	☐
6. Gathers appropriate equipment (1.1, 5.5, 6.1): ■ medication administration sheet ■ medication ■ dry powder inhaler (DPI) ■ eye-dropper or medicine cup ■ sterile saline ■ sterile nebuliser pack ■ tubing and connector ■ oxygen or compressed (wall) air ■ mouthpiece or mask ■ metered dose inhaler device ■ spacer ■ clean disposable gloves	☐	☐	☐	☐	☐
7. Uses the six (or more) rights to administer the medication (1.1, 1.2, 1.3, 1.4, 1.5, 2.2, 3.4, 4.1, 4.2, 4.3, 6.1, 6.2, 6.5, 6.6)	☐	☐	☐	☐	☐
8. Performs hand hygiene (1.1, 3.4, 6.1)	☐	☐	☐	☐	☐
9. Assesses the person prior to administering medication (4.1, 4.2, 4.3, 6.1)	☐	☐	☐	☐	☐
10. Prepares the medication using aseptic technique for a nebuliser (1.1, 6.1)	☐	☐	☐	☐	☐
11. Safely administers medication to maximise its effects and to minimise discomfort (1.1, 3.4, 6.1)	☐	☐	☐	☐	☐
12. Cleans, replaces and disposes of equipment appropriately (3.6, 6.1)	☐	☐	☐	☐	☐
13. Documents relevant information (1.4, 1.6, 2.2, 3.5, 3.7, 6.2, 6.5, 7.3)	☐	☐	☐	☐	☐
14. Demonstrates the ability to link theory to practice (1.1, 3.3, 3.4, 3.5)	☐	☐	☐	☐	☐

Student:

Clinical facilitator: Date:

CHAPTER 45

PARENTERAL MEDICATION

INDICATIONS

Administering parenteral medication means administration of an internal medication not involving the gastrointestinal tract; that is, injecting a medication into a body tissue. Parenteral administration of medication is faster-acting than oral administration, since the drug does not go through the digestive process but is absorbed directly from the tissues into the bloodstream, and then to the target tissues. This bypasses the 'first pass' detoxification processes in the liver, increasing the effectiveness of the medication. Other indications for parenteral administration are when the oral route is unavailable (e.g. nil by mouth, nausea, oral surgery) or when the drug would be destroyed by digestion (e.g. heparin, insulin). Because of the rapid effect and the irretrievable nature of injected medications, the person must be closely monitored for both therapeutic and toxic effects.

The types of parenteral medication are:

- *intradermal (ID)* – an injection into the dermis layer of the skin, often used for allergy testing. It has the slowest absorption rate of the parenteral sites, and minute volumes of potentially allergy-causing medication are administered
- *subcutaneous (SC)* – an injection that places the medication (e.g. insulin, heparin, opioids) into the SC tissue. It is more rapidly absorbed than ID injection, but slower than intramuscular. Only small volumes can be injected; however, larger volumes can be infused over time (see **Clinical Skill 51**)
- *intramuscular (IM)* – an injection that delivers the medication (e.g. antibiotics) into a muscle mass. The muscle sites can take larger volumes and more irritating solutions than either ID or SC sites. The greater blood supply increases the rate of absorption
- *intravenous (IV)* – a type of administration very commonly used for antibiotics or analgesia (see **Clinical Skills 31, 32, 46, 47 and 48** detailing the administration of IV medication)
- *epidural administration* – provides analgesia (commonly a combination of opioids and anaesthetic medications) via a fine catheter inserted directly into the epidural space (see **Clinical Skill 50**)
- *intraarterial, intraosseous, intrapleural, intrathecal* and *intraperitoneal injections* – are other forms of parenteral administration that are not performed by nurses.

Verify the written medication order

Check the medication administration sheet for time, route, dose and medication. Question any unclear or incomplete order or any that seem inappropriate or unreasonable for the person. The facility where you are practising will provide a list of acceptable abbreviations for medication administration. Confusion about medication names is a common source of error. The Australian Commission on Safety and Quality in Health Care (ACSQHC) website has a number of publications that discuss the various errors and how to prevent these.

To question an order, you *must know* the person's diagnosis, the purpose of the medication, the medication's therapeutic effect, any adverse effects, the usual dose, any pertinent nursing implications, and individual factors that alter response to medications (e.g. age, weight, psychological status).

Be aware of any drug or food allergies that the person may have so that potentially harmful substances are not administered (or, if allergy testing, the type of reaction can be anticipated).

EVIDENCE OF THERAPEUTIC INTERACTION

Many people fear or become anxious about injections. Listen to the person's fears and concerns, correct their misapprehensions and explain some of the techniques used to minimise discomfort to help prepare them for the sensations they will feel. Do not tell them the injection will be painless – describe it as a pinch or sting. Discussing the therapeutic effects (and adverse effects they may encounter) helps potentiate the effects of the medication. Gain their consent. They have the right to refuse the injection.

PART 7

DEMONSTRATE CLINICAL REASONING

The key issue is that you recognise the type of injection required and where to inject it. Identify the person and check the six rights of medication administration and for allergies. Provide privacy, position the person for comfort and access the injection site. Assess both the person and the volume of medication to be given. Depending on the injection type (ID, SC, IM), consider the person's muscle mass, body mass index (BMI), access to site, ease of site identification, rotation of sites, type of medication being injected, condition of the person's skin and underlying tissue at the site (see 'Locate and assess the appropriate site') and the person's preferences if possible. Administration of parenteral medication to a child requires special consideration, and a paediatric textbook should be consulted before proceeding.

Provide privacy

Even if the injection site is not located in an intimate position or does not require exposing the body, many people will prefer to have the door closed or their curtains drawn for fear that their response to the injection will cause them embarrassment.

ELDER CARE

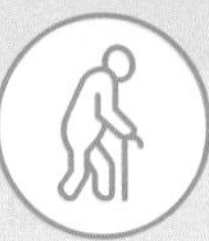

Elderly people have a lower proportion of body water (Walger & Heppner, 2020) and tissue hydration affects the rate of absorption from parenteral medication sites (Usach et al., 2019). Kidney and liver functions decline. Skin becomes thinner, less elastic and prone to tears and bruises injury. There is less fat beneath the skin to cushion the skin (Stephanacci, 2022). Muscle masses atrophy. Consider these physiological changes when giving parenteral medications to elderly people, and handle their skin gently (e.g. pinching up a section to inject, removing the needle at the angle of entry). Watch closely for medication effects, side effects and interactions. Take care with the amount of medication injected into a muscle, as sometimes frail and thin elderly people can take only about 2 mL of fluid.

THE PERSON LIVING WITH SEVERE OBESITY

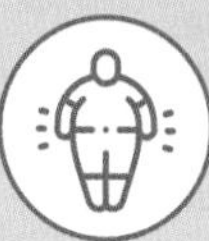

Parenteral medication (IM, SC) in people living with severe obesity is affected by the tissue composition and depth. There is excess adipose tissue at the injection sites, which makes it hard to deposit the medication in the correct tissue. For example, SC injections reach only fat, which has little circulation so allows for little absorption, and IM injections reach either fat or SC tissue rather than muscle. This alters the rate and extent of absorption. Choose the needle length carefully to deposit the medication where it is ordered. If IM is ordered, obtain a longer needle to deposit the medication where it is meant to go. Strohfus, Palma and Wallace (2021) suggest a 38 mm needle for females with a BMI over 25 and in males with a BMI over 35. Potential adverse effects are pain, bruising, haematoma, granulomas, fat necrosis and calcification (Erstad & Barletta, 2022).

It is often very difficult to locate the landmarks you need in people who are severely obese because excess adiposity obscures them. Be persistent in identifying bony landmarks (e.g. iliac crest and greater trochanter). If in doubt, consult a more experienced nurse. Often, severely obese people will have a long-term peripherally inserted IV access device inserted so medications can be given via IV rather than IM or SC. (See **Clinical Skills 15 and 23** for a brief explanation of bariatric issues.)

General concepts of working with therapeutic substances

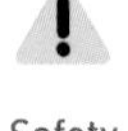

Safety

Please review the general concepts and mechanisms of medication administration presented in **Clinical Skill 37**. The following safety concerns are specific to parenteral medications:

- Inject only medication solutions that are designated 'for injectable use only'. Injecting a solution designed for oral or topical use can result in adverse reactions, from localised (e.g. an abscess) to fatal systemic effects.
- All injections require aseptic technique.
- Never recap the needle on a **used** syringe. To reduce the risk of needle-stick injuries during disposal, ampoules, empty vials, needles and used syringes are discarded in rigid plastic or metal sharps containers. Do not put your fingers into the sharps container. Any needle-stick or sharps injury, whether clean (i.e. while the needle is sterile) or contaminated, must be reported.
- Choose an appropriate injection site to reduce the incidence of injection-related complications. The drug manufacturer will also recommend appropriate sites.

THE SIX RIGHTS OF ADMINISTERING MEDICATION

The six rights are particularly important when administering parenteral medication because of the rapid onset of effects. This leaves little time to intervene if a mistake occurs. Generally, there is a legal requirement for parenteral medication to be checked independently by two registered nurses (RNs), or other healthcare professionals such as a medical officer or an enrolled nurse.

GATHER EQUIPMENT

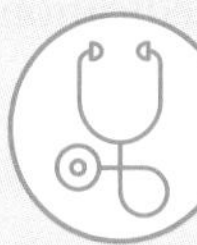

Gathering equipment is an organisational step that helps to create a positive environment for a successful interaction and reduces the risk of errors when preparing medication. It is essential you know the equipment so you are able to choose the correct implements for each injection to minimise discomfort and increase efficiency. Equipment may include the following items:

EQUIPMENT	EXPLANATION
Syringes	• Generally disposable plastic, in a range of sizes from 0.5 mL to 5 mL for injections (and up to 50 mL for IV injections), sterile and packaged individually. Glass syringes are available if the medication to be given is incompatible with plastic • Have three component parts: the calibrated barrel that holds the medication, the plunger that pushes the medication out, and the tip, which connects to the needle • Tips can be plain or Luer Lock; Luer Lock tips are designed for use with a range of connectors as well as for attaching needles • Scales are marked on the barrel of the syringe in both millilitres and tenths of millilitres, or units in an insulin syringe • Insulin syringes come with an attached needle • There are an increasing number of prefilled barrel/needle cartridges (with a compatible syringe/plunger system) in use
Needles	• Made of stainless steel and come with a plastic cap in a sterile package • Are generally disposable • There are three parts to the needle: the hub, which connects to the syringe; the cannula, which is the hollow shaft through which the medication flows; and the bevel, which is the slanted part at the tip of the cannula Needles have three variables: • Length of the bevel – a short bevel is used for IV (although most IV injections are given via an interlock system that does not use needles) and intradermal injections, so the bevel will not become occluded; long bevels are used for SC and IM injections because they are sharper and cause less discomfort • Length of the cannula – ranges from 1 to 5 cm for use with normal injections; some special-purpose needles can be up to 12 cm • Gauge of the cannula – varies from #14 (very large bore) to #28 (very fine bore). The smaller gauges cause less discomfort, but the larger-gauge needles may need to be used if the medication is oily or viscous
Safety syringes	• Developed to reduce the incidence of needle-stick injuries, commonly used • Use either detachable needles or have an inbuilt needle • Either passive or active devices retract the needle into the barrel. Passive retractable needles require you to activate the device (as per the manufacturer's recommendations). Active retractable needle retracts automatically into the barrel of the syringe • New South Wales and Queensland have policies about the use of safety syringes (New South Wales Health, 2018; Queensland Health, 2016)
Ampoules	• Small, single-dose containers of medication made of glass or plastic • The medication is sealed into the container, the neck of which must be broken, twisted off or snapped off to get to the medication. Most glass ampoule necks are prescored so they break cleanly; if not, use a file around the neck of the ampoule to ensure a clean break and an ampoule opener (a tight-fitting cap over the top of the ampoule) to prevent injuries. Break the ampoule neck away from yourself
Vials	• Single- or multi-use glass containers with rubber stoppers • May contain either liquid medication for immediate use or powdered medication that requires reconstitution • The medication is accessed with a filter or drawing up needle through the rubber stopper
Filter needles	To reduce the risk of glass or rubber particulate matter being withdrawn with the medication and inadvertently injected into the person
Alcowipes	To clean vial tops, to cleanse skin before injection, to apply pressure to a puncture site or to wrap around the neck of a glass ampoule to prevent injury when snapping off the neck
Gauze squares	To tend to the puncture site
Injection tray	To transport the filled syringe and needle, the alcowipes or gauze squares and the empty ampoule to the bedside – an organisational tool
Sharps container	• A rigid plastic, metal or glass container used to protect against accidental needle-stick injuries • All used needles, syringes and glass containers are placed in the sharps container as soon as the injection has been given and documented
Clean gloves	To comply with standard precautions and protect both you and the person from cross-contamination

Clinical Skill 37 gives a complete description of the rights of medication administration. In summary, they include:

- *right time* – the first consideration
- *right medication* – verify the validity of the order and then choose from the medications available. Be sure the medication is for parenteral use.
- *right route* – confirm this as noted on the medication administration sheet
- *right dose* – it is imperative to gain a therapeutic level of the medication
- *right person* – it is vital to verify the correct person is receiving the medication
- *right documentation* – must be adhered to.

An additional 'right' for parenteral medication is the right site.

ADMINISTER PARENTERAL MEDICATION

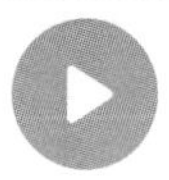
Video

Administering a parenteral medication consists of attending to the rights of medication administration, drawing up the medication, locating and cleaning the appropriate site, inserting the needle and injecting the medication, as discussed in the following sections. Preparation of the injection usually occurs in the medication room (see **Clinical Skill 46** for assessing the preparation area).

Hand hygiene

Hand hygiene (see **Clinical Skill 5**) is an infection-control measure that is crucial during this type of invasive procedure because the person's skin integrity is broken. Clean gloves are used to comply with standard precautions.

Draw up the medication

Choose the appropriate equipment. TABLE 45.1 indicates the usual equipment for each of the administration modes.

Open the syringe and filter needle packages without contaminating their contents. A filter (drawing-up) needle is used if drawing up medications from a glass ampoule or rubber-topped container. Filter needles are blunt and contain a tiny filter, and can only be used for drawing up a medication. Any particles originally drawn up would be deposited in the person if you did not change the needle. To remove the filter needle, use the passive, one-handed technique (scoop the cap and click it onto the needle) or other sharps safety technique required by your healthcare facility. Then remove it from the syringe and discard into the sharps container. It is important to follow the policies and procedures of the healthcare setting to ensure safety (both yours and the person you are injecting). This is an infection-control measure and a comfort measure, and reduces the possibility of drawing up flakes of glass, rubber or plastic into the syringe and injecting them into the person. Erkoc and Yazici (2021) demonstrated that contamination with glass particles decreased by 85 per cent by use of a drawing-up/filter needle. Slow, low-pressure aspiration also decreases the aspiration of glass particles.

Following the drawing up from the vial/ampoule the 'giving' needle (preferably with a built-in safety mechanism) is attached to the syringe to give the medication. Use pre-prepared syringes if possible. Larmené-Beld, Frijlink and Taxis (2019) demonstrated that reconstituting a medication in the clinical area carries a nearly 100-fold increase in risk of contamination over a medication prepared in a pharmacy. Firmly attach the needle and syringe.

Ampoules and vials contain the medication in either liquid or powder form. Their use is described in the following sections.

Vial of liquid

1. Remove the protective cap (this is a dust cover only) of the vial and clean the rubber stopper with an alcowipe (regardless of whether it is opened or unopened) and allow to air dry.

TABLE 45.1 Description of equipment for parenteral administration

EQUIPMENT	INTRADERMAL	SUBCUTANEOUS	INTRAMUSCULAR
Needle length	0.7 to 2 cm	• A 4 to 5 mm needle is appropriate for all SC injections, as longer needles deposit the medication in the muscle (Hirsch & Strauss, 2019) • Tuberculin and often insulin syringes have fine needles already attached • An 'insulin pen' is preferred if feasible	2.5 to 3 cm (needle length depends on the SC fat – those with a BMI of >30 require a longer needle [White, Goodwin & Behan, 2018]). To determine the length of the needle required, pinch the skin at the injection site and select a needle length that is greater than half the width of the skin fold
Needle gauge	25 to 26 gauge	25 to 27 gauge • Tuberculin and often insulin syringes have fine needles already attached	21 to 23 gauge (select the smallest gauge appropriate for the person and the medication for comfort)
Syringe size	1 mL (check that the scale is marked in appropriate increments for the medication dose)	• 100 units/mL (tuberculin syringe for giving small doses, e.g. paediatric doses) • Insulin syringes must be used when administering insulin and have different calibrations based on the dose required	2, 2.5 and 3 mL sizes, as needed and 5 mL to accommodate 3 mL of solution and still be easily used
Volume	0.01 to 0.1 mL	1.5 mL maximum	• Small muscle: 1 mL maximum • Large muscle: 3 mL

2. Remove the cap from the drawing-up needle and draw up air to equal the amount of medication you require.
3. Set the vial on the bench and carefully penetrate the middle of the rubber stopper with the needle, maintaining sterility. Keep the needle above the level of the medication to avoid forming bubbles, which decreases the accuracy of measurement.
4. Inject the air into the vial (creates positive atmospheric pressure so the medication flows out easily).
5. Turn the syringe, needle and vial upright so the syringe markings are at eye level (to increase accuracy) and the needle tip is in the medication.
6. Carefully draw up the required medication. Withdraw the needle, remove it (one-handed scoop and click) and replace it with a fresh needle. Recap the vial.

Reconstituting powder in a vial

1. This involves a procedure similar to the previous one. Initially (after cleansing the top), insert the needle into the vacant space above the powder, remove a quantity of air equal to the amount of diluent to be added.
2. Withdraw the needle.
3. Draw up the designated diluent from its vial or ampoule.
4. Withdraw the needle and insert it back into the powder vial.
5. Turn the powder vial, needle and syringe upright and inject the diluent into the powder vial.
6. Carefully rotate (do not shake) the vial until all of the powder is dissolved.
7. Withdraw the medication as above.

Ampoule of liquid

1. Select an ampoule and remove any medication trapped in the neck by moving it in a circular motion. This creates centrifugal force to overcome the surface tension holding the liquid in the neck. Flicking the upper portion of the ampoule with a fingernail also breaks surface tension.
2. File the neck of the glass ampoule if required, so the break will be clean. Place an ampoule opener around the ampoule neck and snap it off away from you. Twist off the top of the plastic ampoule. Take care that your fingers don't touch the top of the opening and contaminate the ampoule. Sit the open ampoule safely on the bench.
3. Assemble the needle and syringe. Remove the cap from the drawing-up/filter needle (refer to the facility's policy) and insert it into the ampoule without it touching the rim, preventing contamination.
4. Keep the tip of the needle in the fluid, slowly draw back on the plunger until the requisite amount of medication is obtained. The negative pressure in the barrel of the syringe pulls fluid into the barrel. Air is pulled in if the needle tip does not stay below the fluid level. You may need to tip the ampoule slightly on its side to obtain all the medication.
5. Draw back a small amount of air into the barrel to remove all of the medication from the drawing-up needle.
6. Remove the needle from the ampoule, then hold the syringe upright (vertically) and tap the barrel to release any air bubbles trapped by the surface tension of the fluid. Carefully push the plunger to expel all of the air.
7. Check the level to ensure an accurate dose plus a tiny amount extra. If there is excess, very carefully push the plunger until the excess is expelled onto a gauze square or into a sink.
8. Remove the drawing-up needle (one-handed scoop and click) and discard it in the sharps container.
9. Place the administration/giving needle on the filled syringe and expel the air in the cannula of the needle.

Following after any of the three sets of instructions above, place the syringe and still-capped needle, an alcowipe and the empty ampoule or vial (for a final check prior to administering the medication) in the injection tray so they can be easily carried to the bedside. Take the medication administration sheet, clean gloves and sharps container with you.

Locate and assess the appropriate site

Consult with the medical officer for an alternative route to IM medication. Because of the documented adverse effects of IM injections, it is desirable to use other safer routes. The IM route should only be used if the injection is justified. Many antibiotics and analgesics are now given intravenously.

Intradermal injections

Intradermal injections are usually given on the inner aspect of the forearm. The person should be seated or lying in a comfortable position with the forearm of their non-dominant hand exposed, extended and supported comfortably.

LOOK for rashes, bruises or breaks in the skin of the forearm.

LISTEN for any reports of pruritus or pain.

The injection is given approximately 10 to 12 cm above the wrist in an adult. Cleanse the skin with an antiseptic solution and allow to dry. The needle is placed with the bevel upwards and inserted just under the skin at an angle of 5 to 15 degrees. Expect a weal to form at the tip of the needle. Withdraw the needle and wipe the site lightly. Do not press or massage the site. Discard the needle and syringe into the sharps container.

Subcutaneous injections

SC injection sites include the anterior thigh, the abdomen, the outer aspect of the upper arms, the scapular area, and the upper ventrogluteal and dorsogluteal area. These locations have good blood supply. For self-injection, the thigh and the abdomen are most convenient. SC injections are given where there is good circulation. The sites are rotated around the body to assist absorption and minimise discomfort or the formation of lipodystrophy, which is the accumulation of fatty, subcutaneous nodules at an SC injection site caused by repeated use of that site (Gentile et al., 2023; Huang et al., 2023). An injection site chart can assist to rotate sites. The upper arms or the anterior thighs are often used. The abdomen is used for heparin injections. Insulin injections can be rotated around the upper arms, the anterior and lateral thighs, the abdomen and the subscapular area of the back, as well as the broad range of suitable sites. Subcutaneous injections are less painful and less prone to infection, and if an infection occurs, it is generally local, not systemic (Usach et al., 2019).

Consistent use of the same body area (but a different spot within that area to avoid lipohypertrophy) at the same time of day (e.g. thigh at noon, abdomen at bedtime) improves glycaemic control (Cengiz et al., 2022). Gentile et al. (2023) suggest 1 cm between consecutive injections in the same area.

LOOK for depressed or abnormal areas of skin, bruises, multiple fresh puncture sites, broken skin or rashes, and avoid these areas.

LISTEN to reports of pain, numbness at a site or preferences of site, and honour this if possible.

Intramuscular injections

Discuss possible injection sites with the person and use their preferred site, if possible. Look at the electronic medication administration record (eMAR) to determine any contraindications (e.g. myopathies, coagulation disorders following a myocardial infarction [release of skeletal muscle enzymes from the injection trauma complicate the management of an MI], hypovoaemic shock [reduces absorption for the site]) (Polania Gutierrez & Munakomi, 2023).

LOOK at the site for skin breaks or rashes, lesions, tenderness, inflammation or other signs associated with infection. The tissue must be well perfused for best effect, and you should avoid areas with decreased blood flow.

FEEL at the proposed site for the amount of SC fat and muscular atrophy. Palpate SC tissue and underlying muscle mass as applicable to determine if there is induration (hardness) or other contraindications. Take care to choose an appropriate needle length for the individual. A 3.75 cm needle is effective for those with a BMI of 30 or less (Holliday, Gupta & Vibhute, 2019).

For preference, IM injections are given in the ventrogluteal site because there are no great vessels or nerves underlying the gluteus medius and gluteus minimus muscle masses (Vicdan, Birgili & Baybuga, 2019). There is more muscle mass and less fat tissue than over the dorsogluteal site (which is *not* used for IM injections). The *ventrogluteal* site is distant from the perineal area, which is a consideration in those who are incontinent. Research demonstrates that this site is associated with the fewest complications of the IM injection sites. The ventrogluteal muscle is usually in a relaxed state, even in an anxious person, and has less subcutaneous adipose tissue. The ventrogluteal site is suitable for infants over seven months, children and adults. It is safe and results in less pain.

It is located by placing the heel of the hand (nurse's left hand on person's right hip, or the reverse) over the greater trochanter, with the index finger on the anterior superior iliac spine and the middle finger stretched dorsally to just below the iliac crest. The triangle formed by the fingers and the iliac crest is the injection site. Sitting or lying on the side relaxes this muscle. The technique of squeezing the muscle rather than flattening or stretching it is more effective in adults with a BMI of <30 (Davidson & Bertram, 2019).

The *vastus lateralis* site (middle third of the muscle) is the site of choice for IM injection of infants and young children and is safe for adults (Nakajima et al., 2020). Here the muscle is thick and well-developed in even small infants, and there are no major blood vessels or nerves underlying it.

The *deltoid* is a small muscle mass situated on the lateral aspect of the upper arm. It is close to the radial artery and nerve and is not frequently used for IM injections. Medication is absorbed more rapidly from this site (South Eastern Sydney Local Health District [SESLHD], 2022). It is a triangle, the base of which is located three fingerbreadths (2.5 to 5 cm) below the acromial process. The muscle tapers quickly down to a tip on the lateral arm that is in line with the axilla. Relax the muscle by having the arm hang and the hand open.

The *rectus femoris* site is on the anterior aspect of the thigh. This is used occasionally, although some people report severe discomfort when this site is used.

Safety

WARNING: Although the dorsogluteal muscle was a site traditionally used for both adults and children, it is **not safe** and **not to be used** because of the location of the sciatic nerve in some people.

FIGURE 45.1 shows the locations where major parenteral medications are administered.

Perform hand hygiene. Put on clean gloves so any fluid leaks will not contact your skin.

Cleanse the skin

There are many inconsistencies regarding skin cleaning prior to IM and particularly SC injections. For example, the skin is not cleaned with an alcowipe before an insulin or vaccine injection. Follow your facility's practice guidelines.

For any person who is immunocompromised or whose skin is not physically clean, cleanse the skin on the chosen site with an alcowipe, since alcohol

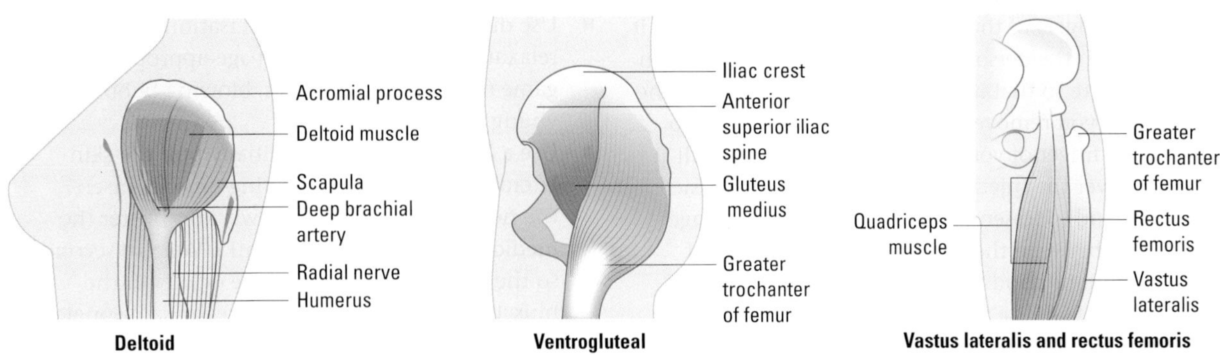

FIGURE 45.1 Locations of major parenteral medication administration: ventrogluteal, deltoid, and vastus lateralis and rectus femoris

and friction remove surface organisms. Use a circular motion beginning at the site and working outwards (for 30 seconds) so that skin flora is not brought back into the site. Allow the site to dry. This maximises the antiseptic effect and reduces irritation during the injection as alcohol irritates the tissue. Place the alcowipe between the third and fourth fingers of your non-dominant hand so that it will be available to support the skin around the puncture site during needle withdrawal. Remove the needle cap and discard it.

Administer the medication

Intradermal injections

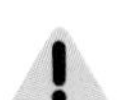

Safety

Pull the skin over the injection site taut with the thumb and index finger of your non-dominant hand. This makes the skin easier to pierce and lessens discomfort. With the syringe supported by four fingers of your dominant hand, the needle parallel to the skin and the bevel up, rest the fingers of your dominant hand on the person's skin to stabilise the syringe. Advance the needle into the skin at an angle of 5 to 15 degrees. The bevel should be under the epidermis and its outline clearly visible. This will ensure the medication is deposited between the dermal layers. Hold the syringe steady with your dominant hand and slowly push the plunger in with the non-dominant hand. Slow injection causes less discomfort as the tissues gradually distend. There will be some resistance. A bleb or weal will appear at the tip of the needle from the fluid pushing the epidermis upwards. When all of the medication is injected, support the tissue with the alcowipe, but do not apply pressure, and withdraw the needle at the same angle it was inserted.

Utilise the needle safety system/discard the *uncapped* needle into the sharps container.

Subcutaneous injections

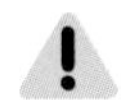

Safety

Hold the alcowipe in your non-dominant hand for later use. Pull the skin over the injection site taut with the thumb and index finger of your non-dominant hand to make it easier to pierce and to lessen discomfort. If the person is thin, pinch up a fold of skin between your thumb and index finger to prevent injecting the medication into the muscle. Hold the syringe like a dart between the thumb and four fingers of your dominant hand to give you control over the movement of the syringe. Stabilise your hand/wrist on the person's skin so that you can control the amount of force and the distance the needle is to be inserted. Quickly insert the needle at a 45- or 90-degree angle, depending on the amount of SC tissue and length of the needle (i.e. at 45 degrees for a thin person so the medication is not introduced into the muscle, or at 90 degrees if there is adequate SC tissue). Remember, skin is only 2 to 2.5 mm thick and a 4 mm needle will deposit the medication into the SC tissue or SC fat where it is readily absorbed (Hirsch & Strauss, 2019). Keep hold of the pinched-up skin held with the non-dominant hand.

Check the policy of the facility regarding aspiration during an SC injection. To aspirate, use your dominant hand to pull back on the plunger while stabilising the syringe with your non- dominant hand. This creates negative pressure in the barrel, so that if the needle has entered a blood vessel, blood will be drawn into the barrel. If this happens, withdraw the needle and discard the needle, syringe and medication and start again, since injecting medication into a vessel could cause harm. According to Valentin (2021), aspirating any medication (including heparin and insulin) given by the SC route to check for blood is no longer necessary, as piercing a blood vessel is extremely rare and could cause the formation of a haematoma.

Stabilise the syringe during injection to reduce movement and discomfort. Slowly inject the medication into the SC tissue so that tissue is distended slowly, minimising pain. Spread the skin around the needle, support the skin with gentle thumb pressure at the puncture site with an alcowipe, but do not massage, and quickly withdraw the needle at the same angle it was inserted to minimise pain. Activate the needle safety feature if available and discard the *uncapped* needle into the sharps container.

Insulin pens with dial-able doses are being used more frequently, as they increase glycaemic control, comfort and confidence (Gorska-Ciebiada, Masierek & Ciebiada, 2020).

Intramuscular injections

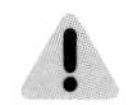
Safety

Hold the swab between the third and fourth fingers of the non-dominant hand or place it on the person's skin just above the injection site so that it will be available to support the skin when you remove the needle. With the thumb and index finger of your non-dominant hand, pull the skin over the injection site taut to make it easier to pierce and to lessen discomfort. Hold the syringe like a dart between the thumb and index finger of your dominant hand to control the movement of the syringe. Stabilise your hand/wrist on the person's skin to control the amount of force and the distance the needle is inserted. Quickly insert the needle at a 90-degree angle. Release the skin and use your non-dominant hand to stabilise the syringe to reduce movement and discomfort.

Valentin (2021) suggests aspiration is not necessary for ventrogluteal, deltoid or vastus lateralis injections. Follow the policy of the facility. Slowly (1 mL per 10 seconds) (Kim & de Jesus, 2021) inject the medication into the muscle tissue so that tissue is distended slowly, minimising pain. Spread the skin around the needle, support the skin at the puncture site with the alcowipe and quickly withdraw the needle to reduce pain.

Activate the needle safety system and discard the needle and the syringe into the sharps container.

Reduce discomfort

The following will help to minimise the pain of injections (and help the person adhere to the therapeutic regimen [Inangil & Inangil, 2020]):

- For IM injections, choose a sufficiently long needle to place the medication deep in the muscle (White, Goodwin & Behan, 2018), with the exception of the deltoid site (deltoid bursa is only 0.8 to 1.6 cm deep [Bancsi, Houle & Grindrod, 2019]).
- Keep the outside of the needle free of solution that may irritate tissue.
- Ask the person to choose the injection site if possible.
- Locate the site using anatomical landmarks. Do not inject when skin is irritated or broken.
- Alternate injection sites to avoid repeated trauma to one area.
- Apply ice to the site for about 30 seconds to numb pain receptors before administering the injection, although some people may find the ice more painful (Jamalinik et al., 2023).
- Inject room temperature liquids – cold ones are more painful (Usach et al., 2019).
- Use an ice-cold needle (0 to 2 °C) to reduce pain (Jancy, 2019).
- Apply pressure to the site for 10 seconds prior to and after administering the injection (Kaplan, Güler & Avşaroğulları, 2023).
- Rhythmically tap the site with your palm (~20 times) just prior to the needle insertion (Rautela, Thomas & Rita, 2020).
- Apply a topical anaesthetic cream up to an hour prior to the injection.
- Use distraction, such as conversation or relaxation techniques, or an age-appropriate game (e.g. electronic games, blowing bubbles for young people).
- Use a Z-track technique. Initially pull the skin laterally away from underlying muscle, insert the needle at 90 degrees, slowly administer the medication (10 seconds per mL). Wait 10 seconds so the medication can disperse evenly in the muscle. Withdraw the needle at the same angle, and then release the skin. The pool of medication is sealed from the needle track and cannot irritate the tissue (Şanlialp Zeyrek et al., 2019). Do not massage the Z-track site. Do not give subsequent injections at the same site.
- For heparin administration, Yılmaz et al. (2020) applied pressure for 10 seconds after withdrawal of the needle to reduce both pain and bruising. Fulmer et al. (2016) add that using a 3 mL syringe with a 25-gauge needle and taking 20 to 30 seconds to inject the medication also reduces bruising and pain.

Tend to the puncture site

Intradermal injections are not massaged because the medication must stay in one place to slow absorption and to give a focal point for a reaction (e.g. allergy, tuberculin testing). SC sites are massaged to help disperse the medication over a larger area for easier absorption. Exceptions are SC heparin and insulin, as massage would increase the rate of absorption and medication action and may cause tissue irritation. IM sites are not massaged, to decrease tissue irritation and damage. Pressure may need to be applied to the puncture site if bleeding occurs due to any cutting of capillaries during the injection.

Post-procedure

Remain with the person for a short time to assess for any adverse effects (e.g. allergy). Assist the person into a comfortable position. Remove your gloves and wash your hands. Ensure the person's possessions and call bell are readily available. Return in 15 to 30 minutes to assess the effects of the medication.

CLEAN, REPLACE AND DISPOSE OF EQUIPMENT

All used syringes, needles, ampoules and empty vials are carefully deposited into the sharps container as soon as possible. This minimises the risk of needle-stick injury to nursing and domestic staff. Alcowipes, gauze squares and gloves are deposited in the contaminated waste bin. The injection tray is washed, dried and returned to its storage place. All stock is replenished as necessary and medications ordered from the pharmacy to ensure a ready supply for the next 24 hours.

DOCUMENTATION

Controlled substances must be signed out of the medication cupboard at the time they are removed (i.e. before they are given) by two registered healthcare professionals.

Sign or initial regularly scheduled medications on the medication administration sheet next to the appropriate timeslot (or use the eMAR for electronic documentation). Chart once-only medications as per the facility's policy. Some injections, such as preoperative sedation or medication, require signatures on the theatre sheet and notation in the progress notes.

Record the person's pre- and post-injection assessment findings (e.g. pain assessment, sedation), plus a notation about its effectiveness within 30 minutes. Report any adverse effects to the shift coordinator and document them in the person's progress notes.

CLINICAL SKILLS ASSESSMENT

Parenteral medication

Demonstrates the ability to effectively and safely administer parenteral medication. Incorporates the *National Safety and Quality Health Service Standards*: 2 Partnering with Consumers, 3 Preventing and Controlling Healthcare-Associated Infection, 5 Comprehensive Care, 6 Communicating for Safety, and 8 Recognising and Responding to Acute Deterioration (ACSQHC, 2021).

Performance criteria	1	2	3	4	5
(Numbers indicate NMBA *Registered Nurse Standards for Practice*)	**(Dependent)**	**(Marginal)**	**(Assisted)**	**(Supervised)**	**(Independent)**
1. Identifies indication (1.1, 3.3, 3.4)	☐	☐	☐	☐	☐
2. Verifies the validity of the written medication order (1.4, 3.4, 6.2, 6.5)	☐	☐	☐	☐	☐
3. Evidence of therapeutic interaction with the person, e.g. gives the person a clear explanation of the procedure (1.4, 1.5, 2.1, 2.2, 3.2)	☐	☐	☐	☐	☐
4. Demonstrates clinical reasoning abilities, e.g. positions the person, obtains the appropriate form of the medication, assesses the person if warranted (1.1, 1.2, 1.3, 4.1, 4.2, 4.3, 6.1)	☐	☐	☐	☐	☐
5. Adheres to the general concepts of working with therapeutic substances (1.1, 1.3, 1.5, 3.3, 3.4, 4.1, 4.2, 4.3, 6.2, 6.5, 6.6)	☐	☐	☐	☐	☐
6. Gathers equipment (1.1, 5.5, 6.1): ■ syringes and needles or safety syringes ■ ampoules or vials ■ filter needles ■ alcowipes ■ gauze squares ■ injection tray ■ sharps container ■ clean gloves	☐	☐	☐	☐	☐
7. Uses the six (or more) rights of medication administration (1.1, 1.2, 1.3, 1.4, 1.5, 2.2, 3.4, 4.1, 4.2, 4.3, 6.1, 6.2, 6.5, 6.6)	☐	☐	☐	☐	☐
8. Performs hand hygiene (1.1, 3.4, 6.1)	☐	☐	☐	☐	☐
9. Draws up the medication using aseptic technique to prepare the medication (1.1, 3.4, 6.1)	☐	☐	☐	☐	☐
10. Locates and assesses the appropriate site (1.1, 6.1)	☐	☐	☐	☐	☐
11. Safely administers the medication to maximise effects and to minimise discomfort (1.1, 6.1)	☐	☐	☐	☐	☐
12. Tends to the puncture site appropriately (1.1, 6.1)	☐	☐	☐	☐	☐
13. Cleans, replaces and disposes of equipment appropriately (3.6, 6.1)	☐	☐	☐	☐	☐
14. Documents relevant information (1.4, 1.6, 2.2, 3.5, 3.7, 6.2, 6.5, 7.3)	☐	☐	☐	☐	☐
15. Demonstrates the ability to link theory to practice (1.1, 3.3, 3.4, 3.5)	☐	☐	☐	☐	☐

Student:

Clinical facilitator: Date:

CHAPTER 46

INTRAVENOUS MEDICATION ADMINISTRATION – VOLUME-CONTROLLED INFUSION SET

INDICATIONS

Intermittent infusion is the intravenous (IV) administration of a small volume of medicated fluid over a short period of time (one to two hours) but longer than a bolus administration. These volume-controlled infusion sets are indicated:

- when a medication does not remain stable for the length of time it takes an entire solution container to infuse
- to administer medications intermittently
- to avoid mixing incompatible medications
- to dilute a medication that is very irritating to the veins
- to deliver medications in precise amounts of liquid (e.g. when the volume administered is critical)
- for use when infusion pumps are not available.

Burette, Buretrol and Volutrol are all volume-control infusion sets that can be attached to the primary fluid container. They have a drip chamber in line and are attached via a giving set to the IV cannula. Many, if not most, volume-controlled medication administration sets are being replaced by pharmacy-prepared secondary administration sets (piggybacks) and smart pumps to reduce the risks of medication error.

Piggyback sets

Secondary administration sets (i.e. piggybacks) are often used for intermittent infusions. Being pharmacy-prepared, in airflow-controlled conditions, they are much less likely to be contaminated (Larmené-Beld, Frijlink & Taxis, 2019). They consist of small bags of IV solution (50 to 250 mL) plus a short giving set with either a micro- or macro-drip chamber. They are used if the medication is incompatible with the primary solution or the medication in the primary bag. The primary line maintains venous access and delivers fluids. Piggyback sets must be hung above the primary bag. There should be a wire extender to lower the primary bag. The piggyback set is attached to the primary line by a Y-connection at a port near to the insertion site.

Secondary administration sets are prepared in the same way as the IV container medication if not pharmacy-prepared (see **Clinical Skill 47**).

Verify the written medication order

A valid, signed medication order from a qualified healthcare provider is a requirement for legal administration of a medication. (See **Clinical Skill 37** for a detailed discussion of verifying a medication order.)

You are responsible and accountable for questioning and clarifying any order that is unclear or incomplete or that seems inappropriate or unreasonable for the person (e.g. a very high dose, the same medication with two different names). Potentially harmful prescribing errors often go undetected (e.g. a mistake in the prescription that the nurse did not identify [Brindley, 2020]). Nurses are partly responsible (along with the physician) if an inappropriate order is followed. To question an order, you *must know* the person's diagnosis, the purpose of the medication, its therapeutic effect, any adverse or toxic effects and the usual dose. Anticipate any pertinent nursing implications (e.g. the patency of the IV line) as well as individual factors that mediate response to medications (e.g. age, weight, psychological factors). Be aware of any drug or food allergies the person has, so potentially harmful substances are not administered.

EVIDENCE OF THERAPEUTIC INTERACTION

Give the person a clear explanation of the procedure. Many people will be apprehensive about receiving medication via an IV. Knowing that there is no additional needle insertion is reassuring. Warn the person that they may experience some vein irritation and offer assistance if this occurs (e.g. warm compresses, mild analgesia). Discuss adverse effects that are common with the medication to be administered and ask the person to alert you to any changes they note. Assess all their complaints. Just because an adverse reaction is unusual or unexpected, do not ignore it – it needs exploration. This will develop the person's trust in the nursing staff.

DEMONSTRATE CLINICAL REASONING

Assess the preparation area

Adequate lighting, ventilation and space are necessary. Preparing IV medications requires Aseptic Non Touch Technique (ANTT), so the area must be scrupulously clean. Preparing any medication requires concentration and freedom from distraction.

Safety: Distraction and interruption are the most common causes of medication error (Manzo et al., 2019). Hang a 'Do not disturb' sign on the door, and wear a brightly coloured vest to discourage interruptions (Linden-Lahti et al., 2019).

Calculate the correct dose (see your pharmacy text for formulae). Mulac, Hagesaether and Granas (2022) found the most common medication errors to be dosage (e.g. 10-fold increase in dose) due to inaccurate calculations (misplaced decimal point; missing, added or misplaced zero). Multiple strengths and different units of a medication contributed to error. However, the most common mechanism producing error was omitting or deviating from double-checking, although they also found that double-checking medication dosage failed to intercept the calculation error to a significant degree. Brindley (2020) suggests the following to minimise error in medication calculation:

- Calculate in a calm, quiet place with minimal distraction.
- Identify the medication using the medication administration record.
- Ensure that the units in the prescription and on the label match.
- Have your calculations double-checked (independently) by a senior nurse.

General concepts of working with therapeutic substances

Please review the general concepts and mechanisms of medication administration presented in **Clinical Skill 37.**

ELDER CARE

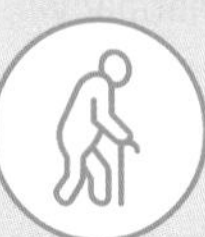

Volume-controlled infusion sets or bolus IV administration may be used more frequently than container-based IV medications for elderly and frail individuals. These people often have chronic and comorbid conditions and volume control infusion reduces the chances of fluid overload (e.g. in congestive cardiac failure, renal failure). They often also have frail, tortuous veins that easily become irritated if the catheter tip is against the vein wall, so secure the cannula so it will not move and watch for early signs (irritation, erythema, slow or irregular drip rate) of irritation or infiltration. Often, signs are minimal due to a reduced inflammatory response.

GATHER EQUIPMENT

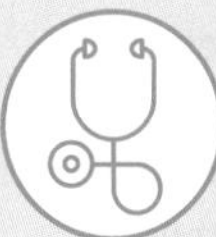

Gathering equipment is an organisational step that helps to create a positive environment for a successful interaction and reduces the risk of errors when preparing medications. It ensures that you have all needed material, boosts the person's confidence and trust in you, and increases your self-confidence. Equipment required includes the following:

EQUIPMENT	EXPLANATION
Medication administration sheet/record	• Use the written medication order to determine the medication and dosage required • Includes the person's name, hospital number, date of birth, doctor and any known allergies are correctly documented • Use to identify the person (against their hospital identification armband) to ensure that the correct medication, dose, time and route are being given to the correct person
Volume-control infusion set (or small-volume IV fluid bag)	• Burette, Buretrol or Volutrol • Attached to the primary fluid container; has a drip chamber in line and is attached via a giving set to the IV cannula
Required medication	• Obtained from stock – usually comes as a vial, sometimes an ampoule • If it requires reconstitution, the recommended sterile diluent will be needed
Sterile syringe	• Required to draw up the medication • Has a valve device or similar if using a needle-free system
Sterile needle (or a needle-free cannula)	Use the smallest gauge reasonable for the viscosity of the medication to minimise damage to the access port seal. A damaged seal allows contamination of the system and requires the entire system to be changed
Alcowipes	To cleanse and disinfect the tops of vials and the latex seal on the medication access port of the burette

EQUIPMENT	EXPLANATION
Medication additive label	• A brightly coloured label with an adhesive back • Complete it with the person's name, hospital number and room number; medication, dose, date and time of administration; and signatures of the preparing and checking nurses • To prevent misidentification of the person and accidental doubling of the dose
Two syringes, needles (if required) and sterile normal saline	• Flushing of the tubing below the burette prior to administration alerts you to patency problems, clears fibrin/biofilm from the tubing • Flushing following administration of a medication clears the residual medication from the line and ensures all of a dose is administered (Keogh et al., 2020)
Injection tray	For transporting the medications, syringes and alcowipes to the bedside
Sharps container	Taken to the bedside so that used needles, glass ampoules and vials can be immediately disposed of, to reduce the chance of needle-stick injuries
Clean gloves	To comply with standard precautions

THE SIX RIGHTS OF ADMINISTERING MEDICATION

IV medications must be checked by two healthcare professionals (registered nurses, medical officers, enrolled nurses).

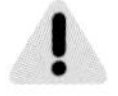
Safety

Vigilance in using the six rights of medication administration reduces errors. **Clinical Skill 37** gives a complete description of the rights of medication administration. In summary, they include:

- *right time* – the first consideration and a frequent source (about 20 per cent) of medication errors
- *right medication* – verify the validity of the order and then choose from the medications in stock. Be cautious – look-alike/sound-alike medication names may be mistaken for each other, causing up to 14 per cent of medication errors (Bryan et al., 2020)
- *right route* – confirm this as noted on the medication administration sheet
- *right dose* – it is imperative to gain a therapeutic level of the medication
- *right person* – it is vital to verify the correct person is receiving the medication
- *right documentation* – must be adhered to.

For IV medication, the *right rate* is extremely important. It is the most frequent source of intravenous medication error (Sutherland et al., 2020).

ADMINISTER A VOLUME-CONTROLLED INTRAVENOUS MEDICATION

Video

Hand hygiene

Hand hygiene (see **Clinical Skill 5**) as well as ANTT is used because the medication goes directly into a vein. Clean hands and clean gloves reduce contamination and protect you from absorbing medications.

Prepare the syringe

Review **Clinical Skill 45** for use of vials and ampoules, and for reconstituting powders. Be aware that IV medication volumes may be large, and consider and record this when calculating the total volume of fluid administered to the person. Assess the medication for compatibility with the fluid that is infusing, its normal dosage, its action and adverse effects, the recommended administration time, and the medication's peak action time. Label the syringe (person's name, medication and dose) for transport.

Prepare a flushing syringe with 10 mL of normal saline (see **Clinical Skill 48** for a discussion of flushing an IV line) (some facilities will have manufacturer-prepared and labelled flushing syringes). Label it, if using a piggyback bag.

Carry the syringe with the medication, the label and the empty ampoule/vial (and the flushing syringe) to the bedside for checking before injecting the medication into the burette.

Administer the medication

Attach a burette

If this is the initial dose using a burette, attach it by inserting the spike of the burette into the solution container and hanging the container on the IV stand (see **Clinical Skill 31**). Open the air vent clamp on the burette to allow air to escape as fluid flows in. Move the roller clamp to just below the drip chamber and clamp it so that the burette chamber can fill before you prime the line. Open the upper clamp and allow 30 mL of fluid into the burette chamber. Close the upper clamp (between the IV bag and the burette) and open the lower one. Gently squeeze the drip chamber and then close the lower clamp. Some drip chambers are damaged if they are squeezed with the lower clamp closed. Release the drip chamber and gently reshape it. It should be half full of fluid. Prime and attach the tubing (see **Clinical Skill 31**). Rickard et al. (2015) suggest replacing the device weekly is sufficient (follow the facility's protocol).

Assess the person

Identify the person (ask, check the identity band against the medication administration sheet). Recheck the six rights of medication administration. Assess the person for baseline vital signs, allergies to medications and their general condition as well as the IV site.

PART 7

LOOK at the IV site for the following: swelling, pallor (blanching), reddened 'tracking' up the vein, slowed infusion rate.

LISTEN to reports of discomfort, burning, tightness, general malaise.

FEEL the IV site area for warm to hot tissue, or cool oedematous area around the insertion site, and/or induration along the vein.

Assess the IV system for patency, kinks and air in the line.

Inject medication into the burette

Perform hand hygiene and put on clean gloves. Use ANTT.

Fill the burette with the required/ordered amount of fluid from the primary bag (usually 50 mL or 100 mL) so the medication is sufficiently diluted and dispersed throughout the fluid in the burette.

Clean the injection port with alcowipes to remove microorganisms. Allow the alcohol to dry to destroy as many microbes as possible. The injection port is designed for multiple punctures or is fitted with a needleless port.

Clamp the inflow line from the primary container to prevent the medication from being further diluted by the solution. Use the slide or roller clamp. Damage occurs to the line if the slide/roller clamp is left in the same position for more than six hours.

Insert the needle into the medication port of the burette. Inject the medication and gently rotate (agitate) the fluid chamber to mix the fluids. To use a needless system, remove the cap on the port and insert the connector using ANTT. Secure it with tape.

Safety

Attach the medication additive label to the burette. This clearly indicates that a medication has been added to the burette. Peel back one side or one corner only and attach that to the burette to reduce the amount of paper tape that sticks to the burette, an important consideration over time. Also, attaching labels over old attachments helps reduce the amount the burette is obscured. Take care not to obscure the measure line.

Re-establish the IV flow and adjust the drip rate by adjusting the roller clamp below the drip chamber. Preferably, use a pump to deliver the desired volume over time as ordered, as rate errors are the most common IV medication error (Sutherland et al., 2020). Allow all of the medication to drain out of the burette.

Remove gloves and perform hand hygiene.

ADMINISTER PIGGYBACK MEDICATION

Obtain the pre-prepared medication in a piggyback format (50 or 100 mL diluent) from pharmacy, or use the steps above, and add the medication ordered to the recommended solution in a piggyback bag. Check the orders for the medication name, dose, amount of solution to be used and timeframe for infusing. Take the piggyback bag (and the medication vial if you have prepared the infusion) for a final check at the bedside.

Assess the person and the IV site and the IV patency.

If using a piggyback system, you should also take the medication vial with you for a final check. If a piggyback set is used, check that the backflow valve on the piggyback system has stopped the flow of the primary solution. If not, clamp the primary line. Then follow this process:

- Spike the piggyback bag with the secondary tubing set using ANTT.
- Half-fill the drip chamber of the piggyback bag.
- Hang the piggyback bag above the main IV bag so gravity helps infuse the fluid (if accessing a IV lock system, there will be no main IV bag and the piggyback bag is set up like a primary IV).
- Scrub the IV tubing port (either closest to the person, or above the IV pump as applicable) with an antiseptic wipe for 15 seconds and connect the piggyback tubing using ANTT.
- Adjust the rate to deliver the medication over the recommended time frame or set the pump to do so. Make sure the piggyback bag has emptied. Cooper, Rassam and Mellor (2018) found that 11 to 20 per cent of antibiotic medication was not given if the piggyback bag was not completely emptied.
- After the solution/medication has infused, backflush the piggyback (according to the policy of the facility) to minimise the need for the connection and disconnection of sets which, in turn, decreases the risk of contamination. Lower the piggyback below the main IV and allow the primary fluid to fill the piggyback tubing up to its chamber. Clamp the piggyback tube. The empty piggyback bag is left clamped until the next dose of medication is due, at which time the empty piggyback is removed and the fresh piggyback bag is spiked and hung.
- Switch to the primary fluid after completing the piggyback. Unclamp the roller, and reset the pump.

Alkazemi et al. (2022), Gregorowicz et al. (2020) and McLauglin et al. (2021) demonstrated the safety, efficacy and savings in equipment and time in using IV push/bolus rather than IV piggyback administration of commonly used medications (antibiotics, anticonvulsants) in critical and emergency departments. With more research into other medications, the use of IV piggybacks will likely reduce.

?

If the piggyback medication is incompatible with the medication/solution in the primary bag, or if the drip rate is slow (e.g. Keep the Vein Open – 20 mL/hour [Doyle et al., 2021]), flush the primary IV tubing with normal saline (NS) before and after administration of the piggyback medication (Keogh et al., 2020).

Post-procedure

Assess the person during administration of the medication and when it is completed. Reopen the inflow on the burette when the medication has been absorbed. The first 10 mL of fluid from the primary bag will flush the line. Reset the rate. Keep the burette partially filled with fluid, even when there is no medication in it, so there is a buffer and the drip chamber does not run dry. Remove the medication additive label when the medication has been completely infused. For a piggyback bag, use the normal saline syringe to flush the line (see **Clinical Skill 48** for a discussion on flushing). Use a pulsatile (push, pause – several times) to empty the line of medication and flush out fibrin to maintain patency (Keogh et al., 2020).

Return within 30 minutes to reassess the person and note their response to the medication.

CLEAN, REPLACE AND DISPOSE OF EQUIPMENT

Place the needles, syringes and vials/ampoules into the sharps container to prevent accidental needle-stick injuries of either the nursing or domestic staff. Piggyback bags are placed in normal waste, as are alcowipes. Perform hand hygiene. Assess needle, syringe and medication stocks and replenish if required so there are sufficient amounts for the next shift's use.

DOCUMENTATION

Sign or initial the timeslot on the medication administration sheet or access the electronic medication administration record (eMAR) to indicate that you administered the ordered dose of medication to the person by the IV route at the designated time. The checking nurse countersigns the medication administration sheet. The effects of the medications, expected or unexpected, are assessed 30 minutes to one hour after administration, and are then documented. Adverse effects should be reported to the shift coordinator and the medical staff, and the remaining doses of the medication withheld. Record the amount of fluid in a piggyback bag (usually 50 or 100 mL) plus the amount of normal saline used to flush the piggyback line on the fluid balance sheet. All of the fluid used to dilute the medication in a burette comes from the primary bag and will be recorded on the fluid balance sheet when the primary bag is complete.

CLINICAL SKILLS ASSESSMENT

Intravenous medication administration – volume-controlled infusion set

Demonstrates the ability to effectively and safely administer intravenous medication via a volume-controlled infusion set. Incorporates the *National Safety and Quality Health Service Standards*: 2 Partnering with Consumers, 3 Preventing and Controlling Healthcare-Associated Infection, 5 Comprehensive Care, 6 Communicating for Safety, and 8 Recognising and Responding to Acute Deterioration (ACSQHC, 2021).

Performance criteria	1	2	3	4	5
(Numbers indicate NMBA *Registered Nurse Standards for Practice*)	(Dependent)	(Marginal)	(Assisted)	(Supervised)	(Independent)
1. Identifies indication (1.1, 3.3, 3.4)	☐	☐	☐	☐	☐
2. Verifies the validity of the written medication order (1.4, 3.4, 6.2, 6.5)	☐	☐	☐	☐	☐
3. Evidence of therapeutic interaction with the person, e.g. gives a clear explanation of the procedure (1.4, 1.5, 2.1, 2.2, 3.2)	☐	☐	☐	☐	☐
4. Demonstrates clinical reasoning abilities, e.g. assesses the person, the IV site and the medication (1.1, 1.2, 1.3, 4.1, 4.2, 4.3, 6.1)	☐	☐	☐	☐	☐
5. Adheres to the general concepts of working with therapeutic substances (1.1, 1.3, 1.5, 3.3, 3.4, 4.1, 4.2, 4.3, 6.2, 6.5, 6.6)	☐	☐	☐	☐	☐
6. Gathers equipment (1.1, 5.5, 6.1) ■ medication administration sheet ■ volume-control infusion set ■ required medication ■ sterile syringe and sterile needle (or a needle-free cannula) ■ alcowipes ■ medication additive label ■ injection tray ■ sharps container ■ clean gloves	☐	☐	☐	☐	☐
7. Uses the six (or more) rights of medication administration (1.1, 1.2, 1.3, 1.4, 1.5, 2.2, 3.4, 4.1, 4.2, 4.3, 6.1, 6.2, 6.5, 6.6)	☐	☐	☐	☐	☐
8. Performs hand hygiene (1.1, 3.4, 6.1)	☐	☐	☐	☐	☐
9. Prepares the syringe with the medication (1.1, 1.4, 3.4, 6.1, 6.2, 6.5)	☐	☐	☐	☐	☐
10. Inserts a burette into a new intravenous fluid bag (if necessary) (1.1, 6.1)	☐	☐	☐	☐	☐
11. Injects the medication into the burette (1.1, 6.1)	☐	☐	☐	☐	☐
12. Attaches the medication additive label (1.1, 1.4, 6.1, 6.2, 6.5)	☐	☐	☐	☐	☐
13. Sets the rate of the intravenous administration (1.1, 1.4, 6.1, 6.2, 6.5)	☐	☐	☐	☐	☐
14. Returns when the medication is absorbed; resets the rate (1.1, 6.1)	☐	☐	☐	☐	☐
15. Cleans, replaces and disposes of equipment appropriately (3.6, 6.1)	☐	☐	☐	☐	☐
16. Documents relevant information (1.4, 1.6, 2.2, 3.5, 3.7, 6.2, 6.5, 7.3)	☐	☐	☐	☐	☐
17. Demonstrates the ability to link theory to practice (1.1, 3.3, 3.4, 3.5)	☐	☐	☐	☐	☐

Student:

Clinical facilitator:

Date:

CHAPTER 47

INTRAVENOUS MEDICATION ADMINISTRATION – INTRAVENOUS CONTAINER

INDICATIONS

Intravenous (IV) medication via continuous (i.e. container) delivery provides a medication at a constant rate over a specific time. It is used to:

- provide a constant level of medication in the blood
- dilute irritating medications for delivery at a continuous and slow rate
- deliver large volumes of fluid and electrolytes or medications.

The pharmacy prepares, labels and delivers many IV medications in IV fluid; however, nurses often also undertake this task. Knowledge of medications, doses and interaction, a positive attitude and careful attention to the processes of preparation and administration reduce intravenous medication error (Márquez-Hernández et al., 2019).

Verify the written medication order

A valid, signed medication order from a physician is a requirement for legal administration of an intravenous medication. See **Clinical Skill 37** for a detailed discussion of verifying a medication order.

You are responsible and accountable for questioning and clarifying any order that is unclear or incomplete or that seems inappropriate or unreasonable for the person (e.g. a very high dose, the same medication with two different names). Potentially harmful prescribing errors often go undetected (Brindley, 2020). Nurses are partly responsible (along with the physician) if an inappropriate order is not identified and is followed. You *must know* the person's diagnosis, the purpose of the medication, its therapeutic effect, any adverse or toxic effects and the usual dose. Anticipate any pertinent nursing implications (e.g. the patency of the intravenous line) as well as individual factors that mediate response to medications (e.g. age, weight, psychological factors). Be aware of any drug or food allergies the person has, so that potentially harmful substances are not administered. Also take into account the hydration status of the person and the potential for over-hydration (e.g. in congestive cardiac failure, renal failure).

EVIDENCE OF THERAPEUTIC INTERACTION

Clearly explain the procedure to the person. Apprehension about receiving medication via an IV can be reduced by reassurance that the IV will only be uncomfortable for a short time during insertion and while being established. Enlist cooperation by discussing the need for IV therapy and medications and educating the person about the purpose of the medication. Discuss common adverse effects of the medication, and ask them to alert you to any changes they note during administration. Warn them that some vein irritation may occur and offer assistance (warm compresses, mild analgesia). Assess all of their concerns and complaints. Just because an adverse reaction is unusual or unexpected, do not ignore it – it needs exploration. This develops the person's trust in the nursing staff.

DEMONSTRATE CLINICAL REASONING

Assess the medication

Assess the medication for compatibility with the infusing fluid; know its normal dose, action and adverse effects, the recommended time for administering the medication and its peak action time. If a second medication is to be added to the fluid, check that it is compatible, not only with the fluid but also with the initial medication.

Assess the person

Assess the person and the IV site before hanging the container. Assess their vital signs. Scan the entire person.

LOOK for signs of malaise or over-hydration – dependent oedema.

LISTEN for shortness of breath, a cough or reports of excess urine output.

FEEL for peripheral oedema.

Long-term viability of a peripherally inserted intravenous cannula is dependent on maintaining its patency. Infiltration, inflammation and thromboembolism are the most common complications (Hontoria-Alcoceba et al., 2023). Assess the IV site for the following:

LOOK for swelling, pallor (blanching), slow flow rate and reddened 'tracking' up the vein.

LISTEN to reports of discomfort, pain, burning and tightness of the insertion site or the vein.

FEEL for coolness or heat and swelling around the insertion site.

Assess the IV system for patency, kinks and air in the line.

Assess the preparation area

Adequate lighting, ventilation and space are needed. Preparing IV medications requires aseptic technique, so the area must be scrupulously clean. Preparing any medication requires concentration and freedom from distraction during the procedure.

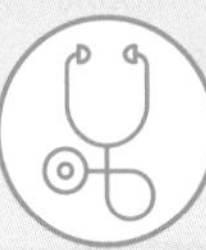
Safety

Distraction and interruption are the most common causes of medication error (Márquez-Hernández et al., 2019). Hang a 'Do not disturb' sign on the door, and wear a brightly coloured vest to help discourage interruptions. Bucknall et al. (2019) found ignoring the other person or head shaking to indicate 'no interruptions' was used by nurses to protect their concentration. Other distractions are unavoidable – finding another nurse to double-check a medication, teaching the person about their medication or advocating for the person all contribute to distracting you from the task.

THE SIX RIGHTS OF ADMINISTERING MEDICATION

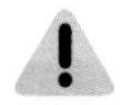
Safety

Two healthcare professionals (registered nurse [RN], medical officer or enrolled nurse) are required to independently check IV medications for accuracy and safety. Modern technology (e.g. bar code medication administration) assists nurses to verify the six rights of medication administration by electronically scanning the person's identification band to confirm the information and cross-match with their electronic medical chart (Hanson & Haddad, 2022).

GATHER EQUIPMENT

Gathering equipment is an organisational step that helps to create a positive environment for a successful interaction and reduces the risk of errors when preparing medication. Equipment required includes the following:

EQUIPMENT	EXPLANATION
Medication administration sheet/eMAR if using the bar code medication administration system	• Together with the written medication order determines the medication and dosage required. Includes the person's name, hospital number, date of birth, doctor and any known allergies are correctly documented • Used to identify the person (against their hospital identification armband) to ensure that the correct medication, dose, time and route are being given to the correct person
Required medication and ordered fluid	• The ready-prepared mixture may come from the pharmacy, or the fluid and medication may be obtained from stock or ordered from the pharmacy • The medication is supplied in either a vial or an ampoule • A powdered medication needs reconstitution with the recommended sterile diluent • The fluid order sheet states which IV fluid is to be used. Check that the medication and the fluid are compatible • Check the bag of fluid as described in **Clinical Skill 31** • Reconstituting medications and preparing the IV are sterile procedures that require aseptic technique
Sterile syringe	• Required to draw up the medication • Should have a valve device or similar if using a needle-free system
Sterile needle or needleless adaptor	Use the smallest gauge needle reasonable for the viscosity of the medication to minimise damage to the access port seal. A damaged seal allows contamination of the system and requires the entire system to be changed
Alcowipes	To cleanse and disinfect the tops of vials and the latex seal/medication port on the medication access of the container
Medication additive label	• A brightly coloured label with an adhesive back • Complete it with the person's name, hospital number and room number; medication, dose, date and time of administration; and signatures of the preparing and checking nurses. This information prevents misidentification of the person and accidental double dosing
Injection tray	For transporting the medications, syringes and alcowipes to the bedside
Sharps container	Taken to the bedside so that used needles, glass ampoules and vials can be immediately disposed of, to reduce the chance of needle-stick injuries
Clean gloves	To comply with standard precautions

However, you will be responsible to know and use the 'rights' of medication administration. **Clinical Skill 37** gives a complete description of the rights of medication administration. In summary, they include:

- *right time* – the first consideration
- *right medication* – verify the validity of the order and then choose from the medications in stock
- *right route* – confirm this as noted on the medication administration sheet
- *right dose* – it is imperative to gain a therapeutic level of the medication
- *right person* – it is vital to verify the correct person is receiving the medication
- *right documentation* – must be adhered to.

The *right rate* is an important addition when IV medications are being administered. Sutherland et al. (2020) found that flow rate was the most common IV medication error.

ADMINISTER INTRAVENOUS MEDICATION

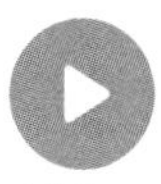

Video

Hand hygiene

Hand hygiene (see **Clinical Skill 5**) as part of Aseptic Non Touch Technique (ANTT) (see **Clinical Skill 7**) is used because the medication goes directly into a vein. Clean gloves protect your hands from contact with medications and comply with standard precautions.

Prepare the solution

Check the compatibility of the solution with the medication. Check its sterility and expiry date (see **Clinical Skill 31**).

Prepare the syringe

Review **Clinical Skill 45** about using vials and ampoules, reconstituting medications and drawing-up injectable medications. Many medication errors are made at this point (diluting varying concentrations of liquids, reconstituting powdered medication [Hermanspann et al., 2019]). Take care, and have your calculations and drawing-up checked. Prepare the medication additive label.

Inject the medication into the fluid container

Identify the injection port into which the medication will be administered. This is different from the IV tubing insertion port. Clean the port with alcowipes to remove microorganisms. Allow the alcohol to dry (to destroy as many microbes as possible).

Insert the needle into the centre of the container's injection port or seat the needleless adaptor onto the syringe and into the medication port. Penetrate the internal diaphragm of the port. Inject the medication slowly. Carefully withdraw the needle and discard into the sharps container. The injection port is self-sealing. Mix the fluids by gently rotating the fluid container, turning it end over end several times.

Attach the giving set and prime the line. Remove your gloves and perform hand hygiene.

Attach the prepared medication additive label (including the signatures of the two nurses) to the container. Pull a corner of the label back and attach the corner only to the container to prevent obscuring the information on the fluid bag. Take the prepared solution to the bedside.

Administer the medication

Check the person's identity using the medication administration sheet or the bar code medication administration system, the medication additive label and their identity band. Ask them their name, if they have any allergies to foods or drugs. Assess them for baseline vital signs and their general condition (e.g. fluid overload, infiltration at the site). Discuss the medication with them (e.g. reason for use, any effects, how long it will take to infuse). Perform hand hygiene and put on clean gloves.

> ?
> If you detect one of the complications, alert a senior nurse and institute measures to assist (e.g. warm compresses for discomfort, determination of the patency of the line). You may need to remove the cannula (for infiltration, inflammation, phlebitis, and non-patency of the line) and have the IV resited (see **Clinical Skill 31**).

Attach the solution container to the existing cannula or spike the medicated fluid bag with the existing giving set, whichever is applicable (see **Clinical Skill 31**). Adjust the roller clamp below the drip chamber to establish the IV flow to the ordered rate, or thread the line through the pump and establish the flow rate. Rate of flow (both using gravity and pumps) is the most common error in medication administration via container (Blandford et al., 2020; Sutherland et al., 2020).

Post-procedure

Safety

Check the medication additive label and the drip rate one more time, tidy up around the bedside (e.g. dispose of the backing of the label) and help the person into a comfortable position. Perform hand hygiene.

Periodically return to monitor the rate of flow and assess the person's reaction to the medication. Ensure the entire contents of the fluid container are absorbed before changing the container to provide the person with the prescribed dose of the medication.

CLEAN, REPLACE AND DISPOSE OF EQUIPMENT

The needles, syringes and vials/ampoules are placed into the sharps container to prevent accidental needle-stick injuries to nursing or domestic staff. Alcowipes are disposed of in the normal waste bin. Perform hand hygiene. Assess needle, syringe and medication stocks and obtain sufficient amounts for the next shift's use. Return the medication administration sheet to its storage position following documentation.

DOCUMENTATION

Sign or initial the timeslot on the medication administration sheet or use the bar code medication administration system to indicate that the ordered dose of the medication was given by the IV route at the designated time. If the medication has been ordered on the fluid sheet (e.g. potassium chloride [KCl]), it is to be signed off there. The checking nurse then countersigns the medication administration sheet. The effects of the medications, expected or unexpected, are assessed 30 minutes to one hour after administration, and are then documented. Adverse effects should be reported to the shift coordinator and the medical staff, and the remaining doses of the drug withheld.

CLINICAL SKILLS ASSESSMENT

Intravenous medication administration – intravenous container

Demonstrates the ability to effectively and safely administer intravenous medication via an intravenous container. Incorporates the *National Safety and Quality Health Service Standards*: 2 Partnering with Consumers, 3 Preventing and Controlling Healthcare-Associated Infection, 5 Comprehensive Care, 6 Communicating for Safety, and 8 Recognising and Responding to Acute Deterioration (ACSQHC, 2021).

Performance criteria	1	2	3	4	5
(Numbers indicate NMBA *Registered Nurse Standards for Practice*)	**(Dependent)**	**(Marginal)**	**(Assisted)**	**(Supervised)**	**(Independent)**
1. Identifies indication (1.1, 3.3, 3.4)	☐	☐	☐	☐	☐
2. Verifies the validity of the written medication order (1.4, 3.4, 6.2, 6.5)	☐	☐	☐	☐	☐
3. Evidence of therapeutic interaction with the person, e.g. gives the person a clear explanation of the procedure (1.4, 1.5, 2.1, 2.2, 3.2)	☐	☐	☐	☐	☐
4. Demonstrates clinical reasoning abilities; assesses the person, the intravenous site and the medication (1.1, 1.2, 1.3, 4.1, 4.2, 4.3, 6.1)	☐	☐	☐	☐	☐
5. Adheres to the general concepts of working with therapeutic substances (1.1, 1.3, 1.5, 3.3, 3.4, 4.1, 4.2, 4.3, 6.2, 6.5, 6.6)	☐	☐	☐	☐	☐
6. Gathers equipment (1.1, 5.5, 6.1): ■ medication administration sheet ■ volume-control infusion set ■ required medication and ordered fluid ■ sterile syringe and sterile needle ■ alcowipes ■ medication additive label ■ injection tray ■ sharps container ■ clean gloves	☐	☐	☐	☐	☐
7. Uses the six (or more) rights of medication administration (1.1, 1.2, 1.3, 1.4, 1.5, 2.2, 3.4, 4.1, 4.2, 4.3, 6.1, 6.2, 6.5, 6.6)	☐	☐	☐	☐	☐
8. Performs hand hygiene (1.1, 3.4, 6.1)	☐	☐	☐	☐	☐
9. Prepares the syringe with the medication (1.1, 1.4, 3.4, 6.1, 6.2, 6.5)	☐	☐	☐	☐	☐
10. Injects the medication into the intravenous container (1.1, 6.1)	☐	☐	☐	☐	☐
11. Attaches the medication additive label (1.1, 1.4, 3.4, 6.1, 6.2, 6.5)	☐	☐	☐	☐	☐
12. Hangs the medicated intravenous bag (1.1, 6.1)	☐	☐	☐	☐	☐
13. Cleans, replaces and disposes of equipment appropriately (3.6, 6.1)	☐	☐	☐	☐	☐
14. Documents relevant information (1.4, 1.6, 2.2, 3.5, 3.7, 6.2, 6.5, 7.3)	☐	☐	☐	☐	☐
15. Demonstrates the ability to link theory to practice (1.1, 3.3, 3.4, 3.5)	☐	☐	☐	☐	☐

Student:

Clinical facilitator: Date:

CHAPTER 48

INTRAVENOUS MEDICATION ADMINISTRATION – BOLUS

INDICATIONS

A bolus intravenous (IV) infusion is the administration of a medication directly into the vein over a short period of time. Bolus infusions are given when:

- the medication is urgently needed by an organ or system, and it does not need to be diluted (as in a volume-controlled burette)
- a peak level is required immediately at the time of administration (e.g. a loading dose [Broyles et al., 2017]) or a rapid effect is required (e.g. severe pain [DiSarno et al., 2023])
- the person is on fluid restrictions as minimal additional fluid is added (Johnson et al., 2023)
- a short-acting medication is used, so it can be titrated according to the person's response (Doyle & McCutcheon, 2015).

The IV bolus is administered directly into:

- the vein following venipuncture
- an existing IV line
- a saline lock device – a cannula placed in situ that is kept patent at the end of the cannula using saline solution (or, rarely, a dilute heparin solution) to prevent clotting.

Bolus medication can also be administered into a central venous catheter.

Some medications are given *bolus*, meaning over a minute or two, rather than via the slower *push* approach. However, these terms are often used interchangeably, and the rate needs to be determined prior to administration (usually three to 10 minutes). The *Australian Injectable Drugs Handbook* currently the 9th edition, 2024 (your university or the facility will have this handbook or a subscription to the website) should be consulted for the rate of administration of any IV medication. Administration of a bolus IV medication is the most hazardous of all types of administration because the entire dose is administered in a short time, the effects are immediate and the drug is irretrievable. Too rapid a rate of infusion could result in a toxic or anaphylactic reaction (Hertig et al., 2018). Some medications cannot be given via the IV bolus – consult the manufacturer's recommendations or check with the pharmacy if you are unsure. There is great potential for medication error and infection control risks when giving an IV bolus – take care.

Verify the written medication order

As for any medication, the written order for the medication, dose, time, route and correct person are verified on the medication order sheet. For an IV bolus dose, two registered professionals must check the medication and dose calculation. You will need to understand the dose, the purpose and therapeutic effect of the medication, the person's diagnosis and any individual factors that may affect their use of the medication (e.g. age, frailty, psychological distress), any adverse effects and any nursing implications (e.g. vein irritation, rate of administration) so you can question an order and anticipate its effects.

EVIDENCE OF THERAPEUTIC INTERACTION

Clearly explain the procedure. Many people are initially anxious about receiving medication via an IV. Advise the person that the adaptor is introduced into an existing IV line, with no need to access another vein, which reassures most people. If the IV is to be established prior to administration, the person will need reassurance and support while the vein is accessed (see **Clinical Skill 31**).

Tell them that they may experience some vein irritation and offer assistance if this occurs (e.g. warm compresses, mild analgesia). Discuss adverse effects common to the medication to be administered and ask the person to alert you to any changes they note. Assess all of their complaints. Just because an adverse reaction is unusual or unexpected, do not ignore it – it needs exploration. This develops trust in nursing staff.

DEMONSTRATE CLINICAL REASONING

ELDER CARE

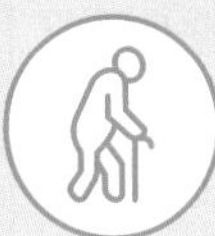

IV bolus medications are usually preferred for elderly people because of the concern about fluid overload in many comorbidities (e.g. congestive cardiac failure, renal failure) found in this vulnerable group. Older adults are at greater risk of developing IV catheter-related complications than younger people. Risk factors include urinary incontinence, haematoma at the insertion site, dressing changes and some medications (e.g. Furosemide) (Gras et al., 2023). Extra suspicion should be used when assessing the catheter site prior to administering an IV bolus/push medication.

THE PERSON LIVING WITH SEVERE OBESITY

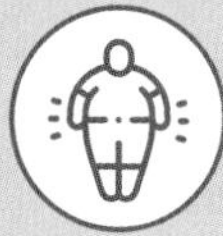

Severe obesity affects the pharmokinetics of medications. 'Normal' doses will probably be titrated to the person's adjusted (from ideal) weight and clinical response (Erstad & Barletta, 2022). Be very careful with the dose calculations as the dose may change frequently.

Assess the preparation area

Adequate lighting, ventilation and space are required. Preparing IV medications requires aseptic technique, so the area must be scrupulously clean and dry. Hand-washing equipment must be available. Preparing any medication requires concentration and you should be free from distraction during the procedure. Distraction and interruption are the most common causes of medication error (Brindley, 2020; Hare, 2020). Hang a 'Do not disturb' sign on the door and wear a brightly coloured vest to discourage interruptions and indicate you are concentrating (Bucknall et al., 2019), or wear a lighted lanyard to alert other staff to not disturb you (Hare, 2020). Perform hand hygiene.

Paparella (2019) found the following unsafe practices were common. Take care to avoid:

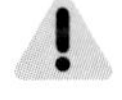
Safety

- using pharmacy or manufacturer pre-prepared medications (excess volume)
- diluting medication that is pre-prepared from either the pharmacy or the manufacturer
- labelling or poorly labelling each syringe, including the flush syringes.

Assess the person

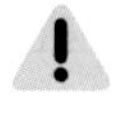
Safety

Check the identity of the person using their identification band and the medication administration sheet (best practice is two nurses checking) or the bar code medication administration system. Recheck the six rights of medication administration. Assess the person for baseline vital signs, allergies to medications, the reason for the medication and their general condition. Assess the IV site for the following (Eau, 2023):

LOOK for infiltration, inflammation, thrombosis or phlebitis – swelling, pallor (blanching), slow flow rate or reddened 'tracking' up the vein.

LISTEN for reports of discomfort, burning, tightness at the insertion site and general malaise.

FEEL for warm to hot skin at site, swelling and fever.

Assess the IV system for patency, kinks and air in the line. Inspect it from the person to the insertion into the container (or the lock device).

Use general concepts and the six rights of medication preparation

Use the information in **Clinical Skills 46 and 47** to prepare and administer an IV bolus medication. IV medications are checked by two registered nurses (RNs) or by an RN and either a medical officer or an endorsed enrolled nurse (check the facility's protocol). In addition to the six rights of medication administration, the right rate is extremely important. The rate of a bolus administration of a medication should conform to the manufacturer's recommendations and be timed with a watch with a second hand (Arthur et al., 2019).

GATHER EQUIPMENT

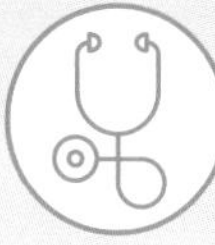

Gathering equipment is an organisational step that helps to create a positive environment for a successful interaction and reduces the risk of errors when preparing medication. It ensures that you have all needed material, boosts the person's confidence and trust in you, and increases your self-confidence. Equipment includes the following items:

EQUIPMENT	EXPLANATION
Medication administration sheet or bar code medication administration system	• Includes the written medication order used to identify the medication, route, time and dosage required • Has the person's name, hospital number, date of birth and doctor on it, and is used during identification to ensure the correct medication, dose, time and route are given to the correct person • The bar code medication administration system has additional checks such as compatibility, appropriateness of the medication, allergies to improve safety of medication administration
Ordered medication	• To be obtained from stock or the ADC – it will be in a vial or sometimes an ampoule (see **Clinical Skill 45** for a discussion of ampoules and vials) • Should come from the pharmacy ready to use; i.e. a single-dose unit. If it is to be reconstituted, you will need a sterile diluent as recommended by the manufacturer for the medication • Only dilute liquid medications as required by the manufacturer (Institute for Safe Medication Practices [ISMP], 2015) • Check that the medication is compatible with the infusing IV fluid and is suitable for bolus injection. You may need to consult the pharmacy
Sterile syringe	• A size larger than the anticipated dose is needed. This allows draw-back on the syringe as a test of IV patency prior to the bolus • Extra syringes will be needed for the flushes
Sterile needleless adaptor (or sterile needle in the smallest gauge reasonable for the viscosity of the medication)	• Used so that the access port seal is damaged as little as possible. The port may be needed as often as hourly in some critically ill people. A damaged seal allows contamination of the system and requires the entire system to be changed, including the cannula • Needles are very infrequently used, as they are more damaging
Alcowipes	To cleanse and disinfect the tops of vials and the latex seal on the medication access port of the IV line
Injection tray	To carry medications, syringes and alcowipes to the bedside
Sharps container	To immediately dispose of needles, glass ampoules and vials. Reduces the chance of needle-stick injuries/cuts from broken glass
Watch with a second hand	Timing of the administration of the medication is crucial. It is essential to time the bolus infusion. Infusion rates vary with the medication – follow the manufacturer's recommendation. Too rapid an injection may precipitate either local reaction or more serious, systemic reactions
Normal saline (NS) in a sterile syringe	• Used to flush both the IV line and the intermittent set before and after administering the medication to prevent any incompatibilities • Effective in preventing occlusion of the cannula, and most facilities use only NS flush following medication administration. Some adhere to the NS flush, medication, NS flush, heparin regimen. Check the facility's policy
Heparin flush solution in a sterile syringe (NB – used much less frequently now)	• Used in some facilities to maintain the patency of intermittent infusion devices, although Sotnikova et al. (2020) found heparin was no more effective than NS in maintaining patency • Standard sterile solutions of dilute heparin (often 50 units per 5 mL) are available • Make sure you do not confuse the heparin flush solution with the more concentrated heparin for subcutaneous (SC) and IV administration
Clean gloves	To comply with standard precautions
Medication labels (or adhesive tape)	To identify the medication, saline (or heparin flush) in the syringe

ADMINISTER A BOLUS INTRAVENOUS MEDICATION

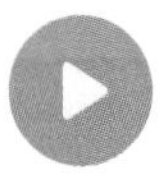

IV bolus medication can be injected into an existing IV line or into a capped (locked) line.

Hand hygiene

Hand hygiene (see **Clinical Skill 5**) removes microorganisms from your hands. It is the most effective preventative measure for cross-contamination, reducing incidences of nosocomial (i.e. hospital- or treatment-acquired) infection. It is also important for this Clinical Skill, as the medication being prepared is administered directly into a vein. Take care in the preparation to maintain asepsis.

Don gloves

Gloves reduce transfer of microorganisms and provide for self-protection since a blood source is being accessed.

Prepare the syringes

Safety

Assess the medication for:

- compatibility with the fluid infusing and the diluent (if used)
- strength/concentration of the solution available
- its normal dosage, action and adverse effects
- the recommended infusion time of the medication
- its peak action time.

Use a pre-prepared medication syringe whenever possible. Ready-to-administer syringes have the correct dose/strength and dilution prepared in the pharmacy or commercially. They eliminate most of the following steps, are safer and are the preferred method of administering IV bolus/push medications (Degnan, Bullard & Davis, 2020). Pre-prepared syringes (either from the pharmacy or the manufacturer) reduce medication errors, as there are fewer steps in their preparation (Hertig et al., 2018). Any manipulation, including dilution, is not only unnecessary but can lead to errors, including compromised sterility, altered potency or stability of the drug, and dose and rate errors (Degnan, Bullard & Davis, 2020). Prefilled sterile syringes with 0.9% NS are available for flushing in many facilities (Lee & Terry, 2021). It will be prescribed as a medication (Royal Children's Hospital Melbourne [RCHM], 2022).

If you must prepare the medication on the unit, the following steps are followed. Prepare the syringe just before administering it. Note: the metal caps on vials are 'dust covers' and do not mean the vial membrane is sterile (ISMP, 2015). Use Aseptic Non Touch Technique (ANTT). Verify your calculations with a registered healthcare professional who has independently calculated the dose. Cleanse the vial membrane with an alcowipe vigorously for 30 seconds and allow to dry. Draw up the undiluted medication, sterile heparin flush (if used) and NS flushes (see **Clinical Skill 45** for more on using vials and ampoules and reconstituting powdered medications). Confirm the medication and dose with a second nurse. Dilute medications *only* if recommended by the manufacturer. Medications are safe and comfortable to give IV bolus/push if the rate of injection is followed (Deutsch, 2020).

The amount of flush NS varies. The RCHM (2022) recommends 2 mL for infants/small children; Deutsch (2020) recommends 10 mL for adults. Parriera et al. (2020) report a research protocol to assess the safety and efficacy of a 'double-barrelled' syringe that has medication in one barrel and flush NS in the other, reducing the need to manipulate the cannula so often. Check the protocol on the unit where you are working. Label the medication (i.e. syringe) with the person's name, time, medication and dose on a piece of adhesive tape or on a medication label provided for this use (ISMP, 2015). Take care not to obscure the calibrations on the syringe containing the medication. Similarly identify the heparin flush (if used) and NS syringes. Attach the needleless adaptor (e.g. interlock) to the syringe if using.

Inject medication into an existing line

Safety

Determine the nature of the solution flowing through the existing line and confirm its compatibility with the medication.

> If the existing IV line is infusing solutions other than those compatible with the medication, do not use it for medication administration. Either a new IV line will have to be established, or the primary IV line flushed with 10 mL of NS before the medication is given (Eau, 2021).
>
> *Never* administer an IV medication through an IV line that is infusing blood, blood products, heparin IV, insulin IV, cytotoxic medications or parenteral nutrition solutions.

Clean the injection/adaptor port with alcowipes vigorously for 30 seconds and allow it to dry. This destroys as many microbes as possible. (The injection port is designed for multiple punctures.) Use the port closest to the person to minimise the amount of medication in the line if an adverse reaction occurs.

Stop the infusion pump if one is being used. Clamp the IV line with the roller clamp or by pinching it just above the access port. This will prevent the medication from going up the line into the solution. Familiarise yourself with the giving sets in use, as many types permit administration of bolus doses without clamping or pinching the line (e.g. anti-reflex sets).

Flushing the IV line determines and enhances patency and increases the life of the peripherally inserted venous cannula (PIVC) by removing fibrin from the lumen of the cannula (Parriera et al., 2020). Fibrin can be the basis of thromboembolism formation. Flushing after medication also delivers the final amount of the prescribed dose (Cooper, Rassam & Mellor, 2018) and removes medication precipitate from the cannula (Ribeiro et al., 2023; Zhu et al., 2020).

For a needleless adaptor:

1. Insert the first NS syringe with the needleless adaptor.
2. Test that the IV cannula is in the vein by drawing back slightly on the plunger of the syringe. Draw back only until a trace of blood appears in the hub of the cannula, so the medication is not in touch with the blood. If it is a small-gauge cannula (e.g. 22 or smaller), no blood may be returned (the tip of the cannula may collapse when negative pressure is applied).
3. Flush the cannula with the NS using a push (about 2 mL at a time [Zhu et al., 2020]), pause, repeat action until the flush amount is used. Remove the NS syringe.
4. Insert the medication syringe with its needleless adaptor. Inject medication at the recommended rate. Many medications must be given over a three- to five-minute time frame or longer to prevent irritation or damage to vein walls by too high a concentration of the medication. Manufacturers

suggest a rate that minimises discomfort. This should be calculated at the same time as the dose is calculated. Time this carefully using a watch with a second hand (ISMP, 2015). Too rapid injection of a medication may damage the vein, causing pain and phlebitis, and requiring the removal and resiting of the cannula, or it may cause rapid 'peak' of the medication with subsequent ill effects. Speed shock manifests as facial flushing, hypotension, irregular pulse, chest pain and even cardiac arrest (Eau, 2023). It is extremely important to know and adhere to the timing of the bolus medication. Remove the medication syringe.

5. Insert the second NS flush syringe with the needleless adaptor and flush the cannula (the first 1 mL to be given at the same rate as the medication to clear the tubing of medication; the remainder of the flush is given according to the comfort of the person). Again, use the pulsatile (push/pause) action. Remove the syringe and adaptor.

If there is no needleless device:

1. Insert the needle attached to the NS flush syringe and aspirate to determine the patency of the cannula.
2. Inject the NS, pulsing it. Remove the NS needle and syringe – removing only the syringe and leaving the needle in situ for the next two syringes increases the risk of contaminating the system.
3. Insert the needle of the medication syringe, inject the medication using the manufacturer's recommended times and using the second hand on your watch for accuracy. Remove the medication needle and syringe.
4. Insert the second NS needle and syringe and flush the line with NS (the first 1 mL to be given at the same rate as the medication to clear the tubing of medication, the remainder of the flush is given using pulses according to the comfort of the person). Remove the NS needle and syringe. (If using, insert the heparin needle and syringe and flush the line with heparin. Remove the needle and syringe.)

On completion of each injection, discard the used needle and syringe into the sharps container to avoid needle-stick injury. Re-establish the flow of the IV by unclamping the line. Reset the IV rate or restart the pump. Remove your gloves and perform hand hygiene.

Inject the medication into the intermittent infusion set

Injecting medication into an intermittent infusion set (bunged or capped lock system) is similar to injecting medication into an infusing IV line. The 'lock' system (e.g. saline lock, IV lock, peripheral lock) is simply an IV cannulae in a peripheral vein that has a short tube, filled with saline and capped to keep the cannula patent for intermittent administration of medications. The IV lock provides rapid access for emergency medications as well as intermittent access for ongoing medication administration. It does not require continuous fluid administration. Observe standard precautions by performing hand hygiene and putting on clean gloves.

1. Clean the port with alcowipes and allow it to dry to remove microorganisms.
2. Insert the needleless adaptor attached to the NS flush syringe into the centre of the access port and aspirate to ascertain the patency of the cannula. Inject the NS using a push-pause-push-pause action to increase turbulence within the cannula and to remove any debris (Zhu et al., 2020). Remove the syringe.
3. Insert the medication syringe/adaptor. Inject the medication over the manufacturer's recommended times using the second hand on your watch to time it. Remove the medication syringe.
4. Administer the second NS syringe by flushing the line with NS, again using the pulsatile action. This should be no faster than the rate the medication is administered and should be done using a 'stop-start' technique to create turbulence in the cannula to remove adhering substances (Zhu et al., 2020). (If using, insert the heparin needle and syringe. Flush the line with heparin.)

In the unlikely event that there is no needleless access to the IV cannula, follow the steps (above) for adding medication and flushes to the capped cannula.

Often people do not receive IV medications frequently, and the intermittent infusion set requires flushing with NS at regular intervals to maintain patency of the line. Keogh et al. (2016) indicate that once every 24 hours is sufficient to maintain patency, although others, such as the RCHM (2022), recommend once per eight hours, while the Australian Commission on Safety and Quality in Health Care (ACSQHC, 2021) recommends leaving the timing to local policy. NS is as effective as heparin. The long interval was proven to be safer, more cost-effective with fewer complications; however, you must follow the policy of the facility regarding the flushing interval and solution.

Often a positive pressure device injection system is used to decrease the incidence of thrombosis formation by preventing the backflow of blood into the catheter. These are attached to peripherally inserted central cannula (PICC) lines. A positive pressure device injection system requires a similar procedure, but a Luer Lock syringe is used and attached to the port by pushing and twisting it into the positive pressure device until there is a tight fit. Flush with NS, remove the syringe and attach the syringe containing the medication and inject it at the recommended rate, then remove the syringe. Finally, flush the line with NS and remove the syringe while still moving the plunger forward. This maintains the positive pressure in the catheter. These devices are only flushed with NS, and the line must not be clamped or have extension sets added, as these negate the anti-reflux action of the device (Hull, Moureau & Sengupta, 2018).

Post-procedure

Observe the person carefully during and after the IV bolus injection for adverse effects. If the injection of the solution has caused discomfort to the vein, offer warm compresses and mild analgesia. The local effects of a few medications given via IV bolus can last for some time. Remove your gloves and perform hand hygiene.

Help the person into a comfortable position. Check that the IV flow rate is correct. Return within a half-hour to assess the effects of the medications.

CLEAN, REPLACE AND DISPOSE OF EQUIPMENT

Place the needles and syringes into the sharps container as soon as they are used to prevent accidental needle-stick injuries. Place vials and ampoules into the sharps container after your final check of medication, strength and dose. Alcowipes and used gloves are disposed of in the normal waste bin. Wash, dry and return the injection tray to its storage place. Assess needle, syringe and medication stocks and obtain sufficient amounts for the next shift's use.

DOCUMENTATION

The administering nurse signs or initials the timeslot on the medication administration sheet/electronic medication administration record (eMAR) indicating that the ordered dose was given to the person by the IV route at the designated time. The RN who checked the medication usually countersigns the medication (as per the facility's policies). Any untoward reactions are to be reported immediately to the shift coordinator and the medical officer because they could be very serious.

CLINICAL SKILLS ASSESSMENT

Intravenous medication administration – bolus

Demonstrates the ability to effectively and safely administer intravenous medication via a push or bolus dose. Incorporates the *National Safety and Quality Health Service Standards*: 2 Partnering with Consumers, 3 Preventing and Controlling Healthcare-Associated Infection, 5 Comprehensive Care, 6 Communicating for Safety, and 8 Recognising and Responding to Acute Deterioration (ACSQHC, 2021).

Performance criteria	1	2	3	4	5
(Numbers indicate NMBA *Registered Nurse Standards for Practice*)	(Dependent)	(Marginal)	(Assisted)	(Supervised)	(Independent)
1. Identifies indication (1.1, 3.3, 3.4)	☐	☐	☐	☐	☐
2. Verifies the validity of the written medication order (1.4, 3.4, 6.2, 6.5)	☐	☐	☐	☐	☐
3. Evidence of therapeutic interaction with the person, e.g. gives the person a clear explanation of the procedure (1.4, 1.5, 2.1, 2.2, 3.2)	☐	☐	☐	☐	☐
4. Demonstrates clinical reasoning, e.g. assesses the person, the IV site and the medication (1.1, 1.2, 1.3, 4.2, 4.3, 6.1)	☐	☐	☐	☐	☐
5 Uses general concepts of medication administration plus six rights (1.1, 1.2, 1.3, 1.4, 1.5, 2.2, 3.3, 3.4, 4.1, 4.2, 4.3, 6.1, 6.2, 6.5, 6.6)	☐	☐	☐	☐	☐
6. Gathers equipment (1.1, 5.5, 6.1): ■ medication administration sheet ■ ordered medication ■ sterile syringe ■ sterile needleless adaptor (or sterile needle in the smallest gauge reasonable for the viscosity of the medication) ■ alcowipes ■ injection tray ■ sharps container ■ watch with a second hand ■ heparin flush solution in a sterile syringe ■ normal saline in a sterile syringe ■ clean gloves ■ medication labels (or adhesive tape)	☐	☐	☐	☐	☐
7. Performs hand hygiene (1.1, 3.4, 6.1)	☐	☐	☐	☐	☐
8. Dons gloves (1.1, 3.4, 6.1)	☐	☐	☐	☐	☐
9. Prepares the syringes with medication, saline and/or heparin (1.1, 3.4, 6.1)	☐	☐	☐	☐	☐
10. Injects the medication into an existing line (1.1, 3.4, 6.1)	☐	☐	☐	☐	☐
11. Injects the medication into the intermittent infusion set (1.1, 3.4, 6.1)	☐	☐	☐	☐	☐
12. Cleans, replaces and disposes of equipment appropriately (3.6, 6.1)	☐	☐	☐	☐	☐
13. Documents relevant information (1.4, 1.6, 2.7, 3.5, 3.7, 6.1, 6.2, 6.5, 7.3)	☐	☐	☐	☐	☐
14. Demonstrates the ability to link theory to practice (1.1, 3.3, 3.4, 3.5)	☐	☐	☐	☐	☐

Student:

Clinical facilitator: Date:

REFERENCES

Abdelhadi, R., Barakat, A. & Lyman, B. (2022). Ch. 7: Enteral and parenteral devices. In P. Goday & C. Walla (eds), *Pediatric nutrition for dietitians.* CRC Press: Taylor and Francis.

Abd-El-Maeboud, K. H., El-Naggar, T., El-Hawi, E. M., Mahmoud, S. A. & Abd-El-Hay, S. (1991). Rectal suppository: Common sense and mode of insertion. *Lancet, 338*(8770), 798–800.

Alhashemi, S., Ghorbani, R. & Vazin, A. (2019). Improving knowledge, attitudes and practice of nurses in medication administration through enteral feeding tubes by clinical pharmacists: A case-control study. *Advances in Medical Education and Practice, 10,* 493–500. https://doi.org/10.2147/AMEP.S203680

Alkazemi, A., McLaughlin, K. C., Chan, M. G., Schontz, M., Anger, K. & Szumita, P. (2022). Safety of intravenous push Levetiracetam compared to intravenous piggyback at a tertiary academic medical center: A retrospective analysis. *Drug Safety, 45,* 19–26. https://doi.org/10.1007/s40264-021-01122-7

American Academy of Ophthalmology (2023). How to put in eye drops. https://www.aao.org/eye-health/treatments/how-to-put-in-eye-drops

Amirthalingam, S., Yi, K. S., Ching, L. T. & Mun, N. Y. (2015) Topical antibacterial and global challenges on resistance development. *Tropical Journal of Pharmaceutical Research, 14*(5). https://doi.org/10.1016/j.sjbs.2017.01.004

Appelbaum, N., Rodriguez-Gonzalvez, C. & Clarke, J. (2020). Ideal body weight in the precision era: Recommendations for prescribing in obesity require thought for computer-assisted methods. *Archives of Disease in Childhood, 105*(5), 516. https://doi.org/10.1136/archdischild-2019-318370

Arthur, J., Reddy, A., Smith, U., Hui, D., Park, M., Liu, D., Vaughan-Adams, N., Haider, A., Williams, J. & Breura, E. (2019). Practices and perceptions regarding intravenous opioid infusion and cancer pain management. *Cancer, 125*(21), 3882–9. https://doi.org/10.1002/cncr.32380

Asad, U., Boothe, D. & Tarbox, M. (2019). Effect of topical dermatologic medications in humans on household pets. *Proceedings (Baylor University Medical Center), 33*(1), 131–2. https://doi.org/10.1080/08998280.2019.1679003

Asthma Australia (2020). *Devices and techniques.* https://asthma.org.au/about-asthma/medicines-and-devices/preventers

Australian Commission on Safety and Quality in Health Care (ACSQHC) (2019). *Electronic medication management systems: A guide to safe implementation* (3rd ed.). Sydney, NSW: ACSQHC.

Australian Commission on Safety and Quality in Health Care (ACSQHC) (2021). *National safety and quality health service standards* (3rd edn). Sydney, NSW: ACSQHC.

Australian Commission on Safety and Quality in Health Care (ACSQHC)/NPS Medicinewise. (2022). Consumer medicine information: Otocomb otic. https://www.nps.org.au/medicine-finder/otocomb-otic-ear-drops

Bancsi, A., Houle, S. & Grindrod, K. (2019). Shoulder injury related to vaccine administration and other injection site events. *Canadian Family Physician, 65*(1), 40–2. https://www.cfp.ca/content/65/1/40

Bayat, A., Aydemir, E., Aydemir, G. & Gencer, H. (2023). Assessment of tear film anomalies in childhood obesity. *Klin Monbl Augenheilkd, 239*(03), 331–7. https://doi.org/10.1055/a-1668-0276

Biran, A., Goldberg, M., Shemesh, N. & Achiron, A. (2023). Improving compliance with medical treatment using eye drop aids. *MDPI Encyclopedia, 3*(3), 919–27. https://doi.org/10.3390/encyclopedia3030065

Bischoff, S., Austin, P., Boeykens, K., Chourdakis, M., Cuerda, C., Jonkers-Schuitema, C., Lichota, M., Nyulasi, I., Schneider, S., Stanga, Z. & Pironi, L. (2022). ESPEN practical guideline: Home enteral nutrition. *Clinical Nutrition, 41*(2), 468–88. https://doi.org/10.1016/j.clnu.2021.10.018

Blandford, A., Furniss, D., Galal-Edeen, G. H., et al. (2020). Intravenous infusion practices across England and their impact on patient safety: A mixed-methods observational study. Southampton (UK): *NIHR Journals Library*; 2020 Feb. (Health Services and Delivery Research, No. 8.7.) Chapter 3, Phase 1: Observed errors and discrepancies in the administration of intravenous infusions. https://www.ncbi.nlm.nih.gov/books/NBK553532

Boyd, K. (2019). *Eye medication mixups.* American Academy of Ophthalmology. https://www.aao.org/eye-health/treatments/eye-medication-mix-ups

Brindley, J. (2020). How to undertake intravenous infusion calculations. *Nursing Standard (2014+), 35*(3), 47–50. https://doi.org/10.7748/ns.2020.e1144

British Association for Parenteral and Enteral Nutrition and The British Pharmaceutical Nutrition Group (n.d.). *Administering drugs via enteral feeding tubes: A practical guide.* http://www.bapen.org.uk/pdfs/d_and_e/de_pract_guide.pdf

Brotto, V. (2020). Administering medications. In *Professional nursing and midwifery practice: A custom compilation for Monash University School of Nursing.* https://books.google.com.au/books?hl=en&lr=&id=X9PWDwAAQBAJ&oi=fnd&pg=PA110&dq=Vanessa+ Brotto+medication+administration

Broyles, B., Reiss, B., Evans, M., McKenzie, G., Pleunik, S. & Page, R. (2017). *Pharmacology in nursing* (Australia & New Zealand 2nd ed.). South Melbourne, VIC: Cengage Learning.

Bryan, R., Aronson, J. K., Williams, A. & Jordan, S. (2020). The problem of look-alike, sound-alike name errors: Drivers and solutions. *British Journal of Clinical Pharmacology, 1*(9). https://doi.org/10.1111/bcp.14285

Bucknall, T., Fossum, M., Hutchinson, A. M., Botti, M., Considine, J., Dunning, T., Hughes, L., Weir-Phyland, J., Digby, R. & Manias, E. (2019). Nurses' decision-making, practices and perceptions of patient involvement in medication administration in an acute hospital setting. *Journal of Advanced Nursing, 75,* 1316–27. https://doi.org/10.1111/jan.13963

Caminati, M., Vaia, R., Furci, F., Guarnieri, G. & Senna, G. (2021). Uncontrolled asthma: Unmet needs in the management of patients. *Journal of Asthma Allergy, 14,* 457–66. https://doi.org/10.2147/JAA.S260604

Cengiz, E., Danne, T., Ahmad, T., Ayyavoo, A., Beran, D., Ehtisham, S., Fairchild, J., Jarosz-Chobot, P., Ng, S., Paterson, M. & Codner, E. (2022). ISPAD Clinical Practice Consensus Guidelines 2022: Insulin treatment in children and adolescents with diabetes. *Pediatric Diabetes, 23*(8), 1277–96. https://pubmed.ncbi.nlm.nih.gov/36537533

Chen, S., Cui, Y., Ding, Y., Sun, C., Xing, Y., Zhou, B. & Liu, G. (2020). Prevalence and risk factors of dysphagia among nursing home residents in eastern China: A cross-sectional study. *BMC Geriatrics, 20,* 352. https://doi.org/10.1186/s12877-020-01752-z

Cheng, K. (2019). Prevention or treatment of human ear pain, itch or vertigo (dizziness) caused by cerumen (earwax) impaction and ear hairs. *Open Science Journal of Clinical Medicine, 7*(2), 52–5. http://www.openscienceonline.com/journal/osjcm

Cleveland Clinic (2019). *Home nebuliser.* https://my.clevelandclinic.org/health/drugs/4254-home-nebulizer

Cleveland Clinic (2023). *Ear drops.* https://my.clevelandclinic.org/health/treatments/24654-ear-drops

Cohrs, J. & Kerns, R. (2020). Using transdermal patches to treat neuropathic pain. *Nursing, 50*(4), 15–16. https://doi.org/10.1097/01.NURSE.0000657076.10174.66

Cooper, D., Rassam, T. & Mellor, A. (2018). Non-flushing of IV administration sets: An under-recognised under-dosing risk. *British Journal of Nursing, 27*(14), S4–S12. https://doi.org/10.12968/bjon.2018.27.14.S4

Crisp, J. & Taylor, C. (eds) (2009). *Potter & Perry's fundamentals of nursing* (3rd Australian ed.). Chatswood, NSW: Mosby Elsevier.

Dall'Oglio, V., Fioril, M., DiCiommo, V., Tiozzo, E., Mascolo, R., Bianchi, N., Degli'Arri, M., Ferracci, A., Gawronski, O., Pomponi, M. & Taponi, M. (2017). Effectiveness of an improvement programme to prevent interruptions during medication administration in a paediatric hospital: A preintervention–postintervention study. *British Medical Journal Open, 7*, e013285. https://doi.org/10.1136/bmjopen-2016-013285

Davidson, K. M. & Bertram, J. E. (2019). Best practice for deltoid intramuscular injections in older adults: Study in cadavers. *Journal of Nursing Education and Practice, 9*(9), 92. https://doi.org/10.543-.jnep.v9n9p92

Degnan, D., Bullard, T. & Davis, M. (2020). Risk of patient harm related to unnecessary dilution of ready-to-administer prefilled syringes, *Journal of Infusion Nursing, 43*(3), 146–54. https://doi.org/10.1097/NAN.0000000000000366

DeLaune, S., Ladner, P., McTier, L. & Tollefson, J. (2024). *Fundamentals of nursing* (Australia and New Zealand 3rd ed.). South Melbourne, VIC: Cengage Learning.

Deutsch, L. (2020). Dilution is no solution. *Nursing, 50*(5), 61–2. https://doi.org/10.1097/01.NURSE.0000659316.76576.58

Di Sarno, L., Gatto, A., Korn, D., Pansini, V., Curatola, A., Ferretti, S., Capossela, L., Graglia, B. & Chiaretti, A. (2023). Pain management in pediatric age. An update. *Acta Biomed, 94*(4), e2023174. https://doi.org/10.23750/abm.v94i4.14289

Dixon, A. & Peters, U. (2018). The effect of obesity on lung function. *Expert Review of Respiratory Medicine,12*(9), 755–67. https://doi.org/10.1080/17476348.2018.1506331

Doyle, B., Kelsey, L., Carr, P., Bulmer, A. & Keogh, S. (2021). Determining an appropriate To-Keep-Vein-Open (TKVO) infusion rate for peripheral intravenous catheter usage. *Journal of the Association for Vascular Access, 26* (2), 13–20. https://doi.org/10.2309/JAVA-D-21-00006

Doyle, G. & McCutcheon, J. (2015) *Clinical procedures for safer patient care.* Open Educational Resource. Vancouver, Canada: University of British Columbia. https://opentextbc.ca/clinicalskills

Dragon, N. (2020). 10 tips to avoid medication errors. *Australian Nursing and Midwifery Journal.* https://anmj.org.au/10-tips-to-avoid-medication-errors/

Earlam, A. & Woods, L. (2020). Obesity: Skin issues and skinfold management. *American Nurse.* https://www.myamericannurse.com/obesity- skin-issues-and-skinfold-management

Eau, C. (2021). Chapter 23 IV therapy management. In K. Ernstmeyer & E. Christman (eds), *Open Resources for Nursing (Open RN); Nursing Advanced Skills* [Internet]. https://www.ncbi.nlm.nih.gov/books/NBK593209

Eau, C. (2023). Chapter 1 Initiate IV therapy. In K. Ernstmeyer & E. Christman (eds), *Open Resources for Nursing (Open RN); Nursing Advanced Skills* [Internet]. https://www.ncbi.nlm.nih.gov/books/NBK594499

Erdinest, N., London, N., Lavy, I., Morad, Y. & Levinger, N. (2021). Vision through healthy aging eyes. *Vision, 5*(4), 46. https://doi.org/10.3390/vision5040046

Erkoc, H. & Yazici, Z. A. (2021), Glass particle contamination threat in nursing practice: A pilot study. *Journal of Advanced Nursing, 77*, 3189–91. https://doi.org/10.1111/jan.14847

Erstad, B. L. & Barletta, J. F. (2020). Drug dosing in the critically ill obese patient: A focus on sedation, analgesia, and delirium. *Critical Care, 24*, 315. https://doi.org/10.1186/s13054-020-03040-z

Erstad, B. L. & Barletta, J. F. (2022). Implications of obesity for drug administration and absorption from subcutaneous and intramuscular injections: A primer. *American Journal of Health Systems Pharmacy, 79*(15), 1236–44. https://doi.org/10.1093/ajhp/zxac058. PMID: 35176754

Estes, M., Calleja, P., Theobald, K. & Harvey, T. (2020). *Health assessment and physical examination* (3rd Australian and New Zealand ed.). South Melbourne, VIC: Cengage Learning.

Eye Practice, The (2020). *Eye drops – all you need to know.* https://www.theeyepractice.com.au/education-advice/eyedrops

Felix, T. C., Borges de Araújo, L., Von Dolinger de Brito Röder, D. & Reginaldo dos, S. P. (2020). Evaluation of vulvovaginitis and hygiene habits of women attended in primary health care units of the family. *International Journal of Women's Health, 12*, 49–57. https://doi.org/10.2147/IJWH.S229366

Fonceca, A., Ditcham, W., Everard, M. & Devadason, S. (2019). Drug administration by inhalation in children. In R. Wilmot, R. Deterding, A. Li, F. Ratjen, P. Sly, H. Zar & A. Bush (eds), *Kendig and Chernick's disorders of the respiratory tract in children* (9th ed., pp. 257–71). Philadelphia, PA: Elsevier. https://research-repository.uwa.edu.au/en/publications/drug-administration-by-inhalation-in-children

Fullington, D., Song, J., Gilles, A., Guo, X., Hua, W., Anderson, C. E. & Griffin, J. (2017). Evaluation of the safety and efficacy of a novel product for the removal of impacted human cerumen. *BMC Ear, Nose and Throat Disorders, 17*, 5. https://doi.org/10.1186/s12901-017-0038-8

Fulmer, M., Karasek, N., Mazzante, R., Briscese, M., Leech, C. & Wapinsky, K. (2016). *Affecting change in the administration of subcutaneous anticoagulation therapy.* Presented 28 October at Lehigh Valley Health Network, Allentown, PA. http://scholarlyworks.lvhn.org/cgi/viewcontent.cgi?article=1794&context=patient-care-services-nursing

Gentile, S., Satta, E., Guarino, G. & Strollo, F. on behalf of the AMD-OSDI Study Group on Injection Technique (2023). Lipodystrophies from insulin injection: An update of the Italian Consensus Statement of AMD-OSDI Study Group on Injection Technique. *Diabetology, 4*(1), 119–27. https://doi.org/10.3390/diabetology4010013

Gibson, P., McDonald, V. & Thomas, D. (2023). Treatable traits, combination inhaler therapy and the future of asthma management. *Respirology, 28*(9), 828–40. https://doi.org/10.1111/resp.14556

Glaucoma Australia (n.d.) *How to instil eye drops.* https://www.glaucoma.org.au/articles/how-to-instil-eye-drops-article

Glaucoma Australia (2023). Eye drops and glaucoma. https://glaucoma.org.au/what-is-glaucoma/glaucoma-treatments/eye-drops-and- glaucoma

Global Initiative for Asthma (2019). *Global strategy for asthma management and prevention.* https://www.ginasthma.org

Gorska-Ciebiada, M., Masierek, M. & Ciebiada, M. (2020). Improved insulin injection technique, treatment satisfaction and glycemic control: Results from a large cohort education study, *Journal of Clinical & Translational Endocrinology, 19.* https://doi.org/10.1016/j.jcte.2020.100217

Government of Western Australia: WA Country Health Service (2019). *Policy: Enteral tubes and feeding – Adult Clinical Practice Standards.* https://www.wacountry.health.wa.gov.au/~/media/WACHS/Documents/About- us/Policies/Enteral-Tubes-and-Feeding---Adults-Clinical-Practice-Standard.pdf?thn=0

Gras, E., Jean, A., Rocher, V., Tran, Y., Katsahian, S., Jouclas, D., Dano, C., Cedile, J., Manar, D., Kassis Chikhani, N., Le Guen, J., Patas D'illiers, C. & Lebeaux, D. (2023). Incidence of and risk factors for local complications of peripheral venous catheters in patients older than 70 years: Empirical research quantitative. *Journal of Clinical Nursing, 32*, 5000–9. https://doi.org/10.1111/jocn.16732

Great Ormond Street Hospital for Children (2020). *How to give your child eye drops.* https://www.gosh.nhs.uk/medical-information/medicines-information/how-give-your-child-eye-drops

Gregorowicz, A., Costello, P., Gajdosik, D., Purakal, J., Petit, N., Bastow, S. & Ward, M. (2020). Effect of IV push antibiotic administration on antibiotic therapy delays in sepsis. *Critical Care Medicine, 48*(8), 1175–9. https://www.ingentaconnect.com/content/wk/ccm/2020/00000048/00000008/art00026

Gwenhure, T. & Shepherd, E. (2019). Principles and procedure for eye assessment and cleansing. *Nursing Times* [online]; *115*(12), 18–20. https://www.nursingtimes.net/clinical-archive/assessment-skills/principles-and-procedure-for-eye-assessment-and-cleansing-28-11-2019

Hagmeyer, L., van Koningsbruggen-Rietschel, S., Matthes, S., Rietschel, E. & Randerath, W. (2023). From the infant to the geriatric patient: Strategies for inhalation therapy in asthma and chronic obstructive pulmonary disease. *Clinical Respiratory Journal, 17*(6), 487–98. https://doi:10.1111/crj.13610

Hanson, A. & Haddad, L. (2022). Nursing rights of medication administration. StatPearls. https://www.ncbi.nlm.nih.gov/books/NBK560654

Hare, R. (2020). *Targeting distraction during medication administration.* Doctoral thesis. St Francis Medical Centre College of Nursing. ProQuest Dissertations Publishing, 2020. 27837325. https://search.proquest.com/openview/dcba140211561e2afac661af34e93a9e/1?pq-origsite=gscholar&cbl=18750&diss=y

Hermanspann, T., van der Linden, E., Schoberer, M., Fitzner, C., Orlikowsky, T., Marx, G. & Eisert, A. (2019). Evaluation to improve the quality of medication preparation and administration in pediatric and adult intensive care units. *Drug, Healthcare and Patient Safety, 11*, 11–18. https://doi.org/10.2147/DHPS.S184479

Hertig, J., Degnan, D., Scott, C., Lenz, J., Li, X. & Anderson, C. (2018). A comparison of error rates between intravenous push methods: A prospective, multisite, observational study. *Journal of Patient Safety, 14*(1), 60–5. https://doi.org/10.1097/PTS.0000000000000419

Hirsch, L. & Strauss, K. (2019). The injection technique factor: What you don't know or teach can make a difference. *Clinical Diabetes, 37*(3), 227–33. https://doi.org/10.2337/cd18-0076

Holliday, R., Gupta, V. & Vibhute, P. (2019). Body mass index: Reliable predictor of subcutaneous fat thickness and needle length for ventral gluteal intramuscular injections. *American Journal of Therapeutics, 26*(1), 72–8. https://doi.org/10.1097/MJT.0000000000000474

Hontoria-Alcoceba, R., López-López, C., Hontoria-Alcoceba, V. & Sánchez-Morgado, A. (2023). Implementation of evidence-based practice in peripheral intravenous catheter care. *Journal of Nursing Care Quality, 38*(3), 226–38. https://journals.lww.com/jncqjournal/abstract/2023/07000/implementation_of_evidence_based_practice_in.5.aspx

Hua, S. (2019). Physiological and pharmaceutical considerations for rectal drug formulations. *Frontiers in Pharmacology, 10*, 1196. https://doi.org/10.3389/fphar.2019.01196

Huang, J., Yeung, A., Kerr, D., Gentile, S., Heinemann, L., Al-Sofiani, M., Joseph, J., Seley, J. & Klonoff, D. (2023). Lipohypertrophy and insulin: An old dog that needs new tricks. *Endocrine Practice, 29*(8), 670–7. https://www.sciencedirect.com/science/article/pii/S1530891X23003865

Hull, G. J., Moureau, N. L. & Sengupta, S. (2018). Quantitative assessment of reflux in commercially available needle-free IV connectors. *Journal of Vascular Access, 19*(1), 12–22. https://doi.org/10.5301/jva.5000781

Hull, R., Garcia, D. & Vazquez, S. (2023). Patient education: Warfarin (beyond the basics). *UpToDate.* https://www.uptodate.com/contents/warfarin-beyond-the-basics

Hutton, K., Ding, Q. & Wellman, G. (2021). The effects of bar-coding technology on medication errors: A systematic literature review. *Journal of Patient Safety, 17*(3), e192–e206. https://doi.org/10.1097/PTS.0000000000000366

Inangil, D. & Inangil, G. (2020). The effect of acupressure (GB30) on intramuscular injection pain and satisfaction: Single–blind, randomised controlled study. *Journal of Clinical Nursing, 29*, 1094–101. https://doi.org/10.1111/jocn.15172

Institute for Safe Medication Practices (ISMP) (2015). *Safe practice for adult IV push medications. A compilation of safe practices from the ISMP Adult IV Push Medication Safety Summit.* http://www.ismp.org/Tools/guidelines/IVSummitPush/IVPushMedGuidelines.pdf

Institute for Safe Medication Practices (ISMP) (2019). *ISMP guidelines for the safe use of automated dispensing cabinets.* ISMP. https://www.ismp.org/resources/guidelines-safe-use-automated-dispensing-cabinets

Institute for Safe Medication Practices (ISMP) (2020). *ISMP Targeted Medication Safety Best Practices for Hospitals.* https://www.ismp.org/guidelines/best-practices-hospitals

Institute for Safe Medication Practices (ISMP) (2022a). *Prevent administration of ear drops into the eye.* https://www.ismp.org/resources/prevent- administration-ear-drops-eyes

Institute for Safe Medication Practices (ISMP) (2022b). *Preventing errors when preparing and administering medications via enteral feeding tubes.* https://www.ismp.org/resources/preventing-errors-when-preparing-and- administering-medications-enteral-feeding-tubes

Ishau, S., Reichard, J. F., Maier, A., Niang, M., Yermakov, M. & Grinshpun, S. A. (2020). Estimated dermal exposure to nebulized pharmaceuticals for a simulated home healthcare worker scenario. *Journal of Occupational and Environmental Hygiene, 17*(4), 193–205. https://search.proquest.com/docview/2384348225?accountid=88802

Ismail, A., El-Azeim, A. & Saif, H. (2023). Effect of aerobic exercise alone or combined with Mediterranean diet on dry eye in obese hypertensive elderly. *Irish Journal of Medical Science.* https://doi.org/10.1007/s11845-023-03387-6

Jamalinik, M., Hasheminik, M., Paivar, B., Khaleghipour, M., Khorashadizadeh, F., Bordbar, R., Lakziyan, R., Siavoshi, M. & Shafigh, N. (2023). Comparative study of the effect of lidocaine spray and ice spray on the pain intensity during intramuscular injection: A randomized clinical trial. *Pain Management Nursing, 24*(2), 229–34. https://doi.org/10.1016/j.pmn.2022.07.009

Jancy, J. (2019). Effect of cold needle on perception of pain during intra muscular injection. *Asian Journal of Nursing Education and Research, 9*(4), 483–7. https://doi.org/10.5958/2349-2996.2019.00101.0

Javidi, H., Nat, P., Patel, R., Barry, R., Rauz, S. & Murray, P. (2020). Adherence to topical medication in patients with inflammatory eye disease. *Ocular Immunology and Inflammation, 16*, 1–6. https://doi.org/10.1080/09273948.2019.1699122

Johnson, T. M., Whitman Webster, L. C., Mehta, M., Johnson, J. E., Cortés-Penfield, N. & Rivera, C. G. (2023). Pushing the agenda for intravenous push administration in outpatient parenteral antimicrobial therapy. *Therapeutic Advances in Infectious Disease, 10.* https://doi.org/10.1177/20499361231193920

Kacker, A., Fraser, M. & Pierce-Smith, D. (2022). Impacted earwax. Cedars-Sinai, The StayWell Company, LLC. https://www.cedars-sinai.org/health-library/diseases-and-conditions/i/impacted-earwax.html

Kaplan, A., Güler, S. & Avşaroğulları, Ö. L. (2023). Comparison of manual pressure and shotblocker on pain and satisfaction in intramuscular injection: A randomized controlled trial. *Sağlık Bilimleri Dergisi, 32*(1), 89–96. https://doi.org/10.34108/eujhs.1123965

Keogh, S., Flynn, J., Marsh, N., Mihala, G., Davies, K. & Rickard, C. (2016). Varied flushing frequency and volume to prevent peripheral intravenous catheter failure: A pilot, factorial randomised controlled trial in adult medical-surgical hospital patients. *Trials, 17*(1), 348. https://doi.org/10.1186/s13063-016-1470-6.

Keogh, S., Shelverton, C., Flynn, J., Mihala, G., Matthew, S., Davies, K., Marsh, N. & Rickard, C. (2020). Implementation and evaluation of short peripheral intravenous catheter flushing guidelines: A stepped wedge cluster randomised trial. *BioMedCentral Medicine, 18*, 252. https://doi.org/10.1186/s12916-020-01728-1

Kessemeier, N., Meyn, D., Hoeckel, M., Reitze, J., Culmsee, C. & Tryba, M. (2019). A new approach on assessing clinical pharmacists' impact on prescribing errors in a surgical intensive care unit. *International Journal of Clinical Pharmacy, 41*(5), 1184–92. https://doi.org/10.1007/s11096-019-00874-8

Kim, J. & de Jesus, O. (2021). *Medication routes of administration.* Treasure Island, FL: StatPearls Publishing. https://europepmc.org/article/MED/33760436/NBK556121#impact

Kollstedt, K., Fowler, S. B. & Weissman, K. (2019). Hospital nurses' perceptions about distractions to patient-centered care delivery. *Medsurg Nursing, 28*(4), 247–50. https://search.proquest.com/docview/2310240707?accountid=88802

Kumar, R., Mehta, P., Shankar, K. R., Rajora, M., Mishra, Y., Mostfav, E. & Kaushik, A. (2022). Nanotechnology-assisted metered-dose inhalers (MDIs) for high-performance pulmonary drug delivery applications. *Pharmaceutical Research, 39*, 2831–55. https://doi.org/10.1007/s11095-022-03286-y

Kunieda, K., Kurata, N., Yoshimatsu, Y., Ohno, T., Shigematsu, T. & Fujishima, I. (2022). A safe way to administer drugs through a nutrition tube: The simple suspension method. *Dysphagia, 37*. https://doi.org/10.1007/s00455-021- 10280-w

Larmené-Beld, K., Frijlink, H. & Taxis, K. (2019). A systematic review and meta-analysis of microbial contamination of parenteral medication prepared in a clinical versus pharmacy environment. *European Journal of Clinical Pharmacology, 75*, 609–17. https://doi.org/10.1007/s00228-019-02631-2

Lee, P. & Terry, J. (2021). Changing practice to using pre-filled syringes for flushing IV cannulas. *British Journal of Nursing, 30*(14), S14–S22. https://www.magonlinelibrary.com/action/showCitFormats?

Leppert, W., Malec-Milewska, M., Zajaczkowska, R. & Wordiczek, J. (2018). Transdermal and topical drug administration in the treatment of pain. *Molecules, 23*(3). https://doi.org/10.3390/molecules23030681

Linden-Lahti, C., Holmström, A., Pennanen, P. & Airaksinen, M. (2019). Facilitators and barriers in implementing medication safety practices across hospitals within 11 European Union countries. *Pharmacy Practice, 17*(4), 1583. https://search.proquest.com/docview/2385295384?accountid=88802

Lister, S., Hofland, J. & Grafton, H. (eds) (2020). *The Royal Marsden manual of clinical nursing procedures* (10th ed.). Oxford, UK: Wiley-Blackwell.

Mahmoud, R., Boshra, M., Haitham, S. & & Abdelrahim, M. (2023). The impact of the clip-tone training device and its smartphone application to pressurized metered-dose inhaler in adult asthmatics. *Journal of Asthma, 60*(2), 227–34. https://doi.org/10.1080/02770903.2022.2043359

Manzo, B. F., Brasil, C., Reis, F., Correa, A. d. R., Simao, D. A. d. S. & Costa, A. (2019). Safety in drug administration: Research on nursing practice and circumstances of errors. *Enfermería Global, 18*(4), 45–56. https://doi.org/10.6018/eglobal.18.4.344881

Márquez-Hernández, V. V., Fuentes-Colmenero, A. L., Cañadas-Núñez, F., Di Muzio, M., Giannetta, N. & Gutiérrez-Puertas, L. (2019). Factors related to medication errors in the preparation and administration of intravenous medication in the hospital environment. *PLOS ONE, 14*(7), e0220001. https://doi.org/10.1371/journal.pone.0220001

Martin, R. (2019). *Foam applicator for in-ear use.* Patent application. https://patents.google.com/patent/US20200061356A1/en

Martyn, J., Paliadelis, P. & Perry, C. (2019). The safe administration of medication: Nursing behaviours beyond the five-rights. *Nurse Education in Practice, 37*, 109–14. https://www.sciencedirect.com/science/article/pii/S1471595317308673

Mayo Clinic (2020a). *Metronidazole (vaginal route).* https://www.mayoclinic.org/drugs-supplements/metronidazole-vaginal-route/before-using/drg-20064738

Mayo Clinic (2020b). *Warfarin side effects: Watch for interactions.* https://www.mayoclinic.org/diseases-conditions/deep-vein-thrombosis/in- depth/warfarin-side-effects/art-20047592

Mayo Clinic (2022). *Warfarin diet: What foods should I avoid?* https://www.mayoclinic.org/diseases-conditions/thrombophlebitis/expert- answers/warfarin/faq-20058443

McAdoo, S. (2022). St. John's wort interactions you should know about. *GoodRX Health.* https://www.goodrx.com/well-being/supplements-herbs/st-johns-wort-interactions

McCormick, R., Robin, A. T., Gluch, J. & Lipman, T. H. (2019). Oral health assessment in acute care pediatric nursing. *Pediatric Nursing, 45*(6), 299–307, 309. https://search.proquest.com/docview/2328559361?accountid=88802

McLaughlin, K., Carabetta, S., Hunt, N., Schuler, B., Ting, C., Tran, L., Szumita, P. & Anger, K. (2021). Safety of intravenous push Lacosamide compared with Intravenous piggyback at a tertiary academic medical center. *Annals of Pharmacotherapy, 55*(2),181–6. https://doi.org/10.1177/1060028020943569

MIMS (2024). Online. https://www.mims.com.au

Mitchell, A. (2019). Administering suppositories: Types, considerations and procedure. *British Journal of Nursing, 28*(80). https://www.britishjournalofnursing.com/content/clinical/administering-a-suppository- types-considerations-and-procedure

Mulac, A., Hagesaether, E. & Granas, A. G. (2022). Medication dose calculation errors and other numeracy mishaps in hospitals: Analysis of the nature and enablers of incident reports. *Journal of Advanced Nursing, 78*, 224–38. https://doi.org/10.1111/jan.15072

Musafiri, J. J. & Daniels, F. (2020). Nursing students' perceptions of clinical learning opportunities and competence in administration of oral medication in the Western Cape. *Curationis, 43*(1). https://doi.org/10.4102/curationis.v43i1.2044

Nakajima, Y., Fujii, T., Mukai, K., Ishida, A., Kato, M., Takahashi, M., Tsuda, M., Hashiba, N., Mori, N., Yamanaka, A., Ozaki, N. & Nakatani, T. (2020). Anatomically safe sites for intramuscular injections: A cross-sectional study on young adults and cadavers with a focus on the thigh. *Human Vaccines & Immunotherapeutics, 16*(1), 189–96. https://doi.org/10.1080/21645515.2019.1646576

Nanno, F., Nell, M. J., Brand, R., Jansen-Werkhoven, T., van Hoogdalem, E. J., Verrijk, R., Vonk, P., Wafelman, Q., Valentijn, A., Frijns, J., Hiemstra, P., Drifthout, J., Nibberling, P. & Grote, J. J. (2020). Ototopical drops containing a novel antibacterial synthetic peptide: Safety and efficacy in adults with chronic suppurative otitis media. *PLOS ONE, 15*(4). https://doi.org/10.1371/journal.pone.0231573

National Asthma Council Australia (2020). *The asthma handbook.* https://www.nationalasthma.org.au/health-professionals/australian-asthma-handbook.

National Asthma Council Australia (2021). *How to use a metered dose inhaler.* https://www.nationalasthma.org.au/living-with-asthma/how-to-videos/how-to-use-mdi

National Library of Medicine (2016). *Drug record: Verapamil.* https://livertox.nlm.nih.gov/Verapamil.htm

New South Wales Health (2018). *Guideline: Workplace health and safety: Blood and body substances occupational exposure prevention.* NSW Health. https://www1.health.nsw.gov.au/pds/ActivePDSDocuments/GL2018_013.pdf

Palmer, D., Robin, A., McCabe, C. & Chang, D. for the Ophthalmic Instrument Cleaning and Sterilization Task Force (2022). Reducing topical drug waste in ophthalmic surgery: Multisociety position paper. *Journal of Cataract & Refractive Surgery, 48*(9), 1073–7. https://doi.org/10.1097/j.jcrs.0000000000000975

Paparella, S. (2019). IV push medication matters: New survey points to slow adoption of best practices. *Journal of Emergency Nursing, 45*(2), 202–5. https://doi.org/10.1016/j.jen.2018.12.011

Parker, R. (2020). Decreasing hospital transfers in skilled nursing: Utilizing a rectal administration catheter for fluid and medication delivery. *The Director: Official Journal of the National Association of Directors of Nursing Administration in Long Term Care, 28*(1). https://nadonathedirector.scholasticahq.com

Parriera, P., Sousa, L., Marques, I., Santos-Costa, P., Braga, L., Cruz, A. & Salgueiro-Oliveira, A. (2020). Double-chamber syringe versus classic syringes for peripheral intravenous drug administration and catheter flushing: A study protocol for a randomised controlled trial. *BioMed Central Trials.* https://doi.org/10.1186/s13063-019-3887-1

Perry, A., Potter, P. & Ostendorf, W. (2019). *Nursing interventions and clinical skills* (7th ed.). Philadelphia, PA: Elsevier.

Polania Gutierrez, J. J. & Munakomi, S. (2023). *Intramuscular injection.* Treasure Island, FL: StatPearls Publishing. https://www.ncbi.nlm.nih.gov/books/NBK556121

Qiao, J. (2023). Medication strategies for the elderly in dermatology. *Frontiers in Medical Science Research, 4*(9), 1–5. https://doi.org/10.25236/FMSR.2022.040901

Queensland Health (2016). *Prevention of needlestick injuries: Recommendations.* https://www.health.qld.gov.au/clinical-practice/guidelines-procedures/diseases-infection/infection-prevention/standard-precautions/sharps-safety/needle-stick-injuries

Rautela, M., Thomas, S. & Rita, P. D. (2020). A true experimental study to assess the effectiveness of Helfer skin tap technique on the level of pain during intramuscular injection of tetanus toxoid among antenatal mothers in a selected hospital of Delhi. *International Journal of Nursing Education, 12*(1), 46–50. https://doi.org/10.5958/0974-9357.2020.00010.0

Reed, P. (2022). Do eye drops expire? *Perry & Morgan Eyecare.* https://perryeyecare.com/do-eye-drops-expire

Ribeiro, G., Campos, J., Camerini, F., Parreira, P. & da Silva, R. (2023). Flushing in intravenous catheters: Observational study of nursing practice in intensive care in Brazil. *Journal of Infusion Nursing, 46*(5), 272–80. https://nursing.ceconnection.com/files/FlushinginIntravenousCatheters- 1694096100729.pdf

Rickard, C., Marsh, N., Webster, J., Gavin, N., McGrail, M., Larsen, E., Corley, A., Long, D., Gowardman, J., Murgo, M., Fraser, J., Chan, R., Wallis, M., Young, J., McMillan, D., Zhang, L., Choudhury, M., Graves, N. & Playford, E. (2015). Intravascular device administration sets: Replacement after standard versus prolonged use in hospitalised patients – a study protocol for a randomised controlled trial (the RSVP trial). *British Medical Journal Open, 5*(2). https://doi.org/10.1136/bmjopen-2014-007257

Rodríguez, R., Curado, M., Pastor, R. & Toribio, J. (2022). Mechanism cleaning of the ear canal. *Inventions, 7*(1), 20. https://doi.org/10.3390/inventions7010020

Rosana, A., Fabiana Bolela, d. S., Mayara Carvalho, G., Pereira, J. R., Laís Rosa Moreno, d. C. & Fernanda Raphael, E. (2020). Quality improvement programme reduces errors in oral medication preparation and administration through feeding tubes. *British Medical Journal Open, 9*(1). https://doi.org/10.1136/bmjoq-2019-000882

Royal Children's Hospital Melbourne (RCHM) (2022). *Peripheral intravenous device management. Clinical Guidelines, RCH.* https://www.rch.org.au/rchcpg/hospital_clinical_guideline_index/Peripheral_Intravenous_IV_Device_Management

Rull, G. (2016). *Eye drugs – prescribing and administering.* https://patient.info/doctor/eye-drugs-prescribing-and-administering

Sachi, M., Saburo, I., Jun, A. & Kazuyoshi, K. (2023). Drugs against metabolic diseases as potential senotherapeutics for aging-related respiratory diseases. *Frontiers in Endocrinology, 14.* https://www.frontiersin.org/articles/10.3389/fendo.2023.1079626

Safer Care Victoria (2019). *Otitis externa.* https://www.safercare.vic.gov.au/sites/default/files/2019-07/Otitis%20externa.pdf

Salama, R., Choi, H., Almazi, J., Traini, D. & Young, P. (2022). Generic dry powder inhalers bioequivalence: Batch–to-batch variability insights. *Drug Discovery Today, 27*(11). https://doi.org/10.1016/j.drudis.2022.103350

Salami, I., Subih, M., Darwish, R., Al-Jbarat, M., Saleh, Z., Maharmeh, M., Alasad, J. & Al-Amer, R. (2019). Medication administration errors: Perceptions of Jordanian nurses. *Journal of Nursing Care Quality, 34*(2), E7–E12. https://doi.org/10.1097/NCQ.0000000000000340

Sanchez, F., Mansberger, S., Kung, Y., Gardiner, S., Burgoyne, C., Jones, E. & Kinast, R. (2020). Novel eye drop delivery aid preferred over traditional eye drop delivery. *Investigative Ophthalmology and Visual Science, 61*(7), 2663. https://iovs.arvojournals.org/article.aspx?articleid=2769760

Şanlialp Zeyrek, A., Takmak, Ş., Kurban, N. K. & Arslan, S. (2019). Systematic review and meta-analysis: Physical-procedural interventions used to reduce pain during intramuscular injections in adults. *Journal of Advanced Nursing, 75,* 3346–61. https://doi.org/10.1111/jan.14183

Savio, R. D., Parasuraman, R., Lovesly, D., Shankar, B., Ranganathan, L., Ramakrishnan, N. & Venkataraman, R. (2020). Feasibility, tolerance and effectiveness of enteral feeding in critically ill patients in prone position. *Journal of the Intensive Care Society.* https://doi.org/10.1177/1751143719900100

Scott, E. (2020). *Process improvement to reduce route of medication administration errors in patients with enteral feeding tubes.* Doctoral Projects. 107. https://scholarworks.gvsu.edu/kcon_doctoralprojects/107

Sheikh, F. (2023). Celebrating cultural diversity and spirituality in long term care facilities. *Diversity, Equity and Inclusion, 14*(4), 14. https://doi.org/10.1016/j.carage.2023.04.007

Shitu, Z., Aung, M. M. T., Kamauzaman, T. H. T., Bhagat, V. & Rahman, A. F. A. (2019). Medication error in hospitals and effective intervention strategies: A systematic review. *Research Journal of Pharmacy and Technology, 12*(10), 4669–77. https://doi.org/10.5958/0974-360X.2019.00804.7

Shukla, M., Shukla, K. & Srivastava, H. (2023). A review on transdermal patches. *World Journal of Pharmacy and Pharmaceutical Sciences, 12*(9), 1250–61. https://www.researchgate.net/publication/371508617_A_Detailed_Review_On_Artificial_Intelligence_In_Pharmacy

Sotnikova, C., Fasoi, G., Efstathiou, F., Kaba, E., Bourazani, M. & Kelesi, M. (2020). The efficacy of normal saline (N/S 0.9%) versus heparin solution in maintaining patency of peripheral venous catheter and avoiding complications: A systematic review. *Materia Socio-Medica, 32*(1), 29–34. https://doi.org/10.5455/msm.2020.32.29-34

South Eastern Sydney Local Health District (SESLHD) (2022). *Guideline: Intramuscular injections in mental health.* https://www.seslhd.health.nsw.gov.au/sites/default/files/documents/SESLHDGL%20076%20-%20Intramuscular%20Injection%20in%20Mental%20Health.pdf

Stephanacci, R. (2022). Changes in the body with aging. *MSD Manual.* https://www.msdmanuals.com/en-au/home/older-people%E2%80%99s-health-issues/the-aging-body/changes-in-the-body-with-aging

Strohfus, P., Palma, S. & Wallace, C. T. (2021). Dorsogluteal intramuscular injection depth needed to reach muscle tissue according to body mass index and gender: A systematic review. *Journal of Clinical Nursing, 31*(5). https://doi.org/10.1111/jocn.16126

Sutherland, A., Canobbio, M., Clarke, J., Randall, M., Skelland, T. & Weston, E. (2020). Incidence and prevalence of intravenous medication errors in the UK: A systematic review. *European Journal of Hospital Pharmacy: Science and Practice, 27*(1), 3. https://doi.org/10.1136/ejhpharm-2018-001624

Takahashi, M., Iwasaki, S., Kawano, T., Ikoma, R., Oka, S., Terasaki, M., Sato, H., Kariya, S. & Takahashi, H. (2023). Efficacy and safety of 1.5% levofloxacin otic solution for the treatment of otitis media in a multicenter, randomized, double-blind, parallel-group, placebo-controlled, phase III study. *Auris Nasus Larynx, 50*(4), 521–33. https://doi.org/10.1016/j.anl.2022.12.013

Talha, M. (2023). Non-compliance. *Biological Times, 2*(6), 30–1. https://biologicaltimes.com

To, T-P., Brien, J-A. & Story, D. A. (2020). Barriers to managing medications appropriately when patients have restrictions on oral intake. *Journal of Evaluation in Clinical Practice, 26*, 172–80. https://doi.org/doi: 10.1111/jep.13139

Townsend, R. (2022). NSAIDs and acetomenophen : Effects on blood pressure and hypertension. https://www.uptodate.com/contents/nsaids- and-acetaminophen-effects-on-blood-pressure-and-hypertension

Tudball, J., Reddel, H., Laba, T., Jan, S., Flynn, A., Goldman, M., Lembke, K., Roughead, E., Marks, G. & Zwar, N. (2019). General practitioners' views on the influence of cost on the prescribing of asthma preventer medicines: A qualitative study. *Australian Health Review, 43*(3), 246–53. https://doi.org/10.1071/AH17030

Tverdohleb, T., Candido, K. D., & Knezevic, N. N. (2019). Topical medications. In A. Abd-Elsayed (ed.), *Pain.* Cham, Switzerland: Springer.

Usach, I., Martinez, R., Festini, T. & Peris, J. (2019). Subcutaneous injection of drugs: Literature review of factors influencing pain sensation at the injection site. *Advances in Therapy, 36*, 2986–96. https://doi.org/10.1007/s12325-019- 01101-6

Usami, O. (2022). Improved inhaler handling after repeated inhalation guidance for elderly patients with bronchial asthma and chronic obstructive pulmonary disease. *Medicine (Baltimore), 101*(35), e30238. https://doi.org/10.1097/MD.0000000000030238

Valentin, V. L. (2021). Injections. In R. Dehn & D. Asprey (eds), *Essential clinical procedures* (4th ed.). Philadelphia, PA: Elsevier.

Vera, M. (2023) Ten rights of drug administration. *NurseLabs: Fundamentals of Nursing.* https://nurseslabs.com/10-rs-rights-of-drug-administration

Vicdan, A., Birgili, F. & Baybuga, M. (2019). Evaluation of the training given to the nurses on the injection application to the ventrogluteal site: A quasi-experimental study. *International Journal of Caring Sciences, 12*(3), 1467–79. https://internationaljournalofcaringsciences.org/docs/17_vicdan_original_12_3%20(2).pdf

Vizzoni, L., Migone, C., Grassiri, B., Zambito, Y., Ferro, B., Roncucci, P., Mori, F., Salvatore, A., Ascione, E., Crea, R., Esin, S. & Prias, A. (2023). Biopharmaceutical assessment of mesh aerosolised plasminogen, a step towards ARDS treatment. *Pharmaceutics, 15*(6), 1618. https://doi.org/10.3390/pharmaceutics15061618

Walger, P. & Heppner, H. J. (2020). Calculated parenteral initial therapy of bacterial infections: Antibiotic treatment in the elderly. *GMS Infectious Diseases, 26*(8), Doc05. https://doi.org/10.3205/id000049

Wang, C., Lodhia, N. & Chan, W. (2021). Obesity is an independent risk factor for fecal incontinence, rectal hyposensitivity and worse health related quality of life. *American Journal of Gastroenterology, 116*, S580. https://doi.org/10.14309/01.ajg.0000778568.48389.2d

White, R. & Bradnam, V. (2017). *Handbook of drug administration via enteral feeding tubes* (3rd ed.). British Pharmaceutical Nutrition Group. London: Pharmaceutical Press. https://rudiapt.files.wordpress.com/2017/11/handbook-of-drug-administration-via-enteral-feeding-tubes-2015.pdf

White, S., Goodwin, J. & Behan, L. (2018). Nurses' use of appropriate needle sizes when administering intramuscular injections. *Journal of Continuing Education in Nursing, 49*(11), 519–25. https://doi.org/10.3928/00220124-20181017-09

World Health Organization (WHO) (2023). *Primary ear and hearing care training manual.* Geneva: World Health Organization. https://apps.who.int/iris/bitstream/handle/10665/366334/9789240069152-eng.pdf? sequence=1&isAllowed=y

Wright, D., Smithard, D. & Griffith, R. (2020). Optimising medicines administration for patients with dysphagia in hospital: Medical or nursing responsibility? *Geriatrics, 5*(1), 9. https://doi.org/10.3390/geriatrics5010009

Yang, J. R., Hidayat, K., Chen, C. L., Li, Y. H., Xu, J. Y. & Qin, L. Q. (2020). Body mass index, waist circumference, and risk of hearing loss: A meta-analysis and systematic review of observational study. *Environmental Health and Preventative Medicine, 25*, 25. https://doi.org/10.1186/s12199-020-00862-9

Yılmaz, D., Düzgün, F., Durmaz, H., Çinar, H. G., Dikmen, Y. & Kara, H. (2020). The effect of duration of pressure on bruising and pain in the subcutaneous heparin injection site. *Japanese Journal of Nursing Science*, e12325. https://doi.org/10.1111/jjns.12325

Yilmaz, O. F., Sarmis, A., Mutlu, M. A., Ersoy, E., Askarova, U. & Oguz, H. (2023). Bacterial contamination of multi-use antibiotic steroid eye ointments and drops. *Graefe's Archive for Clinical and Experimental Ophthalmology, 261*, 1691–700. https://doi.org/10.1007/s00417-023-05977-7

Zhao, L., Song, J., Du, Y., Ren, C., Guo, B. & Bi, H. (2023). Therapeutic applications of contact lens-based drug delivery systems in ophthalmic diseases. *Drug Delivery, 30*(1). https://doi.org/10.1080/10717544.2023.2219419

Zheng, W., Lichtner, V., Van Dort, B. & Baysari, M. (2021). The impact of introducing automated dispensing cabinets, barcode medication administration, and closed-loop electronic medication management systems on work processes and safety of controlled medications in hospitals: A systematic review. *Research in Social and Administrative Pharmacy, 17*(5), 832–41. https://www.sciencedirect.com/science/article/pii/S155174112030406X

Zhu, L., Liu, H., Wang, R., Yu, Y., Zheng, F. & Yin, J. (2020). Mechanism of pulsatile flushing technique for saline injection via a peripheral intravenous catheter. *Clinical Biomechanics, 80*, 105103. https://doi.org/10.1016/j.clinbiomech.2020.105103

PART 8

PAIN MANAGEMENT

49 NON-PHARMACOLOGICAL PAIN MANAGEMENT INTERVENTION – DRY HEAT AND COLD THERAPY

50 PATIENT-CONTROLLED ANALGESIA AND OTHER SYRINGE-DRIVEN MEDICATION

51 SUBCUTANEOUS INFUSIONS

Note: These notes are summaries of the most important points in the assessments/procedures and are not exhaustive on the subject. References of the materials used to compile the information have been supplied. The student is expected to have learnt the material surrounding each skill as presented in the references. No single reference is complete on each subject.

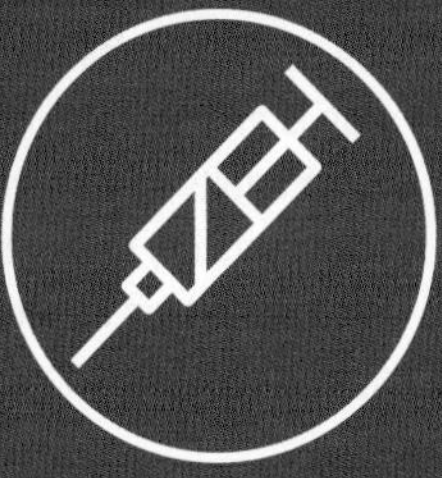

CHAPTER 49

NON-PHARMACOLOGICAL PAIN MANAGEMENT INTERVENTION – DRY HEAT AND COLD THERAPY

INDICATIONS

Thermotherapy is a group of complementary therapies that include localised applications of heat or cold packs to relieve pain through sensory and cutaneous stimulation (Mann, 2016). Many people find thermotherapy has beneficial effects on alleviating pain, muscle spasms and inflammation, and improving circulation (Porritt, 2022). Thermotherapy also includes superficial moist heat fomentations (hot packs), cryotherapy (ice packs), warm paraffin wax and infrared therapy, and faradic baths (Slade, 2023).

Localised heat therapy application

Heat therapy increases tissue temperature and local blood circulation and encourages the rapid removal of inflammatory metabolic products (e.g. prostaglandin, bradykinin and histamine), alleviating pain and promoting healing (Shim, 2014). Heat therapy is categorised as superficial heat therapy or deep heat therapy. Superficial heat, which produces effects to a depth of 1 to 2 cm, has been shown to reduce muscle spasm and pain in people with lower back pain (Picot, 2020).

Localised cold therapy application

Cold therapy (or cryotherapy) involves the application of very low temperatures to the skin surrounding an injury or surgical site (Valdez, 2024). Cold therapy promotes vasoconstriction, which diminishes bleeding; reduces inflammatory processes, cellular metabolism, pain and oedema; and is a useful non-pharmacological intervention for postoperative pain and oedema (Khoshnevis, Craik & Diller, 2015; Valdez, 2024; Watkins et al., 2014). It provokes immediate cutaneous vasoconstriction and diminishes nerve conductivity, which reduces oedema and decreases pain sensations. Cold therapy initially causes hyperaesthesia in the area it is applied; later, numbness and paraesthesia.

Pain assessment

The initial pain assessment (see **Clinical Skill 13**) determines the person's suitability and preference for heat or cold therapy. Age is an important consideration because the very young and older adults tolerate heat poorly. The level of consciousness, neurosensory impairment and degree of debility need to be established, as the person must be capable of recognising and appropriately responding to excessive heat or cold.

Determine the area to be treated and assess skin integrity, as broken skin increases sensitivity to heat and cold (Mann, 2016). Altered circulation (e.g. in people with heart failure, diabetes mellitus or peripheral vascular diseases) reduces circulatory function and heat cannot be dissipated, resulting in local tissue damage. Cold is contraindicated because of vasoconstriction.

Contraindications

Contraindications for heat therapy are:

- a *traumatic injury* (within the first 24 hours) – vasodilatation increases bleeding and oedema
- *active haemorrhage* (or suspected, i.e. internal) or *recent surgery*, because of vasodilatation
- *non-inflammatory oedema* – heat increases capillary permeability
- *acute inflammation* (e.g. appendicitis) – because of increased oedema
- *a localised malignant tumour* – heat accelerates cell metabolism and cell growth and increases circulation – it may accelerate metastasis
- *pregnancy* – heat to the abdomen of a pregnant woman can cause mutation in the foetal germinal cells and affect foetal growth
- *skin disorders* – heat can further damage compromised skin
- *metallic implants* (e.g. pacemaker, joint replacements) – metal is an excellent heat conductor; some heat applications are contraindicated (e.g. diathermy) while others must be used cautiously.

Contraindications for cold therapy are:

- *open wounds* – cold decreases blood supply to the area and could cause tissue damage or delayed healing
- *impaired circulation* – vasoconstriction further impairs nourishment of the tissues; people with Raynaud's disease will have increased arterial spasms
- *cold allergy* or *hypersensitivity* – could result in hives, erythema, muscle spasm, joint stiffness or severe hypertension
- *shivering* – causes increased metabolic rate and a raised temperature.

EVIDENCE OF THERAPEUTIC INTERACTION

Explain to the person what to expect from the procedure; this helps them to relax and maximises the procedure's effect. It also helps gain the person's cooperation and increases trust, and so reduces the time required to initiate the procedure. You should outline the preparation (i.e. skin inspection, pain assessment and application of heat/cold therapy) and indication – that is, that heat/cold may or may not completely eliminate the pain, but it will modify the pain so the person can rest or carry out normal activities of daily living. Also provide a brief explanation of the theory behind the treatment's use.

DEMONSTRATE CLINICAL REASONING

Explain the procedure to the person and gain their consent. Focus on the person's comfort. Conduct an appropriate assessment to determine the person's needs and any contraindications or precautions. Test the affected area for heat sensitivity. You must ascertain the person's pain level and decide with them if they require analgesic pain relief to augment this therapy to increase their comfort levels. Other comfort measures need attention as well. Ask the person if they need to use the toilet and assist them if necessary. Position the person in anatomical alignment, ensuring that the affected area is adequately supported. Attend to associated symptoms, such as nausea, and provision of privacy. Each situation is individual, and holistic nursing care encompasses a broad range of comfort measures.

ADMINISTER HEAT OR COLD THERAPY

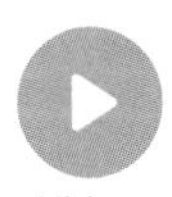

Video

Hand hygiene

Hand hygiene (see **Clinical Skill 5**) removes microorganisms from your hands. It is the most effective preventative measure for cross-contamination, reducing incidences of healthcare-associated infections (HCAIs).

Administer heat therapy

Prepare the hot pack

Preheat the pack according to the manufacturer's instructions. These are generally warmed in hot water or a microwave (clinical; not the kitchen microwave unless provision is made to keep the pack clean). Dry the pack's surface, because moisture conducts heat quickly enough to cause a burn or tissue damage. The temperature must be checked prior to application.

If using a commercially prepared chemical hot pack, follow the manufacturer's instructions for use.

Wrap the pack in a protective cover

Wrap the pack in six to eight layers of towels to increase the person's comfort and safety, and adjust as necessary (Picot, 2020).

Position the person into a comfortable position, only exposing the affected area, and inspect the skin (Slade, 2023). Apply the hot pack with cover in situ on the body part; if the affected area is on a limb, secure the pack in place with a cling-wrap bandage.

The stimulation of thermal receptors declines rapidly in the initial period of treatment. As the tissue adapts to new temperatures, the person might feel that the treatment is ineffective and may request (or get for themselves) hotter packs. However, serious burns or impaired circulation can result if the correct temperatures are not adhered to. For adults who are conscious and not debilitated, the temperature should be 52 °C; for unconscious or debilitated adults or for young children, the temperature should be 46 °C (Foottit, 2021).

Safety

If there is any doubt about the person's safety, you must stay with the person for the therapy's duration (Mann, 2016).

GATHER EQUIPMENT

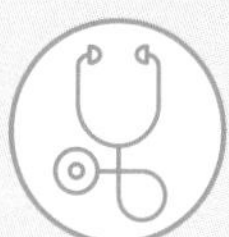

Gathering equipment is an organisational step that helps to create a positive environment for a successful interaction and reduces the person's discomfort and embarrassment. It ensures that you have all needed material, boosts the person's confidence and trust in you, and increases your self-confidence. Equipment required includes:

EQUIPMENT	EXPLANATION
Hot pack	• Used for heat therapy • Warmed in hot water or a microwave • Commercially prepared chemical hot packs are available. These are reusable, provide a consistent heat for a long period of time and are easily 'triggered' to produce a safe level of heat by chemical reaction
Commercial cold pack; or ice chips, a plastic bag and rubber bands	• Used for cold therapy • Usually kept in a refrigerator or freezer • Ice chips can be added to a plastic bag and secured with a rubber band if a commercial cold pack is not available
Towel	• Used in both hot and cold therapy to provide a protective cover (or as per facility's guidelines)
Cling-wrap (or similar) bandage	• Used in both hot and cold therapy to keep the pack in position on a limb

Observe the person's skin. Cease treatment immediately if the person reports any irritation, discomfort or burning sensations; excessive redness and swelling indicate the heat treatment should be stopped (Slade, 2023). Hot packs are generally applied for either 20 minutes, as long as the person desires, or until the hot pack cools (Picot, 2020).

Cold therapy

Prepare the cold or ice pack

Cold packs are usually kept in a refrigerator or freezer. Cool the pack or fill the bag two-thirds full of ice. Fill ice packs to about two-thirds capacity with chips rather than cubes of ice and expel the air from the pack so that the pack more easily conforms to the body part being treated. Firmly secure the stopper or seal with rubber bands to prevent leakage of cold liquid.

Wrap the pack in a protective cover

Wrap the pack in two layers of towel to increase the person's comfort, and safety and adjust as necessary (Picot, 2020). Dry the pack's surface, as moisture conducts cold quickly enough to cause tissue damage.

Position the person comfortably, only exposing the affected part, and inspect the skin (Slade, 2023). Mould the cold pack or bag to the shape of the affected part and apply the covered pack. If positioning the pack on a limb, secure it in place with a cling-wrap bandage.

A person may feel the treatment is ineffective and request, or get for themselves, colder packs. However, serious burns or impaired circulation may result if the correct temperatures are not adhered to. For adults who are conscious and not debilitated, the temperature should be 15 °C; for unconscious or debilitated adults or for young people, the temperature should be 18 °C (Foottit, 2021). Certain body areas are more sensitive to cold; for example, the axillae, the neck and the perineal area. Take care that a pack intended for these areas has a more moderate temperature.

Remove the pack after five to 10 minutes, or earlier if not tolerated (Picot, 2020). Pallor and mottled skin are considered a reaction to a cold application. Reapply the cold pack once the area has returned to normal temperature (Picot, 2020). Reassess by asking the person if the area feels improved.

Monitor the treatment site

Safety

Assess the person's comfort level and skin condition five minutes after applying the treatment. Monitoring may be necessary as often as every five to 10 minutes, depending on the person's ability to report ill effects or their previous response to the treatment.

Assess the pain

Use a pain assessment tool to determine the effectiveness of the intervention. Assess the skin underlying the application following the treatment.

Post-procedure

Perform hand hygiene. Assist the person to a comfortable position. Replace the call bell and anything that was moved during treatment so that it is within reach.

CLEAN, REPLACE AND DISPOSE OF EQUIPMENT

Replacing the equipment is a time-management strategy and a courtesy to colleagues. Remove and discard any disposable items. To reduce cross-contamination, clean the pack as per the manufacturer's guidelines or the protocols of the facility and return it to storage (return cold packs to the refrigerator or freezer). Follow the facility's guidelines regarding pack reuse.

DOCUMENTATION

Include a notation of the time, date, the type of treatment, the location of treatment and its effectiveness. Report any adverse reactions to the team leader.

CLINICAL SKILLS ASSESSMENT

Non-pharmacological pain management intervention – dry heat and cold therapy

Demonstrates the ability to effectively and safely assess and provide heat or cold therapy. Incorporates the *National Safety and Quality Health Service Standards*: 2 Partnering with Consumers, 3 Preventing and Controlling Healthcare-Associated Infection, 5 Comprehensive Care, and 6 Communicating for Safety (Australian Commission on Safety and Quality in Health Care [ACSQHC], 2021).

Performance criteria	1	2	3	4	5
(Numbers indicate NMBA *Registered Nurse Standards for Practice*)	**(Dependent)**	**(Marginal)**	**(Assisted)**	**(Supervised)**	**(Independent)**
1. Identifies indication (1.1, 3.3, 3.4, 4.1)	☐	☐	☐	☐	☐
2. Verifies there are no contraindications (1.4, 1.5, 2.1, 2.2, 3.2)	☐	☐	☐	☐	☐
3. Evidence of therapeutic interaction with the person, e.g. gives the person a clear explanation of the procedure and gains consent (1.4, 1.5, 2.1, 2.2, 3.2)	☐	☐	☐	☐	☐
4. Demonstrates clinical reasoning abilities, e.g. provides privacy, comfort measures and pharmacological pain relief as ordered (1.1, 1.2, 1.3, 2.3, 4.2, 6.1)	☐	☐	☐	☐	☐
5. Gathers equipment (1.1, 5.5, 6.1): ■ hot pack ■ commercial cold pack; or ice chips, a plastic bag and rubber bands ■ towel ■ cling-wrap (or similar) bandage	☐	☐	☐	☐	☐
6. Performs hand hygiene (1.1, 3.4, 6.1), i.e. on entering the person's room; prior to donning gloves to apply hot or cold packs; on procedure completion; following glove removal; and on leaving the person's bed area	☐	☐	☐	☐	☐
7. Prepares the hot or cold pack according to the manufacturer's directions (1.1, 6.1)	☐	☐	☐	☐	☐
8. Wraps the pack in a protective cover (1.1, 6.1)	☐	☐	☐	☐	☐
9. Places the covered pack on the treatment site and secures with cling wrap as necessary (1.1, 6.1)	☐	☐	☐	☐	☐
10. Times the treatment (1.1, 6.1)	☐	☐	☐	☐	☐
11. Assesses the treatment site after five minutes for adverse effects (1.1, 4.2, 6.1)	☐	☐	☐	☐	☐
12. Completes the prescribed treatment and assesses the person's pain (1.1, 1.2, 1.3, 2.3, 4.1, 4.2, 4.3, 6.1)	☐	☐	☐	☐	☐
13. Assists the person to reposition themselves, replaces the call bell and anything moved during procedure to within reach (2.1, 2.2, 4.1, 4.2, 4.3, 6.1)	☐	☐	☐	☐	☐
14. Cleans, replaces and disposes of equipment appropriately (3.6. 6.1)	☐	☐	☐	☐	☐
15. Documents relevant information and reports adverse reactions to the team leader (1.1, 1.4, 1.6, 2.2, 2.7, 3.5, 3.7, 6.1, 6.2, 6.5, 7.3)	☐	☐	☐	☐	☐
16. Demonstrates the ability to link theory to practice (1.1, 3.3, 3.4, 3.5)	☐	☐	☐	☐	☐

Student:

Clinical facilitator: Date:

CHAPTER 50

PATIENT-CONTROLLED ANALGESIA AND OTHER SYRINGE-DRIVEN MEDICATION

INDICATIONS

This Clinical Skill outlines advanced skills that are usually undertaken by second- or third-year students. Direct supervision by a registered nurse (RN) with the required training is required.

Patient-controlled analgesia (PCA) is one aspect of a multimodal approach to pain management that combines analgesics, opioids, adjuvants and regional techniques (Sharma, 2023). PCA is a pain-control method using electronic or disposable infusion devices allowing people to titrate their analgesia to achieve an acceptable level of pain control (Sharma, 2023). PCA is used to manage all types of pain, most commonly acute postoperative pain (see FIGURE 50.1). PCA is usually administered intravenously (IV); however, it may also be given subcutaneously (SC), via the epidural or intrathecal space or regional analgesia (Moola, 2022; Sharma, 2023).

The PCA approach to pain management recognises that only the person can feel the pain and only the person knows how much analgesia will relieve it (Pasero & McCaffery, 2011). PCA is an alternative, safer method for giving IV opioids (usually morphine or fentanyl) in the ward environment. It provides better pain control and greater patient satisfaction than conventional parenteral analgesia (Magtoto, 2022; Moola, 2022). The advantages of PCA over conventional opioid analgesia (intramuscular [IM], SC or IV) administration include that it:

- enables the person to receive relief without delay – they do not need to ask an RN or wait while an RN prepares analgesia
- results in better pain relief by avoiding unwanted peaks and the leading opioid-related adverse effects (sedation, nausea or vomiting)
- avoids pain associated with troughs associated with larger single-dose IM or SC injections
- is able to maintain opioid blood concentrations within the therapeutic range
- increases the person's sense of control postoperatively
- provides prompt management of pain caused by procedures (e.g. physiotherapy, movement, dressing changes)
- decreases the risk of pulmonary complications
- increases mobility (Moola, 2022; Ortega-Arroyo, 2021).

PCA is similar to responsive PRN (pro re nata) dosing in that it requires the person to recognise they are experiencing pain. However, the difference between PCA and PRN dosing is that with PCA the person rather than an RN administers the analgesia (Pasero & McCaffery, 2011).

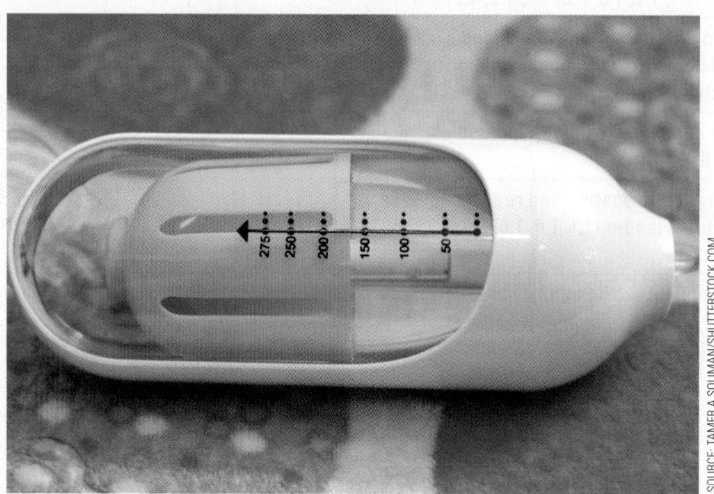

FIGURE 50.1 PCA infusion pump

PCA machines can be pre-programmed to operate in the following three modes:

- *PCA mode only* (demand dose only) – the person receives analgesia only when the PCA demand button is pushed.
- *Continuous (background) infusion* – the person receives a continuous dose of analgesia.
- *Continuous (background) infusion with additional demand analgesia* – the person receives a prescribed continuous dose of analgesia with additional bolus doses on demand (Ortega-Arroyo, 2021).

Patient-controlled epidural analgesia

The patient-controlled epidural analgesia (PCEA) is used in postoperative clinical areas, providing superior efficiency and a lower analgesic dose requirement compared to IV PCAs (Minooee, 2021; Moola, 2022; Ortega-Arroyo, 2021). A PCEA allows the person to initiate epidural doses of opioid, local anaesthetic (LA) or a combination of both. Low LA (e.g. bupivacaine) concentrations block nerve impulses in the smallest diameter of nerve fibres, which include the pain and temperature sensory fibres. The goal of adding low-dose LA to epidural opioids is to provide analgesia and not produce anaesthesia, which allows the person to mobilise if their condition permits (Pasero & McCaffery, 2011).

Morphine is water-soluble and penetrates the dura slowly, giving it a longer onset and duration of action. Fentanyl is lipid soluble and is readily taken up into the systemic circulation, reducing the duration of action (Pasero & McCaffery, 2011). Continuous infusion facilitates prompt dosage adjustment on the basis of the person's response, avoiding the peaks and troughs associated with bolus doses (Moola, 2022; Ortega-Arroyo, 2021).

An epidural catheter is placed into the epidural space to provide pain relief to the abdomen, thorax and lower extremities by enabling medication administration. This decreases the possibility of the adverse effects associated with systemic opioid administration.

If you are assisting with epidural catheter placement (or if you are involved in the ongoing care of a person with PCEA), you must be familiar with the nervous system anatomy. Specifically, the epidural space, as a potential space between the dura mater and the vertebral canal, must be understood.

The epidural space is a 'potential space' filled with vasculature, fat and a network of nerve extensions. There is no free-flowing fluid in the epidural space; a true space is created when fluid or air is injected into it (Tortora & Derrickson, 2020). Opioid diffusion through the dura into the cerebrospinal fluid and then into the spinal cord directly to the site of analgesic action (i.e. receptors in the dorsal horn of the spinal cord) leads to direct regional analgesia, eliminating many opioid systemic adverse effects with minimal effect on motor or sympathetic function (Wagner et al., 2019).

Indications for epidural analgesia include the following:

- pain management after thoracic, major abdominal or lower limb surgery, and elective amputation of a lower limb to prevent or reduce phantom pain (Prabhakar et al., 2014)
- oncologic pain below the T4 dermatome (nipple line) when systemic analgesic routes are no longer an option because of unmanageable and intolerable adverse effects at the anticipated dosages required to achieve adequate analgesia (e.g. sedation/respiratory depression) (Lister, Hofland & Grafton, 2020)
- management of chronic intractable pain in people who experience unacceptable systemic opioid adverse effects, were unsuccessful with treatments of opioids via other routes, or with severe neuropathic pain due to tumour invasion or nerve compression (Lister, Hofland & Grafton, 2020).

Opioids and LA are used as a bolus dose with a designated lockout period, either alone or in conjunction with a continuous background infusion (Magtoto, 2022). PCA is programmed to the person's characteristics, their baseline pain and the type of analgesia prescribed.

Epidural catheter placement and ongoing medical direction is done by those trained and skilled in anaesthesiology. In large regional and metropolitan hospitals, acute pain management teams (e.g. anaesthetists and pain management RNs) are generally available around the clock to facilitate assessment and infusion titration, and to manage complications. The anaesthetist orders the medication, the dose and the delivery method (e.g. intermittent or continuous, lockout time) of the PCA analgesic administration.

Verify the written medication order

A valid, signed order from a qualified healthcare provider is a requirement for legal administration of a medication. A valid order consists of the person's name, hospital or unit record number, date of birth, sex; allergy information; medication/s to be used; initial loading; bolus or incremental dose; dose duration; continuous (background) infusion; lockout duration; medical officer's name and signature; management of possible complications and their management (Moola, 2022). This is usually reviewed daily by the acute pain management team to ensure the person's pain is being well controlled. The correctly completed medication administration sheet is required to identify the person, ensuring the correct medication, dose, time and route is given to the correct person.

You are responsible and accountable for questioning and clarifying any order that is unclear or incomplete, or that seems inappropriate or unreasonable for the person (e.g. a very high dose, the same medication with two different names). Potentially harmful prescribing errors often go undetected (Lister, Hofland & Grafton, 2020). Nurses are responsible (along with the medical officer) if an inappropriate order is followed. To question an order, you *must know* the person's diagnosis, the purpose of the medication, its therapeutic effect, any adverse or toxic effects and the usual dose. You must anticipate any pertinent nursing implications (e.g. dose and delivery method) as well as individual factors that mediate response to medications (e.g. age, weight, renal function). Be aware of any medications or food allergies the person has so potentially harmful substances are not administered.

EVIDENCE OF THERAPEUTIC INTERACTION

Give the person a clear explanation of the procedure. Many people are apprehensive about controlling their pain by using the PCA machine. Teaching the person how the PCA works, what it does, and how to manipulate the pump to control their pain alleviates their anxiety. Stay with the person while they initiate their own treatment, demonstrating they can manage the PCA.

Discuss adverse effects common to the medication/s administered and epidural analgesia. Ask the person to alert nurses to any changes they note during PCA administration. Assess all the person's concerns. Just because an adverse reaction is unusual or unexpected, do not ignore it – it needs exploration. This develops the person's trust in the nursing staff.

DEMONSTRATE CLINICAL REASONING

Patient-controlled analgesia

Assessments prior to PCA consist of baseline vital signs, medication allergies, pain level (see **Clinical Skill 13**) and the person's general condition. The IV site is assessed for inflammation, infiltration, thrombus or phlebitis of the insertion site or the vein.

The medication is assessed for compatibility with the infusing fluid; its recommended dosage, action and adverse effects; the recommended lockout time; and its peak action time. Programming a lockout time or a delay between patient-initiated doses reduces the possibility of the person overdosing (Magtoto, 2022).

PCA is not for everyone. A 'suitable' person is anyone who is happy to take some control over their pain relief, wants to use PCA, and can understand how to use it (Magtoto, 2022). Cognitive assessment is made to determine the person's ability to understand the concept of self-administration and comply with the instructions to use the PCA (Pasero & McCaffery, 2011). Additionally, the person must have the physical ability to manipulate the dose button (Pasero & McCaffery, 2011).

Although the very young and very old may be less likely to successfully manage PCA, it should not be withheld for these reasons. Many children as young as four have coped well with PCA (Slade, 2021). People with language barriers should not automatically be excluded – translators can interpret verbal instructions, and written instructions can be translated into the person's language. A person who becomes confused postoperatively may need to have their PCA discontinued and alternative pain management implemented (Pasero & McCaffery, 2011).

If an opioid is administered, monitor the person for central nervous system depression (e.g. excessive sedation, respiratory depression, apnoea). Reports of nausea and vomiting result from opioid action on the vomiting centre in the brainstem and stimulation of the chemoreceptor trigger zone in the fourth ventricle of the brain. Prophylactic anti-emetics are often used during PCA administration and are recommended to reduce the incidence of nausea and vomiting (Sharma, 2023). Consult with your team leader and medical staff if the person reports nausea or is vomiting, so an effective anti-emetic can be administered.

Patient-controlled epidural analgesia

Additional contraindications for PCEA include people with coagulation disorders, which may cause haematoma formation and spinal cord compression; local sepsis at the proposed epidural injection site, which could lead to meningitis or epidural abscess formation; unstable spinal fracture and people with increased intracranial pressure, who are at risk of herniation if a dural tap occurs (Pasero & McCaffery, 2011).

Vigilance is required when assessing the epidural site to identify clinical manifestations and provide immediate management for the following rare, serious complications:

- infection of the site and epidural space, including epidural abscess
- bleeding into the epidural space, including epidural haematoma
- LA adverse effects such as motor blockade, hypotension and urinary retention (if a urinary indwelling catheter is not in situ).

If the PCA/PCEA pump has been in use for a while, check the battery levels to avoid flat batteries interrupting the administration of medication.

You must understand the pharmacology of the epidural analgesia medication/s, including adverse effects and duration of action. It is also essential that you understand the clinical manifestations of profound motor and sensory blockade or overmedication and the appropriate nursing management of these.

GATHER EQUIPMENT

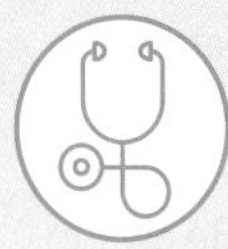

Gathering equipment is an organisational step that helps to create a positive environment for a successful interaction and reduces the person's discomfort and embarrassment. It ensures that you have all needed material, boosts the person's confidence and trust in you, and increases your self-confidence. It also prevents distractions once you have started preparing the medication, which will reduce errors. Equipment required includes:

EQUIPMENT	EXPLANATION
Medication administration sheet	• Determines the medication and dosage required • Includes the person's name, hospital/unit record number, date of birth, sex; allergies; medication/s to be used; initial loading; bolus/incremental dose; dose duration; continuous infusion; lockout duration; medical officer's name and signature; possible complications and their management
Required medication	• To be obtained from stock • Some facilities have pharmacy-prepared medication for PCA. Others require RNs to prepare the PCA syringe • If it needs to be reconstituted, the sterile diluent recommended for the medication and the route of administration are required • Medications are diluted to an ordered concentration, usually with normal saline *For PCEA:* Ensure all medications and diluents are preservative-free
Sterile Luer Lock (interlock) syringe	• If prepared by RN: usually 60 mL, depending on type of syringe driver • Pharmacy-prepared medication will come in a prefilled syringe
Sterile needle +/– filter	Used to draw up medication and diluent as per facility's guidelines
PCA/PCEA pump	An electronically controlled infusion pump delivering intravenous or epidural analgesia when the person presses the button
Syringe driver	• An electrical or battery-operated pump device (sometimes delivering a small amount of medication continuously) with the capacity to deliver small bolus doses of the medication on demand, but with a minimum time (lockout time) between bolus doses • Most are fitted with a key or have an access code to ensure the medication remains secure once placed in the machine. The RN in charge has the key • Various pump types are available – familiarise yourself with those used in the facility in which you are working
Syringe driver extension tubing	• A fine short IV line connecting the syringe in the syringe driver with the existing IV line or epidural access via a needleless Luer Lock device • For a PCEA, a bacterial filter is required
One-way anti-reflux and anti-siphon valves	• Anti-reflux valves prevent opioid backing up into the primary IV line if the IV cannula becomes occluded • An anti-siphon valve placed between the syringe and the person prevents emptying of the syringe by gravity if it is above the person and not correctly fixed in the machine, or if an air leak develops due to a cracked syringe
Medication label	• To adhere to the National standard for user-applied labelling of injectable medicines, fluids and lines a specifically colour-coded adhesive-backed paper (see **FIGURES 50.2** and **50.3**) containing information about the person, the medication amount, volume, concentration, diluent, preparation date and time; who prepared and checked, and the administration route is required to be completed prior to adhering to the medication syringe (Australian Commission on Safety and Quality in Health Care [ACSQHC], 2015) • Medication label is placed so graduations on the syringe scale remain visible • Apply the completed label parallel to the long axis of the syringe barrel, top edge flush with scale (ACSQHC, 2015). • Dedicated continuous infusion lines such as PCEA and PCA infusion require two labels – one for medication (see **FIGURES 50.2** and **50.3**) and one for the line (see **FIGURE 50.4**)
Alcowipes	Used to cleanse and disinfect the tops of vials and the latex seal on the medication access port of the IV line
Injection tray	Used for transporting the medications, syringes and alcowipes to the bedside
Sharps container	Taken to the bedside so that used needles, glass ampoules and vials can be immediately disposed of, to reduce the chance of needle-stick injuries
Clean gloves	Used to comply with standard precautions

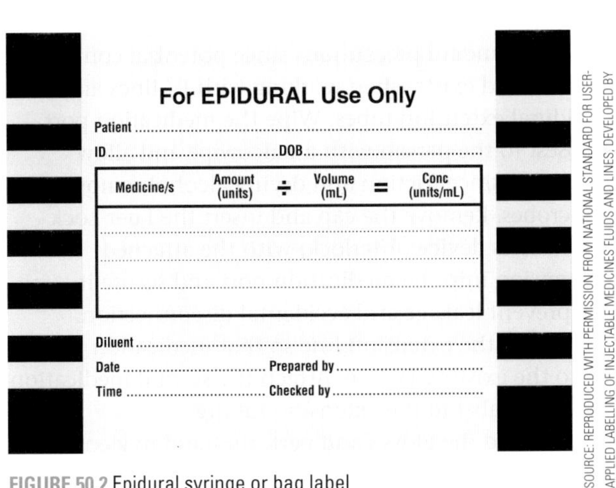

For EPIDURAL Use Only

Patient ....

ID .... DOB ....

Medicine/s	Amount (units)	÷	Volume (mL)	=	Conc (units/mL)

Diluent ....

Date .... Prepared by ....

Time .... Checked by ....

FIGURE 50.2 Epidural syringe or bag label

SOURCE: REPRODUCED WITH PERMISSION FROM NATIONAL STANDARD FOR USER-APPLIED LABELLING OF INJECTABLE MEDICINES FLUIDS AND LINES, DEVELOPED BY THE AUSTRALIAN COMMISSION ON SAFETY AND QUALITY IN HEALTH CARE (ACSQHC). ACSQHC: SYDNEY 2015.

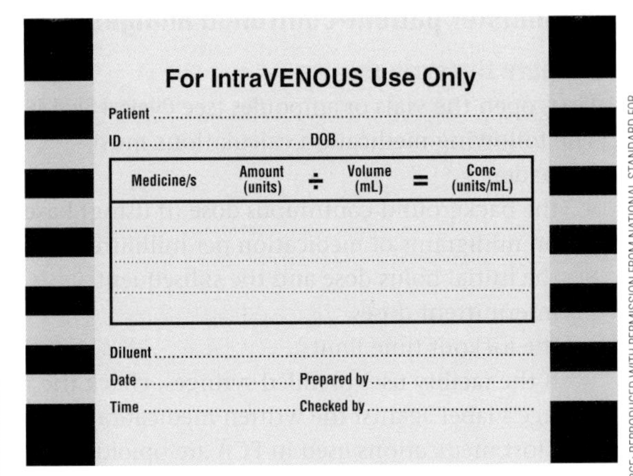

For IntraVENOUS Use Only

Patient ....

ID .... DOB ....

Medicine/s	Amount (units)	÷	Volume (mL)	=	Conc (units/mL)

Diluent ....

Date .... Prepared by ....

Time .... Checked by ....

FIGURE 50.3 Intravenous syringe or bag label

SOURCE: REPRODUCED WITH PERMISSION FROM NATIONAL STANDARD FOR USER-APPLIED LABELLING OF INJECTABLE MEDICINES FLUIDS AND LINES, DEVELOPED BY THE AUSTRALIAN COMMISSION ON SAFETY AND QUALITY IN HEALTH CARE (ACSQHC). ACSQHC: SYDNEY 2015.

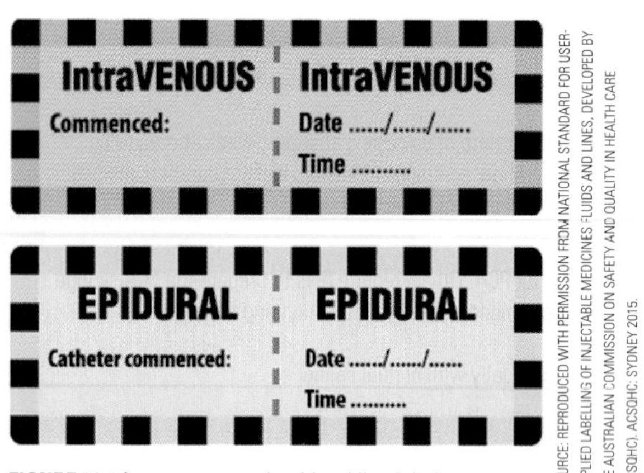

FIGURE 50.4 Intravenous and epidural line label

USE GENERAL CONCEPTS AND THE SIX RIGHTS OF ADMINISTERING MEDICATION

Please review **Clinical Skill 37**, which outlines the general concepts and mechanisms of medication administration and provides a complete description of the rights of medication administration. In summary, the rights include: right time, right medication, right route, right dose, right person and right documentation.

Follow the facility's policy regarding requirements to check the preparation of the medication and attend to its administration because of the schedule of PCA medications.

ADMINISTER PATIENT-CONTROLLED ANALGESIA AND PATIENT-CONTROLLED EPIDURAL ANALGESIA

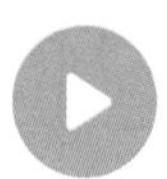

Video

Safety

Hand hygiene

Hand hygiene (see **Clinical Skill 5**) is an infection prevention and control measure. The medication being prepared is administered directly into a vein or the epidural space, so take care to maintain Aseptic Non Touch Technique (ANTT) (see **Clinical Skill 7**).

Administer patient-controlled analgesia

Prepare the syringe

First, open the vials or ampoules (see **Clinical Skill 45**). The following medication calculations must be made:

- the background continuous dose (if using) based on milligrams of medication per millilitre of fluid
- the initial bolus dose and the subsequent intermittent doses
- the lockout time limit.

If the facility uses prefilled syringes, check the syringe's label against the written medication order.

Most medications used in PCA are opioid analgesia, which have a legal requirement to be checked by two RNs (or as per the facility's policy). The syringe is capped without a bung for transport to the bedside. The medication must be labelled with the person's name, hospital number, medication and dose, the type and amount of diluents, time prepared and signatures of the preparing RN and the person checking the medication, on a medication label, or as per the facility's policy.

Unlock the syringe driver and remove the used syringe

The pump device's control is locked, preventing tampering or inadvertent alterations in the settings. Unlock the device and remove the syringe by following the manufacturer's instructions. Usually, the syringe and the extension tubing are removed together and discarded in the sharps container. Follow the facility's policy regarding required procedure for discarding PCA opioids.

Fit a new syringe into the driver

The plunger is held by the driver arm. The driver arm on most models swings out and the new syringe can be slipped into the moulded cradle. The driver arm is then clipped back into place, either over the top of the plunger or with the top of the plunger fitted into a crevice in the driver arm, and the driver arm clicks into place.

Attach and prime the extension tubing

The cap on the syringe is now removed and the extension tube is attached using ANTT. The extension line is primed until a drop of solution appears at the end of the needleless insertion device (Luer Lock). Clamp the extension line.

Set syringe size; confirm continuous dose, bolus dose and delay keys; and lock the syringe driver

The various controls are set using the manufacturer's instructions to regulate the dose, method and lockout time. Each type of pump will differ. Familiarise yourself with the type in use. Lock the syringe driver to activate the pump. Failure to do so will result in the analgesia not being administered (Stephenson, 2022). Smart pumps have the ability to check programmed medication doses against preset limits specific to medication and clinical area (Stephenson, 2022).

Don gloves and attach extension tubing

Follow standard precautions since potential contact with blood exists when working with IV lines and epidural extension tubes. Wipe the medication port closest to the person with an alcowipe and allow it to dry, since friction and drying alcohol remove microbes. Remove the cap and insert the Luer Lock needleless device (interlock) with the attached extension into the medication port and secure it to prevent leakage and accidental disconnection. Unclamp the extension line so that medication flows into the existing IV line. Attach the second medication additive label to the extension tubing.

Discard the gloves and perform hand hygiene.

If required, provide a loading dose for the initial use of PCA. Loading doses are designed to elevate the person's blood level of the medication to a therapeutic level. Some pumps allow a loading dose to be given after the controls have been set; others incorporate a loading dose into the settings of the pump. Again, you need to understand the equipment being used. Administering a loading dose often takes three or four minutes and is usually three to four times the bolus dose.

Assess a person with a patient-controlled analgesia

Maintaining the person's safety is a priority. After the PCA is established, make an overall assessment of the person. Evaluate the person's level of pain (at rest and with activity), sedation score, vital signs (including respiratory rate and SpO_2), infusion rate, nausea and vomiting, constipation, IV site and knowledge of PCA use. See TABLE 50.1 for PCA opioid adverse effects management.

Additionally, check the medication amount delivered against the amount remaining in the syringe, cumulative dose, background infusion rate (if in progress), total demands and good demands, and assess the effectiveness of any intervention for complications and management as per the facility's guidelines. Follow the facility's procedural guidelines.

For the first 24 hours, assessment is required every two hours (or as per the facility's policy). People with high risk (e.g. morbid obesity, sleep apnoea, pulmonary disease) require closer assessment.

The PCA pump settings should be checked against the prescription and recorded at the beginning of your shift, if the person is transferred, and when the syringe or bag is changed.

Administer patient-controlled epidural analgesia

Follow standard precautions since potential contact with blood exists when working with IV lines and epidural extension tubes. Wipe the medication port closest to the person with an alcowipe and allow to dry, since friction and drying alcohol remove microbes.

Remove the cap and insert the Luer Lock with the attached extension into the medication port and secure to prevent leakage and accidental disconnection. Discard the gloves. Unclamp the extension line so that medication flows into the existing IV line.

Attach an 'epidural only' label to the epidural tubing and tape over any ports if a portless system is unavailable. No other solution or medication

TABLE 50.1 PCA opioid adverse effects management

ADVERSE EFFECT	MANAGEMENT

Nausea/vomiting	• Administer anti-emetic; if ineffective, discuss with medical staff the need for additional anti-emetic
	• If nausea seems related to PCA demand, anticipate that medical staff will:
	  • reduce the PCA dose size (if person's requirements are low) or increase the dose duration
	  • change to another opioid
	  • Identify if the person is hypotensive and assess their fluid balance status

Pruritus	• Check if opioid-related (distributed over face and trunk); if the person is disturbed by it, anticipate medical staff will change to fentanyl • Be aware: although naloxone may relieve pruritus in small carefully titrated doses, it may also reverse analgesia, especially if given repeatedly • Antihistamines may be ineffective, as pruritus is thought to be an action on opioid receptors rather than histamine release, and it may increase sedation risk
Excessive sedation/respiratory depression	• Best early clinical indicator of respiratory depression is sedation • Check there is no other reason for sedation – hypovolaemia or sedation given • Sedation score = 2 respiratory rate (RR) ≥ 8 breaths per minute (bpm) bolus dose to be halved • Sedation score = 2 RR < 8 bpm bolus dose halved, person closely monitored and naloxone may be administered • Sedation score = 3 (difficult to rouse or unrousable regardless of RR) PCA ceased and call the acute pain management team or medical emergency team. Anticipate naloxone will be given IV and repeated PRN • Oxygen saturation is monitored at night and during sleep
Urinary retention	• Catheterise – either an 'in/out' or an indwelling catheter
Confusion	• Opioids are not usually the cause or sole cause. Look for causes other than PCA, e.g. hypoxia, sepsis, alcohol or benzodiazepine withdrawal • PCA may need to be ceased if the person is no longer able to manage PCA and alternative analgesia organised
Decreased bowel motility/colicky pain	• Provide anticipatory treatment where possible • Discourage PCA use to cover discomfort resulting from resumption of peristalsis • If pain becomes severe, consider bowel obstruction
Hypotension	• Opioids do not usually cause hypotension • Assess for hypovolaemia or other causes of hypotension

SOURCES: ORTEGA-ARROYO (2021). *PATIENT CONTROLLED ANALGESIA: ACUTE CARE* [EVIDENCE SUMMARY]. JOANNA BRIGGS INSTITUTE EBP DATABASE, JBI@OVID. MAGTOTO, L. S. (2022). *PATIENT-CONTROLLED ANALGESIA: HYPOXEMIA* [EVIDENCE SUMMARY]. JOANNA BRIGGS INSTITUTE EBP DATABASE.

(e.g. antibiotic or total parenteral nutrition) should be given through the epidural catheter. Inadvertent administration of IV solutions can cause serious adverse reactions, including hypotension and cardiovascular collapse.

Label the epidural pump and place it on one side of the person's bed and all other pumps on the other side of the bed, to decrease the risk of mistaking the epidural infusion for an IV infusion system.

A chlorhexidine-impregnated dressing has been shown to be effective in reducing vascular and epidural catheter bacterial colonisation and should be considered (Moola, 2022). Follow the facility's guidelines regarding the dressing type to be used for epidural catheter insertion sites.

The epidural extension tubing is secured to the person's back. There is no evidence regarding which type of epidural securement dressing (e.g. Hyperfix, Tegaderm CHG Chlorhexidine Gluconate IV Securement Dressing, TSD; 3M and 2 pieces Biopatch dressing) best avoids migration or disconnection of the epidural catheter (Moola, 2022). The epidural filter with gauze padding underneath is secured onto the person's shoulder.

Assess a person with patient-controlled epidural analgesia

Maintaining the person's safety is a priority. After the PCEA is established, evaluate the person's pain intensity (at rest and with activity), sedation score, respiratory rate, blood pressure, dermatomes to establish block level, neurovascular assessment for sensation and motor power (see **Clinical Skill 24**), and pruritus.

Assess the epidural catheter site every four to eight hours or as needed. Early identification of an epidural abscess, a rare although serious complication, is important if the person is to recover without neurological injury.

If the person experiences redness, tenderness or increasing diffuse back pain, pain or paraesthesia during epidural injection, induration and swelling, or the presence of exudates, then report it to the team leader.

Monitor the person's urinary output to identify urinary retention or possible early signs of epidural abscess or epidural haematoma. Urinary incontinence, change in bladder function and lack of urination for more than six to eight hours should be reported to the team leader.

Motor loss (e.g. leg numbness or inability to bend knees) or sensory loss in the person's extremities may be an early clinical manifestation of an epidural abscess or haematoma or indicate an excessive LA dose. An epidural haematoma is a rare and serious complication; if undetected, it results in permanent paralysis.

If the person experiences changes in sensory or motor function in extremities, sudden onset of back pain with increasing motor weakness, and loss of bladder and bowel function (incontinence), then report it promptly to the team leader.

The epidural catheter may migrate into a blood vessel or the cerebrospinal fluid, resulting in opioid or LA toxicity. Opioid toxicity causes sedation and respiratory depression. LA toxicity results in circumoral tingling, numbness, twitching, convulsions and apnoea. Lister, Hofland and Grafton (2020) warn that if the epidural catheter migrates into the cerebrospinal fluid, the epidural and LA medications may reach as high as the cranial subarachnoid space. If this occurs, the respiratory muscles and cranial nerves are paralysed, resulting in apnoea, profound hypotension and unconsciousness. Assess the person for tingling around their lips and/or ringing in their ears, as these indicate impending LA toxicity. Skin integrity of the sacrum and heels needs to be monitored every two hours and as needed. Reposition the person as needed. Report any redness or blistering of the skin on the sacrum or heels.

Additionally, the medication amount delivered is checked against the amount remaining in the syringe and the number of attempts. The effectiveness of any interventions for adverse effects is also assessed. Follow the facility's guidelines.

For the first 24 hours, assessment is required every two hours (or as per the facility's policy). People with high risk (e.g. morbid obesity, sleep apnoea, pulmonary disease) require closer assessment.

The PCA pump settings should be checked against the prescription and recorded at the beginning of your shift, if the person is transferred, and when the syringe or bag is changed.

Manage inadequate pain relief

Inadequate analgesia may occur for various reasons, including inadequate loading dose, inadequate use by the person, opioid-related adverse effects, and ineffective PCA prescriptions. The following strategies for inadequate pain relief management can be followed:

- *Reassess the person* – consider alternative causes for new or increased pain, such as haematoma formation, compartment syndrome, leaking anastomosis or nerve injury.
- *Treat opioid adverse effects as required* – the person may be reluctant to use PCA.
- *Review multimodal analgesia* – review if other components of pain management (paracetamol or non-steroidal anti-inflammatory drugs [NSAIDs]) have been given.
- *Inadequate analgesia* – contact the acute pain management team anaesthetist to review the person (Magtoto, 2022; Pasero & McCaffery, 2011).

CLEAN, REPLACE AND DISPOSE OF EQUIPMENT

The extension line needle, syringe and vials/ampoules must be placed into the sharps container to prevent accidental needle-stick injuries to either the nursing or domestic staff. Dispose of alcowipes in the normal waste bin. The injection tray should be washed, dried and returned to its storage place. Assess needle, syringe and medication stocks and obtain sufficient amounts for the next shift's use.

DOCUMENTATION

PCA medication documentation is different from other medication. The RN and the checking nurse sign or initial the time slot on the PCA infusion sheet to indicate that the ordered dose of the medication was initiated at the indicated time. The concentration and dilution of the medication are to be noted. The lockout time must be specified and assessment details noted – pain level and the relief achieved from the medication, sedation score, vital signs, IV and/or epidural site status, amount of solution infused and amount of infusion remaining.

Complications, such as pruritus, reports of nausea and any vomiting, and the person's response to the interventions provided are documented and taken into account to reduce the person's discomfort from the adverse effects.

CLINICAL SKILLS ASSESSMENT

Patient-controlled analgesia and other syringe-driven medication

Demonstrates the ability to effectively and safely care for a person with a PCA. Incorporates the *National Safety and Quality Health Service Standards*: 2 Partnering with consumers, 3 Preventing and controlling healthcare-associated infections, 5 Comprehensive care, 6 Communicating for safety, and 8 Recognising and responding to acute deterioration (Australian Commission on Safety and Quality in Health Care [ACSQHC], 2021).

Performance criteria	1	2	3	4	5
(Numbers indicate NMBA *Registered Nurse Standards for Practice*)	(Dependent)	(Marginal)	(Assisted)	(Supervised)	(Independent)
1. Identifies indication (1.1, 3.3, 3.4, 4.1)	☐	☐	☐	☐	☐
2. Verifies the validity of the written medication order (1.4, 3.4, 6.2, 6.5)	☐	☐	☐	☐	☐
3. Demonstrates clinical reasoning abilities, e.g. assesses the person's ability to manage the patient-controlled analgesia, assesses the person to identify indications, contraindications, and potential complications identified (1.1, 1.2, 1.3, 3.2, 4.1, 4.2, 6.1)	☐	☐	☐	☐	☐
4. Evidence of therapeutic interaction with the person, e.g. gives the person a clear explanation of the procedure (1.4, 1.5, 2.1, 2.2, 3.2)	☐	☐	☐	☐	☐
5. Gathers equipment (1.1, 5.5, 6.1): ■ medication administration sheet ■ required medication ■ appropriate additive label ■ sterile Luer Lock (interlock) syringe ■ sterile needle +/– filter ■ PCA/PCEA pump ■ syringe driver ■ syringe driver extension tubing ■ one-way anti-reflux and anti-siphon valves ■ medication label ■ alcowipes ■ injection tray ■ sharps container ■ clean gloves	☐	☐	☐	☐	☐
6. Uses the six rights and three identifiers to administer the medication (1.1, 1.2, 1.3, 1.4, 1.5, 2.2, 3.4, 4.1, 4.2, 4.3, 6.1, 6.2, 6.5, 6.6)	☐	☐	☐	☐	☐
7. Performs hand hygiene (1.1, 3.4, 6.1), i.e. on entering the person's room; prior to donning gloves to perform procedure; on procedure completion; following glove removal; and on leaving the person's bed area	☐	☐	☐	☐	☐
8. Prepares medication in a syringe and ensures appropriately labelled or obtains the pre-prepared syringe from the pharmacy (1.1, 6.5, 6.6)	☐	☐	☐	☐	☐
9. Unlocks the syringe driver and removes the used syringe (1.1, 6.1)	☐	☐	☐	☐	☐
10. Fits a new syringe into the driver (1.1, 6.1)	☐	☐	☐	☐	☐
11. Attaches and primes the extension tubing (1.1, 6.1)	☐	☐	☐	☐	☐
12. Sets the syringe size, confirms the continuous dose, the bolus dose and the delay keys and locks the syringe driver (1.1, 6.1)	☐	☐	☐	☐	☐
13. Dons gloves and attaches the extension tubing (1.1, 6.1)	☐	☐	☐	☐	☐
14. Provides a loading dose (for the initial use of PCA) (1.1, 6.1)	☐	☐	☐	☐	☐
15. Hands the PCA button to the person and monitors the person (1.1, 3.2, 4.1, 4.2, 4.3, 6.1)	☐	☐	☐	☐	☐
16. Cleans, replaces and disposes of equipment appropriately (3.6, 6.1)	☐	☐	☐	☐	☐
17. Documents relevant information (1.4, 1.6, 2.2, 2.7, 3.5, 3.7, 6.1, 6.2, 6.5, 7.3)	☐	☐	☐	☐	☐
18. Demonstrates the ability to link theory to practice (1.1, 3.3, 3.4, 3.5)	☐	☐	☐	☐	☐

Student:

Clinical facilitator: Date:

CHAPTER 51

SUBCUTANEOUS INFUSIONS

INDICATIONS

Subcutaneous (SC) infusion is an alternative parenteral administration route to intravenous (IV), intramuscular (IM) injection or intermittent SC injections (Aginga, 2021; Pamaiahgari, 2023). SC infusions have a number of advantages over IV treatments, such as bolus, infusion or injection, for people unable to tolerate enteral fluids (Aginga, 2021; Bellman, 2022). SC infusions are associated with fewer complications and offer a wider range of infusion sites.

The SC fluid movement works by osmosis. Fluid moves from an area of high concentration to an area of low concentration, with the sodium-potassium pump creating an osmotic gradient (Saganski & de Souza Freire, 2019).

Continuous subcutaneous infusion (CSCI) may be indicated for people:

- with limited or no venous access
- who are unable to tolerate numerous oral medications
- who are unresponsive to oral symptom control or disease management
- who have a single venous access device and incompatible medications
- whose medications are adaptable to CSCI
- without a functioning gastrointestinal tract
- with diabetes mellitus requiring CSC insulin infusion (CSII) (Aginga, 2021; Bellman, 2022; Pamaiahgari, 2023; Saganski & de Souza Freire, 2019).

CSCI is contraindicated in people with the following conditions:

- occlusive vascular disease
- decreased local tissue perfusion
- hypothermia
- shock
- severe dehydration
- electrolyte imbalances (hyponatraemia, hypokalaemia)
- clotting disorders
- severe heart failure
- generalised oedema
- skin or allergic skin diseases at injection site/s (Aginga, 2021; Bellman, 2022; Pamaiahgari, 2023; Saganski & de Souza Freire, 2019).

As CSCI is safe, effective and cost-efficient, it is a pain management option for people requiring hospice and palliative care (Bellman, 2022; Pamaiahgari, 2023; Saganski & de Souza Freire, 2019). CSCI of opioids provides an option for pain relief, particularly in people with persistent pain unable to take oral medications (Pasero & McCaffery, 2011; Pamaiahgari, 2023). Additionally, CSCI analgesia improves people's quality of life, allows people to be more mobile, and generally provides better pain control than IM injections (Pasero & McCaffery, 2011).

Subcutaneous rehydration therapy (SCRT), originally referred to as 'hypodermoclysis', is indicated for treatment of mild to moderate dehydration. SCRT is used to deliver isotonic IV solutions to people:

- experiencing mild to moderate dehydration and not requiring rapid fluid correction
- with transient dysphagia
- with inadequate oral fluid intake
- in sub-acute settings (particularly frail older adults)
- who are difficult to cannulate (Pamaiahgari, 2023; Saganski & de Souza Freire, 2019).

SCRT is well accepted by children and adults and offers a cost saving when compared with IV therapy (Saganski & de Souza Freire, 2019).

Fluids should infuse slowly (e.g. 50 mL/hr) during the first 30 minutes of SCRT, after which the infusion rate may be increased if the person remains comfortable (Pamaiahgari, 2023). Fluids can be administered at a rate of 20 to 125 mL per hour over 24 hours (Aginga, 2021). In general, SCRT is used to treat short-term reversible fluid deficits only. Generally, no more than 1.5 L is administered per site over 24 hours (Aginga, 2021; Pamaiahgari, 2023). If long-term management is required, IV access should be initiated.

CSII is used to manage a small but growing number of people with diabetes mellitus. The insulin is absorbed more efficiently and the amount required can be reduced by 25 per cent (Bellman, 2022). All people with type 1 diabetes mellitus using CSII should be managed by a specialist diabetes team (Bellman, 2022).

PART 8

EVIDENCE OF THERAPEUTIC INTERACTION

Give the person a clear explanation of the procedure and gain their consent. Many people will be apprehensive about controlling their pain by using the infusion pump. Focus on the person's comfort, their understanding of the CSCI and its role in their pain management. Teach the person how the pump works, what it does and how to manipulate it to control their pain, which will alleviate their anxiety.

Discuss common adverse effects of the medication to be administered, management strategies for these, and ask the person to alert nurses to any changes they note during medication administration. Discuss with the person their options for the management of breakthrough pain.

Discuss optimal needle placement sites that will not interfere with the person's mobility and incorporate their preference for site location.

Assess all of the person's concerns. Just because an adverse reaction is unusual or unexpected, do not ignore it – it needs exploration. This will develop the person's trust in the nursing staff.

DEMONSTRATE CLINICAL REASONING

Assess the person's general condition, their baseline vital signs, allergies to medications, and pain level (see **Clinical Skill 13**). Check the compatibility of the medication with the fluid in which it is to be infused, its normal dosage, action and adverse effects, the recommended infusion time and its peak action time. Assess the person's understanding of the pump.

The insertion site is assessed every two hours for the first eight hours and then twice per shift or according to the facility's policy.

The winged infusion set should be changed every 48 hours or if the insertion site becomes painful (Pamaiahgari, 2023), or according to the facility's policy.

Provide privacy

Privacy reduces anxiety and feelings of embarrassment. Comfort measures such as toileting, positioning, fluids or pain relief increase comfort and minimise disruptions to the procedure. Assist the person into a comfortable position for the procedure.

GATHER EQUIPMENT

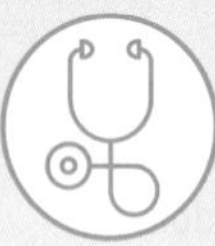

Gathering equipment is an organisational step that helps to create a positive environment for a successful interaction and reduces the person's discomfort and embarrassment. It ensures that you have all needed material, boosts the person's confidence and trust in you, and increases your self-confidence. It also prevents distractions once you have started preparing the medication, which will reduce errors. Equipment required includes:

EQUIPMENT	EXPLANATION
Medication administration sheet	• Used to ascertain the medication and the continuous rate (generally written in mL/hr) and dosage required • Includes the person's name, hospital or unit record number and date of birth; list any allergies and the person's reactions to the allergen; and provide the doctor's name and signature • Used to identify the person to ensure the correct medication, dose, time and route are given to the correct person
Required medication	• Obtained from stock – usually in vial or ampoule • Most facilities require a registered nurse (RN) to prepare the syringe for a SC infusion • Medication is primed in an appropriate syringe, with required extension tubing (an additional syringe with normal saline [NS] may be needed to prime the extension tube)
Recommended sterile diluent	• Required for medication that needs reconstitution • Usually NS • Another registered healthcare professional will need to check the medication preparation
Sterile syringe	• Usually a 10 or 20 mL Luer Lock syringe, depending on the type of pump • Used to prevent inadvertent disconnection or leakage
Sterile blunt drawing needle	Used to draw up medication and diluent
Injection tray	Used to transport the medication containers, the filled syringe and the antiseptic swab to the bedside
Sterile or clean gloves	As per the facility's policy
Sharps container	Taken to the bedside so that used needles, glass ampoules and vials can be immediately disposed of, to reduce the chance of needle-stick injuries
Antibacterial skin preparation	• Such as chlorhexidine or Betadine • Ensure that the person does not have allergies to the skin preparation being used
A small-gauge (25 to 27 gauge) subcutaneous needle	An IV cannula with attached tubing or a subcutaneous infusion catheter designed especially for CSCI (e.g. MiniMed Sof-Set SC needle)
Infusion pump	A pump that delivers fluids
Sterile occlusive transparent dressing	Used to cover the insertion site

EQUIPMENT	EXPLANATION
Subcutaneous medication label	• To adhere to Australian Commission on Safety and Quality in Health Care (ACSQHC) Medication Safety Standard apply the subcutaneous use only adhesive-backed paper (syringe) label (see **FIGURE 51.1**) containing information about the person, medication amount, volume, concentration, diluent, preparation date and time; who prepared and checked, and the administration route is to be completed prior to adhering to the medication syringe (ACSQHC, 2015) • Dedicated continuous infusion lines such as subcutaneous infusion require two labels – one for the medication (see **FIGURE 51.1**) and one for the route of administration (see **FIGURE 51.2**) (ACSQHC, 2015). • Medication label is placed so syringe scale graduations remain visible • Apply the completed label parallel to the long axis of the syringe barrel, top edge flush with scale graduations (ACSQHC, 2015)
Syringe driver	• A small battery-operated pump device that delivers a small amount of medication on a continuous basis, with the capacity to deliver small bolus doses of the medication when purged • Many are fitted into a clear plastic sleeve to protect the pump • There may be a belt attachment to secure and protect the pump when the person is mobile • There are several types of pumps – ensure you are familiar with the pump that is used in the facility
Syringe driver extension tubing	• A fine line allowing for extra movement and ease of placement • Connects to the syringe in the syringe driver with the infusion set
Alcowipes	Used to cleanse and disinfect the tops of vials
Apron and goggles	Used to prevent accidental exposure to blood and body fluids when removing an SC infusion

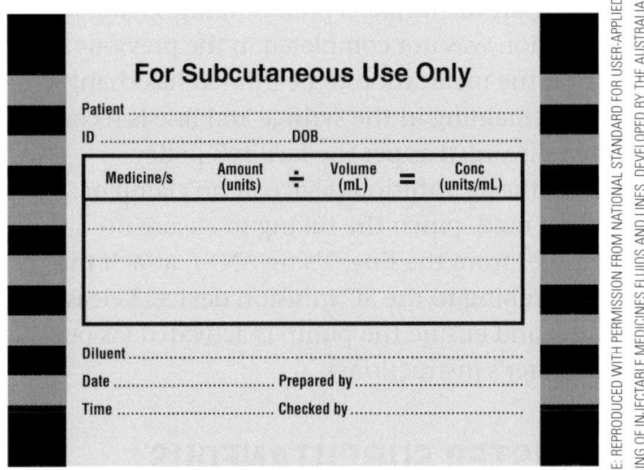
For Subcutaneous Use Only

Patient ....

ID .... DOB ....

Medicine/s	Amount (units)	÷	Volume (mL)	=	Conc (units/mL)

Diluent ....

Date .... Prepared by ....

Time .... Checked by ....

FIGURE 51.1 Subcutaneous syringe label

Subcutaneous Commenced: | Subcutaneous Date ....../....../...... Time ....

FIGURE 51.2 Line label attached to infusion line

USE GENERAL CONCEPTS AND THE SIX RIGHTS OF ADMINISTERING MEDICATION

Please review **Clinical Skill 37**, which outlines the general concepts and mechanisms of medication administration and provides a complete description of the rights of medication administration. In summary, the rights include: right time, right medication, right route, right dose, right person and right documentation.

Prepare the medication and administer it to the person. There is a legal requirement for two RNs or appropriate registered healthcare professionals to both check the medication preparation and attend to its commencement administration because the medications are generally Schedule 8 medications.

ADMINISTER A SUBCUTANEOUS INFUSION

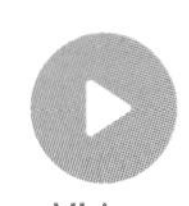
Video

Hand hygiene

Hand hygiene (see **Clinical Skill 5**) should be undertaken as per the facility's policy. Many people receiving analgesia via CSCI are immune-compromised, and sterile gloves should be used as an infection prevention and control measure. The medication and the fluid are going directly into the person's tissue, and care needs to be taken to maintain Aseptic Non Touch Technique (ANTT) during preparation (see **Clinical Skill 7**).

Prepare the syringe

Prepare the medication and dilute it to the required concentration (see **Clinical Skill 45**). Complete the subcutaneous medication only label and adhere it to the syringe. You must calculate the continuous dose based on the milligrams of medication per millilitre of fluid, and the time over which it is to be infused. Most medications used in SC analgesic infusions generally include an opioid analgesia, which is legally required to be checked by two RNs or appropriate registered healthcare professionals.

Prepare the syringe driver

Check the administration rate of the driver, which is generally identified in the bottom right-hand corner. Some drivers allow medication administration on an hourly rate and others deliver the medication on a 24-hourly rate, which can cause confusion for nurses when doing the rate calculations. Confusion over rate settings could result in fatal errors. It is essential that the calculation and flow rate control are specific for the pump to ensure the medication is safely delivered to the person.

Safety

The flow rate on the pump is generally checked by two RNs. Generally, the alarm system on a syringe driver sounds only when the plunger is obstructed, not when the flow is too fast or too slow.

Attach and prime the extension tubing

Perform hand hygiene and don sterile gloves.

The syringe cap must be removed and the extension tube attached using ANTT. The extension line must be primed until the medication appears at the Luer Lock attachment. Clamp the extension line. The medication should be labelled as per the facility's policy (see **FIGURE 51.1**).

Initiate the subcutaneous infusion

Choose infusion sites based on the thickness of the person's SC tissue and their preference. Recommended sites for SC infusion are the lateral aspects of thighs and arms, the chest in males, the abdomen (avoid areas around the waist and pants line and within 5 cm of the umbilicus) or the scapulae (Applegarth, 2021).

Lister, Hofland and Grafton (2020) warn that you should avoid the following:

- lymphoedematous areas and previously irradiated skin areas, as absorption could be impaired and infection may be introduced
- sites over bony prominences, if there is insufficient SC tissue
- sites near a joint, as movement may cause the cannula to become dislodged
- any areas where skin integrity is compromised, inflamed, infected or broken.

Insert the infusion device

Follow standard precautions and facility policy, since there is a risk of contact with body fluid and blood when you are working with SC infusions. Clean the infusion site with an antiseptic swab (as per the facility's policy) using circular motions, and allow the site to dry, since friction and drying alcohol remove microbes.

Hold the needle in your dominant hand and remove the cap. Next, using the thumb and index finger of your non-dominant hand, gently pinch a fold of skin at the injection site and insert the needle of the infusion device gently at approximately 45 to 60 degrees to the surface of the skin. Some pre-packaged needles are shorter than butterfly needles and should be inserted at a 90-degree angle. (Refer to the manufacturer's instructions.)

Release the skinfold and secure the needle with tape

Hold the cannula in position while flushing the device with 1 to 2 mL of NS to ensure cannula patency. If patent, cover the insertion site with an occlusive transparent dressing. This protects the site from infection and allows nurses to visually assess it.

Attach the extension tubing and syringe

Attach the tubing to the infusion device or butterfly using ANTT and insert the syringe into the pump. Unclamp the extension line so the medication will flow into the tubing when the pump is turned on.

Turn on the infusion pump

Each type of pump will differ. Make yourself familiar with the type in use. You can now discard your gloves and perform hand hygiene.

Replace the syringe and remove the used syringe from the pump

The pump device's controls are not locked, but they are generally protected by a plastic case to decrease tampering or inadvertent setting alterations. Remove the device from its case. Remove the syringe and turn it off following the manufacturer's instructions. Usually, the syringe and extension tubing are removed together (depending on the facility's policy on line changes). If the infusion was not completed in the previous 24 hours or if the medication to be infused has changed, any fluid remaining in the syringe and line is recorded and then discarded as per the facility's policy.

Clamp the SC infusion device. If no clamp or butterfly is used, pinch the tubing to ensure no fluid escapes from the line. Using ANTT, attach the extension tubing to the SC infusion device. Release the clamp and ensure the pump is activated (as per the manufacturer's instructions).

ADMINISTER SUBCUTANEOUS FLUID REPLACEMENT

Administer subcutaneous fluids

The technique for administering SC fluids is similar to IV administration. See **Clinical Skill 31** for priming the line and commencing the ordered flow using either the infusion pump or timing with a watch. Once the SC infusion is initiated, the IV line is attached to the infusion cannula. The infusion is commenced by regulating the drip rate as ordered. The rate will depend on the type of solution and the person's infusion indications.

Assess the site before leaving the person and instruct them to inform nurses if the site becomes red or begins to leak. A new site with a new needle must be initiated whenever erythema or leaking occurs.

Monitor the person

After establishing the CSCI, evaluate the person's level of consciousness, comfort level, vital signs (including SpO_2), infusion rate, nausea and vomiting, and fluid status. Examine the site. Confirm the person understands the infusion procedure. Assessment is required every two hours for the first 24 hours. Follow facility policy guidelines for ongoing monitoring of a person with SC infusions.

Discontinue the subcutaneous infusion

Verify the medical order before discontinuing the infusion and establish an alternative method for administering fluids or medication, if necessary, to continue management of the person's illness or pain. Explain to the person why the SC infusion is to be discontinued.

Stop the infusion pump and clamp the infusion line to prevent spillage.

Put on personal protective equipment

As part of standard precautions (and according to the facility's policy), put on clean non-sterile gloves, an apron and goggles to prevent accidental exposure to blood and body fluids.

Gently remove the dressing

Care must be taken to avoid dislodging or removing the needle or damaging the person's skin.

Clean the site with normal saline

Clean the site with NS (follow the facility's policy). If the site is infected, consult with the team leader and medical staff, as you may need to obtain a wound swab for microculture and sensitivity. Cleanse the site with a skin preparation agent, such as chlorhexidine (as per the facility's guidelines). Be sure to check whether the person has an allergy to any skin preparation agents.

Remove the tape from the needle

Remove the tape from the needle, which enables you to remove it at the same angle at which it was inserted. This promotes the person's comfort.

Apply pressure at the site

Apply pressure at the site to prevent fluid leaks, which could cause skin irritation. This also assists in preventing haematoma formation.

Apply a small dry dressing to the site

Apply a small dry dressing to prevent microorganisms entering the puncture site.

Follow the facility's policy for disposing of and documenting any remaining opioid analgesia. Often, this is recorded on the infusion sheet. Another nurse should witness discarding of the remaining medication.

You can now remove your gloves, apron and goggles. Perform hand hygiene.

Post-procedure

Assist the person to a comfortable position, replacing the call bell and anything that was moved during treatment so that it is within reach.

CLEAN, REPLACE AND DISPOSE OF EQUIPMENT

The extension line, syringe and vials/ampoules must be placed into the sharps container to prevent accidental needle-stick injuries to healthcare staff or visitors. Dispose of the antiseptic swab in the normal waste bin. Wash and allow the injection tray to dry; once dry, return it to its storage place. Assess needle, syringe and medication stocks and obtain sufficient amounts for the next shift's use.

DOCUMENTATION

SC infusion and medications are recorded differently to other medication. Nurses sign or initial the timeslot on the medication administration sheet to indicate that the medication was initiated at the indicated time. Document the findings of your assessment of the person's pain level, sedation, vital signs, site status, the volume infused and the remaining volume, on the appropriate assessment charts. Document any reports from the person of localised pain or burning at the injection site and notify your team leader and medical staff. The SC site is to be observed every two to four hours (depending on the facility's policy).

Document and report to your team leader any redness, swelling, leakage or bleeding at the SC insertion site.

The person's response to medication is to be evaluated. Ineffective pain management may indicate the person is not receiving medication into SC tissue (e.g. due to pump malfunction or medication leaking at site). Similarly, report and document in the person's notes if the desired effect of the medication is not achieved or if the person has any adverse reactions to the medication. Document interventions implemented to rectify the person's ineffective pain management and adverse reactions.

CLINICAL SKILLS ASSESSMENT

Subcutaneous infusions

Demonstrates the ability to effectively and safely care for a person with a subcutaneous infusion. Incorporates the *National Safety and Quality Health Service Standards*: 2 Partnering with consumers, 3 Preventing and controlling healthcare-associated infections, 5 Comprehensive care, 6 Communicating for safety, and 8 Recognising and responding to acute deterioration (ACSQHC, 2021).

Performance criteria	**1**	**2**	**3**	**4**	**5**
(Numbers indicate NMBA *Registered Nurse Standards for Practice*)	**(Dependent)**	**(Marginal)**	**(Assisted)**	**(Supervised)**	**(Independent)**
1. Identifies indication (1.1, 3.3, 3.4)	☐	☐	☐	☐	☐
2. Verifies the validity of the written medication order (1.4, 3.4, 6.2, 6.5)	☐	☐	☐	☐	☐
3. Evidence of therapeutic interaction with the person, e.g. gives the person a clear explanation of the procedure (1.4, 1.5, 2.1, 2.2, 3.2)	☐	☐	☐	☐	☐
4. Demonstrates clinical reasoning abilities, e.g. assesses the person's ability to manage the infusion pump, assesses for an appropriate site location, identifies indications, contraindications and potential complications (1.1, 1.2, 1.3, 3.2, 4.2, 6.1)	☐	☐	☐	☐	☐
5. Gathers equipment (1.1, 5.5, 6.1): ■ medication administration sheet ■ required medication ■ recommended sterile diluent ■ sterile syringe ■ sterile blunt drawing needle ■ injection tray ■ sterile or clean gloves ■ sharps container ■ antibacterial skin preparation ■ a small-gauge (25 to 27 gauge) subcutaneous needle ■ infusion pump ■ sterile occlusive transparent dressing ■ medication label ■ syringe driver	☐	☐	☐	☐	☐
6. Adheres to principles of medication administration safety and follows facility medication administration procedural guidelines. Incorporates the six rights and three identifiers to administer the medication (Please review Clinical Skill 37) (1.1, 1.2, 1.3, 1.4, 1.5, 2.2, 3.4, 4.1, 4.2, 4.3, 6.1, 6.2, 6.5, 6.6)	☐	☐	☐	☐	☐
7. Performs hand hygiene (1.1, 3.4, 6.1) i.e. on entering the person's room; prior to donning gloves to perform procedure; on procedure completion; following glove removal; and on leaving the person's bed area	☐	☐	☐	☐	☐
8. Prepares medication in a syringe and ensures appropriately labelled or obtains the preprepared syringe from the pharmacy (1.1, 6.5, 6.6)	☐	☐	☐	☐	☐
9. Dons PPE. Stops the pump and inserts or replaces the syringe in the insertion device (1.1, 6.1)	☐	☐	☐	☐	☐
10. Fits and secures a new syringe into the driver. Resets the pump (1.1, 6.1)	☐	☐	☐	☐	☐
11. Initiates the subcutaneous infusion (1.1, 6.1)	☐	☐	☐	☐	☐
12. Secures the needle and checks it for patency (1.1, 6.1)	☐	☐	☐	☐	☐
13. Connects the infusion device to the extension tubing and syringe, establishes the infusion and sets the rate (1.1, 6.1)	☐	☐	☐	☐	☐
14. Verifies the order for infusion discontinuation; discontinues the subcutaneous infusion (1.4, 3.4, 6.2, 6.5)	☐	☐	☐	☐	☐
15. Performs hand hygiene (1.1, 3.4, 6.1)	☐	☐	☐	☐	☐
16. Dons appropriate PPE. Stops the pump and clamps the infusion line to prevent spillage (1.1, 6.1)	☐	☐	☐	☐	☐
17. Gently removes the dressing to avoid dislodging or removing the needle or damaging the person's skin (1.1, 6.1)	☐	☐	☐	☐	☐
18. Cleans the site with normal saline (follow the facility's policy) (1.1, 6.1)	☐	☐	☐	☐	☐
19. Removes the tape from the needle and removes the needle at the same angle at which it was inserted (1.1, 3.4, 6.1)	☐	☐	☐	☐	☐
20. Applies pressure at the site to prevent fluid leaks (1.1, 3.4, 6.1)	☐	☐	☐	☐	☐
21. Applies a small dry dressing over the site (1.1, 3.4, 6.1)	☐	☐	☐	☐	☐
22. Follows the facility's policy for disposing of and documenting any remaining opioid analgesia (1.1, 3.4, 6.1)	☐	☐	☐	☐	☐
23. Removes PPE and performs hand hygiene (1.1, 3.4, 6.1)	☐	☐	☐	☐	☐
24. Assists the person to reposition, replaces the call bell and anything moved during the procedure to within their reach (1.1, 2.3, 3.2, 4.1, 6.1)	☐	☐	☐	☐	☐
25. Cleans, replaces and disposes of equipment appropriately (3.6, 6.1)	☐	☐	☐	☐	☐
26. Documents relevant information (1.1, 1.4, 1.6, 2.2, 2.7, 3.5, 3.7, 6.1, 6.2, 6.5, 7.3)	☐	☐	☐	☐	☐
27. Demonstrates the ability to link theory to practice (1.1, 3.3, 3.4, 3.5)	☐	☐	☐	☐	☐

Student:

Clinical facilitator: Date:

REFERENCES

Aginga, C. (2021). *Hypodermoclysis: Acute care* [Evidence summary]. Adelaide, SA: Joanna Briggs Institute.

Applegarth, J. (2021). Pain management. In B. Kozier, G. L. Erb, A. Berman, S. Snyder, T. Levett-Jones, T. Dwyer, M. Hales, N. Harvey, L. Moxham, T. Park, B. Parker, K. Reid-Searl & D. Stanley (eds), *Kozier & Erb's fundamentals of nursing* (11th Australian ed.), vol. 3, pp. 1261–303. Frenchs Forest, Australia: Pearson.

Australian Commission on Safety and Quality in Health Care (ACSQHC) (2015). *National standard for user-applied labelling of injectable medicines, fluids and lines*. Sydney, NSW: ACSQHC.

Australian Commission on Safety and Quality in Health Care (ACSQHC) (2021). *National safety and quality health service standards* (3rd ed.). Sydney, NSW: ACSQHC.

Bellman, S. (2022). *Continuous subcutaneous insulin infusion (CSII)* [Evidence summary]. Adelaide, SA: Joanna Briggs Institute.

Foottit, J. (2021). Skin integrity and wound care. In A. Berman, S. Snyder, G. Frandsen, T. Levett-Jones, A. Burston, T. Dwyer, M. Hales, N. Harvey, T. Langtree, L. Moxham, K. Reid-Searl, F. Rolf & D. Stanley (eds), *Kozier & Erb's fundamentals of nursing: Concepts, process, and principles* (11th Australian ed.), Vol. 2, pp. 916–52. Frenchs Forest, NSW: Pearson.

Khoshnevis, S., Craik, N. & Diller, K. (2015). Cold-induced vasoconstriction may persist long after cooling ends: An evaluation of multiple cryotherapy units. *Knee Surgery, Sports Traumatology, Arthroscopy, 23*(9), 2475–83. https://doi.org/10.1007/s00167-014-2911-y

Lister, S., Hofland, J. & Grafton, H. (eds) (2020). *The Royal Marsden manual of clinical nursing procedures* (10th ed.). Oxford, UK: Wiley-Blackwell.

Magtoto, L. S. (2022). *Patient controlled analgesia: Hypoxemia*. [Evidence summary]. Adelaide, SA: Joanna Briggs Institute.

Mann, E. (2016). *Pain: Thermotherapy*. Adelaide, SA: Joanna Briggs Institute.

Minooee, S. (2021). *Labor: Patient-controlled analgesia* [Evidence summary]. Adelaide, SA: Joanna Briggs Institute.

Moola, S. (2022). *Postoperative epidural analgesia (adults): Safety and effectiveness* [Evidence summary]. Adelaide, SA: Joanna Briggs Institute.

Ortega-Arroyo (2021). *Patient controlled analgesia: Acute care* [Evidence summary]. Joanna Briggs Institute EBP Database, JBI@Ovid.

Pamaiahgari, P. (2023). *Dehydration (older people): Hypodermoclysis in residential care* [Evidence summary]. Adelaide, SA: Joanna Briggs Institute.

Pasero, C. & McCaffery, M. (2011). *Pain assessment and pharmacological management*. St Louis, MO: Elsevier.

Picot, E. (2020). *Non-specific low back pain: Superficial heat or cold* [Evidence summary]. Adelaide, SA: Joanna Briggs Institute.

Porritt, K. (2022). *Acute pain management (emergency department): Non-pharmacological interventions* [Evidence summary]. Adelaide, SA: Joanna Briggs Institute.

Prabhakar, A., Mancuso, K., Owen, C., Lissauer, J., Merritt, C., Urman, R. & Kaye, A. (2014). Perioperative analgesia outcomes and strategies. *Best Practice and Research Clinical Anaesthesiology, 28*, 105–15. https://doi.org/10.1016/j.bpa.2014.04.005

Saganski, G. F. & de Souza Freire, M. H. (2019). Safety and effectiveness of hypodermoclysis compared to intravenous fluid infusion for rehydrating children with mild to moderate dehydration: A systematic review protocol. [Systematic Review Protocols] AN: JBI22147.

Sharma, L. (2023). *Administration of PRN analgesia* [Evidence summary]. Adelaide, SA: Joanna Briggs Institute.

Shim, J-M. (2014). The effects of wet heat and dry heat on the gait and feet of healthy adults. *Journal of Physical Therapy Science, 26*(2), 183–5. https://doi.org/10.1589/jpts.26.183

Slade, S. (2021). *Patient controlled analgesia: Pediatric patients (benefits, devices, route of administration, age, drugs)* [Evidence summary]. Adelaide, SA: Joanna Briggs Institute.

Slade, S. (2023). *Rheumatoid arthritis: Thermotherapy* [Evidence summary]. Adelaide, SA: Joanna Briggs Institute.

Stephenson, M. (2022). *Medication safety: Smart infusion pumps* [Evidence summary]. Adelaide, SA: Joanna Briggs Institute.

Tortora, G., & Derrickson, B. (2020). *Principles of anatomy and physiology* (16th ed.). Hoboken, NJ: John Wiley & Sons.

Valdez, F. C. (2024). *Knee osteoarthritis: Superficial heat or cold*. [Evidence summary]. Adelaide, SA: Joanna Briggs Institute.

Wagner, K., Hardin-Pierce, M., Welsh, D. & Johnson, K. (2019). *High-acuity nursing* (7th ed.). Upper Saddle River, NJ: Pearson.

Watkins, A., Johnson, T., Shrewsberry, A., Nourparvar, P., Madni, T., Watkins, C., Feingold, P., Kooby, D., Maithel, S., Staley, C. & Master, V. (2014). Ice packs reduce postoperative midline incision pain and narcotic use: A randomized controlled trial. *Journal of the American College of Surgeons, 219*(3), 511–17. https://doi.org/10.1016/j.jamcollsurg.2014.03.057

PART 9

PERIOPERATIVE CARE

52 PREOPERATIVE CARE

53 POST-ANAESTHESIA CARE AND HANDOVER

54 POSTOPERATIVE CARE

Note: These notes are summaries of the most important points in the assessments/procedures and are not exhaustive on the subject. References of the materials used to compile the information have been supplied. The student is expected to have learnt the material surrounding each skill as presented in the references. No single reference is complete on each subject.

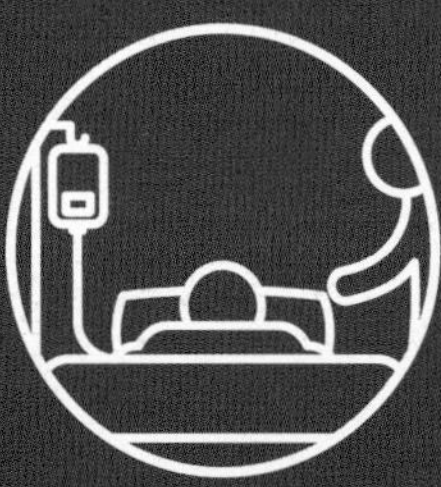

CHAPTER 52

PREOPERATIVE CARE

INDICATIONS

Carefully preparing a person for an operation is an effective strategy. Those who are well prepared:

- understand more about their surgery
- feel more in control of the actions and consequences affecting their care
- experience less postoperative pain and anxiety
- are better motivated for self-care
- require less time in the hospital
- recuperate more quickly.

The type of surgery affects the preoperative care given, the time in which to do it and, sometimes, the actual care. For instance, a person undergoing an elective gall bladder removal has time for a full medical assessment, where any underlying disease or symptom is explored and either eradicated or controlled. They may also attend a preadmission clinic; these are proving helpful in managing expectations and preparing people for the pending hospital care (Roche & Jones, 2021). These individuals will have time to:

- ask their surgeon questions
- engage in preoperative exercises and teaching
- be physically prepared (e.g. for fasting, skin preparation)
- have some of their anxiety allayed preoperatively.

In contrast, in an emergency (e.g. a ruptured appendix) there is little, if any, opportunity for preoperative care, with the exception of basic safety requirements. If it is a day surgery, preparing and admitting the person is done on the same day, which affects the amount and timing of preoperative care.

Preparing the person for surgery also depends on the surgical procedure. Preparing two people, one for a bunionectomy and the other for an abdominal resection, for example, will have elements of similarity, but information given, emphasis on postoperative exercises and physical preparation for these two people will be different.

EVIDENCE OF THERAPEUTIC INTERACTION

Provide information

Providing preoperative information via teaching, video/CD, internet (vetted sites), brochures, pamphlets and skills training is more effective if it is done preadmission. The goal of preoperative teaching and communication is to empower the person. This will enhance their self-efficacy and promote self-care, improve their knowledge and understanding of the processes involved and reduce anxiety. Ultimately, preoperative teaching decreases postoperative complications, assists post-surgical recovery, and decreases postoperative pain (Fernández Fernández et al., 2023). As well, Grondahl et al. (2019) demonstrated the positive effect of preoperative teaching on the person's perception of the quality of care they received. People facing surgery are most concerned about:

- *information* – for example, pain management, getting out of bed, eating and going home
- *psychosocial support* – for example, reassurance and honest information
- *roles and expectations* – for example, desired behaviours such as standing straight
- *skills training* – for example, splinting the incision, and deep breathing.

Provide psychological support

Facing surgery evokes anxiety in most people. Good communication skills draw out the person's concerns and fears to help reduce the stressors of impending surgery. By being available, you provide an opportunity to discuss fears and feelings, all of which are dependent on the individual and are influenced by many factors (e.g. diagnosis and prognosis; proposed procedure; age; educational, cultural and social background; occupation; social support; and family responsibilities). Information and education about the procedure and some of the common concerns reduces the person's psychological stress, anxiety and pain, and improves recovery time (Horn, Kaneshiro & Tsui, 2020).

Answer questions about common concerns, such as:

- What is the surgical procedure and what will it do to my body?
- What happens when I get to the theatre?
- What will happen to me when I am unconscious? Will I feel anything? Will I lose control of my bowels or bladder? Will I say things I would be embarrassed about?
- What will the incision be like? How big will the scar be?
- What will I have to deal with after surgery? Will there be tubes and drips? Will there be blood transfusions?
- Will I have pain when I wake up?
- When will I be able to eat and drink? Will I be sick?
- When will I be able to go home, return to work or return to school?
- Will I be able to lead a normal life? Will I be disfigured?

Answer these questions honestly, factually and completely to the person's level of need and understanding.

> ?
>
> If the questions are beyond your knowledge or need more detail than you can provide, refer questions to a senior nurse as soon as possible and learn from the answers and interaction.

Preoperative anxiety affects about half of people going for surgery. It interferes with the perioperative anaesthetic management (amount of anaesthetic needed, delayed awaking, altered haemodynamics) and overall surgical outcomes (postoperative pain, delayed wound healing, impaired immune system response, increased risk of infection) (Abate, Chekol & Basu, 2020). Compassionate and empathetic listening, as well as preoperative teaching, are excellent nursing interventions to help allay anxiety. Álvarez-García and Yaban (2020) demonstrated the effectiveness of guided imagery in reducing preoperative anxiety and postoperative pain. Ma et al. (2021) found that preoperative anxiety (along with advanced age, alcohol abuse and lower education) predicated postoperative delirium.

Psychosocial difficulties such as depression, isolation and loneliness are addressed to decrease complications such as postoperative confusion following surgery (Ripollés-Melchor et al., 2018). Spiritual needs are considered. You may need to arrange a visit by the person's minister, priest, rabbi, imam or other spiritual adviser if asked to do so. Allaying anxiety is a paramount nursing concern because preoperative anxiety predicts postoperative anxiety, pain and depression (Abate, Chekol & Basu, 2020).

Provide pain management information

Pain is a major fear for most people facing surgery. Reassurance that the pain will be managed effectively assists some people to relax. Others require detailed information about medications to be used, routes, times and effects of the analgesia. Teach them how to use pain assessment tools (see **Clinical Skill 13**) and discuss the use of patient-controlled analgesia (PCA) (see **Clinical Skill 50**) as appropriate. Reassurance that medication addiction is virtually nonexistent when a medication is given appropriately for pain relief will assist some people to utilise the pain management program more comfortably. Individualised pain education has been demonstrated to decrease severe pain and pain frequency postoperatively (Sinderovsky et al., 2023). Preoperative information and teaching was demonstrated to reduce postoperative anxiety levels, the occurrence and frequency of postoperative pain, and the dose and frequency of opioid and non-opioid analgesics required within the first 12 hours postoperative for cardiac surgery (Arpag & Öztekin, 2023).

DEMONSTRATE CLINICAL REASONING

Preoperative assessment

This includes assessing the individual for:

- *medical status* – for example, comorbidities, medications and nutrition
- *mental health* – for example, cognition, mood, anxiety and fears
- *functional capacity* – based on basic and instrumental activities of daily living, gait and balance, and activity/exercise status
- *social circumstances* – for example, support from family and friends, social networks and eligibility for care resources
- *environment* – for example, facilities, comfort and safety at home, potential use of telehealth technology, transport and accessibility of local resources.

Preoperative assessment is vital to the management plan for anyone undergoing a surgical procedure, and helps to acknowledge and treat in advance any condition that may postpone or cancel the surgery or affect their care (White, 2019).

> **ELDER CARE**
>
> 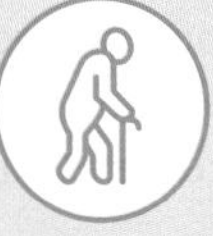
>
> Approximately one-third of the people undergoing surgery are over the age of 65. Older adults carry a higher risk of perioperative morbidity and mortality (Zietlow et al., 2022). Surgery is stressful, and often elderly people do not have sufficient physiological reserves to cope with surgery. They are more prone to postoperative complications, readmissions and longer hospital stays, and are more frequently discharged to long care facilities, compared with adults under age 65 years, making preoperative assessment crucial. Preoperative assessment will include all of the physical parameters (electrocardiography [ECG], urinalysis, blood work, and perhaps X-rays) as well as more comprehensive

assessments (polypharmacy, cognition, frailty, anaemia, loss of muscle mass and tone, nutrition, mobility, self-care ability, social situation, and understanding of their health and the surgery). Carli and Baldini (2021) suggest 'prehabilitation' to prepare the elderly person for the stresses and rigours of surgery (clinical and pharmacologic interventions, preoperative physical, nutritional and mental optimisation) when possible (i.e. elective surgery). Assessment of cognition, dementia, depression and substance abuse alerts the healthcare team to an increased risk of postoperative delirium and pain (Wolfe, Wolfe & Rich, 2020). These authors also advocate for functional assessments (activities of daily living), as these are predictive of post-surgical morbidity and mortality. These actions optimise postoperative functional capacity to improve surgical outcomes.

THE PERSON LIVING WITH SEVERE OBESITY

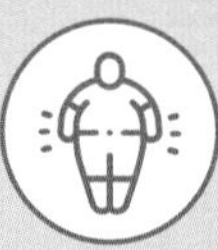

People who are severely obese have additional challenges to face when they have surgery. For them, weight loss surgery is the most common surgical intervention and is often the only method of controlling their weight. Severely obese people have an increased chance of developing many health threats – for example, metabolic syndrome (a triad of hypertension, insulin and cholesterol disorder) – as well as developing respiratory difficulties, cardiovascular disease, obstructive sleep apnoea syndrome, poor wound healing, skin problems, mental illness and osteoarthritis (Carron et al., 2020). The person living with severe obesity will most probably have weeks, if not months, of preparation (for elective surgery) that includes medical management of weight loss, cessation of alcohol and tobacco use, and assessment and stabilisation of any comorbid conditions (cardiovascular problems, ventilation problems, sleep apnoea). Preoperative assessment is thorough, including such assessments as ECG, laboratory tests for diabetes mellitus, circulatory, respiratory, obstructive sleep apnoea and mobility assessment, and liver and renal function studies. Intravenous therapy (IVT) will be established for prophylactic antibiotics and antiemetics, compression (e.g. TED) stockings will be fitted and worn to theatre, and prophylactic anticoagulants ordered (Carron et al., 2020).

Preoperative care focuses on skin preparation, ensuring appropriate equipment is available (i.e. bariatric power-driven bed, ceiling lifts, large theatre bed and trolley) and scouting the path to the theatre to ensure that the trolley will fit through doorways, elevators and around corners. The person may go to theatre in their own bed. (See **Clinical Skills 15 and 23** for a brief explanation of issues faced by people living with severe obesity.)

GATHER EQUIPMENT

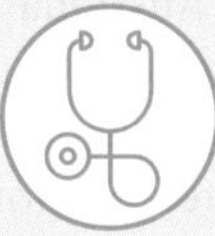

Gathering equipment is an organisational step that creates a positive environment for a successful interaction. It ensures that you have all needed material, boosts the person's confidence and trust in you, and increases your self-confidence. The equipment for preoperative preparation is varied, but includes:

EQUIPMENT	EXPLANATION
Teaching materials	For example, incentive spirometer, thromboembolism deterrent (TED) stockings, brochures
Preoperative checklist	• Lists priority actions to be completed before surgery • Is a time-saving measure

TEACHING TECHNIQUES FOR PREVENTING COMPLICATIONS

Each type of surgery will have unique teaching requirements. Detailed information on various types of surgical teaching is found on the Enhanced Recovery After Surgery Society website. Yuan et al. (2023) demonstrated the effectiveness of one-to-one teaching using information provision (verbal, brochures, video), discussion/questioning with feedback and demonstration/coaching for the various exercises in reducing postoperative complications (see **Clinical Skill 27**).

Respiratory

Respiratory complications in essentially healthy people are increased by factors such as enforced inactivity (reduces ventilation), lack of fluid intake prior to surgery (thickens respiratory secretions), anaesthetic/oxygen inhalation (dries mucous membranes) and postoperative pain (reduces respiratory excursion).

Deep-breathing exercises, incentive spirometry and pursed-lip breathing assist the person to maintain open airways, to inflate the lungs fully and to move secretions up and out of the respiratory tract. Deep-breathing exercises are encouraged hourly for the first two or three days following surgery. Coughing exercises for people who have adventitious breath sounds (not done routinely, and especially not for people with hernia repairs, eye surgery or brain surgery) help to raise secretions so they can be expectorated. Coughing exercises are done as frequently as needed to keep the air passages free of secretions.

Smoking is associated with respiratory complications, surgical site infections, impaired wound healing and death following surgery (An & Wong, 2020). Smokers are advised to abstain from smoking for four weeks ideally but at least 48 hours preoperatively (Enhanced Recovery After Surgery Society, 2020).

Avoiding thrombi and emboli

Blood tends to become more viscous due to such things as fluid restrictions, and positioning during and after surgery, and pools in the lower body due to inactivity/immobility and gravity, trapping blood in the legs. These factors contribute to the formation of thrombi and emboli. Reminders about positioning, such as no prolonged sitting or crossing legs, and not using pillows under their knees, assist to prevent clots forming. Leg exercises promote circulation and prevent clot formation. Attention to the importance of activity and exercise is crucial. Hydration is optimised (Brathwaite, 2023).

Graduated elastic compression stockings (e.g. TED stockings) are thought to prevent thrombi formation by promoting venous flow and reducing stasis, not only in the legs but also in the pelvic veins and inferior vena cava (Molliqaj et al., 2020). TED stockings are fitted on admission to hospital unless contraindicated (e.g. in people with peripheral arterial disease or diabetic neuropathy with significant impairment of tissue oxygenation [Gee, 2019]). Measure the legs and find the correct size of TED stockings before applying the stockings (each leg may require a different size). This helps with adherence and prevents skin complications (e.g. blisters, breaks, erosion) (Prathap & Chitra, 2023).

Mechanical methods, such as intermittent pneumatic compression, are also used to reduce the risk of deep vein thrombosis. You need to become familiar with the devices used in the facility. Pharmacoprophylaxis (e.g. low-dose aspirin or heparin) may be used in conjunction with TED stockings. Teach the person the signs and symptoms of thrombophlebitis and emboli so they can alert the nursing staff early and avert the worst complications.

Activity and exercise

People are supervised in aerobic training and inspiratory muscle training to enhance endurance, strength and functional capacity prior to surgery (Cate et al., 2023). Pain and fear of opening the incision keep many postoperative people inactive. Inactivity contributes to complications that increase the post-surgical convalescent time (e.g. thrombi and emboli, respiratory complications, slow return of bowel peristalsis and reduced gastric emptying). They are encouraged to be active following surgery. They must know they are expected to assist you when they are turned and moved in bed, and in most cases, are expected to get out of bed and walk a short distance eight to 12 hours post-operation, with time out of bed and walking increasing daily.

They need reassurance regarding adequate analgesia and the robustness of the operative site, and to be taught how to splint the incision. Expectations regarding walking upright are made clear prior to the operation and reinforced when the person is sitting and walking. Consider the person's cultural background. Some cultures believe that activity prevents or slows healing.

PERFORM PREOPERATIVE CARE

Video

Hand hygiene

Hand hygiene (see **Clinical Skill 5**) removes transient microorganisms from your hands and prevents cross-infection. Surgery puts the person at extreme risk of invasion by microorganisms, making it imperative that all measures are taken to prevent cross-infection.

Preoperative routine

The preoperative routine involves assessing the person's physical status, preparing the surgical site, completing the checklist (administering the preoperative sedation as ordered) and assisting the person onto the trolley for transport to theatre.

Lab work

Lab work is done according to each individual's need and the surgery to be undertaken (based on a thorough history and physical examination, the person's medical condition and the proposed anaesthesia) (Royal College of Pathologists Australia [RCPA], 2023). Preoperative lab work assesses existing medical conditions, predicts any pre- or postoperative complications and establishes a baseline reference for future comparisons.

Nurses usually schedule the ordered tests and ensure that the test results are on the chart. Preoperative workups may include:

- X-rays and other imaging
- urinalysis
- complete blood count
- type and cross-match as warranted (determine if there have been previous transfusions, or any reactions; find out if the person has objections to receiving blood)
- prothrombin time
- blood chemistry profile
- ECG as necessary
- other tests according to the person's medical history and personal history (liver and renal function studies).

Prepare the surgical site

The site of the surgery is verified visually by the surgeon with an indelible marker and according to the facility's protocol. Most facilities use a three-step verification – when surgery is decided, on admission and during handover just prior to surgery. In addition, the surgical team takes 'time out' to verify the right person, the right procedure and the right site (DeLaune et al., 2024).

The surgical area (an area of skin around the surgical site) is specially prepared preoperatively to reduce contaminating the incision with the microorganisms on the hair or skin. Its extent is usually outlined in the facility's procedure manual. The person showers/bathes their whole body with soap or an antimicrobial solution for at least five minutes with attention to skin folds (groin, axilla) and perianal area (Salazar Maya, 2022).

Shaving the surgical area reduces microorganisms but causes micro-abrasions of the skin and thus more surgical site infections (Salazar & Maya, 2022); therefore, hair in the vicinity of the incision may be clipped prior to surgery and skin preparation done (Seidelman, Mantyh & Anderson, 2023). An electric razor may be used to shave the site or a depilatory cream used two hours prior to surgery (Salazar Maya, 2022).

Different surgeries have different preparation routines. In some, you repeatedly wash the area with antimicrobial soap, swab with antimicrobial solutions and wrap the area in sterile drapes. Povidone-iodine and alcohol formulations or a solution of chlorhexidine gluconate in alcohol scrubbed into the skin with a sterile sponge are currently viewed as the most effective antimicrobial routines (Peristeri et al., 2023). Seidelman, Mantyh and Anderson (2023) found the chlorhexidine gluconate in alcohol superior. Consult the protocol of the clinical facility.

Blood glucose control

Many people scheduled for surgery are diabetic. Assess and aim for optimal blood glucose control pre- and postoperatively to assist in wound healing and reduce the risk of postoperative complications like infection, hyper- or hypoglycaemia, delayed wound healing, prolonged pain, delayed return to work, depression and decreased quality of life (Dale, 2020) (see **Clinical Skill 14**).

Preoperative warming

Perioperative hypothermia affects over 20 per cent (and up to 75 per cent [Wang & Deng, 2023)] of adults undergoing surgery (Kelleci et al., 2023) and has many negative consequences (coagulation disorders, decreased immune functions, prolonged drug clearance, cardiovascular complications, shivering and pain) (National Institute for Health and Clinical Excellence [NICE], 2016). Kelleci et al. (2023) found hypothermia was significantly associated with longer surgical/anaesthesia duration, hospital stays, post-surgical infection and higher intensive care unit (ICU) admissions. Ju et al. (2023) found it was also associated with postoperative delirium.

Preoperative warming is an active measure to raise the temperature of a person to above 36.5 °C (and maintain it throughout the perioperative period) (Bashaw, 2016). Initially, the person is assessed for any factors that might contribute to hypothermia (temperature below 36.5 °C, elderly, low body mass index [BMI], long surgical procedure [Wang & Deng, 2023]). Their temperature is monitored in all phases of perioperative care, and interventions to prevent unplanned hypothermia are used. In the preoperative phase, these standard interventions include warmed blankets, thermal (self-warming, reflective) blankets, or Forced Air Warming Systems in the 30 minutes to one hour prior to surgery. Intra-operatively, the temperature monitoring and external heating are continued, along with the use of warmed fluids (e.g. IVs, irrigation fluid) and a warm ambient temperature in theatre; and post-operatively, the monitoring and external heating are continued.

The checklist

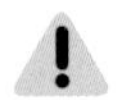
Safety

Most facilities have a checklist of priority actions to be completed before surgery. This reduces time wasted in searching the chart/electronic medication administration record (eMAR) to verify specific actions are complete and ensures all priority actions are addressed.

Identification of the person

Putting a name band on a person's wrist is done on admission. Often an additional name band is placed on the leg in case one band is cut off (follow institutional guidelines). Check the name band with the chart/eMAR and with the person to eliminate misidentification and prevent serious physical and legal repercussions.

Fasting

This is often for a specified time (e.g. six hours for solid food, although clear fluids and carbohydrate drinks are taken up to two hours preoperatively in most facilities [Marsman et al., 2023]). Consult the facility's protocol. It produces an empty and non-active gastrointestinal tract, which prevents aspiration of undigested food if vomiting occurs. Fasting longer than two hours causes dehydration, and increases insulin resistance, nausea and vomiting and distress from hunger (Caalim, 2020). Fasting is minimal in children and is usually not carried out for infants.

Elimination

Elimination of bowel contents (follow surgeon's protocol) reduces the possibility of faecal contamination during abdominal, colorectal or urogenital surgery and postoperative distension and constipation resulting in incisional strain. It is not routine in other surgeries, as it can cause dehydration and does not reduce surgical site infections (Caalim, 2020). Bowel emptying can be accomplished by various measures (e.g. laxatives in the days prior to surgery, a bowel evacuant solution [e.g. polyglycol-electrolyte lavage solution], micro-enema or full enema). Ask the person to void before surgery to reduce discomfort and avoid bladder interference with the procedure.

Valid consent to surgery

You must check if there is valid consent to surgery. It is the surgeon's responsibility to explain the surgery. The person should be able to explain their understanding of the procedure and any reasonable complication (e.g. surgical site infection) (Brunette & Miller, 2023). Confirm it is the person's signature on the consent form. This process complies with legal requirements and ensures the person has understood the surgical procedure.

Consent for blood transfusion

A consent for blood transfusion is attached to the chart if the need is anticipated.

Physical status

Assess physical status – physical assessment, health status, laboratory tests, blood available, special examinations, X-rays, vital signs, weight and height – to reduce surgical risks, avoid complications and prevent unexpected difficulties during and after surgery. For some groups (e.g. over 60 years), specific tests such as an ECG are routinely ordered. These reports are on the chart or accompany the person to theatre (e.g. X-rays).

Vital signs

Vital signs are taken and recorded within an hour of surgery to establish a baseline. Note and report if the temperature is below 36 °C.

Allergies

Any allergies to drugs, food, latex, soap, tape or antiseptic agent are identified. Some allergies may indicate a potential reaction to drugs or substances used during surgery or diagnostic procedures (e.g. allergies to avocado, chestnut or banana are risk factors for latex allergy). Any allergies and the person's reaction are written (usually in red) on an allergy identification band and, as with the identification armband, two are attached to the person. The allergies and reaction are also written in red on the preoperative checklist and medication chart so all members of the multidisciplinary team are aware. Medic alert bracelets are taped in place with clear tape.

Valuables

These are removed and handled according to facility policies (usually sent home) to prevent loss or damage and subsequent legal problems for the facility. Wedding rings are taped with a hypo-allergenic tape; however, they must be removed if there is a danger of the fingers swelling postoperatively (e.g. following mastectomy involving lymphatic node dissection). Other metal jewellery, including any body-piercing jewellery, constitutes a hazard when diathermy is being used. Holm (2022) warns of inadvertent tear or pressure injuries from body-piercing jewellery and other risks (e.g. dislocation and aspiration of tongue jewellery during intubation and possible inability to insert a urinary catheter due to genital piercing) if these are left in situ; the possible loss of the jewellery may also occur.

Shower, bath and/or mouth care

Shower or bath and mouth care are attended to in order to provide comfort and reduce the bacterial load.

Hospital gown, cotton underwear, theatre pants and cap

These are worn to reduce the risk of static electricity, to prevent damage to the person's clothing and to reduce the transfer of microorganisms from the person's hair. Long hair is secured with rubber bands because clips or hairpins might damage the scalp when the person is unconscious. If a woman is menstruating, ensure there is a sanitary pad in place and not a tampon – this prevents infection should the tampon be in situ for more than two hours.

Prostheses and dental work

Prostheses and dental work are removed to protect them from loss or damage. Bridges and dentures can cause choking if left in. Some facilities allow the person to wear dentures to theatre, and the circulating nurse is responsible for their care during surgery.

Glasses or contact lenses

Glasses or contact lenses are removed to prevent loss or damage. Contact lenses can also damage the eye if left in during surgery. If the person's vision is very limited without their glasses, they can be worn to the anaesthetic room (follow the facility's policy). Hearing aids are left in to facilitate communication, reduce anxiety and enable understanding of procedures, then removed after the anaesthesia is in effect and reinserted in the post-anaesthetic care unit.

Cosmetics and nail polish

Removing cosmetics and nail polish enables healthcare personnel to assess circulation (e.g. pallor, flushing, oxygen saturation) and reduces the risk of infection.

Anti-embolism stockings

The TED stockings may be applied and worn throughout surgery. These have proved effective in preventing deep vein thrombosis in moderate-risk surgical patients. They are individually fitted, applied to dry feet and legs prior to surgery and then worn throughout the post-surgical period. Check the neurovascular status of the legs after application (Gee, 2019).

The surgeon or anaesthetist may order other special preoperative procedures (e.g. inserting an indwelling catheter or a nasogastric tube, initiating intravenous therapy or an insulin infusion).

Administer the preoperative medication

Generally, routine preoperative medication is not ordered. The variety of anaesthetic agents and techniques used has reduced the need for sedation. This, combined with the increased attention needed for a sedated person's safety, and minimal benefit from premedication, suggests that caution is required in using these medications.

If preoperative medications are ordered:

- they may be ordered for a specific time or 'on call' – therefore, all preoperative preparation must be done in good time
- an opioid may occasionally be ordered – the person needs to know they will feel relaxed and drowsy and must stay in bed. Raise the side-rails as a reminder and place the call bell in easy reach so assistance is available
- a medication to dry secretions may be ordered – warn the person to expect a dry mouth
- a 'stat' medication (e.g. Ventolin or a prophylactic antibiotic) may be ordered on the person's medication chart with the preoperative medication or when the theatre staff calls for the person.

Routinely taken medications may or may not be given on the morning of surgery. If the person is ordered their routine medications, they are administered with a minimum of water, preferably two hours or more prior to surgery.

Assist the person onto the trolley

The unit nurse who prepares the person accompanies them to theatre. The person may need assistance onto the trolley. Privacy and dignity are maintained. Many facilities prefer that the person (who is able) walks to the theatre, accompanied by the unit nurse. In some facilities, the person is transferred to the operating theatre (OT) in their bed and from their bed to the operating table and back to their bed in theatre, reducing manual handling and discomfort for the person.

Follow the facility's guidelines for preparing and cleaning a bed before sending it to theatre.

Accompany the person to theatre

Walk at the head of the trolley or beside the person and talk to them if they so wish. The paper chart comes with the person and should include:

- all observation charts
- fluid balance and fluid order charts
- blood test results
- blood ordered and available
- pre-anaesthetic assessment
- ECG, possible respiratory function test, X-rays
- an adequate amount of individual identification stickers
- the preoperative checklist signed by the nurse who did the final check, accompanies the person to theatre.

Note: In many facilities, most of this 'paperwork' will be available on the eHealth record and will not physically accompany the person.

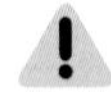
Safety

Labelled containers for dentures, glasses and/or hearing aids are taken with the person to theatre as required.

The unit nurse gives a handover to the perioperative nurse, who identifies the person and verifies the preoperative checklist. Safe nursing care in the operating theatre is contingent on reliable information being given during this handover (Sandelin, Kalman & Gustafsson, 2019).

CLEAN, REPLACE AND DISPOSE OF EQUIPMENT

Change the bed linen in preparation for the return of the person from theatre. Make an open bed. Use protective (waterproof) sheets to protect the mattress. Tidy the bed area so the returning trolley can be moved easily. Depending on the surgery, equipment is brought to the bedside for immediate use on the person's return (see **Clinical Skill 54**).

This preparation is completed as soon as the person has been taken to theatre, to make sure that the room will be ready for their return.

DOCUMENTATION

Theatre and recovery personnel require complete information in the chart or eHealth record (the person will be unable to provide any information to them) so that appropriate decisions are made. The checklist is completed, medication and fluid sheets are signed and clinical notes state the time that the person left the ward for theatre.

CLINICAL SKILLS ASSESSMENT

Preoperative care

Demonstrates the ability to effectively prepare a person for theatre. Incorporates the *National Safety and Quality Health Service Standards*: 2 Partnering with consumers, 3 Preventing and controlling infection, 4 Medication safety, 5 Comprehensive care, and 6 Communicating for safety (Australian Commission on Safety and Quality in Health Care [ACSQHC], 2021).

Performance criteria	1	2	3	4	5
(Numbers indicate NMBA *Registered Nurse Standards for Practice*)	(Dependent)	(Marginal)	(Assisted)	(Supervised)	(Independent)
1. Identifies indication (1.1, 3.3, 3.4)	☐	☐	☐	☐	☐
2. Evidence of therapeutic interaction with the person, e.g. gives the person a clear explanation of the procedure (1.4, 1.5, 2.1, 2.2, 3.2)	☐	☐	☐	☐	☐
3. Provides psychological support (1.1, 1.2, 1.3, 1.5, 2.1, 2.2, 2.3, 2.5, 2.7, 3.2, 6.1, 7.3)	☐	☐	☐	☐	☐
4. Provides pain management information (1.2, 1.3, 2.3, 2.5, 2.7, 3.2, 6.1, 7.3)	☐	☐	☐	☐	☐
5. Demonstrates clinical reasoning; provides information, performs preoperative assessment, provides psychological support, provides pain management information (1.1, 1.2, 1.3, 4.2, 6.1)	☐	☐	☐	☐	☐
6. Gathers equipment (1.1, 5.5, 6.1): ■ teaching materials ■ preoperative checklist	☐	☐	☐	☐	☐
7. Performs hand hygiene (1.1, 3.4, 6.1)	☐	☐	☐	☐	☐
8. Uses appropriate time-management techniques (5.4, 6.1)	☐	☐	☐	☐	☐
9. Teaches techniques for preventing respiratory complications (1.1, 1.3, 1.4, 2.1, 2.2, 2.3, 3.2, 6.1)	☐	☐	☐	☐	☐
10. Teaches techniques for avoiding thrombi and emboli (1.1, 1.3, 1.4, 2.1, 2.2, 2.3, 3.2, 6.1)	☐	☐	☐	☐	☐
11. Promotes activity and exercise (1.1, 1.3, 1.4, 2.1, 2.2, 2.3, 3.2, 6.1)	☐	☐	☐	☐	☐
12. Carries out the preoperative routine, e.g. identification, fasting, elimination, consent signature, valuables (1.4, 2.4, 2.5, 2.7, 3.2, 6.1, 6.2, 6.5, 7.3)	☐	☐	☐	☐	☐
13. Prepares the surgical site (1.1, 6.1)	☐	☐	☐	☐	☐
14. Administers preoperative medication (1.1, 1.3, 1.5, 3.3, 3.4, 4.1, 4.2, 4.3, 6.1, 6.2, 6.5, 6.6, 7.3)					
15. Assists the person onto the trolley and accompanies them to theatre (1.1, 6.1)					
16. Cleans, replaces and disposes of equipment appropriately (3.6, 6.1)					
17. Documents relevant information (1.1, 1.4, 1.6, 2.2, 2.7, 3.5, 3.7, 6.1, 6.2, 6.5, 7.3)	☐	☐	☐	☐	☐
18. Demonstrates the ability to link theory to practice (1.1, 3.3, 3.4, 3.5)	☐	☐	☐	☐	☐

Student:

Clinical facilitator: Date:

CHAPTER 53

POST-ANAESTHESIA CARE AND HANDOVER

INDICATIONS

Following surgery, the person is at great risk in the immediate post-anaesthetic period. Contributing to that risk are:

- the effects of surgery (time, incision, open body cavity, stress, position during surgery)
- anaesthesia and other medications used
- alterations in thermoregulation
- fluid shifts
- airway patency
- cardiovascular complications
- neurological dysfunction.

Nursing care in the Post-anaesthetic Care Unit (PACU) (or Post-anaesthetic Recovery Room – PARR) is dedicated to:

- supporting respiratory and haemodynamic stabilisation following anaesthesia and surgery
- promoting recovery from anaesthesia
- promoting physical comfort and healing
- preventing injury and postoperative complications.

The person remains in the PACU until their physiological status has stabilised. The length of time is individual and depends on the person's surgery, type of anaesthetic and their responses. During this time, carefully and thoroughly monitor them to identify possible complications. This usually entails one-to-one nursing. You must recognise and promptly report any abnormalities in any assessments to the shift coordinator so that further assessment and escalation of care can prevent harm.

EVIDENCE OF THERAPEUTIC INTERACTION

People will display varying degrees of responsiveness, and physical and emotional states, so establishing a rapport with them will gain their confidence and cooperation and aid assessment. Following the final stage of anaesthesia, some people behave in an agitated or emotional and disinhibited manner, at odds with their usual behaviour (emergence delirium) (Heily et al., 2023). This is transient (15 to 30 minutes) and usually forgotten; however, it can be the cause of injury (e.g. incisional, tube or intravenous [IV] tube removal, falls, personnel [Wang et al., 2023]). Use a calm voice and continuous reassurance, and give the person clear explanations of procedures, even if they are unconscious. Hearing is the last sense to leave and the first to return; they may hear your explanation and gain some reassurance from it (Kotomska & Michalak, 2019).

Families should not be forgotten, especially parents of children; inform them that the surgery is completed and their loved one/child is in the recovery room.

DEMONSTRATE CLINICAL REASONING

Caring for someone who is freshly out of surgery demands concentration, vigilance and perception, foreknowledge of the possible complications and existing conditions the person has, and a good understanding of your own abilities and knowledge. This is *situational awareness*, a process nurses use to avert poor outcomes in people whose condition is unstable and can deteriorate quickly. It begins with knowing the person, their diagnosis, what is likely to go wrong and what could go wrong. Following this, *vigilance* is applied, where indications of problems are actively looked for, such as altered vital signs, reduced urine output, poor colour, sweaty skin, saturated dressing or empty IV bag (LOOK, LISTEN, FEEL). Then *perception* is engaged to notice the differences in the person when you assess them, such as increased pain, confusion or being less alert. Notice their environment and equipment. Then use *clinical reasoning* to identify important elements and decide what other cues to look for. From the cues you gather, you can predict what might happen. At this point, you *intervene* if you can (e.g. apply oxygen, give pain relief as ordered) or *communicate* your findings and prediction to a senior colleague who can address the problem (e.g. contact the medical team, initiate a unit protocol for electrocardiograms) as soon as possible.

Most of the care in the PACU is based on situational awareness, and the remainder of the information in this skill discussion reflects that.

ELDER CARE

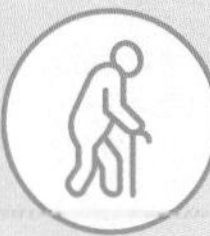

Elderly people endure loss of physiological reserves (cardiovascular, renal, cerebral, respiratory) that affect the way they react to anaesthesia and other medications (e.g. opioids) (Aceto et al., 2023). Note and record/report changes in behaviour, concentration, memory, confusion or delirium. These may be signs of pain, infection or reaction to the medications, and must be treated. Assisting with comfort (positioning, pain relief as ordered) can also help reduce confusion and anxiety.

Remember that pain may be related to pre-existing comorbidities (e.g. arthritis, gout) or to causes other than the surgical procedure (e.g. intubation, positioning on the theatre table), so ask about aches and pains generally, not just incisional pain.

Postoperative delirium is relatively common in elderly people (Assefa et al., 2022). It is a temporary condition causing confusion, disorientation, memory and attention difficulties and being unaware of the environment (American Society of Anaesthesiologists [ASA], 2023). It may occur immediately postoperatively or not start until a few days after surgery, may come and go, and usually disappears after about a week.

THE PERSON LIVING WITH SEVERE OBESITY

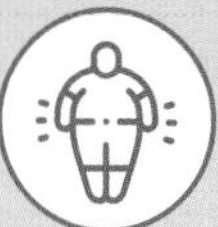

Severely obese people who have had surgery are at an increased risk for:

- airway obstruction from the excess adipose tissue deposits in their neck
- ventilatory problems (atelectasis) because of restricted lung expansion due to pressure on the diaphragm from excess abdominal tissue
- difficulty in clearing anaesthetic medications from their system (making subsequent pain control more complex)
- thromboembolism (Carron et al., 2020; Schlick et al., 2020).

Maya and Galeano (2023) add pressure injuries (sacrum, heels, chin, sternum, trochanter) to this list because of long periods of immobility, and inappropriate weight distribution or support.

Position the severely obese person in a reverse Trendelenburg's position (supine with shoulders higher than feet, ear to sternal notch in same horizontal plane), with adequate strapping to immobilise, padding to prevent the start of pressure injuries and support to prevent neural injuries. Use of oxygen, use of thromboembolism deterrent (TED) stockings, adequate hydration and constant vigilance will help to reduce the poor surgical outcomes associated with severe obesity (Carron et al., 2020). Safeguard your own health by using appropriate equipment and extra assistance when moving a severely obese person. (See **Clinical Skills 15 and 23** for a brief explanation of issues for people living with severe obesity.)

Awareness of anticipated complications

Since there are specific risks for each of the various surgical procedures, you must be familiar with complications that could arise from each one. The very elderly or very young are at greater risk of many complications than a young adult would be. To anticipate complications in each person with a unique medical history or specific condition, you need to know the effects of surgery and/or anaesthesia on these, so research the procedure and any known condition of the person. Diabetes mellitus, impaired vision or hearing, peripheral vascular diseases, a previous cerebrovascular accident, some medications (e.g. benzodiazepines) and tobacco and alcohol intake are examples of conditions that can affect the person's immediate recovery from anaesthesia and surgery. This knowledge allows you to prepare for reasonable eventualities and have sufficient equipment, medications, IV solutions and so on available.

GATHER EQUIPMENT

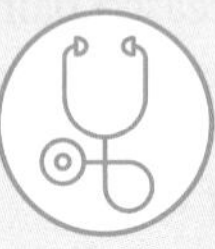

All equipment used must be functioning and at the bedside before the person arrives. The PACU is a short-term critical care area and is generally set out with all of the basic equipment (e.g. airway maintenance, pulse oximetry, non-invasive blood pressure and cardiac monitoring, piped oxygen and suctioning) needed at each individual recovery bay, arranged for ease of access and always clean and in full working order. Become familiar with the essential equipment for respiratory and cardiac support, on the resuscitation trolley (which is usually centrally located). It has additional equipment to that of a general ward. Specific equipment required for an individual (e.g. glucose monitoring equipment) will have to be supplied and tested prior to use.

On arrival, the person who has undergone general anaesthesia will probably be unconscious and require one-to-one nursing. Remain at the bedside and do not leave to obtain forgotten equipment. Anyone who had local or spinal anaesthetic also requires a period of postoperative observation, although the priorities of care will focus on different considerations, such as hypotension, convulsions, dizziness and headaches (DeLaune et al., 2024).

Basic PACU equipment includes the following items:

EQUIPMENT	EXPLANATION
Stethoscope, sphygmomanometer, tympanic or digital thermometer and probe covers, ECG monitor and a watch with a second hand	• To monitor vital signs • Generally, an automatic blood pressure machine is used, although some situations require a manual sphygmomanometer (e.g. shivering or profound bradycardia, power failure and obesity) (Schick, 2019)
IV fluid stand and various solutions	• To hang an IV bag (usually attached to the bed) • During surgery, an intravenous infusion is nearly universally inserted to balance and maintain fluid levels, as well as to provide access routes for intravenous medications
Oxygen equipment	• Tubing, face masks, nasal cannulae, or a T-piece system and full range of oropharyngeal and nasopharyngeal airways can often be required following surgery • The person has been anaesthetised and their respiratory system needs assistance to maintain oxygenation to the tissues. They often return to the recovery area with the endotracheal tube in situ
Pulse oximeter	To monitor oxygen saturation
Suctioning equipment	• A wall unit, regulator, tubing and a range of oral and endotracheal catheters are often required to clear the airway • The depressive effects of anaesthesia and the paralytic medications used can temporarily eliminate or reduce the gag and swallowing reflexes
Dressing supplies	Gauze squares, combines, non-adhesive dressing material and a range of tapes may be needed if the dressing requires reinforcement because of excess bleeding/drainage
Warm blanket/warm air circulator	• To provide comfort and prevent shivering • Altered thermoregulation, the colder ambient temperature of theatre, lying on the cold table and an exposed wound over time contribute to the discomfort felt by the person • Hypothermia (internal temperature below 36 °C) increases cardiopulmonary demand, reduces the reversal of muscle relaxants given in theatre, and can result in cardiac complications as well as surgical site infections (Ashoobi et al., 2023)
Other equipment	As needed and depending on the nature of the surgical procedure (e.g. electro-encephalograph post neurological surgery)

PERFORM POST-ANAESTHESIA HANDOVER AND CARE

Hand hygiene

Hand hygiene (see **Clinical Skill 5**) removes transient microorganisms from your hands and prevents cross-infection. Surgery puts the person at extreme risk of invasion by microorganisms, making it imperative that all measures are taken to prevent cross-infection.

Post-anaesthesia handover

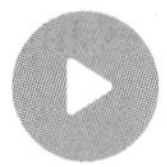
Video

Handover from theatre staff to the post-anaesthetic unit staff is vital. The anaesthetist usually accompanies the person from theatre. During handover, the scrub nurse and PACU nurse assess the person together. A standardised checklist (based on international standards and tailored to the facility) is used to minimise communication errors, increase safety and improve efficiency (Chernyak & Posten, 2022).

The handover report includes at least:

- name, age and language spoken, hospital identification check
- allergies and pre-existing medical conditions (e.g. diabetes mellitus)
- type and extent of the surgical procedure
- preoperative and intraoperative vital signs
- positioning during surgery
- type of anaesthetic used
- time under anaesthesia
- estimated blood loss
- medications and intravenous solutions administered, including reversal medications
- complications if any
- location and type of catheters; urine output
- the presence, position and nature of any arterial devices, drains or packs
- altered sensory or motor functions
- intraoperative events that might affect the postoperative course.

PACU staff need to know what has occurred during surgery. Many events will affect the person during the immediate recovery period from anaesthetic. Any deviations from planned surgery, specific orders left by the surgeon and postoperative standing orders are also discussed. Information about preoperative anxieties (e.g. fear of not coping with the pain) allows appropriate interventions to be taken as the person regains consciousness.

The anaesthetist will also give specific instructions for postoperative care. The information provided in the handover is in the person's notes, but the initial verbal handover ensures no delay in providing immediate care.

Care in the Post-anaesthetic Care Unit

Most of the following activities occur simultaneously or at least in very rapid succession and will depend on the individual's condition. Do not forget to talk to the person, providing information and reassurance that surgery is over while you assess and care for them.

Assess and maintain a patent airway

Assess for airway patency:

LOOK at the rate and depth of respiration and for any accessory respiratory use; check for tracheal tug (i.e. indrawing of skin/tissue at the base of the trachea during inspiration indicating respiratory distress or paralysis of the diaphragm following surgery).

LISTEN for inspiration; noisy respirations, snoring, wheezes and gurgling indicate a partial airway obstruction.

FEEL for movement of expired air.

General anaesthesia depresses many reflexes, including pharyngeal (gag), cough and swallowing reflexes. People usually return to the recovery room with a Guedel's airway in situ. This type of airway forces the tongue forward so it does not block their airway. Leave it in place until the person attempts to, and is able to, remove it by themselves.

> ?
>
> If the Guedel's airway is causing distress and gagging, check with senior staff, after which you may remove it even if the person is not awake or coordinated enough to push it out. Care must be taken to ensure the airway remains patent. Place the person in recovery position (if not contraindicated), support their chin with their neck extended and stay with them.

The person will usually return from theatre in recovery position (side-lying) to protect the airway from secretions and regurgitation, unless there is a specific reason for them to be in a different position. If necessary, support their chin with the neck extended (unless contraindicated). The person will remain in this position until they are fully conscious and able to maintain their own airway. Keep the bed flat if not contraindicated. Elevate the person's upper arm on a pillow to reduce pressure on their chest.

Monitor breath sounds to detect any airway obstruction. Sometimes, verbal stimulation or gentle shaking will awaken a person enough so they can clear their own airway. If not, suction the oropharynx. Use care to avoid damage to the mucosal surfaces, further irritation, initiation of a gag reflex or laryngeal spasm.

Oxygen (humidified) is generally administered continuously during the person's stay in the recovery room. This facilitates gas exchange and helps remove the anaesthetic from their lungs. If an endotracheal tube or laryngeal mask is in position, check whether the cuff or mask is inflated and administer oxygen via a T-piece system. Monitor the person's oxygen saturation with a pulse oximeter. Maintain oxygenation at 95 per cent.

The person may require verbal stimulation to maintain their respiratory rate above 10 since anaesthetics act as a general depressant. Encourage the person to cough and breathe deeply when awake (as appropriate).

Obtain vital signs readings and assess circulatory status

Blood pressure, pulse, temperature and respiratory assessments are done immediately on arrival at the unit and every five to 15 minutes thereafter until the person is stable and returned to the ward. Pulse oximetry is continuous.

LOOK at their colour (lips, conjunctiva, then peripheries); central cyanosis indicates impaired gaseous exchange between the alveoli and pulmonary capillaries; peripheral cyanosis indicates low cardiac output and is associated with shock.

LISTEN for reports of cold, pain or confusion.

FEEL their skin for warmth or moisture.

Haemodynamic instability and altered tissue perfusion occur because of blood pooling during surgery; watch for peripheral vasodilatation, hypothermia and hypovolaemia. Connect the person to the monitoring systems. Cardiac monitors assess the heart rate and rhythm. Apical and peripheral pulses are obtained and compared to preoperative and intraoperative readings. Capillary refill is checked as frequently as the pulse is. Hypoxia can manifest as irritability, restlessness, confusion and/or aggression.

Temperature is monitored initially and then every 30 minutes. Hypothermia can occur in up to half of those returning from surgery (Tu et al., 2023). Hypothermia is due to the anaesthesia (it disrupts basal metabolic rate and thermoregulation [Al-dardery et al., 2023]), the type of surgery, a cold theatre table, the ambient temperature in the theatre and the length/extent of the procedure. It interferes with the effective reversal of muscle relaxants and can be more distressing than postoperative pain (Ashoobi et al., 2023). Shivering may result from a compensatory response or the effects of anaesthetic agents or pain. It can increase oxygen consumption, increasing the risk of hypoxia and ischaemia (Tu et al., 2023).

Although less common, hyperthermia can be a serious complication of surgery. Accidental over-warming during surgery, sepsis or transfusion reactions can cause hyperthermia. An elevated temperature increases oxygen demands, and ventilatory and cardiac workloads. The possibility of malignant hyperthermia (MH), a genetically determined condition, although rare, must always be considered (An et al., 2020) because successful management of MH depends on early assessment and recognition and prompt intervention.

Assess level of consciousness

Observe the person for the return of reflexes (e.g. swallowing, tear secretion, lid reflexes) and response to stimuli using both touch and verbal stimulation (do not shout). Initially, the person will be unable to respond appropriately, but by the time they are ready to be returned to the ward they should be drowsy but easily aroused and able to answer questions fluently. Use the sedation score (e.g. AVPU) for consistency. Frequent stimulation (every five minutes or even more often) may be required. Premedications and anaesthesia can induce a degree of amnesia and disorientation. Reassure the person and orient them to time and place frequently to help alleviate anxiety. Observe for return of movement and sensation, especially if the person has received a regional, spinal or epidural anaesthetic.

Monitor dressings for haemorrhage

Inspect all dressings initially for intactness, strike-through bleeding or drainage, or frank haemorrhage. Check underneath the person's body for any pooling of either blood or drainage, since gravity will assist the liquid to the lowest point. Any haemorrhage or frank bleeding needs to be reported to the shift coordinator and the surgeon immediately. If there is a small amount of drainage or bleeding on the dressing, circle the edge of the bleeding with a pen, note the time on the dressing and monitor any additional bleeding carefully. If necessary, the operative dressing can be reinforced with additional dressing material. Most surgeons prefer that the dressing is left intact for 24 hours and not removed until they are present.

Assess fluid balance

Assessing fluid balance will be ongoing throughout the recovery period to maintain the circulating fluid volume. Initially, note the intravenous infusion solution, the amount remaining to be infused, the rate of flow (verify it is correct) and if further orders are available. The infusion site is assessed for inflammation and infiltration.

Blood transfusions may be required to replace fluid loss during surgery. Follow the policies of the facility to ensure blood compatibility. Infusion rates are adjusted to transfuse blood within four hours (red blood cell rupture [lysis] can occur if the transfusion takes longer than four hours). Consent must be checked (noted on the preoperative checklist) before initiating a blood transfusion (see **Clinical Skill 65**).

A note is made of the urinary output, whether the person is catheterised or not. If catheterised, record the amount of urine in the collection bag hourly, along with its odour, consistency, colour and concentration. A minimum output of 0.5 mL/kg/hr is expected if the cardiovascular system and fluid balance are adequate (Spencer et al., 2020). A fall in the urine output below 0.5 mL/kg/hr is reported to the shift coordinator and the surgeon. If the person is not catheterised, check the height of the bladder since general anaesthesia often affects bladder tone and causes urinary retention.

Postoperative nausea and vomiting

Postoperative nausea and vomiting (PONV) is a common complication following surgery/anaesthesia (30 to 50 per cent of people endure this [Jin, Gan & Bergese, 2020]). It is attributable to several factors: susceptibility – female, non-smoker, history of PONV or motion sickness; surgical procedures such as laparotomy and cholecystectomy; the length of surgery, the use of volatile anaesthesia, and perioperative opioid administration (Jin, Gan & Bergese, 2020). The anaesthetist will generally leave orders for an antiemetic; however, Arslan and Çelik (2023) in a systematic review found the following non-pharmacological nursing interventions to assist in the management of postoperative (up to 24 hours post-surgery) nausea and vomiting: acupuncture, aromatherapy, the oral intake of ginger, listening to music, and educating and visiting.

Other non-pharmacological interventions that can relieve PONV are repositioning and pain relief. Follow the protocol in the facility where you are gaining experience.

Continue to monitor

The person's status is monitored and the information documented on admission, then every five to 10 minutes for the first hour or until stable, and every 15 minutes until discharge from the recovery room. This is a general guideline and may differ in each facility; however, all recovery room monitoring and documentation is frequent.

Inspect and connect drainage tubes

All drainage tubes, including nasogastric tubes, are initially inspected for patency and connected to the appropriate receptacle. Thereafter, their patency (position if applicable) is checked every 10 to 15 minutes and the amount, colour, odour and consistency of the drainage documented on the postoperative chart.

Monitor specific parameters

These assessments will vary depending on the surgery and the person. Some surgical procedures require specific assessments. For instance, musculoskeletal surgery carries a high risk of compartment syndrome. Therefore, any person who has had this surgery has frequent neurovascular observations to determine the peripheral vascular and peripheral neural status (see **Clinical Skill 21**). Similarly, people who have had neurological surgery will require assessment of their neurological functioning (see **Clinical Skill 20**). A person who is a diabetic would have their blood glucose monitored frequently (see **Clinical Skill 14**).

Check the medication chart

Medications for the immediate postoperative period (e.g. analgesia, commencement of patient-controlled analgesia, antibiotics, anti-emetics) are prescribed on the medication administration sheet. Check the orders. Administer them as necessary.

Provide comfort measures

Reassurance is essential for the person's psychological comfort. Repeating that the surgery is finished, what the time is and that the person is safe provides reassurance during the early stages of recovery from anaesthetic.

Comfort measures alter as a person wakens. Pain assessment and relief is important during the postoperative recovery time. Intravenous analgesia (often opioids) is titrated carefully to maintain pain relief. This is based on an assessment of the person's pain intensity, their level of sedation and their respiratory rate. Verbal stimulation can often overcome a person's slow respiratory rate.

Good mouth care is essential during the early post-anaesthetic period as the person has been dehydrated for many hours, had their mouth open for intubation during the procedure and may have been vomiting. Also, many anaesthetics can leave a foul taste in the mouth. Mouth care can be accomplished using mouth swabs (see **Clinical Skill 56**).

Warmth is also essential for comfort and to prevent vasoconstriction and shivering. Cover the person with a warm blanket(s). Reflective blankets are not as effective as forced air warmers but are easier to use (Roshan et al., 2023). Forced air warmers circulate warm air around the person to actively warm them and increase body heating (Roshan et al., 2023). Determine what is used in the facility. Monitor the person's temperature to avoid over-warming them.

Reposition the person every 15 minutes. Assess bony prominences and areas of potential pressure injuries (see **Clinical Skill 59**). The risk of developing pressure injuries is very high until the person's vascular and motor functions return. The person may have lain on the theatre table in one position for several hours and the vascular circulation to specific areas may have been compromised. Relieving pressure from bony prominences assists the circulation. Repositioning provides comfort as well.

Discharge from the Post-anaesthetic Care Unit

Determine the stability of physiological signs prior to transfer to the unit. Use of a flow sheet improves the individual's safety (Moraes et al., 2019). The clinical criteria for discharging a person from the recovery room include, but are not limited to:

- the person is sufficiently conscious (e.g. easily aroused, able to answer simple questions), can maintain their own airway and exhibits protective airway reflexes (e.g. gag reflex, cough)
- respiratory function and good oxygenation are being maintained (e.g. SpO_2 greater than 95 per cent on room air or supplemental oxygen used to maintain saturations above 95 per cent)
- the cardiovascular system is stable with no unexpected cardiac irregularities. The specific values of pulse and blood pressure are within the person's preoperative baseline on consecutive observations
- skin colour and condition are within normal limits
- no persistent or excessive bleeding from the wound or drainage sites; dressing is intact, condition of surgical or procedural site is noted
- those with urinary catheters have an output greater than 0.5 mL/kg/hr; intake and output are within reasonable limits
- all tubes (e.g. cannulae, catheters, drains, nasogastric tubes) are patent
- pain and vomiting are controlled; the anaesthetist has prescribed suitable analgesia/anti-emetic regimens
- body temperature is at least 36 °C
- the person is able to move their limbs; peripheral pulses distal to the surgical site are present
- postoperative complications are resolved or controlled (Schick & Windle, 2021).

Most facilities use a Post-anaesthetic Discharge Scoring System to help determine whether the person is stable enough to return to the unit (or discharged home following day-surgery) – follow the policy of the facility.

CLEAN, REPLACE AND DISPOSE OF EQUIPMENT

Cleaning, replacement and disposal vary with the equipment and disposable materials used for each person. It is imperative that all necessary materials are immediately available at each bedside for use in a possible emergency. Nursing in a one-to-one situation does not permit leaving a vulnerable person to find materials and equipment. It is your responsibility to see that:

- stethoscope earpieces are cleaned (if it is a ward stethoscope), diaphragm is cleaned
- the sphygmomanometer is cleaned or the cuff replaced if there is visible soiling
- there is a thermometer and sufficient probe covers
- the cardiac monitor is cleaned and there are sufficient electrodes in case replacements are needed
- there is an intravenous fluid pole, cannulae and giving sets and commonly used fluids
- all the airway, oxygen and suctioning equipment is present, functioning and clean
- there are sufficient dressing supplies and linen available.

The trolley is stripped, cleaned and made up with fresh linen in preparation for the next person who requires anaesthetic recovery care.

HANDOVER TO WARD STAFF

A thorough handover must be given to the ward staff. They are generally notified when a person is ready to return to the ward. The ward nurse goes to the PACU to assess the person, receive a handover and transfer the person back to the ward, accompanied by an assistant or the PACU staff.

Schick and Windle (2021) state that communication is key in the safe care of people during transition from one area to another and reduces wasted time and staff frustration. The report given at this handover includes the same items addressed on entry to the PACU, plus a summary of the person's stay in the PACU. Special instructions and postoperative orders are reviewed with the ward staff. Together, you need to assess the person's level of consciousness and pain, and their ability to maintain their airway. Check that there are appropriate analgesia, anti-emetic and IV fluid orders and that the postoperative instructions are clearly documented, as the surgeon and the anaesthetist may not be available later due to the operating list. During transfer, most people remain drowsy, so ensure that safety rails are used (or safety belts snugly applied), that trolleys and beds have locked wheels and that transfer from trolley to bed is accomplished with sufficient staff to prevent injury to the person or staff.

DOCUMENTATION

Postoperative Care Unit documentation is made on specific records/flow sheets that are individual to each facility, but based on international standards.

CLINICAL SKILLS ASSESSMENT

Post-anaesthesia care and handover

Demonstrates the ability to effectively and safely provide post-anaesthetic care and deliver a complete verbal handover to or from the recovery. Incorporates the *National Safety and Quality Health Service Standards*: 3 Preventing and controlling healthcare-associated infections, 4 Medication safety, 5 Comprehensive care, 6 Communicating for safety, and 8 Recognising and responding to acute deterioration (Australian Commission on Safety and Quality in Health Care [ACSQHC], 2021).

Performance criteria	1	2	3	4	5
(Numbers indicate NMBA *Registered Nurse Standards for Practice*)	(Dependent)	(Marginal)	(Assisted)	(Supervised)	(Independent)
1. Identifies indication (1.1, 3.3, 3.4)	☐	☐	☐	☐	☐
2. Evidence of therapeutic interaction with the person, e.g. gives a clear explanation of procedure (1.4, 1.5, 2.1, 2.2, 3.2)	☐	☐	☐	☐	☐
3. Demonstrates clinical reasoning, e.g. familiarises self with anticipated complications of the person's surgical procedure (1.1, 1.2, 1.3, 4.2, 6.1)	☐	☐	☐	☐	☐
4. Gathers equipment (1.1, 5.5, 6.1): ■ stethoscope ■ sphygmomanometer ■ thermometer ■ intravenous fluid pole ■ oxygen equipment ■ suctioning equipment ■ dressing supplies ■ warm blanket ■ other equipment as indicated by the person's surgical procedure	☐	☐	☐	☐	☐
5. Performs hand hygiene (1.1, 3.4, 6.1)	☐	☐	☐	☐	☐
6. Receives a verbal handover from the anaesthetist and the theatre nurse (1.1, 2.7, 4.1, 4.2, 4.3, 6.1)	☐	☐	☐	☐	☐
7. Assesses/maintains patency of the airway, level of consciousness, fluid balance (1.1, 4.1, 4.2, 4.3, 6.1)	☐	☐	☐	☐	☐
8. Monitors vital signs, circulatory status and assesses level of consciousness (1.1, 4.1, 4.2, 4.3, 6.1)	☐	☐	☐	☐	☐
9. Inspects and connects drainage tubes, intravenous infusion, oxygen equipment, inspects dressing (1.1, 4.1, 4.2, 4.3, 6.1)	☐	☐	☐	☐	☐
10. Monitors specific parameters (1.1, 4.1, 4.2, 4.3, 6.1)	☐	☐	☐	☐	☐
11. Continues to monitor vital signs, circulatory status, fluid balance (1.1, 4.1, 4.2, 4.3, 6.1)	☐	☐	☐	☐	☐
12. Provides for comfort measures (1.1, 4.1, 4.2, 4.3, 6.1)					
13. Determines the person's stability prior to transfer (1.1, 4.1, 4.2, 4.3, 6.1)					
14. Cleans, replaces and disposes of equipment appropriately (3.6, 6.1)	☐	☐	☐	☐	☐
15. Gives a thorough handover to ward staff (1.1, 2.7, 4.1, 4.2, 4.3, 6.1)	☐	☐	☐	☐	☐
16. Maintains documentation appropriately (1.1, 1.4, 1.6, 2.2, 2.7, 3.5, 3.7, 6.1, 6.2, 6.5, 7.3)	☐	☐	☐	☐	☐
17. Demonstrates the ability to link theory to practice (1.1, 3.3, 3.4, 3.5)	☐	☐	☐	☐	☐

Student:

Clinical facilitator: Date:

CHAPTER 54

POSTOPERATIVE CARE

INDICATIONS

Postoperative care is provided following surgery and stabilisation in the Post-anaesthetic Care Unit (PACU). It includes preventing or recognising common postoperative complications and supporting the person until they regain normal physiological functioning. The effects of anaesthesia and physiological stressors place the person at risk for a variety of physiological alterations. Gao et al. (2024) found anticipatory nursing (i.e. being aware of what happened during surgery and what complications – physical and psychological – may arise) provides appropriate nursing care perioperatively to reduce the incidence of complications and improve surgical outcomes.

Postoperative care is divided into two phases. Initial care occurs in the PACU (or Intensive Care Unit [ICU]). This phase extends until the person has regained consciousness and is physiologically stable (see **Clinical Skill 53**). The second phase is the postoperative convalescent phase, extending from transfer from the PACU to the nursing ward until the person is discharged. This Clinical Skill deals with the second phase. The information contained here is generic and you will need to adapt it to specific situations.

Each facility has policies and procedures for postoperative care. Many surgeons have specific postoperative protocols. Ensure you are familiar with both, preferably before the person goes to surgery, but at least before they return to the unit. This Clinical Skill is written for inpatient postoperative care, and adaptation is required for people undergoing day surgery.

EVIDENCE OF THERAPEUTIC INTERACTION

Reassure the person that surgery is over and they are safely back in their bed. Tell the person (and their family) when you have completed all necessary nursing care. Assure them that you will be checking the person frequently until their condition is stable and this is a routine occurrence post-surgery. Describe how often you will monitor them and the purpose of the equipment being used, since unfamiliar sights provoke anxiety. Tell the family that the person may be drowsy for several hours. Leave the side-rails up and the call bell securely attached and within reach. The surgeon will attend (usually at the end of the theatre day) to inform the person (and family if appropriate) of the outcome of their surgical procedure.

DEMONSTRATE CLINICAL REASONING

Postoperative care begins preoperatively with adequate teaching and support, which are ongoing until the person is transferred to the operating theatre (OT) (see **Clinical Skill 52**).

Prepare for the person's return from the operating theatre

Prepare the person's unit as soon as they leave for the OT, so it is not forgotten during the daily care of others. The bed unit is prepared to receive the person, including the following:

- Clear the room to allow easier manoeuvring of the trolley.
- Use fresh linen to make a postoperative bed (open) to reduce possible contamination of the fresh wound. Provide extra blankets to ensure the person remains warm.
- Add absorption pads to the bed. These can be changed more easily than all the linen (if soiled by blood or antiseptic solutions), meaning less disturbance to the person.
- Adjust the bed to trolley height to help transfer the person from the theatre trolley.
- Clear the top of the bedside locker of personal material for placing equipment onto (e.g. pulse oximeters) in anticipation of an emergent situation.
- Wrap an emesis bag and Guedel's airway in a hand towel and place it on the bedside locker.
- Ensure a sphygmomanometer, stethoscope and pulse oximeter are at the bedside.

ELDER CARE

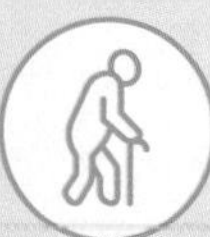

Due to the physiological changes of ageing, altered reaction to pharmacotherapy from renal and hepatic decline, altered neurological functioning and decreased tolerance to stress, elderly people are more prone to postoperative complications (e.g. delirium, dehydration, infections, falls, functional decline, pressure injuries). Care is organised to improve comfort, reduce complications and shorten the length of hospital stay. Care focuses on:

- early ambulation (with assistive devices if necessary) and verticalisation, providing thromboembolism deterrents (antiembolism stockings, TEDs)
- actively assessing cardiovascular, respiratory and cognitive functioning
- providing adequate and timely pain management; management of nausea and vomiting
- promoting oral fluid therapy to decrease time on parenteral fluids, minimising the use of nasogastric tubes, reducing the use of urinary catheters
- early return to optimal nutrition, attention to oral care and use of dentures as needed
- promoting sleep hygiene and minimising restraint use (if used at all)
- supporting the person's ability to self-care and plan for home care
- preventing pressure area injury
- assisting with family participation (adapted from Aceto et al., 2020; Wang et al., 2020; Wolfe, Wolfe & Rich, 2020).

Postoperative delirium (POD) is a frequent complication for elderly people that contributes to their functional decline. POD encompasses confusion, perceptual and cognitive deficits, sleep disturbance, fluctuating levels of consciousness, disorganised thinking and altered attention levels (Jovanovic, Lađevic & Sipetic Grujicic, 2023; Kirfel et al., 2023). It can occur immediately postoperatively, and last from a few hours to five or more days (Kirfel et al., 2023). Wang et al. (2020) found that tailored family-involved care of the person postoperatively decreased POD significantly. Family-involved care encouraged the family to provide much of the non-professional care (assistance with feeding, hygiene, walking, companionship). POD decreased, physical and cognitive functioning was maintained or increased and length of hospital stay shortened.

Communication is key to good care. Avoid using a condescending tone or language (e.g. diminutives such as 'lovey' or 'Gramps'). Treat the elderly person with respect (Kotomska & Michalak, 2019).

THE PERSON LIVING WITH SEVERE OBESITY

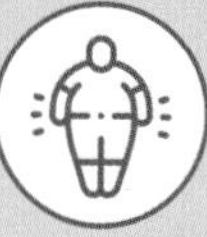

Severely obese people are at high risk of post-operative complications. Open surgery is fraught with wound infection, and keyhole surgery wounds can also become infected. Healthcare education on wound care and identification of potential complications is crucial when people are being discharged early postoperatively (Mackenzie & Nosib, 2023). The severely obese person will likely be transferred to and from theatre on their own bed. If not, a lift and sufficient help will be necessary to move them from the trolley to their bed. The head of the bed will be raised.

Postoperatively, the person will require oxygen saturation assessment continuously (Royal College of Anaesthetists, 2019) due to potential respiratory insufficiency from abdominal adiposity pressing on the diaphragm. Continuous positive airway pressure may be needed. Sleep apnoea is a common problem (Carron et al., 2020). Coughing and deep breathing with abdominal support will assist in removing the anaesthetic gases and mobilising any fluid in the lungs. Skin and wound assessment are imperative – look for signs of pressure injuries and dehiscence due to increased pressure of excess tissue. Wound infections due to poor circulation and underlying chronic diseases (e.g. diabetes mellitus, congestive cardiac failure, hypertension) are common – assess closely for local and systemic signs of infection. Early mobilisation is necessary, as deep vein thrombosis is common due to immobility, poor circulation and increased viscosity of the blood (increased red blood cells [RBCs] due to respiratory insufficiency). The large-sized thromboembolism deterrent (TED) stockings needed must be ordered ahead. Use mechanical and electronic lifts and hoists to help the person to stand, and ensure there are enough staff to safely assist the person to walk. Short walks (a few metres) are all that can be tolerated initially. If the surgery is for gastric banding, the person is assisted to consume 15 to 30 mL of fluids every 15 minutes to minimise nausea and vomiting and maintain hydration. See also **Clinical Skills 15 and 23** for more information on issues of people living with severe obesity.

- Place an IV stand (attached to the bed or free-standing) ready for use.
- Have extra pillows available to support the person in appropriate positions.
- Obtain personal hygiene equipment to meet the person's hygiene needs efficiently.
- Place oxygen supplies (nasal prongs/mask, tubing, an oxygen cylinder if piped oxygen is unavailable) at the bedside.
- Make available the required charting records and flow sheets, such as vital signs, fluid balance and Adult Deterioration Detection System (ADDS) sheets.

Other supplies and equipment are added as required (e.g. suction machines, continuous range of motion machines). Estimate the time the person will return and plan the care of other people, allowing for the extra time needed to care for an acute postoperative person.

PERFORM POSTOPERATIVE CARE

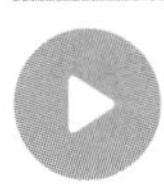
Video

Postoperative care is directed towards preventing the foreseeable complications that can follow surgery and anaesthesia. Individualise care, including attending to pain relief, comfort, allaying anxiety and teaching as needed to decrease negative emotions (fear, anger, depression), pain levels and length of stay, and increase health knowledge and satisfaction with care (Du et al., 2019; Gao et al., 2024).

Situational awareness is important. Vigilance, assessment and monitoring are paramount in assuring the person's safety.

Hand hygiene

Hand hygiene (see **Clinical Skill 5**) is an extremely important standard precaution to reduce the transfer of microorganisms. The post-surgical person is vulnerable to infection because of impaired skin integrity and diminished protective mechanisms in the respiratory system from the effects of anaesthesia.

Immediate postoperative care

Transfer the person to the bed

Safety

If the person returns to the unit on a trolley rather than on their own bed, they are transferred using sufficient staff (and equipment [e.g. mechanical lift if necessary]) to maintain their safety and to minimise muscle strain of the staff. Explain each step before it occurs to reduce the person's anxiety and to coordinate the move. Oxygen is immediately attached to the wall unit or oxygen cylinder to maintain the required flow. Intravenous (IV) fluid is hung on the IV stand (on the same side as the insertion site) to prevent dislodging the cannula if it is left on the trolley pole. Drainage tubes (urine, wound drainage, nasogastric, chest) are identified and attended (e.g. catheter bag is unhooked from the trolley, chest tube drainage is kept upright and often has one staff member responsible for this). The person is moved as a unit, using the trolley sheet, slide sheets and a pat slide to reduce friction and lessen the trauma of the move. Ensure that all drainage tubes are moved with the person.

Assess the postoperative person

Safety

A thorough assessment is performed immediately on return to the unit (see **Clinical Skill 53**). Identify the person (ID band and chart comparison). The person's baseline information and previous medical condition should be known to you from preoperative care. Check the nature of their surgery and any complications that occurred during surgery so that the more likely complications can be anticipated. These will have been covered in the PACU nurse's handover prior to the person's discharge from there. If not already established, initiate the appropriate ADDS flow sheet, an intake and output sheet and other documentation as needed (e.g. Glasgow Coma Scale, Neurovascular Observation sheet).

The assessment includes the following (remember to LOOK, LISTEN and FEEL):

- level of consciousness (reorientate as needed), degree of sedation
- respiratory rate (the most sensitive indicator of postoperative haemorrhage)
- airway patency, breath sounds, respiratory depth and presence of dyspnoea or orthopnoea, chest movement is observed for equal bilateral expansion; note any artificial airway, mechanical ventilator and settings
- blood pressure (cuff or arterial), pulse (apical, peripheral, cardiac monitor pattern) and temperature – hypothermia delays healing and increases the risk of surgical site infection
- oxygen saturation level (pulse oximeter)
- pain assessment
- pressure readings – central venous, arterial blood, pulmonary artery wedge and intracranial pressure as indicated
- position of the person during surgery
- condition and colour of the skin, especially on the area where the person was positioned during surgery
- circulation – peripheral pulses and sensation of extremities as applicable
- condition and location of dressings, and condition of the suture line if no dressing
- type and patency of drainage tubes, catheters and reservoirs as applicable, amount and type of drainage
- muscle strength and response
- pupillary response as indicated
- fluid therapy and hydration, location of cannulae and lines, type, amount and rate of solution infusing
- effects of anaesthesia (general, regional or local)
- level of emotional and physical comfort (e.g. reports of nausea or vomiting)
- postoperative instructions (e.g. a specific position, such as 'elevate leg on Braun pillow') implemented.

If the person is restless, there is something wrong (World Health Organization, 2003).

Position the person

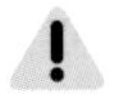
Safety

Place the person in the recovery position (supported on their left side with head extended) to minimise the chances of aspiration (unless contraindicated [e.g. neck surgery]). As consciousness increases and they can protect their own airway, position the person for comfort, maintaining correct body alignment to avoid stressing the incision and to increase comfort and relaxation. Take the surgical procedure and their underlying condition into account.

Check and connect any drainage tubes to the appropriate appliance and maintain patency.

Carry out nursing actions indicated during assessment

Depending on your assessment, specific care is a priority. For example, the dressing may have fresh bleeding and need to be reinforced. If there is just a little blood, mark the extent with a pen and monitor it. If there is a great deal, reinforce the dressing (document and report it to the shift coordinator) and monitor it closely. Early haemorrhage is a common and serious complication occurring as the person's blood pressure returns to normal or becomes hypertensive (e.g. with vomiting), or if a ligature slips or a clot dislodges. Monitor the drains and wound sites for the quantity, quality and nature of drainage.

Monitor fluid intake and output to assess fluid balance. If the person has no indwelling catheter, ask about their need to void. Anaesthetics and analgesia depress the sensation of bladder fullness. Other medications used in the theatre may affect the bladder tone temporarily. Palpate the bladder or calculate bladder volume, using a portable bladder ultrasound scan, to determine urinary retention. Offer a bedpan or urinal, or if more than four hours post-operation and the person is stable, assist to stand at the bedside (or use a commode) to void.

Assess for pain using a 10-point pain scale and careful questioning to determine the source of the pain. Do not assume the pain is due to surgical intervention – it may be due to positioning during surgery or the endotracheal tube or a medical condition (e.g. arthritis). Administer prescribed analgesia and reassess after pain-relieving interventions. Failure to do so signals poor nursing care and can result in higher levels of pain and discomfort. In a postoperative person, the sudden onset of severe pain associated with altered vital signs needs a comprehensive and immediate reassessment of possible complications (e.g. wound dehiscence, pulmonary embolus).

Monitor the person

Safety

It is your professional responsibility to understand the significance of these observations and to keep track of changes. The person's survival may depend on your recognition of the significance of an observation and your decision to call for assistance. Surgical units will have an ADDS chart for the person returning from OT. This assists you to determine any deterioration in observations (the vital signs, pain levels, dressing/drain and drainage assessment and incision assessment, oxygen saturation and fluid status) and guides interventions for any disturbed physiological values. Be sure to assess the person as a whole as well, observing colour, activity level, engagement with others and level of comfort. Other observations are determined by the person's procedure and condition.

Ongoing monitoring occurs according to hospital protocol. Most protocols suggest quarter-hourly observations for one hour, half-hourly observations for two hours, hourly observations for four hours and four-hourly observations for 24 hours as long as the person's condition remains stable. Monitoring is close in the initial 24 hours as changes in baseline measures can reveal the early onset of complications. General postoperative complications of the following systems include:

- *respiratory* – atelectasis, pneumonia, hypoxia, pulmonary embolism
- *cardiovascular* – haemorrhage, hypovolaemic shock, embolism, thrombophlebitis, dysrhythmias
- *gastrointestinal* – abdominal distension from paralytic ileus, constipation, nausea and vomiting
- *genitourinary* – urinary retention, fluid imbalance, acute renal failure (from hypo-perfusion)
- *integumentary* – wound infection, dehiscence or evisceration, pressure injuries
- *nervous* – intractable pain, postoperative cognitive decline in the elderly (postoperative delirium results in increased morbidity).

Complications occur quickly in the early postoperative period. Again, there are specific complications to be aware of for many surgical procedures. The person's condition and the surgery performed determine the assessment criteria to be monitored.

Provide comfort measures

Discomfort is frequent following surgery and anaesthesia. Pain, nausea, anxiety, frequent sleep interruptions, cold and shivering, sore throat from intubation, pressure from lying too long and many other uncomfortable sensations contribute.

Administer pain relief

Providing comfort is one of the most important aspects of nursing care post-surgery because unresolved pain inhibits the immune system, causes the release of catecholamines, respiratory dysfunction (increased secretions and tachypnoea), cardiovascular dysfunction (hypertension and tachycardia), restlessness, anxiety, insomnia and anorexia (Kehlet, 2018), and interferes with recovery by impeding coughing and deep-breathing exercises, mobilisation and nutrition (deBoer, 2020). Pain control/elimination is paramount, as severe acute pain after surgery increases the risk of chronic pain (deBoer, 2020; Horn & Kramer, 2022). Pain is considered the fifth vital sign for assessment. That is, the presence or absence of pain is assessed each time the vital signs are obtained, whenever the person reports pain or after interventions to manage the pain. Do not assume that the pain results from surgery. Sometimes throat pain from the endotracheal tube, or arthritic pain from lying still, or leg cramps are more difficult to bear than the surgical pain. Assess carefully.

Analgesia is administered on a regular schedule for the first 24 to 48 hours postoperatively and then diminished to an as-required pro re nata (PRN) administration. Analgesia is often self-administered by patient-controlled analgesia (PCA-IV), resulting in better pain control and greater satisfaction (Pastino & Lakra, 2023). Newer, multimodal self-administered analgesics (e.g. sublingual sufentanil) offer more pain control. (See **Clinical Skills 13 and 50**.)

Analgesia is administered intravenously, intramuscularly, subcutaneously and, after nausea has diminished, orally or sublingually. Multimodal analgesia is being used more frequently to reduce the use of opioids (Echeverria-Villalobos et al., 2020; Pastino & Lakra, 2023).

> If analgesia is administered, you must assess the effect and the tolerability of the analgesia (e.g. the development of nausea, vomiting, pruritus, sedation, urinary retention) as well as its administration.
> Any unexpected effect of the analgesia requires assessment and attention.

Inform the shift coordinator if insufficient pain relief is obtained.

Administration of analgesia is an important aspect of providing comfort, but it is not the only intervention that is of assistance. Reassure and orient the person, who may be unaware that surgery has been performed, in which case their pain is even more frightening. Maintaining comfort is fostered by distraction, splinting of the incision, positioning, massage of cramped muscles, guided imagery, attention to personal hygiene, activity (e.g. to reduce lower bowel distension), attention to tubing, positional changes or sometimes just by your presence.

Position the person

Positions of comfort are determined by the surgery. Following breast surgery, some relief is obtained from raising the back support 20 to 40 degrees. People with abdominal or gynaecological surgery can be more comfortable lying on their sides. Elevating affected limbs to reduce swelling where appropriate can reduce pain. A semi-Fowler's position is comfortable for those who have had thoracic surgery.

Assist with personal hygiene

Personal hygiene is an important comfort measure. When the person's temperature is normal, and within six hours post-operation, sponge (or bath in a bag) and change the person out of theatre clothes. This removes the antiseptic solution and blood, stimulates the circulation and assists the person to relax. It also provides you with an opportunity to thoroughly inspect the skin and assist the person to actively mobilise. Administer analgesia prior to a sponge bath.

Mouth care is essential because anaesthetics and oxygen dry mucous membranes; nil by mouth (NBM) status for several hours and anaesthetic medications leave an objectionable taste in the mouth. Assist the person to brush their teeth and rinse their mouth (see **Clinical Skill 56**).

Provide warmth

Monitor the person's temperature because of the cold-inducing effects of anaesthesia (decreased metabolic rate, depression of the heat-regulating centre), vasodilatation, the low environmental temperature in the theatre, an open body cavity during surgery and the length of the surgical procedure. Warmth is a comfort measure immediately following surgery. A Bair Hugger or reflective blankets are usually sufficient to restore normal body temperature.

Reorient

Some people require reorientation to place and time following anaesthesia and may need to be told a few times that the surgery is over and they are safe. Having family with them following surgery is important and reassuring.

Encourage postoperative activity and exercise

Movement assists to increase chest expansion, mobilise secretions and promote respiratory function. It also promotes fluid balance, cardiovascular stability and a return of normal gastrointestinal function.

Begin by turning the person with their active assistance every two hours. Remind them about deep breathing/coughing (as indicated), supervise leg exercises hourly and assist them to sit out of bed at the earliest opportunity (incorporating individual circumstances). When the person is sitting at the bedside and/or ambulating, encourage them to keep the thorax in straight alignment, while breathing deeply. The diaphragm is more easily able to expand and the intercostal muscles are used. Sitting or standing enhances ventilation to areas of the lungs that are dependent when the person is supine. This promotes maximal inflation and increases gas exchange. Deep-breathing, coughing and incentive spirometer exercises are done (unless contraindicated [e.g. eye surgery]) two-hourly (have the person splint the incision firmly with a pillow).

TED stockings reduce the incidence of thromboembolism and are fitted individually for most people undergoing surgery (unless contraindicated) (Gee, 2019). TED stockings provide graduated compression to increase velocity of blood flow and increase venous return (contributes to maintaining the intima of the veins and preventing clot formation). If the person is wearing them, check the neurovascular status of their legs and the fit (no wrinkles or roll-overs) two-hourly and remove the stockings at least daily, to clean and inspect the skin. The leg exercises taught preoperatively are encouraged two-hourly. Encourage early ambulation with increased distances each time.

These nursing actions help to prevent postoperative complications (e.g. hypostatic pneumonia, atelectasis, abdominal distension, thrombosis and embolism). They also help the person to become independent and raise their self-esteem.

All postoperative activity is individual and depends on the person's condition and the surgery performed. Knowledge of the surgery/incision helps you to answer questions, reinforce the surgeon's instructions, assist the person to splint the incision and perform the most effective exercises.

Institute fluids, nutrition and elimination patterns

Healing requires appropriate hydration and nutrients. These help the body return to normal functioning. Individuals usually return from the theatre with an intravenous cannula in situ to administer fluids. They are often dehydrated because of the NBM status, fluid loss during surgery, renal retention of sodium and water from stress, and insensible losses caused by high temperatures. They are assessed for electrolyte imbalance. Maintain the IV infusion patency and the rate of the ordered fluid. An IV infusion may be necessary for hours or days, until the person is able to take sufficient fluids by mouth to maintain fluid balance.

Fluid balance includes measuring and recording all fluid intake (IV, blood products, volume expanders, oral and enteral fluids) and output (drainage, stoma drainage, vomitus, nasogastric tube output, bladder irrigations as well as urine). Also observe the nature of all drainage, aspirate and faeces to detect any abnormality following surgery (e.g. a breakdown in anastomosis). Maintain a fluid balance sheet until the person is taking oral fluids freely (2000+ mL/day unless contraindicated) and their voiding pattern has returned to normal (minimum of 1500 mL/day).

A variety of factors are related to postoperative nausea and vomiting (PONV), including anaesthetic agents, opioids, hypotension, abdominal surgery, pain, female, non-smoker and a history of migraine or postoperative nausea and vomiting. PONV can significantly delay recovery and impede convalescence (Kranke, Wilhelm & Eberhart, 2020). Administer intravenous anti-emetics as ordered and monitor their effectiveness. Nutrition is an important consideration perioperatively to counteract the effects of surgery on glucose and protein metabolism (Bongers, Dejong & Dulk, 2020).

Introduce oral fluids cautiously, to reduce the risk of aspiration-related lung injury. Ice chips are offered first because the small quantity of fluid in them is less likely to induce nausea than a larger amount of water. When ice chips are tolerated, clear fluids are offered first as sips, then as desired. Individuals progress to full fluids and onto a normal diet as they tolerate each step.

Often, 'gas cramps' or tympanitis (abdominal distension, gas pains and absence of bowel sounds) becomes a problem from slowed gastrointestinal tract motility from anaesthesia, or handling of the bowel during surgery. Mobilise the person as quickly as possible. Avoid using a straw, and provide clear fluids at room temperature. Gum chewing (sugar free, of course) may help (Douligeris et al., 2023).

Unless contraindicated, a diet high in protein (for tissue repair and healing) and high in carbohydrate (for energy) and vitamins C and D will assist tissue formation. Following major abdominal surgery, a nasogastric tube (NGT) is often in situ to decompress the stomach and to prevent nausea and vomiting. It remains in place until peristalsis returns (bowel sounds present and flatus passed), after which diet progresses through clear fluids to a normal diet. Any further nausea and vomiting indicate abdominal distension and the NGT is reinserted. If the person cannot tolerate an oral diet or if there was preoperative malnutrition, collaborate with a dietitian in the selection of appropriate supplementary drinks or parenteral feeding.

Urinary elimination

Urinary output is measured hourly if the person's condition is unstable. An output of less than 0.5 mL/kg/hr indicates insufficient fluid replacement or an acute renal disease and must be reported to the shift coordinator.

The elimination of urine following surgery is often delayed due to dehydration, or the effects of anaesthetic medications. Epidural or spinal anaesthetics contribute to urinary retention. People usually resume a normal pattern of voiding within eight hours of non-urinary tract surgery, and assuming normal fluid replacement. If not, assess the bladder volume using a portable bladder ultrasound scan or palpate the bladder for fullness. If the bladder is distended, assist the person to toilet, provide privacy and other measures to initiate voiding. An order to catheterise may be necessary.

Some people may need an indwelling catheter (IDC) for 24 to 48 hours, until all medications have cleared the system and bladder tone is restored. Many surgeries require the person to have an IDC inserted in theatre and removed when the surgeon orders. An IDC requires care during insertion (see **Clinical Skill 36**) and ongoing care to minimise the possibility of a bladder infection. Urinary catheters are generally avoided if possible.

Bowel elimination

Bowels are usually sluggish following major surgery due to the combination of fasting, dehydration and medications, and if the bowel is manipulated, peristalsis temporarily ceases. When bowel sounds return, oral intake may resume. It often takes two to three days before bowel function returns to normal after non-abdominal surgery, longer following any manipulation of the bowel. Some people are reluctant to use the Valsalva manoeuvre or 'bear down' to evacuate stool because of the increased incisional pain. Judicious use of analgesia and firm incisional splinting are required (e.g. holding a pillow firmly against the incision). Sometimes, assistance to evacuate the bowels is needed. Initially, oral medications such as psyllium or stool softeners are prescribed, progressing to more irritating medications such as senna-based preparations. Microlax enemas may be ordered.

Wound healing

Healing takes 10 to 14 days after most surgeries. Until the wound is sealed (24 to 48 hours), a dressing is required to protect the tissue from further injury or contamination. Your responsibility includes using strict aseptic technique, keeping the wound clean and dry, assessing for improvement or deterioration and reporting its condition to relevant staff (Boga, 2019). Dressings are often done daily (see **Clinical Skills 67 to 70**) following the surgeon's visit (they will inspect the incision), although this practice is changing with the use of new types of dressings (often left in situ for several days).

Discharge teaching

Planning for discharge commences when the person enters hospital and includes the person's family or significant other. It is dependent on the individual, the surgery performed and the surgeon's protocol. Instructions about self-care and emergency medical care are given verbally and reinforced with written material. Discharge teaching (see **Clinical Skill 27**) includes but is not restricted to:

- guidelines concerning self-care for the specific surgery
- activity and increases in activity
- medication and treatment reviews
- dressing and wound care
- signs of complications and who to contact if they arise
- an appointment for follow-up, with the relevant telephone numbers.

CLEAN, REPLACE AND DISPOSE OF EQUIPMENT

This is ongoing and diverse. Keep the person's bed area clean and tidy. Remove equipment that is no longer required (e.g. Guedel's airway, emesis bag, oxygen masks) and dispose of and replace disposable equipment as necessary. Use the appropriate waste and linen hampers for contaminated materials as necessary. Perform hand hygiene.

DOCUMENTATION

Flow sheets (ADDS) of respiratory rate, temperature, pulse, blood pressure, level of consciousness and oxygen saturation are used to detect the initial signs of deterioration so intervention can be initiated quickly. A notation of each nursing assessment and intervention and the person's response to the intervention is added to the notes or eHealth record when it occurs. Generally, the initial postoperative report includes the following:

- the time the person returned to the ward
- their level of consciousness and orientation
- the vital signs and oxygen saturation
- their level of activity
- their ability to perform effective coughing, deep-breathing and leg exercises
- a pain assessment
- time, type and amount of pain medication administered; its effectiveness, any adverse effects observed
- other interventions to resolve the person's pain and the effectiveness of these
- condition of the dressings and drainage and patency of any drainage devices (e.g. wound drains, chest tubes)
- fluid replacement (type, rate and amount) and fluid balance status
- monitoring equipment (e.g. electrocardiograph), plus a readout, as appropriate.

Documentation will be specific for each type of surgery (e.g. orthopaedic surgery often requires neurovascular observations or a continuous movement machine) and for each facility – or even each unit within a facility. Familiarise yourself with the documentation required.

CLINICAL SKILLS ASSESSMENT

Postoperative care

Demonstrates the ability to effectively and safely care for a person following an operating theatre experience. Incorporates the *National Safety and Quality Health Service Standards*: 2 Partnering with consumers, 3 Preventing and controlling healthcare-associated infections, 4 Medication safety, 5 Comprehensive care, 6 Communicating for safety, and 8 Recognising and responding to acute deterioration (Australian Commission on Safety and Quality in Health Care [ACSQHC], 2021).

Performance criteria	**1**	**2**	**3**	**4**	**5**
(Numbers indicate NMBA *Registered Nurse Standards for Practice*)	**(Dependent)**	**(Marginal)**	**(Assisted)**	**(Supervised)**	**(Independent)**
1. Identifies indication (1.1, 3.3, 3.4)	☐	☐	☐	☐	☐
2. Evidence of therapeutic interaction with the person, e.g. gives the person a clear explanation of the procedure (1.4, 1.5, 2.1, 2.2, 3.2)	☐	☐	☐	☐	☐
3. Demonstrates clinical reasoning, e.g. prepares the environment (1.1, 1.2, 1.3, 4.2, 6.1)	☐	☐	☐	☐	☐
4. Performs hand hygiene (1.1, 3.4, 6.1)	☐	☐	☐	☐	☐
5. Assists with immediate postoperative assessment and care, e.g. transfers the person to bed and attaches in situ equipment (1.1, 4.1, 4.2, 4.3, 6.1, 7.3)	☐	☐	☐	☐	☐
6. Completes required nursing interventions (1.1, 6.1, 6.5)	☐	☐	☐	☐	☐
7. Monitors the person according to hospital protocol (1.1, 4.1, 4.2, 4.3, 6.1)	☐	☐	☐	☐	☐
8. Provides comfort measures (1.1, 4.1, 4.2, 4.3, 6.1)	☐	☐	☐	☐	☐
9. Encourages postoperative activity and exercise (1.1, 4.1, 4.2, 4.3, 6.1)	☐	☐	☐	☐	☐
10. Institutes fluids, nutrition and elimination patterns (1.1, 4.1, 4.2, 4.3, 6.1, 7.1)	☐	☐	☐	☐	☐
11. Provides wound care (1.1, 6.1, 7.1)	☐	☐	☐	☐	☐
12. Implements discharge teaching (1.1, 1.6, 3.2, 6.1)	☐	☐	☐	☐	☐
13. Cleans, replaces and disposes of equipment appropriately (3.6, 6.1)	☐	☐	☐	☐	☐
14. Documents relevant information (1.1, 1.4, 1.6, 2.2, 2.7, 3.5, 3.7, 6.1, 6.2, 6.5, 7.3)	☐	☐	☐	☐	☐
15. Demonstrates the ability to link theory to practice (1.1, 3.3, 3.4, 3.5)	☐	☐	☐	☐	☐

Student:

Clinical facilitator: Date:

REFERENCES

Abate, S., Chekol, Y. & Basu, B. (2020). Global prevalence and determinants of preoperative anxiety among surgical patients: A systematic review and meta-analysis. *International Journal of Surgery Open*, *25*, 6–16. https://doi.org/10.1016/j.ijso.2020.05.010

Aceto, P., Antonelli Incalzi, R., Bettelli, G., Carron, M., Chiumiento, F., Cocione, A., Crucitti, A., Maggi, S., Montorsi, M., Pace, M., Petrini, F., Tommasiino, C., Travucchi, M. & Volpato, S. (2020). Perioperative management of elderly patients (PriME): Recommendations from an Italian intersociety consensus. *Aging Clinical and Experimental Research*, *32*, 1647–73. https://doi.org/10.1007/s40520-020-01624-x

Al-dardery, N., Abdelwahab, O., El-Samahy, M., Seif, A., Mouffokes, A. & Khaity, A. (2023). Self-warming blankets versus active warming by forced-air devices for preventing hypothermia: A systematic review and meta-analysis. *Medicine (Baltimore)*, *102*(18), e33579. https://doi.org/10.1097/MD.0000000000033579

Álvarez-García, C. & Yaban, Z. (2020). The effects of preoperative guided imagery interventions on preoperative anxiety and postoperative pain: A meta-analysis. *Complementary Therapies in Clinical Practice*, *38*, 101077. https://doi.org/10.1016/j.ctcp.2019.101077

American Society of Anaesthesiologists (ASA) (2023). *Post-operative risks: Age*. https://www.asahq.org/madeforthismoment/preparing-for-surgery/risks/age

An, D. & Wong, J. (2020). Improving surgical outcomes and patient health: Perioperative smoking cessation interventions. *Current Anesthesiology Reports*, *10*, 12–18. https://doi.org/10.1007/s40140-020-00370-0

An, X., Wang, Q., Qiu, Y., Zhu, Z., Ma, Z., Hua, W. & Li, X. (2020). Nursing interventions of intraoperative malignant hyperthermia in patients with scoliosis: A report of 3 cases. *Journal of Neuroscience Nursing*, *52*(2), 66–71. https://doi.org/10.1097/JNN.0000000000000496

Arpag, N. & Öztekin, S. (2023). The effect of visits by operating room nurses before cardiac surgery on anxiety and pain management. *Journal of PeriAnesthesia Nursing*. https://doi.org/10.1016/j.jopan.2023.01.022

Arslan, H. & Çelik, S. (2023). Nonpharmacological nursing interventions in postoperative nausea and vomiting: A systematic review. *Journal of PeriAnesthesia Nursing*, *39*(1), 142–54. . https://doi.org/10.1016/j.jopan.2023.06.096

Ashoobi, M., Shakiba, M., Keshavarzmotamed, A. & Ashraf, A. (2023). Prevalence of postoperative hypothermia in the post-anesthesia care unit. *Anesthesia and Pain Medicine*, *13*(5), e136730. https://doi.org/10.5812/aapm-136730

Assefa, M., Chekol, W., Melesse, D., Nigatu, Y. & Bizuneh, Y. (2022). Incidence and risk factors of emergence delirium in elderly patients after general or spinal anesthesia for both elective and emergency surgery. *Annals of Medicine and Surgery*, *84*, 104959. https://doi.org/10.1016/j.amsu.2022.104959

Australian Commission on Safety and Quality in Health Care (ACSQHC) (2021). *National safety and quality health service standards* (3rd ed.). Sydney, NSW: ACSQHC.

Bashaw, M. (2016). Guideline implementation: Preventing hypothermia. *American Operating Room Nurse's Journal*, *103*(3), 304–13. https://doi.org/10.1016/j.aorn.2016.01.009

Boga, S. (2019). Nursing practices in the prevention of post-operative wound infection in accordance with evidence-based approach. *International Journal of Caring Sciences*, *12*(2), 1–8. https://search.proquest.com/docview/2303668811?accountid=88802

Bongers, B., Dejong, C. & Dulk, M. (2020). Enhanced recovery after surgery programmes in older patients undergoing hepatopancreatobiliary surgery: What benefits might prehabilitation have? *European Journal of Surgical Oncology*, *47*(3), 551–9. https://doi.org/10.1016/j.ejso.2020.03.211

Brathwaite, B. M. (2023). Nursing considerations in management of geriatric patients. In P. Petrone & C. E. Brathwaite (eds), *Acute care surgery in geriatric patients*. Cham, Switzerland: Springer. https://doi.org/10.1007/978-3-031-30651-8_56

Brunette, G. & Miller, C. (2023). Is it time to put pressure on informed consent? A view from here. *Journal of Wound, Ostomy and Continence Nursing*, *50*(5), 361–2. https://doi.org/10.1097/WON.0000000000001018

Caalim, A. (2020). *Preoperative and intraoperative interventions for enhanced recovery after gynecological surgery*. University of Maryland PhD dissertation. https://archive.hshsl.umaryland.edu/bitstream/handle/10713/12937/Caalim_Enhanced%20RecoveryAftGynecologicalSurgery_2020.pdf?sequence=1&isAllowed=y

Carli, F. & Baldini, G. (2021). From preoperative assessment to preoperative optimization of frail older patients. *European Journal of Surgical Oncology*, *47*(3 A), 519–23. https://doi.org/10.1016/j.ejso.2020.06.011

Carron, M., Safaee Fakhr, B., Leppariello, G. & Foletto, M. (2020). Perioperative care of the obese patient. *British Journal of Surgery*, *107*(2), e39–e55. https://doi.org/10.1002/bjs.11447

Cate, D., Sabajo, C., Bongers, B. & Slooter, G. (2023). Prehabilitation in elective oncological colorectal surgery enhances preoperative fitness: A single center prospective real-world data analysis. *European Journal of Surgical Oncology*, *49*(2), e139. https://doi.org/10.1016/j.ejso.2022.11.395

Chernyak, M. & Posten, C. (2022). Quality of care improvement: A process to standardize handoff communication between anesthesia providers and post-anesthesia care unit nurses. *Doctor of Nursing Practice Scholarly Projects*, *2*. LaSalle University, Philadelphia, PA, USA. https://digitalcommons.lasalle.edu/dnp_scholarly_projects/2

Dale, A. (2020). *Improving glycemic control for post-orthopedic surgery patients with type 2 diabetes*. Doctoral dissertation, Walden University, ProQuest Dissertations Publishing. 27964708.

deBoer, H. (2020). Post operative multimodal pain management. In D. Ljungqvist, N. Francis & R. Urman (eds), *Enhanced recovery after surgery (ERAS)*. Cham, Switzerland: Springer.

DeLaune, S., Ladner, P., McTier, L. & Tollefson, J. (2024). *Fundamentals of nursing: Standards and practice* (Australia & New Zealand 3rd ed.). South Melbourne, VIC: Cengage Learning.

Douligeris, A., Diakosavvas, M., Kathopoulis, N., Kypriotis, K., Mortaki, A., Angelou, K., Chatzipapas, I. & Protopapas, A. (2023). The effect of postoperative gum chewing on gastrointestinal function following laparoscopic gynecological surgery. A meta-analysis of randomized controlled trials. *Journal of Minimally Invasive Gynecology*, *30*(10), 783–96. https://doi.org/10.1016/j.jmig.2023.06.015

Du, C., Li, H., Qu, L., Li, Y. & Bao, X. (2019). Personalized nursing care improves psychological health, quality of life, and postoperative recovery of patients in the general surgery department. *International Journal of Clinical and Experimental Medicine*, *12*(7), 9090–6. http://www.ijcem.com/files/ijcem0091691.pdf

Echeverria-Villalobos, M., Stoicea, N., Todeschini, A., Fioda-Diaz, J., Uribe, A., Weaver, T. & Bergese, S. (2020). Enhanced recovery after surgery (ERAS): A perspective review of postoperative pain management under ERAS pathways and its role on opioid crisis in the United States. *Clinical Journal of Pain*, *36*(3), 219–26. https://doi.org/10.1097/AJP.0000000000000792

Enhanced Recovery After Surgery Society (2020). *Guidelines*. https://erassociety.org/guidelines/list-of-guidelines

Fernández Fernández, E., Fernández-Ordoñez, E., García-Gamez, M., Guerra- Marmolejo, C., Iglesias-Parra, R., García-Agua Soler, N. & González-Cano-Caballero, M. (2023). Indicators and predictors modifiable by the nursing department during the preoperative period: A scoping review. *Journal of Clinical Nursing, 32*, 2339– 60. https://doi.org/10.1111/jocn.16287

Gao, L., Chen, W., Qin, S. & Yang, X. (2024). The impact of preoperative interview and prospective nursing on perioperative psychological stress and postoperative complications in patients undergoing TACE intervention for hepatocellular carcinoma. *Medicine, 103*(2), e35929. https://doi.org/10.1097/MD.0000000000035929

Gee, E. (2019). The National VTE Exemplar Centres Network response to implementation of updated NICE guidance: Venous thromboembolism in over 16s: Reducing the risk of hospital-acquired deep vein thrombosis or pulmonary embolism (NG89). *British Journal of Haematology, 186*, 782–93. https://doi.org/10.1111/bjh.16010

Grondahl, W., Muurinen, H., Katajisto, J., Suhonen, R. & Leino-Kilpi, H. (2019). Perceived quality of nursing care and patient education: A cross-sectional study of hospitalised surgical patients in Finland. *British Medical Journal Open, 9*, e023108. https://doi.org/10.1136/bmjopen-2018-023108

Heily, M., Gerdtz, M., Jarden, R., Darvall, J. & Bellomo, R. (2023). Anaesthetic emergence agitation after cardiac surgery: An intensive care staff survey. *Australian Critical Care, 36*(5), 832–6. https://doi.org/10.1016/j.aucc.2022.08.081

Holm, R. (2023). Chapter 2: Perioperative nursing assessment and nursing diagnosis. In R. Holm (ed.), *Certified Perioperative Nurse Review*. USA: Springer Publishing.

Horn, A., Kaneshiro, K. & Tsui, B. (2020). Preemptive and preventive pain psychoeducation and its potential application as a multimodal perioperative pain control option: A systematic review. *Anesthesia & Analgesia, 130*(3), 559–73. https://doi.org/10.1213/ANE.0000000000004319

Horn, R. & Kramer, J. (2022). Postoperative pain control. In *StatPearls [Internet]*. Treasure Island (FL): StatPearls Publishing. https://www.ncbi.nlm.nih.gov/books/NBK544298

Ji, B., He, M., Chen, H., Chen, Y., Wang, S., Yang, L., Xu, W. & Shen, N. (2022). Comparison between forced-air and air-free warming on perioperative hypothermia in patients undergoing elective surgery. *Chinese Medical Journal, 135*(19), 2363–5. https://mednexus.org/doi/full/10.1097/CM9.0000000000002145

Jin, Z., Gan, T. & Bergese, S. (2020). Prevention and treatment of postoperative nausea and vomiting (PONV): A review of current recommendations and emerging therapies. *Therapeutics and Clinical Risk Management, 16*, 1305–17. https://doi.org/10.2147/TCRM.S256234

Jovanovic, V., Lađevic, N. & Sipetic Grujicic, S. (2023). Risk factors for the occurrence of postoperative delirium. *Health Care, 52*(4). https://www.doi.org/10.5937/zdravzast52-47258

Ju, J. W., Nam, J., Sohn, J. Y., Joo, S., Lee, J., Lee, S., Cho, Y. J. & Jeon, Y. (2023). Association between intraoperative body temperature and postoperative delirium: A retrospective observational study. *Journal of Clinical Anesthesia, 87*, 111107. https://doi.org/10.1016/j.jclinane.2023.111107

Kehlet, H. (2018). Postoperative pain, analgesia, and recovery: Bedfellows that cannot be ignored. *PAIN, 159*, S11–S16. https://doi.org/10.1097/j.pain.0000000000001243

Kelleci, Y., Abdullayev, R., Cakmak, G., Ozdemir, H., Umuroglu, T. & Saracoglu, A. (2023). Perioperative hypothermia and associated factors: A prospective cohort study. *JARSS, 31*(4), 339–48. https://jag.journalagent.com/anestezi/pdfs/JARSS_31_4_339_348.pdf

Kirfel, A., Jossen, D., Menzenbach, J., Mayr, A. & Wittmann, M. (2023). Occurrence of postoperative delirium and the use of different assessment tools. *Geriatrics, 8*(1),11. https://doi.org/10.3390/geriatrics8010011

Kotomska, M. & Michalak, A. (2019). Communication and perioperative care of elderly patients. *Polish Journal of Public Health, 129*(2), 55–60. https://doi.org/10.2478/pjph-2019-0013

Kranke, P., Wilhelm, W. & Eberhart, L. (2020). Management of postoperative nausea and vomiting (PONV). In O. Ljungqvist, N. Francis & R. Urman (eds), *Enhanced recovery after surgery*. Cham, Switzerland: Springer.

Ma, J., Li, C., Zhang, W., Zhou, L., Shu, S., Wang, S., Wang, D. & Cha, X. (2021). Preoperative anxiety predicted the incidence of postoperative delirium in patients undergoing total hip arthroplasty: a prospective cohort study. *BioMedCentral: Anesthesiology, 21*, 48. https://doi.org/10.1186/s12871-021-01271-3

Mackenzie, C. & Nosib, H. (2023). Managing obesity in gynaecological surgery. *Obstetrics, Gynaecology & Reproductive Medicine, 33*(7), 197–202. https://doi.org/10.1016/j.ogrm.2023.04.003

Marsman, M., Kappen, T., Vernooij, L., van der Hout, E., van Waes J. & van Kiej, W. (2023). Association of a liberal fasting policy of clear fluids before surgery with fasting duration and patient well-being and safety. *Journal of the American Medical Association, 158*(3), 254–63. https://doi.org/10.1001/jamasurg.2022.5867

Maya, A. & Galeano, S. (2023). Nursing care related with surgical position. *Investigacion and Educacion en Enfermia, 41*(1). https://doi.org/10.17533/udea.iee.v41n1e03

Molliqaj, G., Robin, M., Czarnetzki, C., Daly, M. J., Agostinho, A. & Tessitore, E. (2020). Perioperative management: Surgical site infection prevention, DVT prophylaxis, and blood loss management. In E. Tessitore, A. Dehdashti, C. Schonauer & C. Thomé (eds), *Surgery of the cranio-vertebral junction*. Cham, Switzerland: Springer. https://doi.org/10.1007/978-3-030-18700-2_8

Moraes, K., Riboldi, C., Silva, K., Maschio, J., Stefani, L., Travares, J. & Wegener, W. (2019). Transfer of the care of patients with low risk of mortality in postoperative: Experience report. *Revista Gaucha de Enfermagem, 40*, (spe)e20180398. https://doi.org/10.1590/1983-1447.2019.2018039

National Institute for Health and Clinical Excellence (NICE) (2016). *Clinical Guideline CG65: The management of inadvertent perioperative hypothermia in adults having surgery*. https://www.nice.org.uk/guidance/cg65

Pastino, A. & Lakra, A. (2023). Patient-controlled analgesia. In *StatPearls [Internet]*. Treasure Island (FL): StatPearls Publishing. https://www.ncbi.nlm.nih.gov/books/NBK551610

Peristeri, D., Nour, H., Ahsan, A., Abogabal, S., Singh, K. & Sajid, M. (2023). Alcohol-containing versus aqueous-based solutions for skin preparation in abdominal surgery: A systematic review and meta-analysis. *Journal of Surgical Research, 291*, 734–41. https://doi.org/10.1016/j.jss.2023.06.011

Prathap, K. & Chitra, B. (2023). Assessment of incidence of deep vein thrombosis in patients with malignancy undergoing surgery. *International Journal of Academic Medicine and Pharmacy, 5*(4), 1340–4. https://academicmed.org/Uploads/Volume5Issue4/269.%20[1266.%20JAMP_Mohamed%20Ali_QR]%201340-1344.pdf

Ripollés-Melchor, J., Carli, F., Coca-Martínez, M., Barbero-Mielgo, M., Ramirez-Rodriguez, J. & Garcia-Erce, J. (2018). Committed to be fit: The value of preoperative care in the perioperative medicine era. *Minerva Anestesiologica, 84*(5), 615–25. https://doi.org/10.23736/s0375-9393.18.12286-3

Roche, D. & Jones, A. (2021). A qualitative study of nurse-patient communication and information provision during surgical pre-admission clinics. *Health Expectations, 24*, 1357–66. https://doi.org/10.1111/hex.13270

Roshan, M., Jafarpoor, H., Shamsalinia, A., Fotokian, Z. & Hamidi, S. (2023). Effects of a forced-air warming system and warmed intravenous fluids on hemodynamic parameters, shivering, and time to awakening in elderly patients undergoing open cardiac surgery. *Annals of Cardiac Anaesthesia*, *26*(4), 386–92. https://doi.org/10.4103/aca.aca_20_23

Royal College of Anaesthetists (2019). *Guidelines for the provision of anaesthetic services in postoperative care.* https://www.rcoa.ac.uk/gpas/chapter-4

Royal College of Pathologists Australia (RCPA) (2023). *Pre-operative assessment.* https://www.rcpa.edu.au/Manuals/RCPA-Manual/Clinical-Problems/P/Pre-operative-assessment

Salazar Maya, Á. M. (2022). Nursing care during the perioperative within the surgical context. *Investigación y Educación en Enfermería*, *40*(2), e02. https://doi.org/10.17533/udea.iee.v40n2e02

Sandelin, A., Kalman, S. & Gustafsson, B. Å. (2019). Prerequisites for safe intraoperative nursing care and teamwork – operating theatre nurses' perspectives: A qualitative interview study. *Journal of Clinical Nursing, 28,* 2635–43. https://doi.org/10.1111/jocn.14850

Schick, L. (2019). Assessment and monitoring of the peri-anesthesia patient. In J. Odom-Forrem (ed.), *Drain's perianesthesia nursing: A critical care approach* (7th ed.). St Louis, MO: Elsevier.

Schick, L. & Windle, P. (eds) (2021). *Peri-anesthesia nursing core curriculum: Preprocedure, Phase I and Phase II Nursing.* St Louis, MO: Elsevier.

Schlick, C. J. R., Liu, J. Y., Yang, A., Bentrem, D., Billimoria, K. & Merkow, R. (2020). Pre- operative, intra-operative, and post-operative factors associated with post-discharge venous thromboembolism following colorectal cancer resection. *Journal of Gastrointestinal Surgery, 24,* 144–54. https://doi.org/10.1007/s11605-019-04354-2

Seidelman, J., Mantyh C. & Anderson, D. (2023). Surgical site infection prevention: A review. *Journal of the American Medical Association, 329*(3), 244–52. https://doi.org/10.1001/jama.2022.24075

Sinderovsky, A., Grosman-Rimon, L., Atrash, M., Nakhoul, A., Saadi, H., Rimon, J., Birati, E., Carasso, S. & Kachel, E. (2023). The effects of preoperative pain education on pain severity in cardiac surgery patients: A pilot randomized control trial. *Pain Management Nursing, 24*(4), e18–e25. https://doi.org/10.1016/j.pmn.2023.02.003

Spencer, D., Kim, D., de Virgilio, C., Grigorian, A. & Nahmias, J. (2020). Postoperative decreased urine output. In C. de Virgilio & A. Grigorian (eds), *Surgery: A case based clinical review.* Cham, Switzerland: Springer. https://doi.org/10.1007/978-3-030-05387-1_40

Tu, Q., Zhou, R., Wan, Z., Chen, S., Yang, Q. & Que, B. (2023). Perioperative administration of dexamethasone to prevent postoperative shivering: a systematic review and meta-analysis of randomized controlled trials. *Journal of International Medical Research, 51*(8). https://doi.org/10.1177/03000605231187805

Wang, J. & Deng, X. (2023). Inadvertent hypothermia: A prevalent perioperative issue that remains to be improved. *Anaesthesiology and Perioperative Science, 1,* 24. https://doi.org/10.1007/s44254-023-00022-6

Wang, K., Cai, J., Du, R. & Wu, J. (2023). Global trends in research related to emergence delirium, 2012–2021: A bibliometric analysis. *Frontiers in Psychology, 14* (Sec. Consciousness Research). https://doaj.org/article/2350e1943ce04378bc7b0b9543ea2844

Wang, Y., Yue, J., Xie, D., Carter, P., Quan-Lei, L., Gartaganis, S., Chen, J. & Inouye, S. (2020). Effect of the tailored, family-involved hospital elder life program on postoperative delirium and function in older adults: A randomized clinical trial. *Journal of the American Medical Association Internal Medicine, 80*(1), 17–25. https://doi.org/10.1001/jamainternmed.2019.4446

White, B. (2019). *Impact of a pre-admission center on 30-day readmissions and day of surgery cancellations for patients undergoing elective spine surgery.* Manuscript: University of Connecticut – Storrs. https://scholar.google.com/scholar?as_ylo=2016&q=surgical+pre+admission+clinics&hl=en&as_sdt=0,5

Wolfe, J., Wolfe, N. & Rich, M. (2020). Perioperative care of the geriatric patient for noncardiac surgery. *Clinical Cardiology, 43*(2), 127–36. https://doi.org/10.1002/clc.23302

World Health Organization (2003). *Postoperative management.* Geneva: WHO. https://www.who.int/surgery/publications/Postoperativecare.pdf

Yuan, Z., Gao, L., Zheng, M., Ye, X. & Sun, S. (2023). Effect of multimodal health education combined with the feedback method in perioperative patients with lung cancer: A randomised controlled study. *Patient Preference and Adherence, 17,* 413–20. https://doi.org/10.2147/PPA.S394826

Zietlow, K., Wong, S., Heflin, M., McDonald, S., Sickeler, R., Devinney, M., Blitz, J., Sagoo- Deenadayalan, S. & Berger, M. (2022). Geriatric preoperative optimization: A review. *American Journal of Medicine, 135*(1), 39–48. https://doi.org/10.1016/j.amjmed.2021.07.028

PART 10

ASSISTING WITH PERSONAL HYGIENE, SKIN INTEGRITY AND MOBILISING

55 BED BATH OR ASSISTED SHOWER

56 ORAL CARE, HAIR CARE, NAIL CARE AND SHAVING

57 ASSISTING A PERSON TO REPOSITION

58 ASSISTING A PERSON TO MOBILISE

59 PRESSURE AREA CARE – PREVENTING PRESSURE INJURIES

Note: These notes are summaries of the most important points in the assessments/procedures and are not exhaustive on the subject. References of the materials used to compile the information have been supplied. The student is expected to have learnt the material surrounding each skill as presented in the references. No single reference is complete on each subject.

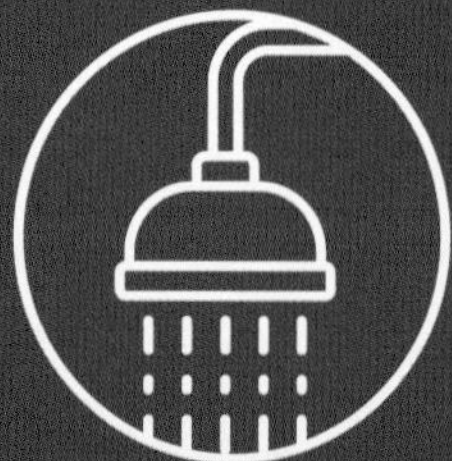

CHAPTER 55

BED BATH OR ASSISTED SHOWER

INDICATIONS

When someone cannot attend to their personal hygiene needs independently, due either to their physical/psychological condition or to limitations placed on them by their treatment, you will need to assist. Skin cleanliness is essential to health and wellbeing, to maintenance of skin integrity and to help people feel refreshed and comforted (Veje et al., 2019). Many nurses underestimate the importance of good skin care to health and wellbeing. Heague, Dyson and Cowdell (2023) state that good hygiene care is a fundamental nursing responsibility.

Bathing removes perspiration, skin oils, dead cells and bacteria, and prevents body odour. It is an important daily hygiene habit when a person is ill or hospitalised. It increases circulation, enhances muscle tone and promotes relaxation and a feeling of wellbeing (Goldenhart & Nagy, 2022). Bathing also provides an excellent opportunity to assess the person and to establish and extend a therapeutic relationship.

Showering is generally the preferred method of bathing, as long as the person is able to stand or sit on a chair safely in the shower. An assisted shower means that you shower the person on a chair.

A *bed bath* is given when the person is physically unable to get out of bed or when treatment precludes the possibility of movement (e.g. traction). Bed baths range from a complete sponge of the person to an assisted sponge, where the person is able to wash when provided with the equipment, with minimal assistance from you.

EVIDENCE OF THERAPEUTIC INTERACTION

Clearly explain the procedure to gain the person's cooperation and empower them. Ask about and honour their preferred items for a shower/bath, their use of soap or not, and their need for ritual. This increases the extent of the therapeutic relationship and demonstrates caring. The bath time is often an excellent time to become better acquainted with the person and to develop and extend the therapeutic relationship. Talking with the person is also a distraction that reduces embarrassment during the bath. It is often the longest contact that you have with the person during the day. Take this opportunity to assess the person physically, emotionally and psychosocially. People appreciate nurses who respect their emotional, psychological and cultural needs, their dignity and individuality (Bagnasco et al., 2019). Bath time is also a good time to assess the person's knowledge and conduct health teaching. Bed bathing can often be seen as intrusion and can give emotional discomfort as people see it as a sign of loss of their independence (Groven et al., 2020). Be sensitive.

DEMONSTRATE CLINICAL REASONING

As a nurse, you are a role model and you use your body to accomplish your work. Practising good personal hygiene (frequent bathing, deodorant use, neat uniform), keeping your hair short or restrained if long (hair is full of bacteria [Fernandez, 2019]), washing your hands after you touch your hair, keeping your nails short and smooth and practising good dental hygiene demonstrate clinical awareness of yourself and your impact on others.

Personal hygiene of people who are hospitalised is an important aspect of fundamental care. Mody et al. (2019) found that the hands of people in hospital become contaminated with multidrug-resistant organisms (e.g. MRSA) within a short time of admission. Ensuring that each person is able, knowledgeable about and is provided with the necessary equipment for hand hygiene is crucial in reducing hospital-acquired infections.

ELDER CARE

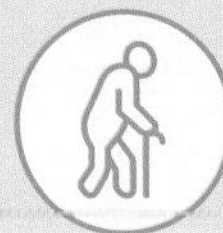

Hospitalisation decreases the functional capacity of elderly people in just a few days. Assisting the older adult to care for themselves wherever possible assists them to maintain their activities of daily living and return to function following discharge. Assess for xerosis, pruritis, skin tears, cracks and fissures in the skin. Use pH neutral cleansers and apply moisturising cream twice daily (Heague, Dyson & Cowdell, 2023). Take care with fragile skin, support joints as they are being cleansed, dry the skin well and moisturise all over. Use the time for the important human interaction needed (Bastos et al., 2019).

THE PERSON LIVING WITH SEVERE OBESITY

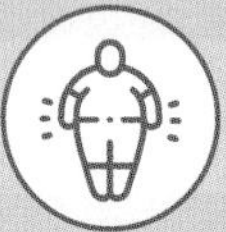

Equipment needed for the severely obese person is described in **Clinical Skill 15**. Mechanical lifts are important to protect your health.

The skin physiology and its barrier effects are altered in severe obesity (Hirt et al., 2019), and its condition is of great concern; pressure areas and injury are likely because the person moves little due to their obesity, and the extra weight increases the pressure on dependent parts of their bodies (e.g. exacerbated by lying on tubes, wrinkles in the linen). As well, circulation is poor to the skin. Skin folds are prone to excoriation and bacterial or fungal infections as the combined immobility and excess weight restrict movement and prevent appropriate self-care hygiene measures. Reduced peripheral circulation makes skin prone to breakdown and leads to the development of infection. Perspiration is greater than normal because of the increased ratio of body mass to skin area, increasing the chances of skin breakdown.

Check all areas of the body where skin overlaps skin – in the groin, perineal areas, behind the knees, under the abdominal apron, under the breasts (both genders), under the arms and under the chin. Move and wash, rinse and dry folds of flesh, use cotton cloth (e.g. washcloth) in skin folds. The person is encouraged to do what they can – they will need reach aids and help with inaccessible areas. Incontinence may be a problem due to pressure on the bladder and bowel from intra-abdominal adipose tissue and decreased mobility. Keep the perineal skin folds clean and dry. (See **Clinical Skills 15 and 23** for a brief explanation of bariatric issues.)

Assess the person

Assessment before starting personal hygiene is important to prevent contravening orders, assuming a higher level of activity than is possible or disregarding personal preferences.

LOOK at the person's notes or care plan for the treatment regimen, activity orders, diagnosis and any orders specific to hygiene. Observe them for activity intolerance, decreased strength or endurance or limited movement.

LISTEN to the person for reports of pain, other symptoms, level of sedation, perceptual or cognitive impairment, neuromuscular impairment, depression or severe anxiety.

Safety

A holistic approach to personal hygiene is needed, as it is affected by age, level of dependence, biological, psychological, sociocultural, environmental and politico-economic factors. Do not impose your own standards of personal hygiene or even assume these will be the same as the person's. Each person is a cultural being and their beliefs and values need to be acknowledged for their psychological comfort and to foster trust in you (Farias et al., 2020).

Discuss hygiene needs and preferences with the person (e.g. preferred toiletries, time of day, or any cultural or religious practices to observe [Bastos et al., 2019]). Ask if a traditional bed bath, a bath-in-a-bag or a shower is preferred (Veje et al., 2019). Santos et al. (2020) found no difference in energy expenditure or clinical variation between the various types of personal hygiene. Respect these preferences while maintaining privacy and dignity at all times. Such supplies as personal soap, bath gel, emollient creams and personal sponges mean a great deal to an individual's feeling of control.

Check on the availability and location of needed supplies or special equipment. During each step in the process, you need to ensure the correct manual-handling technique and/or equipment is used to reduce the risk of injuring the person or yourself.

Safety

Preparation

Clear the area of obstacles and draw the curtains/close the doors to ensure a safe and private environment. Privacy is important since most aspects of personal hygiene are private because of exposure of body areas and the intimate nature of the routines. Adjust the bed height to reduce strain on your back, as reaching over the person and twisting makes back muscles vulnerable to injury. Use the bed's brakes. The room should be comfortably warm and without draughts, as the person will have large areas of their body exposed and wet during washing and will easily become chilled. Determine their ability to assist and discuss how much of the bathing they wish to do by themselves and in private (partial or assisted bed bath). Position the person to facilitate bathing. For example, bathing in bed is easier if the person is supine and towards the near edge of the bed, to make reaching over and turning them easier. Offer the person a bedpan or urinal before beginning the bed bath to reduce interruptions and increase comfort.

GATHER EQUIPMENT

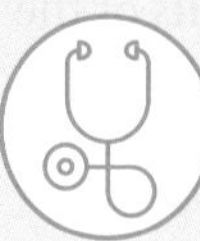

Gathering equipment is a time-management strategy. Completing this procedure efficiently helps to create a positive environment, reduces the person's embarrassment, boosts the person's confidence, comfort and trust in you and increases your self-confidence. Equipment will include the following, depending on whether you are performing a bed bath or an assisted shower:

EQUIPMENT	EXPLANATION
Bath blanket	To maintain dignity and warmth during a bed bath or assisted bath
Basin and warm water	• Clean the basin with hot soapy water before use • Fill to three-quarters with warm water (43 to 46 °C), which is most effective for removing oils, bacteria and debris. Test on the inner aspect of your wrist • Confirm the comfort of the temperature with the person if possible
Shower chair or bath bed	Used if the person is weak or cannot sit in a chair for the shower
Plastic sheets and tape	To protect venipuncture sites or dressings
Soap or a no-rinse cleanser	Emulsifies the skin oils and helps remove debris
Towels	Two or three are needed to dry the person and keep the bed linen dry as well
Washcloths (preferably disposable)	• To wash and rinse the skin • A bath-in-a-bag kit is often used, and is more effective than the traditional water-based bed bath, reduces infections and is often better received by the person (Groven et al., 2020)
Clean clothing	Helps the person feel more comfortable, maintains body cleanliness and boosts self-esteem
Preferred emollient creams, deodorants	Assists the person to feel fresher and boosts self-esteem
Clean linen and a hamper	Required to change the bed and maintain cleanliness following a bath

PERFORM A BED BATH OR ASSISTED SHOWER

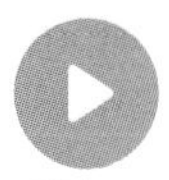

Video

Hand hygiene

Hand hygiene (see **Clinical Skill 5**) removes microorganisms from your hands. It is the most effective preventative measure for cross-contamination, reducing incidences of nosocomial (i.e. hospital- or treatment-acquired) infection.

Personal protective equipment

Use a plastic apron to prevent wetting and soiling your uniform and to prevent the spread of infection. Wear clean gloves as there will be contact with body fluids, including saliva.

Perform a bed bath

Prepare the person

One or two nurses, depending on the condition of the individual, carry out bed bathing. Arrange the equipment on the over-bed table in order of use for efficiency (take care: people in some cultures object to anything on the over-bed table other than food and personal items). Assist the person onto the near side of the bed. Lower the side-rails, since you will be in constant attendance. Replace top linen with a bath blanket by placing the fan-folded bath blanket over the sheet. Ask the person to hold the top of the bath blanket, then pull the sheet and the bottom of the bath blanket to the bottom of the bed. This prevents exposure. Remove and fold the bed linen for reuse or dispose of it in the linen hamper. Remove the person's gown under the bath blanket to prevent exposure. Discard hospital clothing in the linen hamper, or if personal clothing, into a private laundry bag. Remove glasses and hearing aids (if any). Tell the person you will replace these as soon as their face/ears are clean.

Wash the person

Place a towel to protect the bed linen while washing each body part so the person's bed remains dry. Use a washcloth folded into a mitt, with the first third on your palm, second third around the back of your hand, final third on your palm. The excess cloth is folded up over your fingers and palm and tucked under the initial wraps so there are no loose ends dragging over the person to annoy or chill them. To prevent discomfort, use a damp, not dripping, washcloth, which still ensures thorough washing and rinsing. Change the water frequently (i.e. as it cools or becomes murky) to ensure warmth and adequate rinsing and reduce the risk of cross-contamination. Not leaving the soap in the bath water will help it remain clearer.

Use long, firm (moderate pressure) strokes from the distal to the proximal to aid in venous return and to create friction (do not rub vigorously). This removes dirt, oil and microorganisms and is more relaxing and comfortable than short, light strokes. An exception is if the person has a venous thrombosis, in which case long, firm strokes are contraindicated for the affected limb. Pay particular attention to areas where skin lies on skin, such as the axilla, under breasts, abdominal folds, buttock folds and groin. These areas quickly become irritated if left damp or soapy, and microorganisms grow readily in these areas.

Expose, wash, rinse and thoroughly pat dry the body one part at a time to prevent chilling and embarrassment. Support large joints (e.g. elbows, knees) when the limb is elevated for washing, rinsing and drying. Encourage the person to assist in any aspect they are capable of doing. People often prefer to cleanse their own hands and face and perineal and anal areas. The following order is generally used, but it may need to be adapted to individual needs:

- eyes – inner to outer canthus, clean corner of the washcloth, no soap
- face, neck and ears – check the person's preference for soap on the face. Return glasses/hearing aids
- far arm and hand – soak their hand in the basin
- near arm and hand – soak their hand in the basin
- chest and axillae
- abdomen and groin
- far thigh, leg and foot – soak their foot in the basin
- near leg and foot – soak their foot in the basin
- back – assist them to a side-lying position, facing away
- genital and anal areas.

Use the guide for perineal care as outlined in **Clinical Skill 33** to complete the genital area. Replace the bottom sheet with fresh linen. Apply deodorant, emollient cream and talcum powder, as the person prefers. (Take care with talcum powder and aerosol deodorants as some people react strongly to these respiratory irritants.) Assist them to dress in fresh clothing. Perform hand hygiene.

> ?
> If one extremity or side of the person has decreased range of motion (e.g. paralysis, intravenous insertion site, incision, dressing, bandage, cast), dress the affected side first to more easily manipulate clothing over the body part.

Post-procedure

Replace the bath blanket with the clean top sheet (by the same method used to remove the top sheet, above) and discard the bath blanket in the linen hamper. Add additional linen as required. Position the person for comfort and leave the side-rails up, lower the bed and place the call bell within reach and replace anything moved prior to the bed bath. Perform hand hygiene.

Alternative method: bath-in-a-bag kit

Use of a *bath-in-a-bag kit* differs little from the traditional bed bath. It contains a number of disposable washcloths moistened with a non-rinse emollient cleanser. The entire bag is to be warmed in the microwave according to the manufacturer's instructions and brought to the bedside. Clip a plastic bag to the bed for used wipes. Perform hand hygiene and put on gloves. Use a fresh washcloth for each area described in the method for a traditional bed bath. Again, use moderate pressure and long strokes to remove dirt without causing friction or irritation (Konya et al., 2023). Place the used wipe in the plastic bag (Goldenhart & Nagy, 2022). The skin dries in a few seconds without towelling so the benefits of the emollient are maximised. Matsumoto et al. (2019) suggest use of a bath-in-a-bag kit is a cost-effective, evidence-based alternative that is as effective at cleansing as soap and water but better preserves the skin, reduces infections and is satisfactory to nurses and to the people being bathed. Apply emollient creams routinely to moisturise dry skin. Remove your gloves and perform hand hygiene.

Perform an assisted shower

Prepare the area

If the person requires minimal assistance, an assisted shower may be done, or you may need to shower them, depending on their condition. Gather all equipment and linen and take it to the shower stall so the shower can be completed without interruption, reducing chilling and tiring of the person. Place a non-slip mat on the floor of the shower (so neither you nor the person will slip).

Prepare and position the person

Safety

Perform hand hygiene and use personal protective equipment (PPE). Remove and carefully store spectacles and hearing aids. Cover any incisions or venipuncture sites with waterproof material and firmly tape it to prevent contamination of the site during the shower. Note that many facilities encourage the showering of intact and healing post-surgical incisions 48 or more hours after surgery. Tap water and showers have been demonstrated to be safe and effective wound treatments for clean, sutured surgical wounds (Copeland-Halperin et al., 2020).

If the person is mobile, escort them to the shower stall. For privacy, place a 'Do not disturb' sign on the shower door. Regulate the water temperature to between 43 and 46 °C (ask the person to test for comfort) before assisting the person into the shower stall. Assist them to a stool or direct to use handrails to provide support as appropriate. If they can be left alone, remain close, maintain privacy and provide assistance if required. Alert them to the call bell in case weakness or problems develop during the shower.

For the person who needs assistance

Transfer the person to the shower chair or bath bed. Cover them and transport them to the shower stall. Ensure privacy and water temperature as above. Use a hand-held shower head and direct the shower spray in a downward stream from the feet up to the neck. Shower their face only if requested. If they request a spray of water on their face, spray downwards so that water is not forced up the nostrils or into the eyes, or cover the shower rose with a washcloth so water streams rather than sprays. Wash the face with the washcloth formed into a mitt (see 'Perform the bed bath' for how to form a mitt). Wash eyes first, then face, neck and ears. Find out their preference for soap/

bath gel on their face. Thoroughly lather the body parts with a washcloth then remove the soap/bath gel with the water stream. Proceed from the neck downwards and finish with the perineal and anal areas. Rinse thoroughly to prevent irritation from residual soap.

After-shower care

Assist the person to a towel-covered chair. If using a bath bed, drain the residual water away. Pat the person dry rapidly, using two or three towels, since the entire body surface is wet and exposed, leading to chilling by convection. Take particular care to dry between body folds (e.g. between toes, between fingers, under breasts, axillae, abdominal folds and groin) to prevent irritation from moisture between body surfaces. Remember to dry the back and buttocks if the person is using a shower chair or bath bed. Return their spectacles/hearing aid. Apply deodorants, emollient creams and talcum powder as preferred. Assist the person to dress, comb or brush their hair. Return them to their bed or room and assist them to a position of comfort. The person is assisted with facial shaving, oral care and in applying make-up as appropriate (see **Clinical Skill 56**). Remove gloves and perform hand hygiene.

Remember, too, that hearing aids and spectacles need cleaning to ensure these prostheses are in good working order and free from debris and contaminants.

CLEAN, REPLACE AND DISPOSE OF EQUIPMENT

Leave equipment in a usable condition for the next nurse as both a time-management strategy and a courtesy to other staff. Perform hand hygiene and put on gloves. Clean the shower stall according to hospital policy; this usually means you wipe down the surfaces, the non-slip mat, the stool, the shower chair or the bath bed with an antiseptic solution to prevent cross-infection. Dry water spills to reduce the risk of falls, and remove all personal or hospital items such as linen and soap.

Basins are a demonstrated source of hospital-acquired infection. Basins are scrubbed out with an antiseptic, sterilised and thoroughly dried. If basins are used, they are most often individual and returned to the person's bedside locker. Follow hospital protocol. If a bath in a bag is used, the wipes are sealed in their plastic disposal bag and placed in the general rubbish. Do not flush the wipes down the toilet or hopper, as they contain synthetics (plastic) and are not biodegradable (Spencer & Kelly, 2019). Place all soiled hospital linen in the linen hamper for laundering. Personal clothing is to be placed in the person's laundry bag for the family to launder. Remove gloves and perform hand hygiene.

DOCUMENTATION

Notes will include time and date, procedure, response and a notation of any areas of skin breakdown. Some hospitals do not require that personal hygiene be recorded in the nursing notes. Follow the hospital policy. Any relevant information gleaned during the bath or shower is passed on either verbally or in writing so that the healthcare team remains informed.

CLINICAL SKILLS ASSESSMENT

Bed bath or assisted shower

Demonstrates the ability to effectively perform a bed bath or assisted shower. Incorporates the *National Safety and Quality Health Service Standards*: 2 Partnering with consumers, 3 Preventing and controlling healthcare-associated infections, 5 Comprehensive care, and 6 Communicating for safety (Australian Commission on Safety and Quality in Health Care [ACSQHC], 2021).

Performance criteria	1	2	3	4	5
(Numbers indicate NMBA *Registered Nurse Standards for Practice*)	(Dependent)	(Marginal)	(Assisted)	(Supervised)	(Independent)
1. Identifies indication (1.1, 3.3, 3.4)	☐	☐	☐	☐	☐
2. Evidence of therapeutic interaction with the person, e.g. gives the person a clear explanation of the procedure, incorporates the person's preferences (1.4, 1.5, 2.1, 2.2, 3.2)	☐	☐	☐	☐	☐
3. Demonstrates clinical reasoning abilities, e.g. provides privacy, alters bed height, attends to environmental temperature, positions the person (1.1, 1.2, 1.3, 1.5, 4.1, 4.2, 4.3, 5.1, 6.1)	☐	☐	☐	☐	☐
4. Assesses the person for their ability to self-care (1.1, 4.1, 4.2, 4.3, 6.1)	☐	☐	☐	☐	☐
5. Gathers equipment as determined by the procedure (1.1, 5.5, 6.1): ■ bath blanket ■ basin and warm water, bath kit or soft towel kit ■ shower chair or bath bed ■ plastic sheets and tape ■ soap or a no-rinse cleanser ■ towels ■ washcloths (preferably disposable) ■ clean clothing ■ preferred emollient creams, deodorants ■ clean linen and a hamper	☐	☐	☐	☐	☐
6. Performs hand hygiene (1.1, 3.4, 6.1)	☐	☐	☐	☐	☐
7. Dons personal protective equipment (1.1, 3.4, 6.1)	☐	☐	☐	☐	☐
8. Carries out the hygiene measure required (bed bathing or assisted shower) (1.1, 2.1, 3.2, 6.1, 7.1, 7.2)	☐	☐	☐	☐	☐
9. Cleans, replaces and disposes of equipment appropriately (3.6, 6.1)	☐	☐	☐	☐	☐
10. Documents relevant information (1.1, 1.4, 1.6, 2.2, 2.7, 3.5, 3.7, 6.1, 6.2, 6.5, 7.3)	☐	☐	☐	☐	☐
11. Demonstrates the ability to link theory to practice (1.1, 3.3, 3.4, 3.5)	☐	☐	☐	☐	☐

Student:

Clinical facilitator: Date:

CHAPTER 56

ORAL CARE, HAIR CARE, NAIL CARE AND SHAVING

INDICATIONS

Many conditions may contribute to a person's inability to attend to their own personal hygiene needs. Among these are impaired vision, extreme frailty, immobility, paralysis, confusion, dementia, severe depression or unconsciousness.

Oral care is necessary to assess the mouth, maintain the integrity of the oral mucosa, teeth and gums, and to hydrate the mucous membranes, and is a very important comfort measure. It minimises the risk of oral infection and pneumonia (Klompas et al., 2022; Okubo, Hoshi & Kondo, 2023). A clean mouth assists in nutritional intake by stimulating the appetite. People usually accomplish their own oral care with some assistance. Oral care includes care of dentures.

Hair care (i.e. shampooing and maintenance) maintains the integrity of the hair and scalp, improves circulation, provides a sense of wellbeing and improves self-confidence.

Shaving a man's face is a variation of hair care, promoting comfort and contributing to self-confidence and self-worth. Always ask men with beards or moustaches if they want them trimmed, washed or brushed (if they are unable to do it themselves), as these are intensely personal and often religiously or culturally dictated hygiene practices (Gancheva, 2019). Some Sikh men, for instance, never shave their beard and keep it rolled and netted (Mooney, 2015).

Nail care removes detritus from under nails and is an important aspect of prevention of autoinfection. Long, ragged nails can cause injury, so cutting and smoothing them is a safety measure as well as a comfort measure.

All these hygiene measures offer an opportunity to observe and assess the person, to extend the therapeutic relationship and to provide person-centred care (Jakobsson et al., 2019).

EVIDENCE OF THERAPEUTIC INTERACTION

Discuss personal hygiene needs and preferences with the person. Toiletries (e.g. personal shampoo and conditioner, toothpaste, mouthwash, shaving cream and aftershave) mean a great deal to the person's feelings of control. Check the availability and location of supplies needed or special equipment. Honour their preferred items for personal care, shaving and so forth, and uphold their rituals as much as possible – this improves the therapeutic relationship. Clearly explaining the procedure gains their cooperation.

DEMONSTRATE CLINICAL REASONING

Privacy is important because of the intimate nature of hygiene routines. Alter the bed height to reduce personal strain on the back, as reaching over the person and twisting makes your back muscles vulnerable to injury. Provide a comfortably warm room, free of draughts, as a large area is exposed and wet during shampooing and the person can easily become chilled.

Proper positioning helps when providing for hygiene needs. For example, bed shampoos require the person to remain supine near the edge of the bed to rinse their hair. For oral care, help the person into a semi-Fowler's or upright position (as condition permits) if conscious, or a side-lying position if unconscious to prevent aspiration of fluid. Shaving is done with the man upright if possible.

Assess the person

Assessment is important to prevent contravening orders, assuming a higher level of activity than is possible or disregarding the person's preferences. Over time, hygiene support needs change as the person's independence grows or deteriorates (King et al., 2019).

LOOK at the person's chart/care plan for the treatment regimen, activity orders, diagnosis and any orders specific to the person's hygiene. Assess them for:

- activity intolerance
- decreased strength and endurance
- neuromuscular impairment
- fine and gross motor movement.

LOOK to the person for reports of:

- pain and other symptoms
- level of sedation
- perceptual or cognitive impairment
- depression or severe anxiety.

ELDER CARE

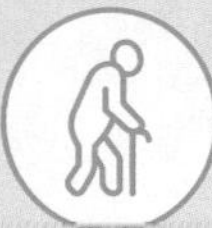

Elderly people (those over 75) in Australia have poor oral health, with 60 per cent suffering from gum disease (e.g. gingivitis and periodontitis) and one-third being edentulous (National Dental Care, 2023). This is a basic contributor to malnutrition. One aspect of the nursing role is teaching oral health care (e.g. importance of brushing/flossing, use of fluoride toothpaste, avoiding the use of lemon and glycerine swabs as they dry the mucous membranes of the mouth [Bhagat et al., 2023], increase the acidity of saliva, cause irreversible softening of tooth enamel, including erosion and exhaust salivary mechanisms [Puntillo et al., 2014]).

THE PERSON LIVING WITH SEVERE OBESITY

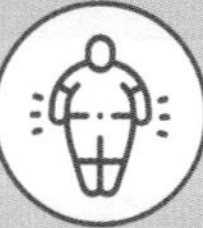

Obesity has been identified as a considerable risk factor for peridontal disease – chronic inflammation, gastric reflux and perhaps insulin resistance are the suspected mechanisms. People living with severe obesity need excellent oral care and information sharing (oral hygiene, use of fluoride, reduced refined carbohydrate diet, avoidance of acidic foods) to reduce the incidence of periodontal disease and the subsequent complications (e.g. pneumonia) (Young, 2022).

Their medical condition may alter their hygiene. For example, chemotherapy can cause alopecia (i.e. hair loss), and shampooing with a pH-neutral shampoo is recommended for anyone at risk of this; clotting disorders would require the use of a soft toothbrush or simply a mouthwash and preclude shaving with a razor.

Social, cultural and religious factors need consideration when attending to hair care. Some cultures or religions do not permit hair washing or brushing. Some Hindu women use combing, brushing and scented oils to cleanse the hair. Others require the hair to be covered, including some Muslim, Orthodox Jewish and Sikh women; some Sikh men cover their hair with a turban (Sherrow, 2023). Similarly, in some religions and cultures facial hair is significant and is never removed without the person's or their relatives' consent (Gancheva, 2019). The appearance and condition of a person's hair provides information on their physical and emotional status, individuality and feelings of worth, and their ability to care for themselves.

GATHER EQUIPMENT

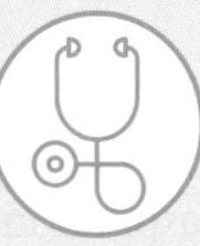

Gathering equipment is an organisational step that helps to create a positive environment for a successful interaction. It ensures that you have all needed material, boosts the person's confidence and trust in you, and increases your self-confidence. While gathering the equipment, you can mentally rehearse the procedure. Gather the following equipment, depending on the task you are to perform:

SKILL	EQUIPMENT
Oral care	• Towel • Toothpaste, toothbrush, dental floss or floss sticks or interdental brushes and mouthwash • Kidney/emesis basin • Glass of cool water • (As needed) denture cup, denture cleanser, oral suction equipment and washcloth
Hair care	• Preferred shampoo and conditioner • Towels • If a bed shampoo is required, add a jug with warm water, a basin, a bed trough, a plastic sheet for protecting the bed, and extra towels
Shaving	Either an electric razor (personal; at bedside), or basin, towel, safety razor and shaving soap • Check chart for medications/disease that influence the choice between safety or electric razor (e.g. anticoagulants, thrombocytopenia, depression, confusion and oxygen administration) • Some facilities only allow personal electric razors or battery rechargers that are checked by biomedical engineering staff for safety; check the facility's policy
Nail care	• Towel • Basin with warm water • Clippers or scissors • Orange stick and a nail file or emery board

PERFORM ORAL CARE, HAIR CARE, NAIL CARE AND SHAVING

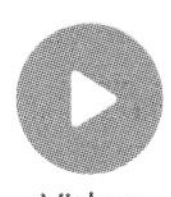
Video

Hand hygiene

Hand hygiene (see **Clinical Skill 5**) removes microorganisms from your hands. It is the most effective preventative measure for cross-contamination, reducing incidences of nosocomial (i.e. hospital- or treatment-acquired) infection. Perform hand hygiene prior to and following contact with the person or their immediate environment. Encourage the person to use frequent hand hygiene and provide the equipment to reduce infection rates (Mody et al., 2019). Education of this and other infection control measures (e.g. coughing/sneezing etiquette, not touching a surgical site or intravenous insertion site) empowers people to assist in the prevention of infection transmission (Hammoud et al., 2020).

Personal protective equipment

Personal protective equipment is an infection-prevention measure. Gloves protect you from contact with body fluids and saliva, and plastic aprons prevent wetting and soiling of your uniform.

Perform oral care

If able, the person can attend to their own oral care. If they are incapacitated, the oral care is up to you. National Dental Care (2023) states that oral care is not a grooming issue but one of infection prevention and disease control. Your attitude to oral care (e.g. believe white clean teeth are an asset) influences your willingness to undertake oral care (Zimmerman et al., 2020). Be aware that research demonstrates that inadequate oral hygiene may cause diseases with serious consequences for general health (Honkavuo, 2019). Vázquez-Reza et al. (2023) report people with periodontitis (inflammation of the gums) are at nearly twice the risk for developing Alzheimer's disease and ischaemic stroke. The biological mechanisms is the low-grade inflammation affecting the intima of vessels and structures of the brain. Systemic disease, polypharmacy and dry mouth contribute to dental problems (Bhagat et al., 2023).

Assess the oral cavity using oral screening tools to evaluate oral hygiene needs or identify the need for a dentist to attend and assist with oral health care (Honkavuo, 2019). Mouth ulcers caused by dentures are pressure injuries and need specialised care (Doshi & Jones, 2019). This persistent trauma is a common cause of oral ulcers; however, other causes include systemic disorders (e.g. gastrointestinal malfunction, cancer, immunologic abnormalities or cutaneous diseases) (Tiwari et al., 2023).

Teeth are brushed at least twice daily (after each meal is optimal) to remove debris and to inhibit colonisation of microorganisms. Anyone who is undergoing chemotherapy or radiation therapy that causes structural change to their oral mucosa needs vigilant oral care (follow the additional treatment regimen provided by the oncology unit) to prevent mucosal damage. Electric toothbrushes are more effective than manual brushing, removing more plaque and are easier to use (Li, Liu & Peng, 2023). Mouth swabs are not effective in removing plaque or oral debris, and can be dangerous (Woon, 2019).

Prepare the person

Position the person upright (as condition permits) to simulate the normal situation. Place a towel over their chest and shoulders to protect clothing from splashes and dribbles. Place a curved basin under the chin to catch the expelled fluid.

Floss the person's teeth

Floss, unless contraindicated (e.g. thrombocytopenia, anticoagulant therapy), by using a floss stick or wrapping about 45 cm of floss around your two middle fingers, with a space of 4 cm left between the fingers. Insert the floss between two teeth and guide to the gum line. Move the floss up and down on the side of each tooth to remove debris and plaque the toothbrush is unable to reach. Replace the floss stick (or turn the floss from one middle finger to the other) as it becomes frayed or soiled, as clean, intact floss is most efficient. Floss between all upper and lower teeth to help prevent periodontal disease (Lin et al., 2020). Flossing is complete when the outside margin of the last tooth is finished. Take care that the person does not bite as a reflex.

Use of an interdental brush is easier and as effective as floss. If the facility or person has interdental brushes, use one to clean between each pair of teeth. Insert it at the gumline, rotate it and draw it back and forth several times. If there is debris, rinse the brush after removing it from between the teeth. They are reusable, and should be thoroughly rinsed and stored in their own sheath between uses.

> ?
> If the interdental brush breaks during use, take a new interdental brush and push the broken portion out from between the teeth. Push it from the inside towards the buccal cavity to prevent inadvertent aspiration or swallowing of the broken section. Remove the section with your (gloved) fingers.

Brush the person's teeth

Wet a soft to medium toothbrush with cool water and apply a small amount of toothpaste. Ask the person to keep their mouth open and, holding the toothbrush at a 45-degree angle, cleanse every surface of the teeth. Use small, circular movements of the toothbrush. Starting at the junction of the teeth and gums, work towards the crown. Use light pressure to avoid injury. Clean the inside, outside and flat surfaces of upper and lower teeth. Add fresh water by either asking the person to sip from the water glass or repeatedly dipping the toothbrush in the water. They spit out the excess toothpaste solution into the emesis basin as it accumulates; if they are unable to spit, use suction. Help the person to rinse with mouthwash after brushing and flossing. This removes any remaining debris and leaves the mouth feeling refreshed. Provide the person with a tissue or towel to wipe their mouth. When providing oral care, assess the person's teeth, dentures and bridges for cracks, sharp edges or missing teeth; and check the gums and mucous membranes.

Perform denture care

Denture care is undertaken daily when the person is unable to care for their own dental work. Either you or the person, if able, remove the dental plates or bridges. If you remove them, use a clean washcloth over a gloved hand to grasp the plate or bridge. The cloth increases friction to facilitate removal and reduces the risk of dropping an expensive item.

Remove the bottom denture first. Remove both dentures by grasping the plate at the front teeth with the thumb and second finger. Slowly rock the plate slightly to release the suction securing it. When loose, lift the plate and turn slightly so one side is lower than the other. This helps to remove the denture without stretching the lips. To avoid damaging or breaking a partial denture/bridge, do not hold the clasps but apply equal pressure on the border of each side of the denture/bridge. Assess the gums for signs of pressure.

Assist the person to rinse their mouth with a preferred mouthwash. Still using the washcloth, hold the dental plate/bridge over a padded basin (use a second washcloth and half fill the basin with water) for safety and remove debris by thoroughly brushing with warm water, and toothpaste if desired. Dissolve a cleaning agent in tepid water in the denture cup (labelled with the person's name). Do not use a glass as the cleaning fluid may be mistaken for a drink. Add the denture/bridge and leave overnight to freshen and disinfect the plastic or metal (Doshi & Jones, 2019). Finally, rinse the denture/bridge and return it to the person using a clean, dry washcloth.

Perform hair care

While the person is in the shower

Washing a person's hair can be incorporated into a shower. Ask the person to tip their head backwards and direct the water stream from the front of the hair backwards to prevent water running over the face. Wet hair thoroughly and lather with the preferred shampoo using the pads of your fingers to massage the scalp, increasing circulation. Rinse well from the forehead backwards with the head tipped back. Remove all traces of shampoo to prevent irritation. Wrap the hair in a towel and gently dry it using short patting movements to prevent damage to the hair shaft.

While the person is in bed

A bed shampoo is done if the person is unable to get out of bed. Use a trough designed for bed shampoos or construct a trough from plastic sheets and towels. To begin, assist the person to the side of the bed and place the trough under their head and neck. The tail of the trough runs off the side of the bed and empties into a basin so that used water is not spilled. Place a small pillow, protected with a waterproof sheet and a towel, under the person's shoulders to increase comfort. Place a damp washcloth over the person's eyes to prevent soapy water entering them.

Use a jug with warm (40 °C) water to wet the hair. Use the person's preferred shampoo and the pads of your fingers to massage their scalp, increasing circulation. Rinse their hair, paying particular attention to the nape of the neck where it is difficult to rinse. Wrap and dry the hair as above and remove the bed trough. This is a skill in itself – do not be discouraged if you must change the person's bed linen as well.

When their hair is towelled dry, style it according to their preference. Take into consideration their ability to care for their hair (e.g. long hair is less likely to mat and tangle in a bed-bound person if it is braided). Hair is thoroughly brushed daily to stimulate scalp circulation, to remove loose hairs, scalp flakes and debris and to arrange the style.

Perform nail care

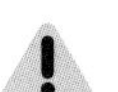
Safety

Either you or the person can care for their nails. Usually, nail care follows the shower or bath since the nails have soaked and softened. Soak the hands or feet, thoroughly dry the skin and assess the nails and skin. Use an orange stick (or similar implement) to carefully pare the debris from under each nail. This may be done while the person is still soaking their nails. Nail edges may require smoothing – feel each one with your index finger. Smooth with the nail file or emery board so there are no jagged edges to catch on clothing, linen or skin.

If the nails are long, and the person agrees, use the clipper to remove the excess nail. Cut the nail straight across. Smooth with the file or emery board. Take care the nail is not cut too short by the lateral folds, so the person does not develop ingrown nails. Toenails especially are trimmed straight across.

Some people have chronic medical conditions that preclude cutting nails – especially toenails – which is left to experts (i.e. podiatrists). For example, peripheral vascular disease and diabetes mellitus both leave the person vulnerable to infection and slow healing if an inadvertent injury occurs. Check the person's chart for contraindications before you cut their toenails.

Apply emollient lotion to keep the skin soft and supple, prevent nail brittleness and hangnails (Kaur et al., 2020). Perform hand hygiene.

Perform a shave

Being clean shaven is important to many males – it improves self-image and makes them feel more dignified (Ette & Gretton, 2019). Sometimes men will need assistance with shaving, or you may need to shave them. Occasionally, a woman may need assistance to shave her legs or underarms. Determine their usual routine (e.g. electric [if permitted by the facility] or safety razor) and bring the equipment to the bedside. Use personal shavers or razors only. Shaving is usually done following the bath. Removing skin oil helps to raise the hair shaft, facilitating its removal. Help the man into an upright position, if possible, since this is the usual position he would assume. Observe his face for lesions, raised moles and birthmarks, and avoid these during shaving to prevent injury. Perform hand hygiene and put on clean gloves in case of nicks to the skin.

Safety

For a safety razor, lather the face with the preferred shaving preparation or soap. Hold the skin taut with your non-dominant hand. With the razor at a 45-degree angle, use short strokes to shave in the direction of the hair growth to promote a closer shave without skin irritation. Rinse the razor between each stroke to keep the cutting edge clean. Start at the top of hair growth and work down to the neck. Be careful to preserve any established moustache or sideburns. Ask him to extend his neck to increase tautness of skin and facilitate hair removal. When the hair has been removed, rinse the area to remove excess lather and hair and to prevent irritation. Apply his choice of aftershave, which acts as an antiseptic on micro-abrasions and feels refreshing. If the shaving is difficult or painful, apply warm towels to the face for 15 minutes, apply more shaving cream and use a fresh blade to reduce discomfort.

> If you inadvertently nick the person, assess the extent of the cut and apply pressure to the area to stop the bleeding. If the cut is more than a nick or the bleeding does not stop after a few minutes, report it to the shift coordinator. Follow the facility's policy on incident reporting.

An electric shaver is used in the same manner on dry skin; that is, the skin is held taut and the razor is moved in the direction of hair growth and from the top downwards. Following the shave, most men rinse their skin and apply aftershave lotion. Electric shavers are contraindicated if the man is receiving oxygen therapy. Oxygen supports combustion and an electric source could supply a spark to start a fire.

Remove gloves and perform hand hygiene.

CLEAN, REPLACE AND DISPOSE OF EQUIPMENT

Safety

Shampoo, conditioner and bath gel bottles are dried and returned to the person's locker for future use. These are personal property and are treated as such. Dispose of razor blades in a sharps container for safety. Electric razors are opened and brushed out (over a newspaper or paper towel) with the brush supplied. The brushings are then folded into the paper and disposed of. Oral care equipment is thoroughly cleaned and returned to the person's locker for future use. Toothbrushes have been shown to harbour organisms such as group A beta-haemolytic streptococci, staphylococci, candida and pseudomonas (Passarelli Mantovani et al., 2019). Plastic covers over toothbrushes increase the humidity and encourage microbial growth. Leave toothbrushes to air dry (Khan et al., 2023). Clean the emesis basin and return it to storage, either in the person's locker or in a utility room, depending on the hospital's practice. Denture cups remain at the person's bedside, empty when not in use and placed somewhere safe while in use. Communal clippers or nail files are washed and dried before storage to prevent cross-infection. Emery boards are not cleanable and therefore are individual and kept in the person's locker. Perform hand hygiene.

DOCUMENTATION

Hygiene measures are usually not specifically documented in detail unless there are findings or observations to report.

CLINICAL SKILLS ASSESSMENT

Oral care, hair care, nail care and shaving

Demonstrates the ability to perform oral care, shaving, hair care and nail care for a dependent person. Incorporates the *National Safety and Quality Health Service Standards*: 2 Partnering with consumers, 3 Preventing and controlling healthcare-associated infections, 5 Comprehensive care, and 6 Communicating for safety (Australian Commission on Safety and Quality in Health Care [ACSQHC], 2021).

Performance criteria	1	2	3	4	5
(Numbers indicate NMBA *Registered Nurse Standards for Practice*)	(Dependent)	(Marginal)	(Assisted)	(Supervised)	(Independent)
1. Identifies indication (1.1, 3.3, 3.4)	☐	☐	☐	☐	☐
2. Evidence of therapeutic interaction with the person, e.g. gives the person a clear explanation of the procedure (1.4, 1.5, 2.1, 2.2, 3.2)	☐	☐	☐	☐	☐
3. Demonstrates clinical reasoning abilities, e.g. provides privacy, alters bed height, attends to environmental temperature, positions the person (1.1, 1.2, 1.3, 1.5, 2.3, 4.1, 4.2, 4.3, 5.1, 6.1)	☐	☐	☐	☐	☐
4. Assesses the person's ability to self-care (1.1, 2.3, 4.1, 4.2, 4.3, 6.1, 6.5)	☐	☐	☐	☐	☐
5. Gathers equipment as determined by the procedure (1.1, 5.5, 6.1)	☐	☐	☐	☐	☐
6. Performs hand hygiene (1.1, 3.4, 6.1)	☐	☐	☐	☐	☐
7. Dons personal protective equipment (1.1, 3.4, 6.1)	☐	☐	☐	☐	☐
8. Carries out the hygiene measure (oral care, hair care, nail care and shaving) (3.2, 6.1, 7.1, 7.2)	☐	☐	☐	☐	☐
9. Cleans, replaces and disposes of equipment appropriately (3.6, 6.1)	☐	☐	☐	☐	☐
10. Documents relevant information (1.1, 1.4, 1.6, 2.2, 2.7, 3.5, 3.7, 6.1, 6.2, 6.5, 7.3)	☐	☐	☐	☐	☐
11. Demonstrates the ability to link theory to practice (1.1, 3.3, 3.4, 3.5)	☐	☐	☐	☐	☐

Student:

Clinical facilitator: Date:

CHAPTER 57

ASSISTING A PERSON TO REPOSITION

INDICATIONS

Positioning in bed promotes comfort, provides proper body alignment and prevents some complications of immobility. Scheduled repositioning of bed- or chairbound people is effective in reducing the occurrence of pressure injuries. The inactive or immobile person may only get exercise during position changes, so these occur two-hourly to prevent circulatory damage, disuse syndrome and to assess skin condition and provide skin care.

The skills for moving and turning people are important to prevent injury to both you and the person. You need to know them before positioning someone in bed.

Repositioning of a dependent person is often a requisite of care. It can also be hazardous to your health. A 'no lifting' policy has been implemented in hospitals to reduce the number of injuries to both nurses and the people in their care. Facilities provide handling equipment, including hoists, friction-reducing (slide) sheets, transfer boards, walking belts, adjustable-height beds and sometimes baths, to promote the individual's and your safety. It is unsafe to lift weights of 20 kg. Spinal and shoulder muscle injury result from repositioning heavy people without sufficient assistance and equipment (Wiggermann, Zhou & McGann, 2020). Follow the facility's policies and use the provided equipment.

EVIDENCE OF THERAPEUTIC INTERACTION

Explain what will be done and why to increase the person's cooperation. Tell them what you will do, their expected or desired behaviour, and any signals to be used to synchronise actions (e.g. 'on the count of three') to increase the effectiveness of the efforts. One person leading the position change ensures a coordinated effort between staff.

DEMONSTRATE CLINICAL REASONING

Determine the need for assistance

Refer to the care plan, manual-handling documentation and risk assessment for information on the individual's needs and the assistance required for repositioning. If these are unavailable, assess before attempting to reposition the person. Some people can assist a great deal, while others are totally dependent. Assess each situation to minimise risk and exertion and to maximise effectiveness. Do not hesitate to obtain assistance if there is doubt about your ability to move a person with safety for yourself and the person.

Principles of good body mechanics

Safety

The following principles of good body mechanics were adapted from McCaw (2022) and Physiopedia (n.d.). Use these principles to protect your back:

- Maintain a good posture: feet shoulder-width apart; 'tailbone' tucked in with a slight outward tilt of your pelvis (tighten the muscles of your buttocks); shoulders back and chest lifted; chin up with your jaw level and relaxed. Check your posture throughout the day.
- Use your longest and strongest muscles to provide the energy needed for the task. The long, strong muscles of arms, legs and hips are less prone to strain and injury than are smaller muscles forced to work beyond their capacity. Back injury is a painful, common nursing injury that is slow to heal and partially preventable by using proper body mechanics.
- Use your internal girdle and make a long midriff (stand tall) to protect the muscles of the abdomen and pelvis. This prevents slouching and utilises muscles properly to prevent strain and injury to the abdominal wall. Tighten the internal girdle by contracting abdominal and gluteal muscle groups.
- Your base of support is enlarged in the direction the movement will occur. To do this, move your front foot forward when pushing and your back foot backwards when pulling (facing the object) or the front foot forward if facing away from the object.
- Bend your knees, flex your hips and keep your back straight when lifting an object rather than bending over from your waist with straight knees. This brings your long, strong thigh muscles into use

ELDER CARE

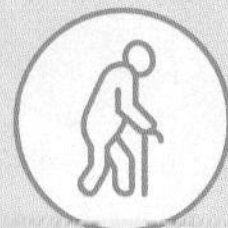

Elderly people tend to stay in bed for a number of reasons: pain, fatigue and weakness; difficulties with tubes, catheters and intravenous lines; and unwillingness to bother the busy staff and concerns about dignity (e.g. flimsy gowns, messy hair). Letting the person do as much as they can for themselves to safely turn, reposition, move in bed and get out of bed assists their ability to maintain activities of daily living and functional capacity (de Oliveira et al., 2023). Take care: the elderly person may overestimate their abilities and underestimate the effects of staying in bed (e.g. vertigo when upright, loss of strength).

THE PERSON LIVING WITH SEVERE OBESITY

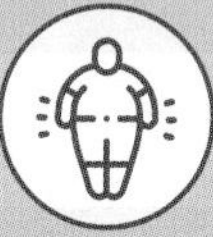

Moving the person living with severe obesity starts with a sound knowledge of the physical logistics and safety requirements. It also requires caring for the person's dignity and comfort. It is a team effort. Communication to coordinate movement is essential to safe and confident care of the severely obese person (Sousa et al., 2023). Encourage the person to assist with the move where they can (e.g. crossing their arms or holding onto a support) to involve them in their care. Listen to their preferences and to their fears to engender trust. Make sure there is sufficient clear space so there is no danger of tripping or entangling equipment (e.g. hoists) and you know how to use the equipment. Mentoring as well as specialised equipment and knowledge are required to keep the person (and you) safe during mobilisation and repositioning. Some of the specialised equipment you may be required to use includes:

- ceiling hoists
- large slide sheets
- portable mechanical and electronic lifts
- power-driven beds and wheelchairs that can accommodate the excess weight
- slide sheets, boards and other transfer equipment.

See also **Clinical Skills 15 and 23** for a brief explanation of issues for people living with severe obesity.

and keeps the weight of the object lifted close to your centre of gravity to improve balance.

- Centre the line of gravity over the base of support. (Keep the work as close to your body as possible.) Lower the side-rail on the side of the bed closest to you to reduce reaching.
- Turn your feet, not your back, if a change of direction is necessary. This avoids twisting and stretching muscles during work – movements that strain muscles. Face in the direction of movement to prevent twisting of the spine and ineffective use of muscle groups.
- Rest muscles between periods of exertion. Muscles that are overused or misused build up chemicals accentuating fatigue. Muscles work more effectively by resting them occasionally after working them strenuously.
- Keep the work area at a comfortable height. When body alignment and balance are easier to maintain, muscle strain is reduced.
- Use smooth, even movements to prevent jerkiness and strain on muscles. Jerky movements are uncomfortable for the person. This is accomplished by contracting your gluteal, abdominal, leg and arm muscles before the move to prepare them for action.

Wear closed-heel, flat shoes with non-slip soles to prevent slips and falls.

Your sleep position (this also applies to the person you are caring for) also contributes to avoiding back injury and pain and contributes to maintaining a healthy spine. Use a firm mattress, sleep on your side or back, use a pillow between your knees when side-lying and under your knees when lying on your back, and use a pillow that keeps your head in alignment with your spine (Türkmen et al., 2023).

Assess the person

Assessment determines the level and type of assistance the person requires. Identify the person's level of dependence:

- *independent* – can perform the transfer/reposition safely without a nurse's assistance
- *partial assist* – can perform the transfer/reposition safely with a nurse's assistance or the use of assistive devices
- *dependent* – cannot perform the transfer/reposition safely without the use of assistive devices.

LOOK at the person's height and weight (a person who is more than 110 to 120 kg requires specific bariatric equipment); the weight-bearing capacity of the person (full, partial or none); their bilateral upper extremity strength (Full? Yes or no); their level of cooperation and comprehension:

- *cooperative* – may need prompting but can follow instructions
- *unpredictable or varied* – behaviour changes frequently, is uncooperative or unable to follow simple instructions.

Assess yourself: a one-person assist (partial assist) involves anyone requiring stand-by assistance, cueing or a lift of *less than* 20 kg of the person's weight. A minimum of two staff and assistive devices are needed if 20 kg or more needs to be lifted, or if the person is unpredictable in the amount of assistance needed.

Check the weight restrictions on all lifting devices. Identify conditions that could affect the repositioning technique (e.g. surgical incision, IVs and drains, fragile skin, pressure area development or pressure injuries, postoperative restrictions on positioning). Review appropriate use of equipment or algorithms to determine the equipment required to safely move the person. Determine the number of staff needed to reposition the person safely based on individual assessment. Document the level of assistance and devices required on the person's care plan.

Identify positions available

Several positions are available to promote the person's physical, physiological and psychological wellbeing. Various conditions and diseases (e.g. fractures, paralysis, lung disease and congestive cardiac failure) preclude moving people into some positions. Common positions include supine, left or right lateral, semi- or high Fowler's and, occasionally, prone.

The person's level of consciousness and ability to assist and comply with instructions may alter positioning. For example, an unconscious person is not positioned in a high Fowler's position (they could not maintain that position) or in a supine position (risk of aspiration of saliva and mucus).

Tubes, incisions, drains and intravenous (IV) lines alter the turning/positioning procedure. Support the body to maintain its natural contours, symmetry and alignment. Positioning is often used to provide the starting point to maximise the benefits of other interventions (e.g. a range of motion and breathing exercises), comfort, optimal rest and rehabilitation to facilitate recovery, prevention of injury (e.g. pressure injury, neural compression, contractures) or to assist the person to access their environment (DeLaune et al., 2024). Positioning is especially important in the operating theatre as the person cannot protect themselves and can easily develop a pressure injury or neural damage from sustained pressure (Brunette & Miller, 2023).

Preparation

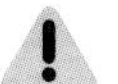
Safety

Draw curtains and/or close the door to ensure privacy. Anticipate the need for slide sheets for turning and repositioning the person by placing these on the bedside locker. Remove any obstacles (e.g. chairs, overbed table). Lock the bed wheels to prevent the bed from moving during the procedure as a safety action for both you and the person. Place the bed in a horizontal position (as the person's condition permits). Raise the bed to an appropriate and comfortable height for moving the person. Lower the side-rail on the near side, so that reaching over the person will not strain your muscles. As a safety precaution, keep the opposite side-rail up if that side is unattended. Move tubing, drains and collecting apparatus to facilitate position changes. Utilise extra staff and available lifting equipment as per facility policy.

ASSIST THE PERSON TO REPOSITION

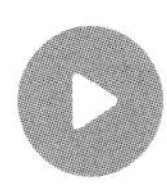
Video

Hand hygiene

Hand hygiene (see **Clinical Skill 5**) removes microorganisms from your hands. It is the most effective preventative measure for cross-contamination, reducing incidences of nosocomial (i.e. hospital- or treatment-acquired) infection.

Position the person

Move the person to the side of the bed opposite to the way they will be turning. If they cannot do this themselves, the assistance of another nurse will be required. Partnered turns are safer for both the person and the nurses (Budarick, Lad & Fischer, 2020). You can move the person using a slide sheet or manually in stages by first moving their head and shoulders while another nurse moves their hips and back; then align their legs and feet.

GATHER EQUIPMENT

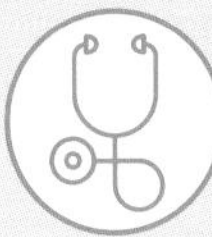

Gathering equipment ensures that you have all needed material, boosts the person's confidence and trust in you, and increases your self-confidence. While gathering the equipment, you can mentally rehearse the procedure. Equipment required includes:

EQUIPMENT	EXPLANATION
Friction-reducing (slide) sheets	• Placed under the person from the head to below the buttocks, and used to slide the person up in bed • Use of slide sheets to move or reposition an incapacitated person reduces nurses' musculoskeletal injury and pain (Higuchi, Takahashi & Tomita, 2023). Slide sheets are used for one individual (i.e. not shared). Check it for tears before use.
Lifting devices: lifts or hoists	• Used with heavy or totally incapacitated people • Check that it can safely move the weight of the person and the sling is an appropriate size • Use as instructed to prevent injury to the person, to you and to other nursing staff • Most slings are made to be left under the person without causing injury (Alperovitch-Najenson et al., 2019)

EQUIPMENT	EXPLANATION
Pillows	• Used to provide padding in front of the headboard to protect the head during moves, provide support for various body parts during the move, and support the person in the new position to relax muscles • Pillows are reasonably effective in maintaining lateral body angle and head/neck alignment for immobilised people (Türkmen et al., 2023)
Other support devices: hand splints, sandbags, wedge pillows, trochanter rolls, fluidised positioner	Used as necessary to maintain body alignment and functional positioning

Position the person with a slide sheet

Most slide sheet position changes require two nurses. Place one (folded in half) slide sheet under the person by turning them one way, insert the slide sheet with a folded edge below their buttocks, or two slide sheets one on top of the other, turn the person the other way and pull the slide sheet(s) through. Turn them onto their back again to finish.

Position the person manually (no slide sheet)

This is not recommended, but may not be avoidable. To centre the person in bed, stand next to the bed and slide your hands under the person's shoulders and neck. Assume a wide stance with one foot next to the bed and the other about 60 cm back. Flex knees and put your weight onto the leg closest to the bed. Contract gluteal and abdominal muscles and shift your weight onto your back foot, pulling the person's head and shoulder (then hips and back as a second step) using your own body weight to reduce muscle strain. Align their legs and feet.

Turn the person

Put the opposite side-rail up to reduce the risk of falling. Stand on the side of the bed towards which the person will turn and undertake the following:

1. Tell the person what you will be doing. Insert the slide sheet.
2. If the person is to be *turned to a prone position*, turn their near arm with the palm upwards, so they can roll over that arm; or, if the person will *remain on their side*, move the near arm away from the body.
3. Place the far arm with the palm towards the thigh to maximise your control of the arm.
4. Turn the head away from the direction of the move so the person does not roll onto their face.
5. Flex or cross the far knee over the near knee to facilitate the move.
6. Grasp the far slide sheet at the shoulder and hip, to provide support for the entire back. Use your wrist to hold the person's arm steady.
7. Assume a wide stance with one foot next to the bed and the other about 60 cm back. Flex your knees and put your weight onto the leg closest to the bed.
8. Contract gluteal and abdominal muscles and shift your weight onto your back foot, pulling the person's shoulder and hips (with the slide sheet) using your own body weight to reduce muscle strain. Support the person's head and extremities in positions of proper body alignment and comfort.
9. To complete the turn to prone, shift your hand position to the front of the shoulders and hips and continue to turn the person until they are prone.
10. Move the person to the centre of the bed, because a 180-degree turn will move them near the edge of the bed.
11. Remove the slide sheets. Adjust alignment and support the person with pillows as necessary for comfort.

Various sizes and shapes of pillows or fluid positioners (gel-filled shapes) can be used to keep bony prominences (e.g. knees) apart, to support limbs in alignment with joints (e.g. arm and elbow with shoulder) and to keep the person in position (e.g. behind the shoulder, back and hips in a side-lying position). When the person is repositioned and comfortable, replace the side-rail, fasten the call bell to the bedclothes within easy reach and return the bed to its original level.

Move the person up in bed

Position the person

Two nurses are generally required to move a person up in bed. Place a pillow at the top of the bed to act as a 'bumper' and to prevent injury if the move is further than planned. Place the slide sheet(s) under them. Ask the person to fold their arms over their chest to prevent squeezing their arms between the slide sheet and their torso. If the person is able, ask them to flex their knees to prevent their legs from pulling across the bed during the move.

Move the person

Once the person is positioned, undertake the following:

1. Tell the person what is being done, and what they are expected to do.
2. Each nurse firmly grasps the top slide sheet at the person's upper back with one hand and at the level of the buttocks with the other hand.
3. Face the head of the bed and assume a broad stance with your legs slightly flexed at the knee and hip to increase the base of support and to facilitate a smooth weight shift. Place your weight on the back leg in preparation for the move.

4. Ask the person to raise their head by putting their chin on their chest and exhaling. This reduces the friction to be overcome, and exhaling prevents the Valsalva manoeuvre, which, if used, can stress the heart.
5. Contract your pelvic muscles to prevent muscle strain and carefully shift weight from your back leg to your front leg, keeping your back and arms straight, and pulling the slide sheet towards the head of the bed. This provides the additional force of your body weight, decreasing the work of muscles.
6. Once the person is positioned, remove the slide sheets.

When the person is supine, positioning is important to maintain comfort and to prevent complications. Trochanter rolls (small firm pillows) or appropriate fluid positioners can be used below the hip joint to prevent external rotation. The heels can be lifted off the bed with small pillows placed under the knees and along the length of the calf. Neck alignment and positioning is important for comfort. Pillows of varying size and firmness are tried until a combination is found that promotes comfort.

Use a hoist to reposition the person

Hoists are used for people unable to bear weight or who are too heavy to safely move manually. The person may need to be moved out of bed, out of a chair or lifted off the floor following a fall. Determine that the hoist can safely move the weight of the person and that it is in working order. There are a number of hoists available, each with their own specific sling, and their own safety requirements. You must be familiar with those used in your clinical facility.

Ensure there is adequate room for the hoist itself, as well as space to manoeuvre the hoist for the repositioning or transfer. Check the wheels are locked on the bed and raise the bed to the high position. Hoist moves require two nurses. Explain the procedure to the person, and then undertake the following steps:

1. Place the person in a supine position with the bed flat (or as low as the person can tolerate) and the side-rails down, and roll the person away from you towards the other nurse. Position the sling under the person (according to the manufacturer's guidelines).
2. Roll the person towards you so the other nurse can pull the sling through. Straighten the sling and roll the person into a supine position. If the person is to be seated in a chair, place the base of the hoist under the bed on the same side of the bed as the chair is positioned.
3. Lock the wheels of the hoist.
4. Attach the straps from the sling to the swivel bar ensuring they are even, which allows for equal distribution of the person's weight. Ask the person to cross their arms over their chest or hold onto the swivel bar.
5. Follow the manufacturer's instructions for raising the person from the bed. Some hoists are battery operated; others require pumping of the lift handle to raise the person clear of the bed.
6. When the person is clear of the bed, release the brakes on the hoist and reposition the person over the bed to allow for position change.
7. Once the person is correctly positioned, lower the hoist and remove the sling straps from the swivel bar. Most slings are designed to remain under the person (if not soiled or wet). To remove the sling, roll the person on their side, tucking half of the sling under, roll them over the tucked sling and remove it.

If sitting the person in a chair, one nurse guides the person in the hoist until they are over the chair, while the other nurse ensures the person's feet are protected from any bumps. Align the person over the chair and slowly lower them into the chair (according to manufacturer's instructions). The second nurse guides them into the chair using the 'handles' on the back of the sling. Remove the straps from the bar and move the hoist out of the way.

Ensure the person is comfortable and place the call bell within easy reach. Perform hand hygiene. (Note: the reverse method is used to return the person to bed.)

CLEAN, REPLACE AND DISPOSE OF EQUIPMENT

Return the hoist to the appropriate storage area. Follow the facility's policy for charging the batteries to ensure they remain charged and the hoist is available for use when needed. This is a time-management strategy and a courtesy to fellow nursing staff.
If slings or slide sheets are soiled, place those in the contaminated linen skip as per the facility's guidelines. Perform hand hygiene.

DOCUMENTATION

Relevant information, including time and date, procedure, response and any areas of skin breakdown, are to be recorded. Document the level of assistance and devices required on the person's care plan. Some hospitals do not require that movement and turning be recorded in the nursing notes/eHealth record. Follow the facility's policy. Any relevant information gleaned during the move is passed on, verbally and in writing, so the healthcare team remains informed.

CLINICAL SKILLS ASSESSMENT

Assisting a person to reposition

Demonstrates the ability to effectively and safely assist a person to reposition. Incorporates the *National Safety and Quality Health Service Standards*: 2 Partnering with consumers, 3 Preventing and controlling healthcare-associated infections, 5 Comprehensive care, and 6 Communicating for safety (Australian Commission on Safety and Quality in Health Care [ACSQHC], 2021).

Performance criteria	1	2	3	4	5
(Numbers indicate NMBA *Registered Nurse Standards for Practice*)	**(Dependent)**	**(Marginal)**	**(Assisted)**	**(Supervised)**	**(Independent)**
1. Identifies indication (1.1, 3.3, 3.4)	☐	☐	☐	☐	☐
2. Evidence of therapeutic interaction with the person, e.g. gives the person a clear explanation of the procedure (1.4, 1.5, 2.1, 2.2, 3.2)	☐	☐	☐	☐	☐
3. Demonstrates clinical reasoning abilities, e.g. determines positions available to the person, secures the bed (1.1, 1.2, 1.3, 1.5, 2.3, 4.1, 4.2, 4.3, 5.1, 6.1)	☐	☐	☐	☐	☐
4. Assesses the person's level of assistance required (2.3, 4.1, 4.2, 4.3, 6.1)	☐	☐	☐	☐	☐
5. Utilises principles of efficient body mechanics (1.1, 3.1, 6.1)	☐	☐	☐	☐	☐
6. Gathers equipment (1.1, 5.5, 6.1): ■ slide sheets ■ lifting devices: lifts or hoists ■ pillows ■ other support devices: hand splints, sandbags, wedge pillows, trochanter rolls	☐	☐	☐	☐	☐
7. Performs hand hygiene (1.1, 6.1)	☐	☐	☐	☐	☐
8. Moves the person up in bed (1.1, 6.1)	☐	☐	☐	☐	☐
9. Positions the person in a side-lying position (1.1, 6.1)	☐	☐	☐	☐	☐
10. Positions the person using a hoist (1.1, 3.1, 6.1)	☐	☐	☐	☐	☐
11. Cleans, replaces and disposes of equipment appropriately (3.6, 6.1)	☐	☐	☐	☐	☐
12. Documents relevant information (1.1, 1.4, 1.6, 2.2, 2.7, 3.5, 3.7, 6.1, 6.2, 6.5, 7.3)	☐	☐	☐	☐	☐
13. Demonstrates the ability to link theory to practice (1.1, 3.3, 3.4, 3.5)	☐	☐	☐	☐	☐

Student:

Clinical facilitator: Date:

CHAPTER 58

ASSISTING A PERSON TO MOBILISE

INDICATIONS

People requiring assistance to mobilise are those who are:

- suffering from paralysis or weakness
- frail – resulting from protracted time in bed of a few days or more
- debilitated from illness or following surgery
- immobile from lower limb treatment measures.

Assisting with mobilisation is the most effective nursing measure to prevent postoperative complications. Mobilisation guidelines and a positive staff attitude encourage early mobilisation (Anekwe et al., 2020). Initial mobilisation of anyone who has had cerebrovascular accidents, paralysis, brain damage, an amputation or some musculoskeletal disorders (e.g. total hip replacement) requires specialised assistance provided by a physiotherapist or a nurse with specialised knowledge. For a person who has been immobilised, regaining the ability to walk is a morale boost.

Prolonged immobility can have severe consequences, including: constipation, urinary retention, altered tissue perfusion, pressure injuries, hypostatic pneumonia, osteoporosis, renal calculi and deep vein thrombosis. Even in the intensive care unit, early mobilisation is a proven safe intervention that reduces complications, including social isolation, pressure injuries, deep vein thrombosis and ventilation associated pneumonia, and improves self-esteem (Wang et al., 2020). Heng et al. (2020) demonstrate that people need knowledge and encouragement to mobilise safely.

EVIDENCE OF THERAPEUTIC INTERACTION

A clear, thorough explanation of the importance of mobilisation helps to improve engagement and reduce anxiety. Explain the procedure (the distance to be walked, the assistance the person can expect). This helps them to assess their own strength and ability. Instruct them to alert you to any fatigue or pain. Most are somewhat unsure about leaving the safety of their bed and venturing out on limbs that feel very shaky. A calm, confident manner, plenty of sincere reassurance and physical support assist the person to take their first steps.

DEMONSTRATE CLINICAL REASONING

Identify safety considerations

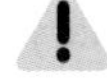

Safety

You must assess an immobile person before attempting to assist them to walk.

LOOK at their care plan for particular instructions. For example, following coronary artery bypass surgery, the person cannot use their arms to push up from a bed or chair and needs to support their chest wound by crossing their arms over their chest. Activity tolerance, strength, orthostatic hypotension, coordination and balance are considered.

LISTEN to any reports of weakness, faintness or pain that might interfere with mobilisation.

Before the person can mobilise, assess their abilities and carry out a preparation program. This may take a few minutes or be undertaken over several days.

Ensure any walking aids (e.g. cane, crutches, walker) are on the preferred side of the bed for easy access.

Assess then implement strengthening exercises

Assess the person's current musculoskeletal condition (see **Clinical Skill 24**).

Encourage muscle strength and range of motion with gradual progression to an active range of motion; for example, isometric exercises, such as quadriceps exercises, to resistance exercises.

Encourage sitting balance by initially positioning the person in a high Fowler's position, assisting them to sit at the edge of the bed, feet supported

ELDER CARE

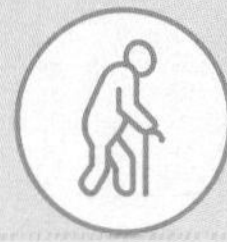

Ageing is generally associated with a loss of muscle mass, strength and reduced balance and frailty. Thus, older adults are at greater risk of falling and injuring themselves, whether at home or in the hospital (Martínez-Velilla et al., 2019). Dowling et al. (2023) state that 30 per cent of adults over 65 years of age fall annually, with up to half of these falls resulting in some harm.

Deconditioning is caused by prolonged immobility (e.g. bed rest following a stroke or hip replacement). It results in functional decline and increases the development of frailty and sarcopenia (Swinnerton & Price, 2023).

To reduce falls in the elderly population, implement the following recommendations (Moreland, Karkara & Henry, 2020): risk assessments for falls on admission; improving strength, gait and balance; modifying medications (e.g. decreasing hypnotics, benzodiazepines); treating vitamin D deficiency and osteoporosis; screening and rectifying vision; and home/room modifications (e.g. remove loose rugs, use of soled slippers). Heng et al. (2020) add educating the person about the causes and prevention of falls.

Since falls and their resultant injuries are extremely common among older adults, considerably increasing both morbidity and mortality in this age group (Pepera et al., 2023), maintaining and increasing elderly people's mobility positively affects their functional and cognitive abilities and quality of life (Tasheva et al., 2020). Exercise programs (in addition to walking), including strength and balance training, flexibility exercises and gait retraining, have proved to decrease the functional decline associated with hospitalisation.

THE PERSON LIVING WITH SEVERE OBESITY

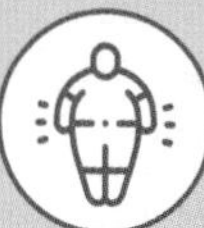

The excess mass of the severely obese person requires more energy to move, reducing their exercise capacity. As well, the muscle strength in their legs may not be sufficient to move their weight for any distance (Sabol et al., 2020). Assess the person's level of mobility and their independence (Hales, Curran & de Vries, 2018). Assisting the severely obese person to mobilise requires bariatric equipment as well as extra staff assistance. Preconditioning with isometric exercises assists the person to mobilise. A ceiling hoist or lift may be required to assist them onto their feet, and a purpose-built walker will be required that can carry the person's weight (severely obese people often bring the bariatric walker from home). Short walks (4 to 5 m) may be necessary to start. Have extra helpers, with one following behind with an appropriately sized wheelchair in case of fatigue. Ensure the person has sufficient covering for modesty and sturdy footwear. (See **Clinical Skills 15 and 23** for a brief explanation of issues with severely obese people.)

on a stool, until no dizziness or swaying is noticed/reported. Monitor their blood pressure to assess for orthostatic hypotension.

Encourage standing balance. Assist the person to stand at the bedside (unless contraindicated), allowing them to hang on to the bedside. Gradually they will stand unassisted. Standing balance means they can keep their trunk still and move their extremities without swaying. Some people require tilt tables if they are extremely deconditioned, severely obese or have very poor balance or endurance.

The next goal is weight shifting, where the person can move their weight from one leg to the other or from one side of their body to the other without losing balance.

The person may require thromboembolism deterrent (TED) stockings to be applied before mobilising. Postoperatively, a pain assessment and adequate analgesic cover are needed before initial mobilisation. Encourage the person to void prior to ambulating.

Remain close to the person. Schedule rest periods, as ambulation increases activity and fatigue. Initial exercise and mobilisation periods are short, gradually increasing in time and distance as their tolerance increases. As well, some people are monitored postoperatively (e.g. cardiac surgery) for heart rate and respiratory rate periodically during mobilisation. Elevated (over baseline by 20 beats per minute) heart and respiratory rates indicate the need for rest.

The person should wear well-fitted shoes with good support and non-skid soles; if such shoes are not available, bare feet are preferable to socks or stockings because they may slip. Silicone dots on socks reduce slipping.

Consider environmental factors. Handrails give the person a sense of security. Dry floors (and if waxed, a non-slip wax used) free of clutter (e.g. electrical cords, scatter rugs, magazines, newspapers) are safest.

Consider medical equipment (e.g. intravenous [IV] tubing, urinary catheters, chest drains, wound drains) when assisting the person to get out of bed and walk. Wheeled IV poles are useful to help with balance (if the IV pole is difficult to wheel, you can push it at the person's walking pace). Cloth bags to carry urinary catheters or drainage apparatus increase mobility. If possible, raise the height of the bed so the person's hips are level or higher than their knees when their feet are on the floor to reduce the effort of standing for the person.

Safety

Know your own strength and ability. If unsure, recruit another nurse to assist as an occupational health and safety precaution as well as a safety measure for the person you are moving. If the person is unstable or very weak, ask an assistant to follow with a wheelchair, keeping pace with the person. Assistive devices are available for use as necessary. Inspect the assistive device to ensure that the rubber tips are not worn or show signs of poor tread, that the frame is stable, that the hand grips are secure and complete, and that the metal tubing is not bent, cracked or damaged (DeLaune et al., 2024). If specific aids are needed (e.g. crutches or a particular type of walker), a physiotherapist or a nurse with specialised knowledge or experience selects the appropriate aid and carries out a training program.

Use a falls risk-assessment tool (FRAT), such as the one devised by Health Victoria (Victorian Government, 2015). These consider such variables as history of previous falls, medications being taken, cognitive and psychological factors, history of risk taking, continence and orientation, all of which can impact the person's risk for falling.

Recommend an exercise program (e.g. tai chi, social dance or other group-based program for increased socialisation) to increase functional mobility, flexibility and strength (Pepera et al., 2023).

In short, assess:

- the task, the environment and any equipment required
- your physical ability (e.g. previous injury, small size) and need for assistance
- the physical (muscle strength), cognitive (understand instructions) and mental (cooperative or not) capabilities of the person being assisted
- your ability to dynamically assess the risks (increasing weakness, feeling faint; or your increasing fatigue) during the move (Brusco et al., 2023).

GATHER EQUIPMENT

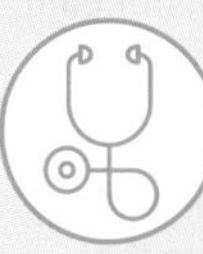

Gathering equipment ensures that you have all needed material, boosts the person's confidence and trust in you, and increases your self-confidence. While gathering the equipment, you can mentally rehearse the procedure. The following devices may be needed:

EQUIPMENT	EXPLANATION
Safety/walking belt	• A heavy leather belt that the person wears snugly around their waist. You walk beside the person, grasping the belt in the middle of the back and at the side. If they become dizzy or lose their balance, you can steady them with the belt. The person is assessed by a physiotherapist, who recommends how and when to use a walking belt (Miller, Rockefeller & Townsend, 2020) • These are no longer recommended in some states, as they may contribute to injuries to the nurse and to the person if a fall occurs
Canes	• Promote a feeling of security • Provide extra stability for anyone who has one weak leg but can bear weight on both legs • The tip has a non-skid rubber surface for safety • The top curve (hand grip) is held in line with the hip joint of the *unaffected leg*, with the person's elbow slightly flexed (15 to 30 degrees) • The cane is moved forward while the affected and unaffected legs support the person simultaneously. The person moves the affected leg past the cane while the cane and the unaffected leg bear the weight. The cane is moved forward, and the affected leg and the cane take the weight while the unaffected leg is moved forward • Two points of support are always present
Walkers	• Provide four points of support, give a wide base and provide the most security of all the assistive devices • The person places the walker in front of them and steps forward. The walker is then moved forward. The top is level with the hands when the elbows are flexed between 15 to 30 degrees • Usually constructed of aluminium, since they must be lightweight • Some have wheels on the front legs to ease movement • Some have modified underarm extensions to support people who have upper-extremity limitations
Crutches	• Used when 'no', 'single-leg' or 'modified' weight bearing is allowed • Upper-body strength and arm control are needed to use 'underarm' crutches. Wrists, hands and shoulders, not the axillae, support the weight. Pressure on the axillae can cause irreversible nerve damage • Forearm or elbow crutches are often used for longer-term assistance • Measured for each individual and fitted by a trained professional • Different gaits are used for different types of weight bearing • Gait pattern is determined by the physician or physiotherapist and is usually taught to the person by that professional
Knee walkers	• An alternative to crutches for anyone who cannot bear weight on one lower limb (ankle, foot) • Four-wheeled scooters have an elevated pad where the person kneels on their injured leg and uses their uninjured leg to propel themselves. Stairs cannot be negotiated with a knee walker

ASSIST WITH MOBILISATION

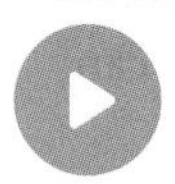
Video

Assisting a person to walk requires assessment skills, attention to safety and patience.

Hand hygiene

Hand hygiene (see **Clinical Skill 5**) removes microorganisms from your hands. It is the most effective preventative measure for cross-contamination, reducing incidences of nosocomial (i.e. hospital- or treatment-acquired) infection.

Assist the person to walk

Prepare the person

Prepare the person to stand upright. Sit them up in bed, move them to the bed edge with feet over the edge to 'dangle' for at least a minute. Place the mobile IV pole (as necessary) at the head of the bed so it does not interfere with standing. Other tubes and drains need to be accounted for – urinary catheter bags are emptied, remain below the level of the bladder and can be placed in a cloth bag for discretion. A Hemovac may be suspended with an elastic band attached with a safety pin to the clothing. If the person has a chest drainage system, a second nurse is needed to keep the underwater system upright and without tension on the chest tubes. Walking aids are within easy reach.

Assist the person to walk

Assist the person to stand upright. Assess for signs and symptoms of orthostatic hypotension (dizziness, light-headedness, sudden tachycardia). If these symptoms occur, return them to bed and monitor their blood pressure and pulse. When they feel secure standing, assist them to walk. It will be a slow process at first. Progressive assistance may be needed. A second nurse may need to follow with a wheelchair in case of weakness or dizziness. Initially assist the person by using a walking or safety belt (as appropriate in the facility). Steady the person until they gain confidence. When the person is competent and confident walking with the safety belt, it can be removed. Walking with you is the next step. Accompany them, as they walk. This provides additional confidence and you can assess their fatigue or alterations in physical parameters. Help them to manage IV poles or other devices. Urge them to use handrails as a safety measure.

Assist a weak or dizzy person to the nearest chair or bed. Despite best efforts (assessment, environmental and personal safety interventions), people do fall. Unfortunately, there is no consistent agreement in Australia and New Zealand regarding assisting the person to fall (Whitby & McLachlan, 2014). 'Assisted falls' occur when there is someone present who is able to control the person's descent to the floor/ground (Venema et al., 2019) and ease the effects of the fall (Bargmann & Brundrett, 2020). Many facilities prefer that the healthcare personnel allow the person to fall, removing obstacles and protecting their head as necessary (Whitby & McLachlan, 2014); others suggest an assisted fall (Brigham and Women's Hospital, 2020), if possible. You will need to follow the facility's protocol if the person begins to faint or fall (so know it before you assist a person to walk).

> ?
>
> If it is acceptable to assist someone to fall, assess your ability to help them, and if able, broaden your base of support by moving the outside leg further out and back. Then support the person under the axillae, bringing them backwards so their weight rests on your hip. The person can be supported like this for a short time or slid down your leg and lowered into a horizontal position on the floor until help arrives. Chu (2014) suggests that severely obese people who are dizzy and fall cannot be safely lowered to the floor without endangering the assisting nurse, and recommends that protecting their head is the most that can be done.

While the person is initially using a walker, cane or crutches, remain with them to ensure their safety and their ability to undertake the activity. Following this, their progress needs to be assessed and documented periodically.

DOCUMENTATION

Documenting mobilisation includes the distance walked, the time taken, assistance required and the person's response to mobilisation (including falling episodes). For some people, body posture, a description of the gait, activity intolerance (e.g. dizziness, tachycardia, shortness of breath), the amount of support required, and blood pressure and respiratory rate following ambulation are important to note.

CLINICAL SKILLS ASSESSMENT

Assisting a person to mobilise

Demonstrates the ability to effectively and safely assist a person to mobilise. Incorporates the *National Safety and Quality Health Service Standards*: 2 Partnering with consumers, 5 Comprehensive care, and 6 Communicating for safety (Australian Commission on Safety and Quality in Health Care [ACSQHC], 2021).

Performance criteria	1	2	3	4	5
(Numbers indicate NMBA *Registered Nurse Standards for Practice*)	(Dependent)	(Marginal)	(Assisted)	(Supervised)	(Independent)
1. Identifies indication (1.1, 3.3, 3.4)	☐	☐	☐	☐	☐
2. Evidence of therapeutic interaction with the person, e.g. provides a clear explanation of the procedure (1.4, 1.5, 2.1, 2.2, 3.2)	☐	☐	☐	☐	☐
3. Demonstrates clinical reasoning, e.g. identifies safety considerations, completes a musculoskeletal assessment (1.1, 1.2, 1.3, 1.5, 4.1, 4.2, 4.3, 5.1, 6.1)	☐	☐	☐	☐	☐
4. Gathers equipment and assistive devices as required (1.1, 5.5, 6.1): ■ safety/walking belt ■ canes ■ walkers ■ crutches ■ knee walkers	☐	☐	☐	☐	☐
5. Performs hand hygiene (1.1, 6.1)	☐	☐	☐	☐	☐
6. Assists the person to walk (3.2, 4.1, 4.2, 4.3, 6.1)	☐	☐	☐	☐	☐
7. Documents relevant information (1.1, 1.4, 1.6, 2.2, 2.7, 3.5, 3.7, 6.1, 6.2, 6.5, 7.3)	☐	☐	☐	☐	☐
8. Demonstrates the ability to link theory to practice (1.1, 3.3, 3.4, 3.5)	☐	☐	☐	☐	☐

Student:

Clinical facilitator: Date:

CHAPTER 59

PRESSURE AREA CARE – PREVENTING PRESSURE INJURIES

INDICATIONS

A pressure injury (PI) – previously known as a pressure sore, decubitus ulcer or bedsore – is localised damage to the skin and underlying soft tissue due to prolonged pressure that occurs in vulnerable people and the unattended. These are usually over a bony prominence or are related to a medical or other device, and any part of the body that is under prolonged pressure may be damaged (e.g. positioned on a folded ear, lying on oxygen tubing, or pressure from the ear stems of heavy glasses). They can present as intact skin or an open ulcer, and may be painful. PIs begin in the deep subdermal tissues between the bones and the skin

The three contributing forces of PIs are as follows:

- *Pressure* – high pressure causes damage in as little as 30 minutes, although slight pressure can cause the same damage over a long period. Tissue tolerance, intensity and duration of the pressure all contribute to the development of a pressure injury (Royal Children's Hospital Melbourne [RCHM], 2019). Pressure compresses the tissues between the bone and the surface and occludes the blood vessels. Compression also prevents lymph fluid drainage, which causes increased interstitial fluid and waste build-up and contributes to pressure injury (Boyko, Longakerm & Yang, 2018). The sustained pressure initiates an inflammatory process (caused by cell deformation and reperfusion), which causes localised oedema in the sub-epidermis, as the superficial layers of the skin are less susceptible to pressure-induced injury (McLaren-Kennedy et al., 2023). If the pressure is relieved in a timely manner, blood rushes into the ischaemic tissue, causing a period of hyperaemia. The flush of fresh blood delivers vital oxygen and nutrients to the area to restore the viability of the tissue. If pressure is prolonged, ischaemia develops into necrosis, resulting in tissue breakdown. (See a fundamentals text for a discussion of the various stages of PI.)
- *Shear force* – the mechanical force of pressure applied parallel to the plane of the body, which contributes to the development of PIs. For example, when the person slides down in the bed, the muscle and deep fascia move in the direction of the slide, but the skin is held relatively still by the frictional forces between it and the bed. Ischaemia occurs because the distortion of soft tissue and capillaries occludes blood flow.
- *Friction* – contributes to PIs by abrading and breaking the skin and beginning the erosion. A moist environment (e.g. incontinence, excessive sweating) increases the effects of friction and pressure to amplify the problem.

The tolerance of soft tissue for pressure and shear is affected by microclimate, nutrition, perfusion, comorbidities and tissue condition (Persaud-Jaimangal, Ayello & Sibbald, 2020).

Risk factors

Risk factors that predispose an individual to the development of PIs have long been known. These include:

- *Demographic factors* – advanced age or very young babies (e.g. premature infants) because of thin and fragile skin. Residential or community care agencies demonstrate higher incidences of PIs.
- *Physiological factors* – decreased level of consciousness, poor nutritional status with a high or, more often, a low body mass index (BMI) (Boyko, Longakerm & Yang, 2018), inadequate hydration, smoking and elevated body temperature.
- *Psychological factors* – such as altered mental status, depression and confusion, contribute to immobility.
- *Pathological factors* – such as peripheral vascular disease, renal disease, malignancies, impaired circulation, diabetes mellitus, cerebral vascular accidents, and para- and quadriplegia.
- *Functional factors* – sensory impairment, incontinence, lack of mobility and prolonged inactivity.
- *Environmental factors* – hyperthermia from resting on plastic or other hard surfaces (e.g. theatre tables), pressure from casts or tubing (e.g. catheters or nasal prongs), prolonged exposure to moisture, creases in bed linen or foreign objects (e.g. buttons or catheters) trapped under limbs. Medical device–related PI account for 10 per cent of PIs and develop faster than non-medical device–related PIs (Cooper et al., 2020).

Pressure injuries cause a great deal of severe pain, take a long time to heal, impact on sleep and mood, cause infection, and adversely affect rehabilitation, mobility and quality of life. Most pressure injuries are preventable (Tervo-Heikkinen et al., 2023). Determining the risk of developing a pressure injury must be followed by measures to prevent such an occurrence (such as pressure relieving mattresses, pressure relieving dressings). These are discussed briefly below.

Healthcare system cost

Not only are PIs painful, slow to heal and decrease quality of life, but they are costly to the healthcare system. In 2018–19, the Australian Commission on Safety and Quality in Health Care identified nearly 2700 hospital-acquired PI in public hospitals with an average in-hospital cost of A$56 000 (ACSQHC, 2020). Besides the actual treatment cost of material and nursing hours, other costs include hospital bed costs, increased lengths of stay, laboratory costs, multidisciplinary consults, the loss of individual productivity and diminished quality of life.

The ACSQHC (2018) reports that some large metropolitan and regional hospitals have managed to reduce the incidence of hospital-acquired PI to 9.8/10 000 admissions by providing preventative care. PI development indicates the care given to the individual was not tailored to that person, not instituted promptly on admission and was not of a high quality. Many factors affect this, such as staff–patient ratios, acuity levels and levels of health-carer education. Some health insurers do not pay for treatment of PIs because they are iatrogenic (caused by the healthcare system) and preventable (ACSQHC, 2020). Employing excellent pressure area care (PAC) is therefore an economic as well as a health imperative. The ACSQHC sets PI prevention as one of the national health service standards, underlining the importance of this clinical problem (ACSQHC, 2018).

Pressure area care

PAC reduces tissue damage caused by prolonged pressure, shearing forces and friction on the skin and tissue that overlay bone near to the surface (e.g. heels, sacrum, ischial tuberosities). PAC is indicated for anyone who cannot reposition themselves or when there is constant pressure on a body part (e.g. a prosthesis).

EVIDENCE OF THERAPEUTIC INTERACTION

Person-centred care improves outcomes, and more so when the person is actively involved in the decision making for their care. Discuss with the person (and/or their carers or visitors) the importance of prevention or treatment of PIs and how they can help. Teach individuals and their carers:

- the risk factors
- how to assess – where to inspect, what to look for; mirrors can assist in viewing difficult areas
- preventative measures – good support surfaces, regular repositioning, good skin care and adequate hydration/nutrition (Li et al., 2023).

Vulnerable people are often repositioned very frequently (every one to two hours around the clock). Excellent explanation of the reasoning behind the need to reposition as well as reminders to them will assist the person to cooperate with you. Enlist the person and their family to help identify and prevent PI. Ledger et al. (2020) demonstrated that factors influencing an individual to adhere to a pressure injury regimen were individual and often constantly changing, such as physical ability, daily routines, roles and responsibilities, competing priorities and day-to-day challenges. There was a link between the individual's involvement in decisions and subsequent adherence to prevention strategies. These authors also found that pain or discomfort was a major concern for the person, and contributed to restricting adherence to certain prevention strategies such as moving and repositioning.

DEMONSTRATE CLINICAL REASONING

Select an appropriate assessment tool

The facility will have selected a single risk-assessment scale appropriate to the person and the facility. It is consistently used so that all healthcare workers become familiar with the scoring and its importance to the care of the person. Validated risk-assessment scales (e.g. Norton and Braden scales), used on admission, periodically in long-term care and when changes occur, are reliable indicators of an individual's risk of developing a PI. The RCHM (2019) uses the child-specific Glamorgan risk-assessment scale. There is a point of care risk assessment tool, the sub-epidermal moisture scanner device that is used in addition to clinical examination and judgement to determine the relative amount of oedema in the sub-epidermis of vulnerable positions (e.g. sacrum, heels, hips) (McLaren-Kennedy et al., 2023). It can identify pressure injuries beneath intact skin earlier than visual inspection can (Gefen & Ross, 2020). Use any risk-assessment scale with clinical assessment and judgement to provide optimum predictive effect as soon as the person is admitted (Tervo-Heikkinen et al., 2023). Brunette and Miller (2023) warn of the largely overlooked incidence of postoperative pressure area development if the person has been in surgery for three hours or more, and state it can take 24 to 72 hours to manifest.

Determining the risk of developing a pressure injury must be followed by measures to prevent such an occurrence (such as pressure-relieving mattresses, pressure-relieving dressings). These are discussed briefly below.

ELDER CARE

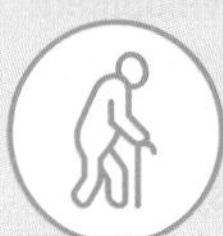

As mentioned above, older age, frailty, thin, fragile skin and reduced mobility are all risk factors for pressure injury formation. These factors plus others, including comorbidities (diabetes, peripheral vascular disease, incontinence), dehydration, malnutrition and polypharmacy, increase the incidence of PI in elders. Frequent visual inspection of possible PI sites, scrupulous hygiene and increased mobility (repositioning) are important factors in preventing PI in this most vulnerable group.

THE PERSON LIVING WITH SEVERE OBESITY

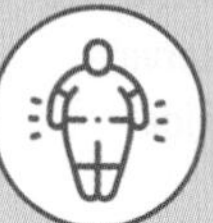

Severe obesity increases the incidence of PI, so the condition of the skin is of great concern. Very obese individuals are generally less mobile, have added pressure on their dependent parts due to the excess adipose tissue, have poor circulation, especially to the skin, and suffer from excess perspiration, and possibly faecal and urinary incontinence followed by skin excoriation. Skin folds are prone to excoriation and bacterial or fungal infections as the combined immobility and excess weight restrict movement and prevent appropriate self-care hygiene measures. Reduced peripheral circulation makes skin prone to breakdown and leads to the development of infection. Frequently check all areas of the body where skin overlaps skin – in the groin, perineal areas, behind the knees, and under the abdominal apron, breasts (both genders), arms and chin. The PI mechanisms specific to this group include increased difficulty repositioning, increased tensile pressure on skin, greater sweat production (due to adipose tissue insulating the body, trapping heat, increasing the core temperature), increased skin folds (where heat and moisture build up, fostering fungal and bacterial growth) and impaired microcirculation (leading to poor oxygenation) (Anderson & Shashaty, 2021).

Foreign objects, such as catheter tubing, a pen or a mobile phone, can get trapped between skinfolds or under a limb or tissue mass, initiating device-related PIs. As well, leaning on the bed rails, a chair arm or wheelchair foot/calf rests can lead to pressure injury. Immobility may itself initiate PIs on heels or sacrum. Provide floating heels as indicated and help patients turn and reposition (Earlam & Woods, 2020). Attend to personal hygiene, keeping skin folds clean and dry. Check frequently for trapped catheter tubing and other potential PI-initiating objects. (See **Clinical Skills 15 and 23** for a brief explanation of issues for people living with severe obesity.)

PERFORMING PRESSURE AREA CARE

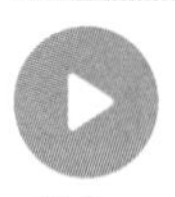

Video

Pressure area care is a combination of assessment and preventative measures. It continues throughout care, and additional measures are implemented if a pressure area is identified as a pressure injury.

> ?
>
> If you think a PI is developing, the facility's protocol for PI care must be implemented and your findings need to be reported immediately. If a PI does develop, care is complex. It involves risk (re)assessment, more frequent skin assessment, provision of excellent nutrition (consult a fundamentals textbook), more frequent repositioning, total offloading of pressure to the injury site, wound cleansing, debridement and moist wound healing practices (see **Clinical Skills 67, 69 and 70**), pain management (see **Clinical Skills 50 and 76**) and education of healthcare professionals, family and the individual (see **Clinical Skill 27**). The PI will need to be graded (see a fundamentals text for staging and care of the PI) and an incident form completed (per the facility's policy). Continue with PAC for any other at-risk areas.

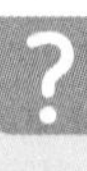

> If the wound is non-healing, the TIME assessment is used to assess the wound and determine the problem:
>
> **T**issue non-viability
> **I**nfection/Inflammation
> **M**oisture imbalance
> **E**dges – not advancing or undermining.
>
> The person is assessed holistically (physical, social, economic and cultural aspects are assessed), a multidisciplinary team (physician, dietitian, physiotherapist and social worker, as necessary) involved, the wound is assessed and the elements impeding healing are treated. The process and the wound are evaluated (Moore et al., 2019).

Hand hygiene

Hand hygiene (see **Clinical Skill 5**) is the cornerstone of infection control and is especially necessary when tending to vulnerable people. Wear clean gloves to protect yourself from body fluids.

GATHER EQUIPMENT

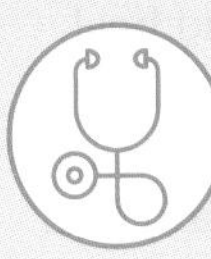

Equipment needed is dependent on the person and the resources of the facility. Some of the equipment you will need for PAC includes:

EQUIPMENT	EXPLANATION
Basin, soap-free cleanser and water, a washer and a towel or cleansing wipes	• To cleanse and dry the skin • Moisture and altered pH from incontinence and faeces exacerbate the development of PIs; remove it promptly • For those who perspire continuously, rinse and dry their skin as often as two-hourly • Clean linen will be required • Most facilities provide disposable cleansing wipes that incorporate a moisturiser and do not require drying
Emollients	Creams that increase the suppleness and elasticity of dry skin
Sheepskin boots, pillows, gel positioners	Used to elevate the heels off the surface of the bed, between legs when side-lying
Pressure-relieving mattresses, pillows and seat cushions	• Constructed of foam material that redistributes the weight and thus the pressure over a wider area to reduce the compression forces over bony prominences. These do not eliminate the need for frequent repositioning. Sacral or occipital foam rings (donuts) only increase the pressure on the area (Gefen, 2021) and should not be used. Fluidised positioners for the occiput are safer • Custom-contoured polyurethane cushions for people in wheelchairs reduce the pressure put on the ischial tuberosities
Alternating pressure mattresses or overlays	Uses an air-pumping system through soft tubes to change the pressure on each part of the body several times an hour
Continuous low-pressure mattresses	Contain air or fluid (similar to a water bed) to redistribute pressure, so that no point on the body is compressed against the skeleton
Mechanical lifting devices	Reduce the shearing and friction produced when moving a person in the bed or a chair

Assess the person

Use the risk-assessment tool

Initial assessment includes:

- clinical history (e.g. age, chronic disease, previous PI, vascular problems, comorbidities, immuno-compromised)
- PI risk scale (validated)
- clinical skin assessment (inspect – don't just ask)
- psychosocial assessment (e.g. smoking, alcohol use, exercise)
- mobility and activity assessment
- nutritional and hydration assessment (note both undernourishment and obesity)
- continence assessment (both urinary and faecal)
- cognition and perception (e.g. paralysis, lack of sensation, unconsciousness) assessment
- assessment of extrinsic factors (e.g. medical devices, shear, friction, moisture, pressure).

Use a validated assessment tool (e.g. Braden, Norton, Waterlow, Glamorgan). Use the facility's recommended risk-assessment tool appropriately and at predetermined and consistent intervals (prescribed by the facility's protocols) based on the susceptibility of the person. In long-care facilities, an admission assessment is done, then again at 48 and 72 hours, then quarterly or if the person's condition changes. Institute PAC for anyone at risk within 24 hours of admission (ACSQHC, 2018).

Assess the skin over identified pressure areas

Skin inspections are carried out at each repositioning according to the person's condition (as frequently as

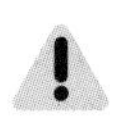

Safety

two-hourly). Look for evidence of moisture or faeces on the skin and clean these promptly; apply a barrier cream. The areas that are most at risk are the tissues overlying bony prominences. These areas depend on the position in which the person is placed and include but are not limited to: heel; big toe; sole; medial and lateral malleolus; patella; lateral, medial and posterior knee; greater trochanter; sacrum; ischial tuberosities; iliac crest; scapula; spinous processes; occipital prominence; ear; shoulder; elbow; chin and nose. The sacrum/coccyx area accounts for 20 to 41 per cent of PIs and the heels for 16 to 27 per cent. Medical equipment can contribute to PIs (e.g. nasal cannula at the nares and behind the ear; endotracheal tubes at the corner of the mouth). Be aware that these medical devices can also cause PIs to the mucous membranes. Be suspicious and actively look/listen/feel for changes.

LOOK at the skin overlying bony prominences or other pressure areas:

- for erythema, which indicates that prolonged pressure has been applied to that area. Compare the area to areas not under pressure to identify skin changes. Use a good light (not fluorescent – natural light or a pen light work best)
- for shiny, tight-looking skin
- for a difference in colour and blanching with firm pressure from your fingertips (i.e. tissue turning

white – the normal finding). Non-blanchable erythema is predictive of PI development (Shi et al., 2020). Blanching and non-blanching are difficult to see in those with darker skin. For people with dark skin, view the area from different angles (look for dark purple or maroon colour) (Black et al., 2023).

LISTEN to reports of pain (ask!) at the pressure site and generally, which may interfere with mobility and repositioning. Provide pain relief as necessary. Ask how long they have been in this position – the longer it is the more suspicious of pressure damage you should be.

FEEL any visually suspicious area for changes in temperature (warmth [use the back of your hand]), for altered texture (i.e. indurated or boggy/spongy or oedematous tissue) and moisture.

These findings (i.e. erythema, non-blanching or changes in dark skin, heat, oedema or induration) mean that a PI has already started, and PAC will be increased and documentation formalised.

New technology (the sub-epidermal moisture scanner) detects the presence of micro-oedema caused by the death and resultant inflammation of the area to identify pressure injuries beneath intact skin earlier than visual inspection can (Gefen & Ross, 2020).

Regularly provide PAC for identified areas

Perform hand hygiene and wear clean gloves.

PAC means providing good support, repositioning, skin cleansing, and attention to details as well as the skin assessment (see 'Assess the person'). Assess the skin at specified intervals – from daily for young, mobile people, more frequently for those at risk (e.g. six to eight hours).

Place the person on a pressure-spreading mattress or underlay. Constant low pressure or alternating pressure mattresses and pads for chairs are recommended (National Pressure Ulcer Advisory Panel [NPUAP], European Pressure Ulcer Advisory Panel [EPUAP] & Pan Pacific Pressure Injury Alliance [PPPIA], 2019). Use of these pressure-relieving devices is an effective strategy, and discussion with more senior nurses is useful. The use of medical-grade sheepskin increases comfort and reduces shear forces, but has not been demonstrated to be any more effective than foam (e.g. egg crate mattress) in reducing the incidence of PI formation (Greenwood, 2020).

The heels can be lifted off the bed, with foam pillows placed under the calf of the legs and the leaving the heels suspended (floating heels). The knees should be supported and slightly flexed. Hyperextension of the knee can reduce popliteal blood flow to the calf and heel and reduce venous return, which may increase the incidence of deep vein thrombosis (Langemo, 2017). Heel pressure offloading devices and foam heel dressings are available for people who cannot maintain their calves on the pillow.

A new technology, a five-layer foam dressing with a silicone border, is beginning to be used to prevent PI in vulnerable people. It reduced sacral and heel PIs by 30 to 70 per cent in acute hospital care, is cost-effective relative to paying for treatment of PIs and in terms of quality of life, and is being assessed in long-term care (Padula, Chen & Santamaria, 2019; Thomas-Tharakan, 2023).

Repositioning remains the cornerstone of PAC. Moving the person off the bony prominence relieves pressure. Do not position them onto the damaged area. A documented regimen that takes into account their medical condition, rest and sleep, mealtimes and visiting hours as much as possible ensures the position changes are done at appropriate intervals. Expert opinion differs as to the timing, with most recommending two-hourly, and some leaving the timing to your assessment of the person's condition. Anyone who is incontinent, uncomfortable or has poor circulation or nutrition, fragile skin, or decreased cognition or sensation is repositioned more frequently than two-hourly. The accepted standard for a compromised person is half-hourly repositioning. Take care not to drag the person when repositioning. Use slide sheets or a lift if necessary.

Manipulate the elements of the person's environment. For example, changing the bed elevation within less than 30 degrees assists in reducing pressure. The 30-degree side-lying position is effective because it eliminates pressure from both the sacrum/coccyx and heels. The individual can be stabilised in this position using pillows behind their back and between their legs. It does create a load on the lower malleolus, which will need frequent assessing (Woodhouse et al., 2019).

Keeping the skin clean and dry is integral to preventing pressure sores. For some, this means washing – with a pH-balanced skin cleanser, not soap – and patting dry the skin and changing linen as frequently as necessary. Moisturise the skin if it is dry. Humidify dry air to prevent drying of skin. Use a barrier cream if the person has increased risk from sweating, incontinence. Attention to details, such as keeping the bed linen tight and wrinkle-free, avoiding 'waterproof' bedding next to the skin, making sure that a person's ear is not folded over when they are turned onto the side, and padding or using layered foam dressings under cheek lengths and/or earpieces of oxygen tubing, will reduce the pressure damage to those body parts. Massage is not recommended, as it further damages compromised tissues (NPUAP, EPUAP & PPPIA, 2019).

Remove your gloves and perform hand hygiene.

CLEAN, REPLACE OR DISPOSE OF EQUIPMENT

Perform hand hygiene and wear clean gloves.

Wash out and disinfect basins. Rinse and leave upside down to dry to prevent biofilm development. Sheepskins and other pressure devices, such as foam mattresses, sheepskin boots and elbow pads, are bagged separately prior to going to the laundry for processing. Clean pressure mattresses and continuous low-pressure mattresses according to the manufacturer's instructions when no longer needed.

Remove your gloves and perform hand hygiene.

DOCUMENTATION

Note relevant information, such as the development of areas of erythema (location, extent) or changed health status and mobility. Sharing this information with colleagues increases compliance with PAC protocols and provides a baseline against which to measure future changes. If a pressure area develops into an injury, it will need more extensive assessment and documentation.

CLINICAL SKILLS ASSESSMENT

Pressure area care – preventing pressure injuries

Demonstrates the ability to assess for and implement timely measures to prevent pressure-related tissue damage. Incorporates the *National Safety and Quality Health Service Standards*: 2 Partnering with consumers, 3 Preventing and controlling healthcare-associated infections, 5 Comprehensive care, 6 Communicating for safety, and 8 Recognising and responding to acute deterioration (ACSQHC, 2021).

Performance criteria	1	2	3	4	5
(Numbers indicate NMBA *Registered Nurse Standards for Practice*)	(Dependent)	(Marginal)	(Assisted)	(Supervised)	(Independent)
1. Identifies indication (1.1, 3.3, 3.4)	☐	☐	☐	☐	☐
2. Evidence of therapeutic interaction with the person and their carers, e.g. discusses the importance of prevention, how they can help, and teaches strategies to them; gives clear explanation of procedures (1.4, 1.5, 2.1, 2.2, 3.2)	☐	☐	☐	☐	☐
3. Demonstrates clinical reasoning abilities, e.g. selects and uses a single risk-assessment scale appropriate to the person and the facility, is able to address related bariatric issues (1.1, 1.2, 1.3, 1.4, 4.2, 6.1)	☐	☐	☐	☐	☐
4. Identifies and gathers appropriate equipment (1.1, 5.5, 6.1): ■ basin, warm water, washer, soap-free cleanser, towel ■ moisturising lotion ■ clean linen as necessary ■ protective devices (e.g. sheepskin pads, elbow and heel protectors)	☐	☐	☐	☐	☐
5. Performs hand hygiene (1.1, 3.4, 6.1)	☐	☐	☐	☐	☐
6. Identifies risk factors (1.1, 4.1, 4.2, 4.3, 7.1)	☐	☐	☐	☐	☐
7. Utilises the risk-assessment tool appropriately and at predetermined intervals (1.1, 4.1, 4.2, 4.3, 7.1)	☐	☐	☐	☐	☐
8. Assesses the identified pressure areas and overlying skin regularly (1.1, 4.1, 4.2, 4.3, 7.1)	☐	☐	☐	☐	☐
9. Regularly provides appropriate care for the identified areas (3.2, 6.1)	☐	☐	☐	☐	☐
10. Cleans, replaces and disposes of equipment appropriately (3.6, 6.1)	☐	☐	☐	☐	☐
11. Documents relevant information and care provided (1.1, 1.4, 1.6, 2.2, 2.7, 3.5, 3.7, 6.1, 6.2, 6.5, 7.3)	☐	☐	☐	☐	☐
12. Demonstrates the ability to link theory to practice (1.1, 3.3, 3.4, 3.5)	☐	☐	☐	☐	☐

Student:

Clinical facilitator: Date:

REFERENCES

Alperovitch-Najenson, D., Weiner, C., Ribak, J. & Kalichman, L. (2019). Sliding sheet use in nursing practice: An intervention study. *Workplace Health & Safety: Promoting Environments Conducive to Well-Being and Productivity, 68*(4), 171–81. https://doi.org/10.1177/2165079919880566

Anderson, M. & Shashaty, M. (2021). Impact of obesity in critical illness. *Chest, 160*(6), 2135–45. https://doi.org/10.1016/j.chest.2021.08.001

Anekwe, D., Milnera, S., Bussieres, A., Marchiec, M. & Spahija, J. (2020). Intensive care unit clinicians identify many barriers to, and facilitators of, early mobilisation: A qualitative study using the Theoretical Domains Framework. *Journal of Physiotherapy, 66*(2), 120–7. https://doi.org/10.1016/j.jphys.2020.03.001

Australian Commission on Safety and Quality in Health Care (ACSQHC) (2018). *Hospital acquired complication 1: Pressure injury.* Sydney: Author. https://www.safetyandquality.gov.au/sites/default/files/migrated/SAQ7730_HAC_Factsheet_PressureInjury_LongV2.pdf

Australian Commission on Safety and Quality in Health Care (ACSQHC) (2020). *Preventing pressure injuries and wound management.* https://www.safetyandquality.gov.au/sites/default/files/2020-10/fact_sheet-preventing_pressure_injuries_and_wound_management_oct_2020.pdf

Australian Commission on Safety and Quality in Health Care (ACSQHC) (2021). *National safety and quality health service standards* (3rd ed.). Sydney, NSW: ACSQHC.

Bagnasco, A., Dasso, N., Rossi, S., Catania, G., Zanini, N., Aleo, G., Watson, R., Hayter, M. & Sasso, L. (2019). Unmet nursing care needs on medical and surgical wards: A scoping review of patients' perspectives. *Journal of Clinical Nursing, 29,* 347–69. https://doi.org/10.1111/jocn.15089

Bargmann, A. & Brundrett, S. (2020). Implementation of a multicomponent fall prevention program: Contracting with patients for fall safety. *Military Medicine, 185*(Supplement 2), 28–34. https://doi.org/10.1093/milmed/usz411

Bastos, S., Gonçalves, F., Bueno, B., Silva, G., Ribeiro, K. & Brasil, V. (2019). Bed-bath: The care-omitting behavior of the nursing team. *Review of Fundamental Care, 11*(3), 627–33. https://doi.org/10.9789/2175-5361.2019. v11i3.627-633

Bhagat, V., Hoang, H., Crocombe, L. A. & Goldberg, L. (2023). Australian nursing students' perception, knowledge, and attitude towards oral healthcare of older people and associated factors: a national cross-sectional survey. *BioMedical Central Nursing, 22,* 190. https://doi.org/10.1186/s12912-023-01366-x

Black, J., Cox, J., Capasso, V., Bliss, D., Delmore, B., Iyer, V., Massaro, J., Munro, C., Pittman, J. & Ayello, E. (2023). Current perspectives on pressure injuries in persons with dark skin tones from the National Pressure Injury Advisory Panel. *Advances in Skin & Wound Care, 36*(9), 470–80. https://doi.org/10.1097/ASW.0000000000000032

Boyko, T., Longakerm, M. & Yang, G. (2018). Review of the current management of pressure ulcers. *Advances in Wound Care, 7*(2), 57–67. https://doi.org/10.1089/wound.2016.0697

Brigham and Women's Hospital (2020). *Patient safety measures: Patient falls.* https://www.brighamandwomens.org/about-bwh/quality/patient-safety-measures/patient-falls

Brunette, G. & Miller, C. (2023). Is it time to put pressure on informed consent? A view from here. *Journal of Wound, Ostomy and Continence Nursing, 50*(5), 361–2. https://doi.org/10.1097/WON.0000000000001018

Brusco, N., Haines, T., Taylor, N., Rawson H., Boyd, L., Ekegren, C., Kugler, H., Dawes, H., Radia-George, C., Graven, C. & Hill, K. (2023). In Australian hospitals and residential aged care facilities, how do we train nursing and direct care staff to assist patients and residents to move? A national survey. *Australian Health Review, 47,* 331–8. https://doi.org/10.1071/AH22296

Budarick, A. R., Lad, U. & Fischer, S. L. (2020). Can the use of turn-assist surfaces reduce the physical burden on caregivers when performing patient turning? *Human Factors, 62*(1), 77–92. https://doi.org/10.1177/0018720819845746

Chu, V. (2014). *Bariatric patients: Manual handling.* Adelaide, SA: Joanna Briggs Institute.

Cooper, K., McQueen, K., Halm, M. & Flayter, M. (2020). Prevention and treatment of device-related hospital-acquired pressure injuries. *American Journal of Critical Care, 29*(2), 150–4. https://doi.org/10.4037/ajcc2020167

Copeland-Halperin, L., Reategui Via y Rada, M., Levy, J., Shank, N., Funderburk, C. & Shin, J. (2020). Does the timing of postoperative showering impact infection rates? A systematic review and meta-analysis. *Journal of Plastic, Reconstructive & Aesthetic Surgery, 73*(7), 1306–11. https://doi.org/10.1016/j.bjps.2020.02.007

de Oliveira, M., Padovez, R., Serrao, P., de Noronha, M., Cezar, N. & de Andrade, L. (2023). Effectiveness of physical exercise at improving functional capacity in older adults living with Alzheimer's disease: A systematic review of randomized controlled trials. *Disability and Rehabilitation, 45*(3). https://doi.org/10.1080/09638288.2022.2037744

DeLaune, S., Ladner, P., McTier, L. & Tollefson, J. (2024). *Fundamentals of nursing: Standards and practice* (Australia & New Zealand 3rd ed.). South Melbourne, VIC: Cengage Learning.

Doshi, M. & Jones, V. (2019). Denture hygiene: Safety issues with denture care. *British Dental Journal, 226*(2). https://doi.org/10.1038/sj.bdj.2019.13

Dowling, L., McCloskey, E., Cuthbertson, D. J. & Walsh, J. (2023). Dynapenic abdominal obesity as a risk factor for falls. *Journal of Frailty and Aging, 12,* 37–42. https://doi.org/10.14283/jfa.2022.18

Earlam, A. & Woods, L. (2020). Obesity: Skin issues and skinfold management. *American Nurse.* https://www.myamericannurse.com/obesity-skin-issues-and-skinfold-management

Ette, L. & Gretton, M. (2019). The significance of facial shaving as fundamental care. *Nursing Times, 115*(1), 40–2. https://insights.ovid.com/nrtm/201901000/00006203-201901000-00054

Farias, D., de Almeida, M., Gomes, G., Lunardi, V., Queiroz, M., Nörnberg, P. & Lourenção, L. (2020). Beliefs, values and practices of families in the care of hospitalized children: subsidies for nursing. *Revista Brasileira de Enfermagem, 73*(suppl 4). https://doi.org/10.1590/0034-7167-2019-0553

Fernandez, S. (2019). Does long hair belong in a clinical setting? *Nursing, 49*(8), 53–5. https://doi.org/10.1097/01.NURSE.0000558098.51162.da

Gancheva, I. (2019). Some aspects of everyday hygiene of Christians and Sunni Muslims in Bulgaria: 'Clash' of two religious and cultural systems. *The Worlds.* https://www.researchgate.net/profile/Magdalena_Slavkova/publication/338402081_Slavkova_Maeva_Erolova_Popov_Eds_Between_the_Worlds_People_Spaces_and_Rituals_e-ISSN_2683-0213/links/5e12cab3299bf10bc3929005/Slavkova-Maeva-Erolova-Popov-Eds-Between-the-Worlds-People-Spaces-and-Rituals-e-ISSN-2683-0213.pdf#page=173

Gefen, A. (2021). The aetiology of medical device-related pressure ulcers and how to prevent them. *British Journal of Nursing, 30*(15), S24–S30. https://www.magonlinelibrary.com/doi/abs/10.12968/bjon.2021.30.15.S24

Gefen, A. & Ross, G. (2020). The subepidermal moisture scanner: The technology explained. *Journal of Wound Care, 29*(Sup2c), S10–S16. https://doi.org/10.12968/jowc.2020.29.Sup2c.S10

Goldenhart, A. & Nagy, H. (2022). Assisting patients with personal hygiene. In *StatPearls [Internet].* Treasure Island (FL): StatPearls Publishing. https://www.ncbi.nlm.nih.gov/books/NBK563155

Greenwood, C. E. (2020). *An exploration of the use of devices for the prevention of heel pressure ulcers in secondary care: A realist evaluation* (Doctoral dissertation, University of Leeds). https://etheses.whiterose.ac.uk/28530

Groven, F., Zwakhalen, S., Odekerken-Schroder, G., Tan, F. & Hamers, J. (2020). *The effects of washing without water versus the traditional bed bath with water and soap on comfort and physical demands: Protocol of a cross-over randomized trial.* Research Square. https://doi.org/10.21203/rs.2.16771/v1

Hales, C., Curran, N. & de Vries, K. (2018). Morbidly obese patients' experiences of mobility during hospitalisation and rehabilitation: A qualitative descriptive study. *Nursing Praxis in New Zealand, 34*(1), 20–31.

Hammoud, S., Amer, F., Lohner, S. & Kocsis, B. (2020). Patient education on infection control: A systematic review. *American Journal of Infection Control, 48*(12), 1506–15. https://doi.org/10.1016/j.ajic.2020.05.039

Heague, M., Dyson, J. & Cowdell, F. (2023). Barriers and facilitators to delivering everyday personal hygiene care in residential settings: A systematic review. *Journal of Clinical Nursing, 32*, 3102–16. https://doi.org/10.1111/jocn.16413

Heng, H., Jazayeri, D., Shaw, L., Kiegaldie, D., Hill, A. & Morris, M. E. (2020). Hospital falls prevention with patient education: A scoping review. *BMC Geriatrics, 20*, 1–12. https://doi.org/10.1186/s12877-020-01515-w

Higuchi, D., Takahashi, Y. & Tomita, Y. (2023). Effects of slide sheet use and bed position on muscle activities in the low back and extremities: A pilot experimental simulation study. *Workplace Health & Safety, 71*(10), 491–8. https://doi.org/10.1177/21650799231155626

Hirt, P., Castillo, D., Yosipovitch, G. & Keri, J. (2019). Skin changes in the obese patient. *Journal of the American Academy of Dermatology, 81*(5), 1037–57. https://doi.org/10.1016/j.jaad.2018.12.070

Honkavuo, L. (2019). Oral health in the shadow of clinical nursing and caring science. *International Journal of Caring Sciences, 12*(2), 674–83. https://www.internationaljournalofcaringsciences.org/docs/10_honkavuo_original_12_2.pdf

Jakobsson, S., Ringström, G., Andersson, E., Eliasson, B., Johannsson, G., Simren, M. & Jakobsson Ung, E. (2019). Patient safety before and after implementing person-centred inpatient care: A quasi-experimental study. *Journal of Clinical Nursing, 29*, 602–12. https://doi.org/10.1111/jocn.15120

Kaur, I., Jakhar, D., Singal, A. & Grover, C. (2020). Nail care for health care workers during COVID-19 pandemic. *Indian Dermatology Online Journal, 11*, 449–50. http://www.idoj.in/text.asp?2020/11/3/449/284095

Khan, S., Syed, F., Khalid, T., Farheen, N., Javed, F. & Kazmi, S. (2023). An updated systematic review on toothbrush contamination: An overlooked oral health concern among general population. *International Journal of Dental Hygiene, 00*, 1–11. https://doi.org/10.1111/idh.12740

King, J., O'Neill, B., Ramsay, P., Linden, M., Darweish Medniuk, A., Outtrim, J. & Blackwood, B. (2019). Identifying patients' support needs following critical illness: A scoping review of the qualitative literature. *Critical Care, 23*, 187. https://doi.org/10.1186/s13054-019-2441-6

Klompas, M., Branson, R., Cawcutt, K., Crist, M., Eichenwald, E. C., Greene, L., Lee, R., Maragakis, L., Powell, K., Priebe, G., Speck, K., Yokoe, D. & Berenholtz, S. M. (2022). Strategies to prevent ventilator-associated pneumonia, ventilator-associated events, and nonventilator hospital-acquired pneumonia in acute-care hospitals: 2022 update. *Infection Control & Hospital Epidemiology, 43*(6), 687–713. https://www.cambridge.org/core/services/aop-cambridgecorecontent/view/A2124BA9B088027AE30BE46C28887084/S0899823X22000885a.pdf/div-class-title-strategies-to-prevent-ventilator-associated-pneumonia-ventilatorassociated-events-and-nonventilator-hospital-acquired-pneumonia-in-acute-carehospitals-2022-update-div.pdf

Konya, I., Nishiya, K., Shishido, I., Hino, M., Watanabe, K. & Yano, R. (2023). Minimum wiping pressure and number of wipes that can remove dirt during bed baths using disposable towels: a multi-study approach. *BMC Nursing, 22*, 18. https://doi.org/10.1186/s12912-022-01162-z

Langemo, D. (2017). *Heel pressure ulcers: 2014 international pressure ulcer prevention & treatment guidelines.* National Pressure Ulcer Advisory Panel. https://www.swrwoundcareprogram.ca/Uploads/ContentDocuments/Heel%20Pressure%20Ulcer%202014%20International%20Pressure%20Ulcer%20Prevention%20and%20Treatment%20Guidelines.pdf

Ledger, L., Worsley, P., Hope, J. & Schoonhoven, L. (2020). Patient involvement in pressure ulcer prevention and adherence to prevention strategies: An integrative review. *International Journal of Nursing Studies, 101*. https://doi.org/10.1016/j.ijnurstu.2019.103449

Li, J., Zhu, C., Liu, Y., Li, Z., Sun, X., Bai, Y., Song, B., Jin, J., Liu, Y., Wen, X., Cheng, S. & Wu, X. (2023). Critical care nurses' knowledge, attitudes, and practices of pressure injury prevention in China: A multicentric cross-sectional survey. *International Wound Journal, 20*(2), 381–90. https://doi.org/10.1111/iwj.13886

Li, M., Liu, J. & Peng, P. (2023). Efficacy analysis of different toothbrush designs on plaque and gingivitis in human factors. *Highlights in Science, Engineering and Technology, 47*, 250–9.

Lin, J., Dinis, M., Tseng, C., Agnello, M., He, X., Silva, D. & Tran, N. (2020). Effectiveness of the GumChucks flossing system compared to string floss for interdental plaque removal in children: A randomized clinical trial. *Scientific Reports, 10*, 3052. https://doi.org/10.1038/s41598-020-59705-w

Martínez-Velilla, N., Casas-Herrero, A., Zambom-Ferraresi, F., Sáez de Asteasu, M., Alejandro, L., Arkaitz, G., García-Baztán, A., Alonso-Renedo, J., González-Glaría, B., Gonzalo-Lázaro, M., Apezteguía Iráizoz, I., Gutiérrez-Valencia, M., Rodríguez-Mañas, L. & Izquierdo, M. (2019). Effect of exercise intervention on functional decline in very elderly patients during acute hospitalization: A randomized clinical trial. *JAMA Internal Medicine, 179*(1), 28–36. https://doi.org/10.1001/jamainternmed.2018.4869

Matsumoto, C., Nanke, K., Furumura, S., Arimatsu, M., Fukuyama, M. & Maeda, H. (2019). Effects of disposable bath and towel bath on the transition of resident skin bacteria, water content of the stratum corneum, and relaxation. *American Journal of Infection Control, 47*(7), 811–15. https://doi.org/10.1016/j.ajic.2018.12.008

McCaw, P. (2022). *Body mechanics in nursing.* https://study.com/learn/lesson/body-mechanics-principles-importance.html

McLaren-Kennedy, A., Chaboyer, W., Carlini, J. & Latimer, S. (2023). Use of point-of-care subepidermal moisture devices to detect localised oedema and evaluate pressure injury risk: A scoping review. *Journal of Clinical Nursing, 32*, 5478–92. https://doi.org/10.1111/jocn.16630c

Miller, H., Rockefeller, K. & Townsend, P. (2020). International round table discussion: Do gait belts have a role in safe patient handling programs? *International Journal of Safe Patient Handling & Mobility, 7*(3), 116–21. https://www.wyeastmedical.com/wp-content/uploads/2020/01/Gait-Belt-Peer-Review-Article.pdf

Mody, L., Washer, L., Kaye, K., Gibson, K., Saint, S., Reyes, K., Cassone, M., Mantey, J., Cao, J., Altamimi, S., Perri, M., Sax, H., Chopra, V. & Zervos, Z. (2019). Multidrug-resistant organisms in hospitals: What is on patient hands and in their rooms? *Clinical Infectious Diseases, 69*(11), 1837–44. https://doi.org/10.1093/cid/ciz092

Mooney, N. (2015). The impossible hybridity of hair: Kesh, gender and the third space. In K. A. Jacobsen & K. Myrvold (eds), *Young Sikhs in a global world: Negotiating traditions, identities and authorities*, p. 97. Farnham, UK: Ashgate.

Moore, Z., Dowsett, C., Smith, G., Atkin, L., Bain, M., Lahmann, N., Schultz, G., Swanson T., Vowden, P., Weir, D., Zmuda, A. & Jaimes, H. (2019). TIME CDST: An updated tool to address the current challenges in wound care. *Journal of Wound Care, 28*(3), 154–61. https://www.researchgate.net/publication/331579294_TIME_CDST_an_updated_tool_to_address_the_current_challenges_in_wound_care

Moreland, B., Kakara, R. & Henry, A. (2020). Trends in nonfatal falls and fall-related injuries among adults aged ≥65 years: United States, 2012–2018. *MMWR: Morbidity and Mortality Weekly Report, 69*, 875–81. https://doi.org/10.15585/mmwr.mm6927a5

National Dental Care (2023). *The importance of oral health for older Australians.* https://www.nationaldentalcare.com.au/article/the-importance-of-oral-health-for-older-australians

National Pressure Ulcer Advisory Panel, European Pressure Ulcer Advisory Panel & Pan Pacific Pressure Injury Alliance (NPUAP, EPUAP & PPPIA) (2019). *Prevention and treatment of pressure ulcers: Quick reference guide* (2nd ed.). Emily Haesler (ed.). Osborne Park, WA: Cambridge Media. http://www.npuap.org/wp-content/uploads/2019/08/Quick-Reference-Guide-DIGITAL-NPUAP-EPUAP-PPPIA-Jan2016.pdf

Okubo, R., Hoshi, S-I. & Kondo, M. (2023). Cost effectiveness of professional and mechanical oral care for preventing pneumonia in nursing home residents. *Journal of the American Geriatric Society, 71*(3), 756–64. https://pubmed.ncbi.nlm.nih.gov/36334034

Padula, W. V., Chen, Y. H. & Santamaria, N. (2019). Five-layer border dressings as part of a quality improvement bundle to prevent pressure injuries in US skilled nursing facilities and Australian nursing homes: A cost-effectiveness analysis. *International Wound Journal, 16*, 1263–72. https://doi.org/10.1111/iwj.13174

Passarelli Mantovani, R., Sandri, A., Boaretti, M., Grilli, A., Volpi, S., Melotti, P., Burlacchini, G., Lleò, M. M. & Signoretto, C. (2019). Toothbrushes may convey bacteria to the cystic fibrosis lower airways. *Journal of Oral Microbiology, 11*(1), 1647036. https://doi.org/10.1080/20002297.2019.1647036

Pepera, G., Krinta, K., Mpea, C., Antoniou, V., Peristeropoulos, A. & Dimitriadis, Z. (2023). Randomized controlled trial of group exercise intervention for fall risk factors reduction in nursing home residents. *Canadian Journal on Aging/La Revue Canadienne Du Vieillissement, 42*(2), 328–36. https://doi.org/10.1017/S0714980822000265

Persaud-Jaimangal, R., Ayello, E. & Sibbald, R. (2020). Ch 28: Preventing pressure injuries and skin tears. In M. Boltz, E. Capezuti, D. Zwicker & T. Fulmer 2020 (eds), *Evidence-based geriatric nursing protocols for best practice*. New York: Springer Publishing Company.

Physiopedia (n.d.). *Injury prevention and body mechanics*. https://www.physio-pedia.com/Injury_Prevention_and_Body_Mechanics

Puntillo, K., Arai, S., Cooper, B., Stotts, N. & Nelson J. (2014). A randomized clinical trial of an intervention to relieve thirst and dry mouth in intensive care unit patients. *Intensive Care Medicine, 40*(9), 1295–302. https://doi.org/10.1007/s00134-014-3339-z

Royal Children's Hospital Melbourne (RCHM) (2019). *Clinical guidelines: Pressure injury prevention and management*. https://www.rch.org.au/rchcpg/hospital_clinical_guideline_index/Pressure_Injury_Prevention_and_Management/#Pressure%20Injury%20Development

Sabol, V., Kennerly, S., Alderden, J., Horn, S. & Yap, T. (2020). Insight into the movement behaviors of nursing home residents living with obesity: A report of two cases. *Wound Management and Prevention, 66*(5), 18–29.

Santos, V., Dourado dos Anjos, L., Paixão, C., Silva, T., Begot, I., Barbosa, C., Guizilinni, S. & Moreira, R. (2020). Myocardial oxygen consumption in the bed bath and shower bath in patients with acute coronary syndrome. *Intensive and Critical Care Nursing, 60*, 102895. https://doi.org/10.1016/j.iccn.2020.102895

Sherrow, V. (2023). *Encyclopedia of hair: A cultural history*. Bloomsbury Publishing USA.

Shi, C., Bonnett, L., Dumville, J. & Cullum, N. (2020). Nonblanchable erythema for predicting pressure ulcer development: A systematic review with an individual participant data meta-analysis. *British Journal of Dermatology, 182*, 278–86. https://doi.org/10.1111/bjd.18154

Sousa, A. D., Baixinho, C. L., Presado, M. H. & Henriques, M. A. (2023). The effect of interventions on preventing musculoskeletal injuries related to nurses work: Systematic review. *Journal of Personalized Medicine, 13*(2), 185. https://doi.org/10.3390/jpm13020185

Spencer, M. & Kelly, L. (2019). Cleaning up the mess: Could a new type of patient bath basin turn the tide of HAIs? *Infection Control Today*. https://www.infectioncontroltoday.com/view/cleaning-mess-could-new-type-patient-bath-basin-turn-tide-hais

Swinnerton, E. & Price, A. (2023). Recognising, reducing and preventing deconditioning in hospitalised older people. *Nursing Older People, 35*(2), 34–41. https://doi.org/10.7748/nop.2023.e1396

Tasheva, P., Vollenweider, P., Kraege, V., Roulet, G., Lamy, O., Marques-Vidal, P. & Méan, M. (2020). Association between physical activity levels in the hospital setting and hospital-acquired functional decline in elderly patients. *JAMA Network Open, 3*(1), e1920185. https://doi.org/10.1001/jamanetworkopen.2019.20185

Tervo-Heikkinen, T., Heikkilä, A., Koivunen, M., Kortteisto, T., Peltokoski, J., Salmela, S., Sankelo, S., Ylitörmänen, T. & Junttila, K. (2023). Nursing interventions in preventing pressure injuries in acute inpatient care: A cross-sectional national study. *BMC Nursing, 22*, 198. https://doi.org/10.1186/s12912-023-01369-8

Thomas-Tharakan, S. (2023). *Silicone foam dressing and preventative care impact on hospital-acquired pressure injuries*. Doctoral Thesis, Grand Canyon University. https://www.proquest.com/openview/e9962132e134bd83a44f19d96bd40c50/1? pq-origsite=gscholar&cbl=18750&diss=y

Tiwari, A., Neha Gupta, N., Singla, D., Swain J., Gupta, R., Mehta, D. & Kumar, S. (2023). Artificial intelligence's use in the diagnosis of mouth ulcers: A systematic review. *Cureus*. https://doi.org/10.7759/cureus.45187

Türkmen, C., Esen, S. Y., Erden, Z. & Düger, T. (2023). Comfort and support values provided by different pillow materials for individuals with forward head posture. *Applied Sciences, 13*(6), 3865. https://doi.org/10.3390/app13063865

Vázquez-Reza, M., Custodia, A., López-Dequidt, I. & Leira, Y. (2023). Periodontal inflammation is associated with increased circulating levels of endothelial progenitor cells: A retrospective cohort study in a high vascular risk population. *Therapeutic Advances in Chronic Disease, 14*. https://doi.org/10.1177/20406223231178276

Veje, P., Chen, M., Jensen, C., Sørensen, J. & Primdahl, J. (2019). Bed bath with soap and water or disposable wet wipes: Patients' experiences and preferences. *Journal of Clinical Nursing, 28*, 2235–44. https://doi.org/10.1111/jocn.14825

Venema, D. M., Skinner, A. M., Nailon, R., Conley, D., High, R. & Jones, K. (2019). Patient and system factors associated with unassisted and injurious falls in hospitals: An observational study. *BioMedicalCentral Geriatrics, 19*, 348. https://doi.org/10.1186/s12877-019-1368-8

Victorian Government (2015). Falls Risk Assessment Tool. https://www.health.vic.gov.au/publications/falls-risk-assessment-tool-frat

Wang, J., Ren, D., Liu, Y., Wang, Y., Zhang, B. & Xiao, Q. (2020). Effects of early mobilization on the prognosis of critically ill patients: A systematic review and meta-analysis. *International Journal of Nursing Studies, 110*, 103708. https://doi.org/10.1016/j.ijnurstu.2020.103708

Whitby, L. & McLachlan, C. S. (2014). Inconsistent approach to providing care worker assistance to the falling patient. *Ergonomics Australia, 1*(3), 1–4.

Wiggermann, N., Zhou, J. & McGann, N. (2020). Effect of repositioning aids and patient weight on biomechanical stresses when repositioning patients in bed. *Human Factors*. https://doi.org/10.1177/0018720819895850

Woodhouse, M., Worsley, P., Voegeli, D., Schoonhoven, L. & Bader, D. (2019). How consistent and effective are current repositioning strategies for pressure ulcer prevention? *Applied Nursing Research, 48*, 58–62. https://doi.org/10.1016/j.apnr.2019.05.013

Woon, C. (2019). Brushing up on oral care. *Kai Tiaki: Nursing New Zealand, 25*(6), 18–19. https://search.proquest.com/docview/2264565604?accountid=88802

Young, M. (2022). Obesity and the dental team. *British Dental Journal Team, 9*, 8–10. https://doi.org/10.1038/s41407-022-0823-0

Zimmerman, S., Wretman, C., Ward, K., Tandan, M., Sloane, P. & Preisser, J. (2020). Fidelity and sustainability of Mouth Care Without a Battle and lessons for other innovations in care. *Geriatric Nursing, 41*(6), 878–84. https://doi.org/10.1016/j.gerinurse.2020.06.002

PART 11

RESPIRATORY SKILLS

60 OXYGEN THERAPY VIA NASAL CANNULA OR VARIOUS MASKS

61 OROPHARYNGEAL AND NASOPHARYNGEAL SUCTIONING

62 ARTIFICIAL AIRWAY SUCTIONING

63 TRACHEOSTOMY CARE

64 CHEST DRAINAGE SYSTEM ASSESSMENT AND MANAGEMENT

Note: These notes are summaries of the most important points in the assessments/procedures and are not exhaustive on the subject. References of the materials used to compile the information have been supplied. The student is expected to have learnt the material surrounding each skill as presented in the references. No single reference is complete on each subject.

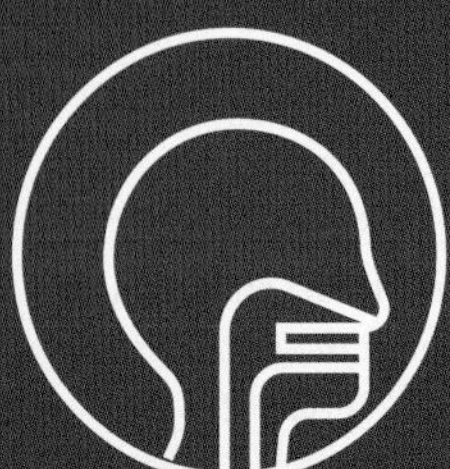

CHAPTER 60

OXYGEN THERAPY VIA NASAL CANNULA OR VARIOUS MASKS

INDICATIONS

Oxygen is a tasteless, odourless and colourless gas that constitutes 21 per cent of normal air. For effective oxygen delivery to the tissues, the following factors are required:

- sufficient oxygen supply in the inspired air
- sufficient ventilation to ensure oxygen is delivered to the alveoli
- adequate cardiac output to carry the oxygenated blood to the tissues
- adequate haemoglobin levels to carry sufficient oxygen in the blood
- immediate release of oxygen from the haemoglobin molecule
- ability to diffuse into the tissues (Marieb & Hoehn, 2019).

The main indication for acute oxygen therapy is the presence of tissue hypoxia. This may occur because of arterial hypoxaemia (i.e. inadequate arterial oxygen content), defined as an oxygen saturation of less than 90 per cent or an oxygen tension (PaO_2) of less than 60 mmHg. This can result from:

- impaired gas exchange in the lung
- inadequate alveolar ventilation
- a shunt allowing venous blood into the arterial circulation (Kydonaki & Parke, 2024).

An arterial blood gas measurement helps you to discriminate between these possibilities.

Failure of the oxygen–haemoglobin transport system may result in tissue hypoxia in the absence of arterial hypoxaemia. This can result from a reduced oxygen-carrying capacity in blood (e.g. anaemia or carbon monoxide poisoning) or reduced tissue perfusion (e.g. shock) (Marieb & Hoehn, 2019).

Acute oxygen therapy has the potential to improve health outcomes and save lives when used appropriately, but may cause harm if used inappropriately. Successful treatment of tissue hypoxia requires early recognition and correction of contributing factors (Sivapuram, 2022a).

In Australia, oxygen is not allocated a poison schedule number within the *Standard for the Uniform Scheduling of Medicines and Poisons* criteria (Therapeutic Goods Administration, 2017). As an unscheduled substance, there is no legislative requirement for supplemental oxygen to be prescribed by a medical practitioner in Australia.

Registered nurses (RNs) can initiate oxygen therapy when a person's oxygen saturation is outside their acceptable parameters. Policies vary between health facilities; however, many require medical staff to order the amount, concentration, delivery method and duration of supplemental oxygen, and the target range for minimum and maximum oxygen saturation values (SpO_2). Oxygen therapy should be decreased if saturation is above the target range and eventually discontinued as the person recovers. As with any alterations in a person's care or condition when managed within an interdisciplinary approach, inform the medical staff when a person's supplemental oxygen is commenced or altered (Sivapuram, 2022a).

While no specific contraindications exist for acute oxygen therapy when clinical indicators are present, care should be taken when administering uncontrolled oxygen to people who are carbon dioxide retainers (Porritt, 2022a). Oxygen administration may depress respiratory drive in people with chronic carbon dioxide retention, whose stimulus to breathe is a decreased partial pressure of oxygen in arterial blood (PaO_2). Careful monitoring of these people for hypoventilation is required during oxygen therapy.

Oxygen therapy should be administered to achieve normal or near-normal SpO_2 (**s**aturation of **p**eripheral arterial blood with **o**xygen) of 94 to 98 per cent for all acutely ill people, and 89 to 92 per cent for those at risk of hypercapnoeic respiratory failure and certain chemotherapy (e.g. bleomycin leading to oxygen-induced lung damage) (Fong, 2021a; Sivapuram, 2022a). Following certain chemotherapeutic agents (e.g. bleomycin), a person may be vulnerable to pulmonary toxicity with resulting fibrosis and/or emphysema (Fong, 2021a). In acute situations, inadequate oxygen therapy accounts for more deaths and permanent disability than high oxygen concentrations.

The onset of acute respiratory distress can be rapid and severe. You need to be alert to changes in the person's baseline and assessment trends. When a person is acutely distressed, immediately assess their airway, breathing and circulation. If compromised, call for help and start cardiopulmonary resuscitation. If their airway is patent, a focused respiratory assessment should be conducted immediately, focusing on clinical manifestations highlighting altered respiratory function.

In a person spontaneously breathing with an intact airway, hypoxia is initially managed with low-flow oxygen via a nasal cannula (up to 6 L/min) or face mask (up to 15 L/min) (Rose & Paulus, 2024) (see **Clinical Skill 19**). See TABLE 60.1 for a list of clinical indicators of altered respiratory function.

Oxygen toxicity may result from prolonged exposure to high oxygen levels. It is unclear what amount or duration of oxygen delivery is required to cause oxygen toxicity (Porritt, 2022a). Where possible, avoid long periods (24 hours or more) of oxygen therapy above 50 per cent to reduce oxygen toxicity (Rose & Paulus, 2024). See TABLE 60.2 for oxygen toxicity manifestations.

Oxygen therapy is commonly used in people with acceptable oxygen saturations with acute myocardial infarction, although there is no evidence of benefit and some potential for harm from unfavourable haemodynamic and metabolic changes (Sivapuram, 2022a; Swe, 2021). Oxygen is indicated to maintain arterial oxygen saturation between 94 and 96 per cent (Sivapuram, 2022a).

Regular assessment and monitoring are required to identify the person's clinical supplementary oxygen requirement (Sivapuram, 2022a).

Review the written order

Policies vary between health facilities; however, many require medical staff to order the amount, concentration, delivery method and duration of supplemental oxygen, and the target range for minimum and maximum oxygen saturation values (SpO_2). Check the policy of the facility.

TABLE 60.1 Clinical manifestation of altered respiratory function

CLINICAL MANIFESTATIONS	ONSET
CENTRAL NERVOUS SYSTEM	
• Sudden increased restlessness and agitation (hypoxia) • Sudden decrease in level of responsiveness, increased lethargy (hypercapnia) • Coma	Early or late Early or late Late
RESPIRATORY SYSTEM	
Changes in breathing pattern: • Respiratory rate greater than 30 per minute • Respiratory rate less than 10 per minute • Shallow or irregular breathing	 Early Late Early or late
Increased dyspnoea on exertion	Early
Increased dyspnoea at rest	Late
Increased orthopnoea	Late
Development of or increased adventitious breath sounds	Early or late
Accessory muscle use: • Shoulder elevation, intercostal muscle retraction • Use of scalene and sternocleidomastoid muscles	 Late Late
Unable to speak in sentences – pauses for breath between words	Late
CARDIOVASCULAR	
Changing trends in vital signs (temperature, pulse, blood pressure): increasing trends indicate compensation occurring; decreasing trends indicate decompensation occurring: • Mild hypertension • Hypotension	 Early Late
Increased cyanosis or duskiness (especially buccal mucosa and lips)	Late
Cool, clammy skin	Late
OTHER	
Diaphoresis	Late
Decreased urinary output	Late
Unexplained fatigue	Late
Pain	Late
Results from diagnostic and laboratory studies: haemoglobin, haematocrit, complete blood count, arterial blood gases (ABG), pulmonary function studies	Early or late

SOURCES: MARIEB, E. N. & HOEHN, K. (2019). *HUMAN ANATOMY AND PHYSIOLOGY* (11TH ED.). GLENVIEW, IL: PEARSON; SIVAPURAM, M. S. (2022A). *ACUTE MEDICAL PATIENTS: OXYGEN THERAPY.* ADELAIDE, SA: JOANNA BRIGGS INSTITUTE.

TABLE 60.2 Oxygen toxicity manifestations

CENTRAL NERVOUS SYSTEM	RESPIRATORY SYSTEM
• Nausea and vomiting • Anxiety • Visual changes • Hallucinations • Tinnitus • Vertigo • Malaise • Hiccups • Paraesthesia • Seizures	• Decreased pulmonary ventilation • Dyspnoea • Copious sputum production • Reduced vital capacity • Cough • Substernal chest pain • Nasal stuffiness • Tracheal irritation • Irreversible lung fibrosis

SOURCES: MARIEB, E. N. & HOEHN, K. (2019). *HUMAN ANATOMY AND PHYSIOLOGY* (11TH ED.). GLENVIEW, IL: PEARSON; ROSE, L. & PAULUS, F. (2024). VENTILATION AND OXYGEN MANAGEMENT. IN L. AITKEN, A. MARSHALL & T. BUCKLEY (EDS), *ACCCN'S CRITICAL CARE NURSING* (5TH ED.), PP. 521–66. CHATSWOOD, NSW: MOSBY.

EVIDENCE OF THERAPEUTIC INTERACTION

Stay with the person, as difficulty breathing is often associated with feelings of impending death, exacerbating anxiety. Use gentle, confident movements, a calm voice and closed questions requiring a brief yes or no answer, to assist the person to relax. Assist the person to assume a forward-leaning 'tripod' position to help maximise chest expansion, improving oxygenation and reducing their panic. Maintain eye contact and encourage the person to slow their breathing through pursed lips. This keeps their airway open longer, slowing their respiratory rate and encouraging deeper breaths. Slowing your own respiratory rate down is sometimes effective.

DEMONSTRATE CLINICAL REASONING

Position the person

Explain to the person their need for oxygen therapy (Sivapuram, 2022a). Position the person comfortably to assist them to breathe easier. Positioning depends on the person's condition and level of consciousness. A semi-Fowler's position assists a person to breathe easier by moving the abdominal contents away from the diaphragm. The orthopnoeic position (i.e. sitting upright with arms bent and elbows supported on an over-bed table, or arms braced against the knees when sitting out of bed) is also effective as it lifts the shoulder girdle, allowing for greater lung expansion. Some people are more comfortable sitting in a chair. The recovery position is necessary for an unconscious person to prevent aspiration or the soft palate from obstructing the airway.

Assess oxygen concentration

Reducing the risk of oxygen toxicity is an important aspect of nursing care when administering oxygen therapy. When the person is stable on oxygen therapy (PaO_2 greater than 80 per cent or SpO_2 greater than 95 per cent), their oxygen concentration should be gradually reduced and their oxygen requirements reassessed daily by measuring PaO_2 or SpO_2 on room air after 10 minutes off oxygen (Fong, 2021b).

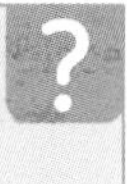

If the person's PaO_2 is greater than 65 mmHg or their SpO_2 is greater than 92 per cent, discuss stopping oxygen therapy with the medical staff (Fong, 2021b).

OXYGEN DELIVERY SYSTEM

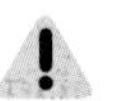

Safety

The oxygen concentration a person breathes can be increased by supplemental oxygen described as a concentration (expressed as a percentage) or the fraction of inspired oxygen (FiO_2; expressed as a decimal). For example, room air has an oxygen concentration of 21 per cent or a FiO_2 of 0.21; supplemental oxygen concentration ranges from 22 per cent to 100 per cent (FiO_2 of 0.22 to 1.0).

Low-flow systems deliver oxygen via small-bore tubing. The exact FiO_2 is dependent on the person's inspiratory flow rate, respiratory rate, tidal volume and respiratory pause, and oxygen delivery device factors, including oxygen flow rate, mask/reservoir volume, air vent size and tightness of fit (Rose & Paulus, 2024).

High-flow systems deliver all the gas in precise amounts. The ratio of oxygen to the room air required during ventilation does not vary with the person's respiratory status or effort.

Oxygen therapy delivered through a nasal cannula may be better tolerated due to increased comfort and freedom over masks. However, a mask may be required if a higher oxygen flow rate is required (Sivapuram, 2022a). See TABLE 60.3 for an overview of commonly used oxygen delivery systems.

A study by Eastwood et al. (2015) highlighted that nurses used only physiological measures such as SpO_2 levels when determining the therapeutic effectiveness of supplementary oxygen. However, people's compliance with oxygen therapy was based on device comfort and their ability to maintain activities of daily living as well as the therapeutic effect. Eastwood et al. also advise nurses to consider using different devices at different times to optimise physiological effects, to improve oxygen therapy management, and to optimise safety and improve outcomes.

TABLE 60.3 Commonly used oxygen delivery devices

OXYGEN DELIVERY DEVICE	LPM	FiO_2	COMMENTS
LOW FLOW			
Nasal cannula	0.25–6	0.22–0.44	• Oxygen concentrations of 24 to 44 per cent obtained • Plastic tube extending across the face, with short (0.6 to 1.5 cm) projections curving into the nostrils • Oxygen inhaled depends on room air and the person's breathing pattern • Inexpensive, comfortable, generally well tolerated • Allows the person to eat, drink, and talk • Difficult to maintain position; prongs easily drop out • Either an elastic strap or an extension of the plastic face tube fits around the person's ears and under their chin to secure it • High flow rates (> 5 L/min dry nasal membranes) may cause frontal sinus pain • Respiratory distress increases flow demand, reducing FiO_2 to alveoli • Mouth breathing and talking can render a nasal cannula ineffective
Simple mask	5–8	0.35–0.55	• Requires at least 5 L/min flow to prevent expired air accumulation in mask • Discomfort from the tight seal required between face and mask may lead to the person being unable to tolerate the mask • Heat radiating from face, nose and mouth is confined • Must be removed to eat or drink • Regularly wash and dry underneath mask • Assess for pressure injury on top of ears from elastic straps – use padding to reduce risk
Partial rebreather	6–10	0.50–0.70	• For short-term (24-hour) oxygen therapy for those requiring higher oxygen concentrations • Reservoir bag conserves oxygen. Flow must be sufficient to keep reservoir bag from deflating upon inspiration • Ensure reservoir does not kink, which results in bag deflation • Mask is lightweight and easy to use • Discomfort can lead to the person being unable to tolerate the mask • Not recommended for people with chronic obstructive pulmonary disease (COPD) • Not to be used with a nebuliser
Non-rebreather	6–10	0.70–1.0	• Mask needs to fit firmly • Flow must be sufficient to keep reservoir bag from collapsing or deflating during inspiration. Make sure valves open during expiration and close during inhalation, preventing FiO_2 decreasing • Closely monitor the person, as intubation may be necessary
HIGH FLOW			
Venturi mask	Variable	0.24–0.50	• Can deliver precise high flow rates (24, 28, 31, 35, 40 and 50 per cent); see manufacturer's instructions for precise flow and corresponding FiO_2 • Mask is helpful in administering constant low oxygen concentration to people with COPD; do not occlude air entrainment ports • Discomfort may lead to the person being unable to tolerate the mask

SOURCES: MARIEB, E. N. & HOEHN, K. (2019). *HUMAN ANATOMY AND PHYSIOLOGY* (11TH ED.). GLENVIEW, IL: PEARSON; ROSE, L. & PAULUS, F. (2024). VENTILATION AND OXYGEN MANAGEMENT. IN L. AITKEN, A. MARSHALL & T. BUCKLEY (EDS), *ACCCN'S CRITICAL CARE NURSING* (5TH ED.), PP. 521–66. CHATSWOOD, NSW: MOSBY; SIVAPURAM, M. S. (2022A). *ACUTE MEDICAL PATIENTS: OXYGEN THERAPY*. ADELAIDE, SA: JOANNA BRIGGS INSTITUTE.

Face masks

All face masks have similar disadvantages. Skin irritation caused by face masks means that facial skin care is necessary. They are hot and confining, and they require a tight seal, which is uncomfortable and claustrophobic. Face masks cannot be used while eating or drinking or during personal hygiene, and make talking and hearing difficult. For these reasons, you must be attentive to the person's needs. Masks are not suitable for long-term use.

Humidification

Humidification may be required for some people, especially those with a tracheostomy or laryngeal stoma and those who have difficulty clearing airway secretions. Assess the person to determine whether they would benefit from humidification. However, humidification should be considered for people receiving oxygen therapy in the following circumstances:

- if the flow rate exceeds 4 L per minute or the oxygen concentration exceeds 35 per cent for more than 24 hours
- in people with a tracheostomy (see **Clinical Skill 63**)
- in people with cystic fibrosis, bronchiectasis or a chest infection retaining thick secretions or having difficulty expectorating
- if the person reports discomfort due to dryness of oxygen therapy.

There are two main active humidification methods: cold humidifiers (e.g. Aquapak system, which can have an external heater added) and heated humidifiers (e.g. Fisher and Paykel). The humidification device depends on the person's clinical situation. For a person self-ventilating with an intact upper airway, a cold or heated Aquapak is generally adequate.

GATHER EQUIPMENT

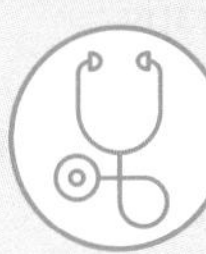

Gathering equipment is an organisational step that helps to create a positive environment for a successful interaction. It ensures that you have all needed material, boosts the person's confidence and trust in you, and increases your self-confidence. While gathering the equipment, you can mentally rehearse the procedure. Equipment may include the following items:

EQUIPMENT	EXPLANATION
Flow meter	• Regulates oxygen output from the oxygen source in litres per minute (L/min) and measures flow rates via a cylindrical tube or a round gauge. Both are calibrated in L/min • Check manufacturer's instructions for individual flow meters regarding where to read the ball (i.e. centre or top of ball), or dial (on Perflow brand) when setting the flow rate • Some may deliver greater than maximum flow indicated if the ball is set above the highest amount • Regulate oxygen flow by turning the knob until the appropriate output is reached • Adjust the flow meter to the ordered concentration or L/min before placing the delivery device onto the person
Oxygen source: wall outlet	• Supplied from large central tanks from which oxygen is delivered under low pressure • Set the flow meter to 'off', to prevent oxygen loss. Push the prongs of the meter unit firmly into the wall outlet. As the unit engages, there is a loud click. If you hear a hissing noise, remove and try again
Oxygen source: cylinder	• Come in a variety of sizes for hospital and home use • Is under high pressure and requires a pressure regulator for oxygen therapy administration at a safe and desirable rate • The flow meter is attached to the pressure regulator • Check the oxygen level before, during and after use
Oxygen tubing	• Specifically designed for use with oxygen equipment • Each end is reinforced with a thicker nipple, which is attached to the metal or plastic adaptors on the flow meter or the delivery device • Oxygen tubing is disposable and is usually distinguished by a pale green tint
Humidifier	• Required in certain circumstances (see the section 'Humidification') • Various devices are available; be familiar with those used in the facility and follow manufacturer's instructions
Pulse oximeter	Used to monitor the effectiveness of oxygen administration to maximise the benefit to the person (see **Clinical Skill 12**)
Safety signs	Alert the person, visitors and staff that oxygen is in use
Personal protective equipment (PPE)	Includes clean gloves and a plastic apron

For a person self-ventilating via a tracheostomy on oxygen, a heated system is preferable. For people with tracheostomy not requiring oxygen, a heat moisture exchange device (Swedish nose) is appropriate (Rose & Paulus, 2024).

SAFETY PRECAUTIONS FOR OXYGEN USE

Safety

Safety precautions are necessary because oxygen facilitates explosive combustion. The recommended safety precautions include:

- placing cautionary signs such as 'No smoking' or 'Oxygen in use' on the person's door, bed and on the oxygen equipment
- advising the person and visitors about oxygen hazards (e.g. electric razors, hair dryers)
- using only appropriately earthed, hospital-inspected and tagged electrical equipment to prevent the occurrence of short circuits/sparks
- avoiding the use of materials that generate static electricity (e.g. synthetics and wool)
- avoiding volatile or flammable materials use (e.g. oils, grease, alcohol, ether, nail polish remover and petroleum-based products such as Vaseline near oxygen use (Joanna Briggs Institute, 2020).

ADMINISTER OXYGEN THERAPY VIA NASAL CANNULA OR VARIOUS MASKS

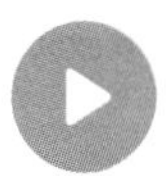

Video

Hand hygiene

Hand hygiene (see **Clinical Skill 5**) removes microorganisms from your hands. It is the most effective preventative measure for cross-contamination. Put on appropriate PPE.

Apply the appropriate oxygen delivery device

- *Nasal cannula (prongs)* – position to curve towards the nares where oxygen is directed upwards into the nose. Fit the plastic tubing over the person's ears and under their chin and tighten the toggle until the tubing is comfortably snug. On some prongs, an elastic strap is fitted over the head and tightened to keep these snug rather than tight on the face.
- *Simple face mask* – set oxygen flow to a minimum of 5 L before placing the mask over the nose and mouth. Adjust the nose clip and the elastic band to ensure a snug fit, so that oxygen does not escape from around the mask.

- *Partial rebreather mask* – check that the mask is functioning. If the reservoir totally collapses during expiration, increase the flow rate.
- *Non-rebreather mask* – check the functioning of the non-rebreather mask.
- *Venturi mask* – as shown in FIGURE 60.1, select the adaptor (on some models, set the dial) to give the required oxygen concentration. Connect the adaptor to the mask's wide corrugated tubing. Slip the humidification sleeve over the adaptor to ensure the air entrainment ports are not blocked by bed linen and that room air can flow in to dilute the oxygen to the correct concentration. Attach the oxygen tubing to the narrow end of the adaptor. Apply the mask as above.

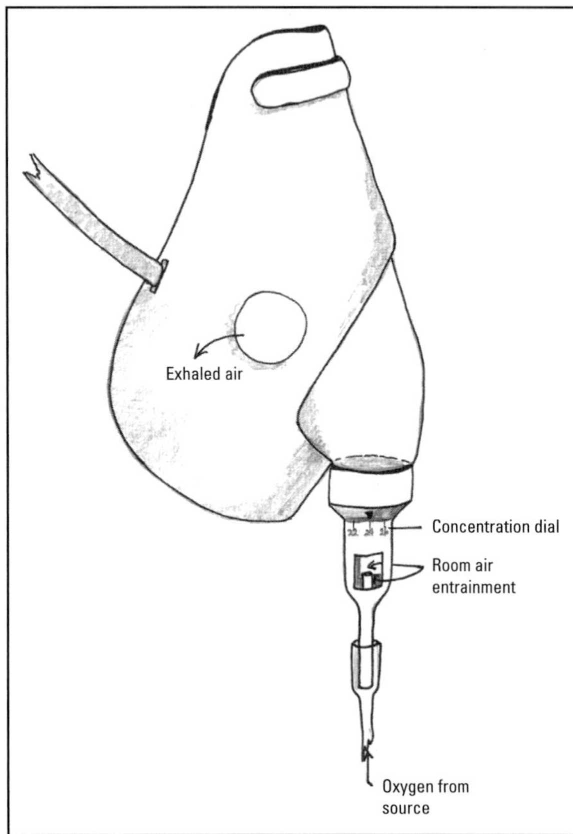

FIGURE 60.1 A Venturi mask that permits the administration of an exact amount of O_2

Explain to the person the importance of leaving the delivery device in place at all times so the flow of oxygen is unimpeded. Advise them to ask for assistance if they feel dyspnoeic and instruct them not to adjust the flow rate themselves.

Remove PPE and perform hand hygiene to prevent cross-contamination.

Assess the person during therapy

Stay with the person until their breathlessness is resolved and they are comfortable with the oxygen delivery device; many people find initial mask use distressing. Assess the person's oxygenation status during this initial time and at least every 15 to 30 minutes, including pulse oximetry, pulse and respiratory rate, work of breathing, lung sounds, accessory muscle use, skin and mucous membrane colour, and anxiety level. This can be extended to every four to eight hours, depending on the person's condition and their response to oxygen therapy.

Skin colour reflects a person's respiratory status and tissue perfusion. Hypoxia can be detected by skin colour change. However, the nature of skin colour varies with the person's natural skin colour (Aginga, 2021; Kydonaki & Parke, 2024). Begin your assessment by examining the person's palms, soles, tongue, palate, oral mucosa, conjunctiva, sclera and nail beds, as these are the areas of least pigmentation (Aginga, 2021). Cyanosis in people with dark skin pigmentation can be recognised by a bluish tint to the conjunctiva or palms, a greyish white colour around their lips or tongue, or a maroon tinge to the nail beds (Aginga, 2021). Ensure oxygen saturations remain within the person's target levels (see **Clinical Skill 19**).

Inspect nasal prongs and nares for mucous encrustations. Clean the prongs with water-dampened cotton applicators. If the nares are encrusted, gently remove the crusting and apply a water-soluble lubricant. Check the placement of the prongs frequently because they are easily displaced. With all face masks, attend to the skin to prevent pressure injury and deterioration because of the constant heat and irritation from the plastic, humidity and pressure. The skin is to be cleaned, dried and assessed at least four-hourly.

Provide oral fluids and mouth care as required.

If a humidifier is being used, check that it is operational.

Once the person's condition is stable, their ability to tolerate reduced or no oxygen therapy is evaluated regularly. The oxygen concentration is gradually reduced, and the person is trialled on room air after 10 minutes off oxygen. Remain with the person during this trial and assess their respiratory status.

Nasal cannulae are used for people with masks during mealtimes so oxygen therapy is not interrupted.

Oxygen tubing for an ambulatory person needs to be long enough so they can move about the room without disconnecting their oxygen. For trips beyond the reach of the tubing, a portable cylinder must be attached.

Inspect equipment regularly

It is important to ensure system integrity and compliance with the ordered concentration of oxygen. Check the flow meter to see if adjustments are needed, check tubing to ensure it is completely connected and not kinked, check masks or prongs to ensure correct positioning and proper working order, and check humidifiers for water and temperature levels. With some Venturi masks, the large-bore tubing connecting the humidifier to the mask needs to be checked for water accumulation and emptied frequently to prevent bacterial colonisation. Wash face masks daily or as required with warm water. Change the mask and tubing according to the facility's protocol.

Post-procedure

Assist the person to a comfortable position and replace the call bell and anything moved during the procedure so that it is within their reach.

CLEAN, REPLACE AND DISPOSE OF EQUIPMENT

Clean the oxygen flow meter and the wall attachment as per the facility's guidelines. Discard the oxygen face mask, tubing and humidifier in the clinical waste bin.

DOCUMENTATION

Note relevant data on initiating oxygen therapy. In the person's progress notes, you should document the time, date, assessment data, oxygen concentration and/or flow rate, delivery method, humidification, the person's response, any adverse effects and nursing interventions to address these.

CLINICAL SKILLS ASSESSMENT

Oxygen therapy via nasal cannula or various masks

Demonstrates the ability to effectively and safely provide oxygen therapy. Incorporates the *National Safety and Quality Health Service Standards*: 2 Partnering with consumers, 3 Preventing and controlling healthcare-associated infections, 5 Comprehensive care, 6 Communicating for safety, and 8 Recognising and responding to acute deterioration (Australian Commission on Safety and Quality in Health Care [ACSQHC], 2021).

Performance criteria	1	2	3	4	5
(Numbers indicate NMBA *Registered Nurse Standards for Practice*)	**(Dependent)**	**(Marginal)**	**(Assisted)**	**(Supervised)**	**(Independent)**
1. Identifies the indication; reviews the medical order (1.1, 3.3, 3.4)	☐	☐	☐	☐	☐
2. Evidence of therapeutic interaction with the person, e.g. provides the person with a clear explanation of the procedure (1.4, 1.5, 2.1, 2.2, 3.2)	☐	☐	☐	☐	☐
3. Demonstrates clinical reasoning abilities, e.g. positions the person, determines the administration mode (e.g. nasal prongs, non-rebreather), FiO_2 required, early signs of respiratory distress or oxygen toxicity (1.1, 1.2, 1.3, 1.5, 4.1, 4.2, 4.3, 5.1, 6.1)	☐	☐	☐	☐	☐
4. Gathers equipment (1.1, 5.5, 6.1): ■ flow meter ■ oxygen source: wall outlet/cylinder ■ oxygen tubing ■ humidifier ■ pulse oximeter ■ safety signs ■ personal protective equipment	☐	☐	☐	☐	☐
5. Attends to safety precautions (3.4, 6.1, 6.5)	☐	☐	☐	☐	☐
6. Performs hand hygiene; dons appropriate personal protective equipment (1.1, 3.4, 6.1)	☐	☐	☐	☐	☐
7. Applies the appropriate oxygen delivery device (1.1, 3.4, 6.1)	☐	☐	☐	☐	☐
8. Assesses and evaluates the person's response to oxygen therapy at regular intervals (4.1, 4.2, 4.3, 6.1, 7.1, 7.2)	☐	☐	☐	☐	☐
9. Regularly inspects equipment (1.1, 3.4, 6.1)	☐	☐	☐	☐	☐
10. Ensures the person is comfortable post-procedure and that the call bell is within easy reach (4.1, 4.2, 4.3, 6.1)	☐	☐	☐	☐	☐
11. Cleans, replaces and disposes of equipment appropriately (3.6, 6.1)	☐	☐	☐	☐	☐
12. Documents relevant information (1.1, 1.4, 1.6, 2.2, 2.7, 3.5, 3.7, 6.1, 6.2, 6.5, 7.3)	☐	☐	☐	☐	☐
13. Demonstrates the ability to link theory to practice (1.1, 3.3, 3.4, 3.5)	☐	☐	☐	☐	☐

Student:

Clinical facilitator: Date:

CHAPTER 61

OROPHARYNGEAL AND NASOPHARYNGEAL SUCTIONING

INDICATIONS

Oropharyngeal and nasopharyngeal suction is intended to stimulate a cough to remove excess secretions and/or aspirate secretions unable to be spontaneously removed by the person from their upper airway (Ahmed & Eid, 2022). Pharyngeal suctioning should only be undertaken when other less invasive techniques (e.g. assisted cough) were unsuccessful, and when the person's secretions are causing physiological deterioration or distress. The need for suctioning is often indicated by conditions that reduce a person's ability to protect their airway, such as:

- neuromuscular or neurological impairment
- decreased swallowing ability or dysphagia
- ineffective cough
- oral trauma or maxillofacial surgery
- assisted respiratory ventilation.

Suction may also be used when secretions are required for diagnosis.

EVIDENCE OF THERAPEUTIC INTERACTION

Introduce yourself and inform the person of your designation. Explain the procedure to the person. Clarify any immediate concerns to help allay fears, and subsequent increases in the person's blood pressure and heart rate (Ahmed & Eid, 2022). Provide a clear explanation of the procedure's purpose and the sensations the person may feel. This reduces anxiety (which is generally high because of the difficulty in breathing) and enables the person to assist where possible. People need to be told it is an uncomfortable procedure and they may gag, cough or sneeze for a short while during or after the procedure. If possible, arrange with the person a signal by which they can communicate they want to stop; it will reduce their anxiety and make the procedure less frightening if they feel they have some control.

DEMONSTRATE CLINICAL REASONING

Assess the person

Suctioning should never be considered a routine procedure. Its frequency should be determined by an individual systematic respiratory assessment (see **Clinical Skill 19**). Indications a person requires suctioning include:

- audible or visible secretions in the upper airway
- reduced/absent breath sounds on auscultation
- ineffective or weak coughing
- desaturation despite increased oxygen requirements
- raised respiratory rate and increased work of breathing
- collection of sputum specimens (Deakin, 2019).

When suctioning is indicated, no absolute contraindications exist and failure to suction can prove more detrimental than potential adverse reactions. Suctioning should be performed by staff with experience and knowledge of risks involved (Ahmed & Eid, 2022). Caution is required in people with:

- severe coagulopathy and/or unexplained haemoptysis
- laryngospasm (stridor)
- acute neck, facial or head injury (particularly basal skull fractures or cerebrospinal fluid leakage via the ear)
- severe bronchospasm
- recent oesophageal or tracheal anastomoses, or tracheooesophageal fistula.

Potential hazards of pharyngeal suctioning include suction-induced hypoxaemia, mucosal damage, vasovagal stimulation and raised intracranial pressure. See TABLE 61.1 for potential complications and nursing management.

TABLE 61.1 Potential pharyngeal suctioning complications

POTENTIAL COMPLICATION	CAUSES AND MANAGEMENT
Distress	• Suction may be very uncomfortable for the person • Nasopharyngeal suction should only take place if absolutely necessary • Careful explanation and reassurance are essential
Suction-induced hypoxia	• Caused by the catheter reducing the airway and decreasing the person's oxygen supply during the procedure • Discontinue suctioning until the person's condition stabilises, unless the person's condition is deteriorating due to secretions in airway • Provide supplemental oxygen • Assess pulse oximetry and vital signs • Administer pre-oxygenation prior to suctioning using an appropriately sized catheter • Avoid prolonging the suction procedure to prevent this
Soft-tissue damage	• Includes epistaxis, mucosal damage and ulceration • Caused by the catheter passing • Use appropriate suction pressures • Carefully select the correct catheter size to help prevent this • If person continues to bleed, stop suction and discuss with the medical team
Gagging or vomiting	• Caused by touching the posterior pharyngeal wall with a suction catheter • Careful technique reduces risks • Position the person correctly before the procedure to limit the aspiration risk if vomiting occurs
Vasovagal stimulation	• Causes bradycardia and hypotension, and is most common in haemodynamically unstable individuals caused by hypoxaemia or vagus nerve irritation • Discontinue suctioning until the person's condition stabilises, unless the person's condition is deteriorating due to secretions in the airway • Provide supplemental oxygen • Assess pulse oximetry and vital signs • Gently introduce the catheter to the correct depth to prevent this
Infection	• Can be introduced during nasopharyngeal suction • A clean technique must be used – it is recommended best practice to use Aseptic Non Touch Technique (ANTT) • Perform hand hygiene and wear appropriate personal protective equipment (PPE)
Atelectasis	• Caused by the vacuum • Ensure the correct suction pressure is used
Laryngospasm	• Rare; this condition is an emergency • If the person stops breathing during suctioning and the catheter feels stuck and cannot be withdrawn, the medical emergency team should be called • Laryngospasm may be relieved by gentle positive pressure ventilation using an Ambu bag (bag valve mask) • Intubation may be necessary
Raised intracranial pressure (ICP)	• An increase in blood pressure increases ICP • ICP rises if the person coughs, vomits or becomes hypoxic • If any of the potential complications persist in a neurologically unstable person, these may cause further instability

SOURCES: AHMED, E. I. & EID, R. (2022). *OROPHARYNGEAL SUCTIONING: SAFE AND EFFECTIVE PRACTICE*. ADELAIDE, SA: JOANNA BRIGGS INSTITUTE; PORRITT, K. (2022A). *ENDOTRACHEAL SUCTIONING (ADULT, PEDIATRIC AND NEONATAL): FREQUENCY AND DURATION* [EVIDENCE SUMMARY]. ADELAIDE, SA: JOANNA BRIGGS INSTITUTE. *AUSTRALIAN GUIDELINES FOR THE PREVENTION AND CONTROL OF INFECTION IN HEALTHCARE*. COMMONWEALTH OF AUSTRALIA. RETRIEVED FROM HTTP://WWW.NHMRC.GOV.AU.

Position the person

Where possible, position the person to ensure their airway is open, either in high side-lying or sitting upright. Suctioning can be accomplished in any position; however, people are often more comfortable in semi- or high Fowler's position, which aligns the airway and aids in maximal lung expansion. The person's head should be turned towards you for oral suctioning or with the neck hyperextended for nasal suctioning (unless contraindicated). These positions help insert the catheter and prevent aspiration of secretions.

An unconscious person is positioned laterally facing you. This position protects their airway by assisting secretions to drain from the pharynx and prevents aspiration as the tongue then falls forward.

Sometimes, people benefit from other measures, such as postural drainage, chest percussion, assistance with coughing, or ordered medications such as bronchodilators, expectorants, opioids or antihistamines. Considering other appropriate measures also displays clinical reasoning abilities.

GATHER EQUIPMENT

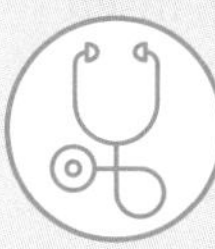

Gathering equipment is an organisational step that helps to create a positive environment for a successful interaction. It ensures that you have all needed material, boosts the person's confidence and trust in you, and increases your self-confidence. While gathering the equipment, you can mentally rehearse the procedure. It is essential that you have both knowledge of and experience in setting up and using suctioning equipment prior to actual care.

Various suction machines are available. Familiarise yourself with the facility's procedural guidelines and equipment. Test all equipment to make sure it is functioning before use to ensure safe nursing care.

The following equipment is required:

EQUIPMENT	EXPLANATION
Suctioning apparatus	• Either a portable machine or a wall unit with a regulator that produces a vacuum, which is the negative pressure used to suction • The regulator is set to various amounts of negative pressure. The recommended suction pressures are listed in **TABLE 61.2**; note that sources vary, and these are average recommendations • Includes a receptacle to contain the secretions collected. Most are disposable closed-system and are changed when three-quarters full or when the person is discharged • Non-disposable receptacles are cleaned and disinfected every 24 hours, although may need to be emptied and cleaned more frequently, depending on the amount of suctioning required • Place 50 mL of water in the receptacle before use to reduce the stickiness of the secretions and make cleaning the container easier (follow the facility's policy)
Suction tubing	• Attaches the catheter to the suction machine • Needs to be about 2 m long to accommodate position changes and manipulation during the procedure • An adaptor is attached to the end to receive the suction catheter. Attach one end to the suction apparatus and the other close to the person
Sterile Y-suctioning catheter	• A soft, flexible tube used to access nasal and oral cavities • Vary in size, but should be the smallest size possible to facilitate secretion removal and allow air entry around the catheter during suctioning • Prevents a sudden drop in functional residual capacity and reduces the risk of atelectasis • Distal end generally has two or three holes in case the distal hole becomes blocked • Use the thumb port at the proximal end to apply and control suction pressure of between 80 and 120 mmHg (Ahmed & Eid, 2022) • See **TABLE 61.2** for suggested suction catheter sizes and recommended suction pressures
Yankauer suction catheter	• A rigid, angled plastic or metal suction catheter with one large hole and several small eyelets on the distal end for removing secretions • Used when secretions are copious, thick and viscous, or for vomitus • Used only for the oral cavity and the external nares
Water-soluble lubricant	Used to reduce friction and ease entry of the catheter tip into the nasopharynx
Tap water, sterile water or normal saline (NS)	• Used between suction passes to clean the tubing of tenacious secretions and to increase suctioning's efficiency • Also lubricates the tip of the catheter to ease passage • Follow the facility's procedural guidelines for the solution used
Sterile or non-sterile gloves	• Required to reduce transmission of microorganisms and to protect you from bodily secretions • Oral and oropharyngeal suctioning using a Yankauer or a Y-suction catheter is a clean procedure requiring clean gloves, as the oropharynx and nasopharynx are not considered sterile (Ahmed & Eid, 2022) • Sterile gloves are required for nasotracheal suctioning (Deakin, 2019) • Follow the facility's procedural guidelines
Personal protective equipment (PPE)	• Used as necessary • A face shield or goggles protect your eyes, nose and mouth from accidental contamination by sprayed body fluids during excessive coughing or sneezing • A plastic apron protects your clothing from being contaminated • Gloves
Pulse oximeter	Used if the person's condition requires monitoring
Oxygen	Used as indicated by the person's condition and their response to suctioning
Oropharyngeal or nasopharyngeal airway	• Used as indicated • Facilitates the passage of the suction catheter, improving secretion clearance • Nasopharyngeal airways are contraindicated in people with suspected head injuries
Waterproof sheet	Placed on the person's chest and pillow to protect the bed linen and clothing from soiling with secretions
Waterproof disposal bag	Used when any piece of disposable equipment is discarded

PART 11

PERFORM OROPHARYNGEAL AND NASOPHARYNGEAL SUCTIONING

Video

Hand hygiene

Hand hygiene (see **Clinical Skill 5**) removes microorganisms from your hands. It is the most effective preventative measure for cross-contamination.

Personal protective equipment is worn to protect staff from splash-back, spills and spray if the person coughs (National Health and Medical Research Council [NHMRC], 2019).

Pre-procedure preparation

1. Explain the procedure to the person and position them comfortably (see 'Position the person').
2. Oxygenate the person if required.
3. Turn the suction device on. If it is not already connected, attach one end of the suction tubing to the suction port or machine. Set the regulator to the desired setting (see TABLE 61.2 for suction pressure). Check that the suction is functioning by suctioning a small amount of water from a container.
4. Position the disposal bag within your reach for easy disposal of used items.
5. Perform hand hygiene and put on the required PPE. Insert the oropharyngeal or nasopharyngeal airway, if indicated.

Attach the catheter tip

Open the sterile suction catheter at the connection end and attach it to the suctioning tubing. Remove the suction catheter from the package without touching the catheter's tip. Occlude the proximal port with the thumb of the non-dominant hand to ensure that the equipment is functioning correctly before commencing the procedure. For nasopharyngeal suctioning, apply a water-soluble lubricant to the catheter's distal end.

Enter the nasal cavity

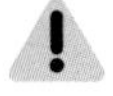
Safety

The nasal cavity is entered first because it harbours the least number of microorganisms. Determine the catheter length needed to reach the pharynx by measuring the distance between the person's nose tip and their earlobe (4 to 8 cm for an infant, 8 to 12 cm for a child and 13 cm for an adult). Grasp the suction catheter by that distance from the distal tip.

Remove the person's oxygen mask or nasal cannula with your non-dominant hand. Advise the person you are going to insert the catheter and ask them to take a deep breath. Without suction applied, as the person inhales with their neck extended if possible, insert the catheter tip gently along the nasal floor. Direct it slightly towards the ear to the desired distance, to avoid the nasal turbinates. Do not force the catheter. If resistance is met, try the other nostril.

Apply suction

Suction is applied by occluding the suction port. Encourage the person to cough. Slowly and gently withdraw the catheter. Apply suction for five to 10 seconds. Assess the amount, colour and consistency of the suctioned fluid. Observe the person for any signs of distress during suctioning. The entire procedure should take 15 seconds to avoid removing excessive air from their airways, causing hypoxia.

Replace oxygen delivery if applicable. Allow the person to rest for 30 seconds. Assess the person for any cardiovascular, respiratory or neurological compromise. Encourage them to cough between suctioning to raise tracheal secretions to the pharynx where these can be suctioned. Clean the lumen of the catheter by suctioning water, until the catheter is clear.

Reassess the need for repeat suctioning. Observe the person for alterations in cardiopulmonary status. Allow one to two minutes before repeating procedure. The entire process should last less than five minutes to avoid distressing the person or decreasing oxygenation. Evaluate the person's response to the procedure. Auscultate the person's lungs and compare with the respiratory assessment before suctioning. Assess the person's respiratory and pulse rates, colour and SpO_2. Ask the person if breathing is improved and whether all secretions were removed.

Enter the oropharynx

Remove the patient's oxygen mask if it is in situ. Ask the person to open their mouth, providing assistance as necessary. A Yankauer sucker is commonly used for oropharyngeal suctioning (Ahmed & Eid, 2022). Introduce the catheter gently along the roof of the mouth until it reaches their pharynx (back of the mouth/nose).

A nasal cannula can remain in place. Without the suction on, advance the catheter about 10 to 15 cm along the gum line to reduce triggering the gag reflex. Follow the facility's procedural guidelines.

Again, apply suction as discussed, only on withdrawal; remove the contents of the oropharynx until the airway sounds clear.

TABLE 61.2 Suction pressure

	WALL UNIT (mmHg)	PORTABLE UNIT (mmHg)	CATHETER SIZE (FRENCH)
Infants (less than 1 year)	60–80	2–5	5–8
Children (1–8 years)	80–120	5–10	8–10 (usually for children under 10 years of age)
Adults (over 8 years)	120–150	10–15	12–18 (generally recommended for adults)
Older adults (older than 75 years)	80–120	5–10	8–10 (for frail older adults)

Post-procedure

Assist the person to a comfortable position, replacing the call bell and anything moved during the procedure so that it is within their reach.

CLEAN, REPLACE AND DISPOSE OF EQUIPMENT

Wrap the suction catheter around your gloved dominant hand. Peel the glove off to envelop the catheter and dispose of it in the waterproof bag. Rinse the suction tubing as needed by inserting the end of the tubing into the used water container. Dispose of the water, the container and the wrappings in the bag. Remove the non-sterile gloves and dispose of them in the bag. Close the bag and place it into the contaminated waste bin.

Place the suction tubing and the Yankauer suction catheter in a clean and dry area for reuse. Generally, these are changed daily. (Follow the facility's protocol.)

Remove remaining PPE and perform hand hygiene. Replace used equipment to ensure an adequate supply when the person requires suctioning again.

DOCUMENTATION

Document: the date and time; initial assessment; procedure; amount, colour, consistency and odour of secretions; and the person's response to the procedure and breathing status following suctioning, and any adverse responses to suctioning and nursing interventions to address these. Report to your team leader any adverse responses or deterioration in the person's condition.

CLINICAL SKILLS ASSESSMENT

Oropharyngeal and nasopharyngeal suctioning

Demonstrates the ability to effectively and safely care for a person requiring oropharyngeal and nasopharyngeal suctioning. Incorporates the *National Safety and Quality Health Service Standards*: 2 Partnering with consumers, 3 Preventing and controlling healthcare-associated infections, 5 Comprehensive care, 6 Communicating for safety, and 8 Recognising and responding to acute deterioration (Australian Commission on Safety and Quality in Health Care [ACSQHC], 2021).

Performance criteria	1	2	3	4	5
(Numbers indicate NMBA *Registered Nurse Standards for Practice*)	(Dependent)	(Marginal)	(Assisted)	(Supervised)	(Independent)
1. Identifies indication (1.1, 3.3, 3.4)	☐	☐	☐	☐	☐
2. Evidence of therapeutic interaction with the person, e.g. provides the person a clear explanation of the procedure (1.4, 1.5, 2.1, 2.2, 3.2)	☐	☐	☐	☐	☐
3. Demonstrates clinical reasoning abilities, e.g. assesses and correctly positions the person, selects the correct catheter size (1.1, 1.2, 1.3, 1.5, 4.1, 4.2, 4.3, 5.1, 6.1)	☐	☐	☐	☐	☐
4. Gathers equipment (1.1, 5.5, 6.1): ■ suction apparatus, tubing and connector ■ suction catheter (e.g. Yankauer) ■ water (as per facility's guidelines) ■ personal protective equipment (PPE) (including non-sterile gloves) ■ waterproof sheet ■ other equipment as required (e.g. pulse oximetry, oxygen)	☐	☐	☐	☐	☐
5. Performs hand hygiene and puts on clean gloves and additional personal protective equipment as required (1.1, 3.4, 6.1)	☐	☐	☐	☐	☐
6. Turns suction device on and sets regulator to the desired setting (6.1)	☐	☐	☐	☐	☐
7. Attaches the catheter tip to the suction tubing (6.1)	☐	☐	☐	☐	☐
8. Advises the person when inserting the catheter and asks the person to take a deep breath (6.1)	☐	☐	☐	☐	☐
9. Maintains clinical observation of the person during the procedure (4.1, 4.2, 6.1)	☐	☐	☐	☐	☐
10. Enters the nasal cavity (6.1)	☐	☐	☐	☐	☐
11. Enters the oropharynx (6.1)	☐	☐	☐	☐	☐
12. Applies suction and asks the person to cough (1.1, 6.1)	☐	☐	☐	☐	☐
13. Reassesses the person and evaluates the person's response and the effectiveness of the procedure (2.2, 2.3, 4.1, 4.2, 4.3, 6.1, 6.5)	☐	☐	☐	☐	☐
14. Cleans, replaces and disposes of equipment appropriately (3.6, 6.1)	☐	☐	☐	☐	☐
15. Documents relevant information (1.1, 1.4, 1.6, 2.2, 2.7, 3.5, 3.7, 6.1, 6.2, 6.5, 7.3)	☐	☐	☐	☐	☐
16. Demonstrates the ability to link theory to practice (1.1, 3.3, 3.4, 3.5)	☐	☐	☐	☐	☐

Student:

Clinical facilitator: Date:

CHAPTER 62

ARTIFICIAL AIRWAY SUCTIONING

INDICATIONS

Suctioning is the aspiration of secretions, blood or vomit through a tube. Tracheal suctioning is an important airway management component in people unable to independently expectorate secretions.

Although the formation of biofilm makes the internal lumen of an airway tube decrease substantially after a few days of intubation, suctioning should be performed *only* when clinically indicated to maintain artificial airway patency (Porritt, 2022a; Mbinji, 2022a; Rose & Paulus, 2024). Performing only when clinically indicated reduces the risk of airway trauma, hypoxaemia, atelectasis and infection risks (Porritt, 2022a; Rose & Paulus, 2024). Indications include:

- the person is unable to cough effectively to clear retained secretions
- the person is unable to maintain airway patency due to an obstruction of sputum, vomit or blood
- sudden respiratory distress, including increased ventilator airway pressure; deteriorating oxygenation (PaO_2 or SpO_2 suddenly decreases); or increases or decreases in heart rate, respiration rate or blood pressure
- the need to collect secretions for diagnostic purposes (Porritt, 2022a).

The three common methods of suctioning are as follows:

- *Open tracheal suctioning* – requires ventilation equipment to be disconnected and the suction catheter inserted into the open end of the endotracheal tube or tracheostomy tube.
- *Semi-closed suctioning* – involves a suction catheter being passed through a swivel connector with a self-sealing rubber flange.
- *Closed tracheal suction system* – consists of a multiple-use catheter enclosed within a sterile plastic sleeve. An 'in-line' catheter is attached between the artificial airway and the ventilator circuit. 'In-line' suctioning is particularly useful for people requiring high levels of inspired oxygen or positive-end expiratory pressure (PEEP) (Rose & Paulus, 2024).

There are two suction methods, based on the catheter suction depth selected during the procedure: deep and shallow. Shallow suction (in which the catheter is advanced to the end of the artificial airway) is preferable if the person is awake and has an effective cough (Porritt, 2022a). Deep suction (in which the catheter is fully advanced to the carina and then withdrawn 1 cm before applying suction) must be used with caution as it may cause tracheal trauma or coughing, increasing intracranial pressure (Porritt, 2022a). Secretions in peripheral airways are not and should not be directly removed by artificial airway suctioning.

EVIDENCE OF THERAPEUTIC INTERACTION

Safety

To reduce the person's anxiety and to promote the person's understanding, assistance and cooperation, talk with the person about their need for suctioning, consequences of not suctioning, and clearly explain the purpose of the procedure, and the sensations the person can expect. Explain to the person that suctioning is uncomfortable and may cause coughing and briefly increase shortness of breath. Also highlight the importance of the person assisting with secretion removal by coughing during the procedure. Relatives may prefer to leave during the procedure; if so, inform them afterwards of the person's response to suctioning.

People with endotracheal or non-fenestrated tracheostomy tubes are not able to speak, so provide them with communication aids (paper and pencil, communication boards).

If the person has a fenestrated outer tube, ensure the plain inner tube is in situ, rather than just the fenestrated tube (see **Clinical Skill 63**).

Suctioning via a fenestrated tube allows the suction catheter to pass through the fenestration, causing tracheal wall trauma (Lister, Hofland & Grafton, 2020).

Remember to assess the person for inadequate oxygenation or ventilation and clinical manifestations of suctioning complications during and after suctioning. Suctioning should be terminated if cardiac dysrhythmias, haemodynamic instability or significant decreases in oxygenation occur (Wagner et al., 2019).

DEMONSTRATE CLINICAL REASONING

The clinical decision to suction a person's airway is based on a systematic analysis and a thorough respiratory assessment (see **Clinical Skills 12 and 19**).

LOOK at the person's colour, respiratory rate, depth and effort; for any accessory respiratory use; and chest expansion – symmetrical or asymmetrical.

LISTEN to the person's description of breathlessness, dyspnoea, anxiety or reports of pain; for air entry – good, fair or poor; and any adventitious sounds.

FEEL for movement of expired air.

See TABLE 62.1 for assessment guidelines prior to, during and after suctioning.

Knowledge of the person's medical condition and history is important because some conditions (e.g. chronic pulmonary diseases, stroke and dehydration) increase the risk of airway obstruction. Assess the person's respiratory and oxygenation status over the previous 24 hours to help distinguish an acute episode from chronic deterioration.

Ensure the person's oxygenation remains between 94 and 98 per cent for most adults, and between 88 and 92 per cent if there is a risk of hypercapnia/type II respiratory failure during the procedure.

This procedure is potentially painful and anxiety-provoking. Prior to suctioning, consider the person's potential complications and contraindications. See TABLE 62.2 for suctioning complications and hazards.

People with thoracic or abdominal incisions or injuries will benefit from effective pain management and splinting of their chest or abdomen, if appropriate.

Position the person for best cough effort and lung clearance. Suctioning can be accomplished in any position. However, people are often more comfortable in semi- or high Fowler's position if they are able. Additional measures can assist in moving secretions from peripheral airways, such as postural drainage, chest percussion, assistance with coughing, and bronchodilators or expectorant medications.

Humidification is essential for people with an endotracheal or a temporary tracheostomy, because the tube bypasses the humidification processes that occur in the upper airways. Lack of humidification increases the viscosity of mucous secretions, depresses ciliary function and mucociliary transport. These in turn increase infection risk, impair secretion removal and cause microatelectasis (Wagner et al., 2019). Adequate systemic hydration (i.e. oral, nasogastric or intravenous) ensures pulmonary secretions remain easy to suction or expectorate. Inadequate humidification can lead to major airway obstruction or artificial airway blockage (see **Clinical Skill 61**).

TABLE 62.1 Assessment guidelines prior to, during and after suctioning

ASSESSMENT	DESCRIPTION

Respiratory assessment	• Breath sounds
	• Oxygen saturation and, if available, arterial blood gases (ABG)
	• Skin colouring
	• Mucosal colouring
	• Pulse oximetry
	• FiO_2
	• Respiratory rate and pattern
	• Work of breathing
	• Cough characteristics (effective or non-effective)
	• Sputum characteristics:
	  ◦ amount: small, moderate, large or copious
	  ◦ consistency: thick or thin
	  ◦ colour: clear, creamy, yellow or green
	  ◦ odour
	• Ventilator parameters:
	  ◦ peak inspiratory pressure and plateau pressure
	  ◦ tidal volume
	  ◦ pressure, flow and volume graphics, if available
	  ◦ FiO_2

Haemodynamic assessment	• Temperature • Pulse or heart rate • Blood pressure (if indicated and available) • Electrocardiogram (if indicated and available)
Intracranial pressure	• If indicated and available

SOURCES: PORRITT, K. (2022A). *ENDOTRACHEAL SUCTIONING (ADULT, PEDIATRIC AND NEONATAL): FREQUENCY AND DURATION* [EVIDENCE SUMMARY]. ADELAIDE, SA: JOANNA BRIGGS INSTITUTE; ROSE, L. & PAULUS, F. (2024). VENTILATION AND OXYGEN MANAGEMENT. IN L. AITKEN, A. MARSHALL & T. BUCKLEY (EDS), *ACCCN'S CRITICAL CARE NURSING* (5TH ED.), PP. 521–66. CHATSWOOD, NSW: MOSBY.

TABLE 62.2 Suctioning complications and hazards

SYSTEM	COMPLICATION/HAZARD	PEOPLE AT RISK
Respiratory	• Hypoxia/hypoxaemia • Atelectasis • Trauma to tracheal tissue and/or bronchial mucosa • Bronchoconstriction/bronchospasm	• Decreased or absent cough reflex • Acute pulmonary haemorrhage • Acute lung injury • PEEP dependent • High O_2 requirements • Reactive airways
Cardiac	• Hypertension • Hypotension • Cardiac dysrhythmias – bradycardia	• Unstable cardiovascular system • Vagal nerve stimulation
Neurological	• Changes in cerebral blood flow • Increased intracranial pressure (ICP)	• Unstable/high ICP • Spinal cord injury with autonomic dysreflexia
Haematological		• Coagulopathy – platelets • < 20; INR >2.5
Infection prevention	• Increased lower airway microbial colonisation	• Immunocompromised

SOURCES: PORRITT, K. (2022A). *ENDOTRACHEAL SUCTIONING (ADULT, PEDIATRIC AND NEONATAL): FREQUENCY AND DURATION* [EVIDENCE SUMMARY]. ADELAIDE, SA: JOANNA BRIGGS INSTITUTE; ROSE, L. & PAULUS, F. (2024). VENTILATION AND OXYGEN MANAGEMENT. IN L. AITKEN, A. MARSHALL & T. BUCKLEY (EDS), *ACCCN'S CRITICAL CARE NURSING* (5TH ED.), PP. 521–66. CHATSWOOD, NSW: MOSBY.

GATHER EQUIPMENT

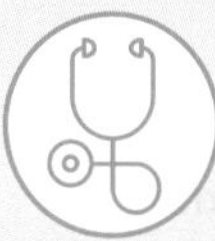

It is essential for safety that you have both knowledge of and experience with setting up and using suctioning equipment prior to using it on a person. Familiarise yourself with the equipment available at the facility. At the commencement of each shift, ensure that all essential emergency equipment is available and in working order to avoid adverse incidents.

The necessary equipment includes the following:

EQUIPMENT	EXPLANATION
Tracheostomy emergency equipment	Must be present and checked prior to initiating suctioning and include: • Ambu bag and an appropriately sized mask (in case of accidental extubation) • Spare tracheostomy tubes in the same size and one size smaller • Stitch cutter if the tracheostomy tube is sutured in place • Tracheal dilators • 10 mL syringe to inflate the tracheostomy tube (TT) cuff • Scissors • Stethoscope to auscultate air entry and lung sounds • Cuff pressure manometer to monitor cuff pressure – not part of emergency equipment, but should be available (see **Clinical Skill 63**)
Suctioning apparatus	• Either a portable machine or a wall unit with a regulator • The regulator can be set to various negative pressure amounts required for suctioning. Atelectasis is a risk if suction pressure is too high • See 'Suctioning apparatus' for further detail
In-line closed suction system	To be connected to endotracheal or tracheostomy tube suction unit, for use during the closed-suction method
NS (10 to 20 mL) in a syringe	• Used to cleanse suction tubing during the closed-suction method • Suction source
A sterile bottle of water	• Label 'suction' with the opening date and time • Changed every 24 hours to minimise the growth of bacteria • When using an open or semi-closed suction method, pour water into a bowl and suction it to clear the tubing of tenacious secretions and to maintain suctioning efficiency. It also lubricates the catheter tip to ease passage • Follow facility lubrication guidelines
Gloves (sterile and non-sterile)	• Used to reduce the transmission of microorganisms and to protect you from bodily secretions • Single packaged sterile gloves are generally used when suctioning. If these are available, use one sterile glove and one non-sterile glove. If these are not available, use one pair of sterile gloves
Personal protective equipment (PPE)	• Protects you from splash injury if the person has copious secretions or violent coughing in response to suctioning • Face shield or goggles and a mask protect your eyes, nose and mouth • Plastic apron protects your uniform from accidental contamination by sprayed body fluids during excessive coughing or sneezing

EQUIPMENT	EXPLANATION
Waterproof sheet	Place on the person's chest and the pillow to protect the bed linen and their clothing from secretions
Waterproof disposal bag	Used when disposable equipment is discarded
Ambu bag and oxygen	Required to pre-oxygenate the person prior to applying suction and for use in an emergency
Stethoscope	Used to assess air entry and lung sounds
A Yankauer suction catheter	Used for oral suctioning
Oral care equipment	Used to provide mouth care following suctioning

SUCTIONING APPARATUS

TABLE 62.3 lists recommendations. Note that sources vary, and these are average recommendations.

TABLE 62.3 Recommended suction pressure

AGE	WALL UNITS	PORTABLE UNITS
Infants (less than 1 year)	60–80 mmHg	2–5 mmHg
Children (1–8 years)	80–120 mmHg	5–10 mmHg
Adults (over 8 years)	120–150 mmHg	10–15 mmHg
Older adults (older than 75 years)	80–120 mmHg	5–10 mmHg

Porritt (2022a) recommends using the lowest possible suction pressure during endotracheal suctioning, usually 80 to 120 mmHg for adults.

Many facilities use closed-wall suction units, which include a disposable collection unit to reduce infection risks. These are changed every 48 to 72 hours (as per the facility's policy), when full, and between patients.

Portable suction apparatus includes a receptacle to contain the secretions collected. If a glass receptacle is used, clean and disinfect it every 24 hours; they may need to be emptied and cleaned more frequently. To reduce secretion stickiness and to make cleaning easier, place 50 mL of water in the receptacle before use.

Generally, two lengths of suction tubing are required: one attaches to the suction source and the other goes to the suction catheter. Suction tubing needs to be a large-bore, non-collapsible plastic tubing about 2 m long to accommodate position changes and manipulation during the procedure. Tubing is changed every 24 hours to prevent the growth of microorganisms. An appropriate adaptor is fitted onto the end of the tubing to which the suction catheter is attached.

Suction catheters are soft, flexible tubes used to access nasal and oral cavities. These have several openings along the distal end and a thumb port on the side of the proximal end to control the application and amount of suction. Multi-holed suction catheters cause fewer traumas to the tracheal mucosa. Suction catheters vary in size; for example, French 5 to 8 (for infants), 8 to 10 (usually for children under 10 years of age and for frail older adults) and 12 to 18 (generally recommended for adults).

Safety

There is consensus in the literature (Porritt, 2022a; Rose & Paulus, 2024) that suction catheters should be as small as possible, yet large enough to facilitate secretion removal. A catheter that is too large causes trauma, hypoxaemia and atelectasis; one that is too small is ineffective. Generally, it is recommended that the suction catheter should occlude less than half of the internal lumen of the artificial airway (Porritt, 2022a; Rose & Paulus, 2024).

PREOXYGENATE THE PERSON

Safety

Consider preoxygenation if suctioning causes a clinically important reduction in the individual's oxygen saturation with suctioning. Preoxygenation is generally delivered with 100 per cent oxygen for at least 30 seconds prior to and after the suctioning procedure and is recommended to prevent a decrease in the person's oxygen saturation (Porritt, 2022a; Rose & Paulus, 2024). Porritt (2022a) concludes that preoxygenation with 100 per cent oxygen reduces the occurrence of suction-induced hypoxaemia by 32 per cent. Refer to the facility's policy, as ventilated people or those receiving supplementary oxygen are often preoxygenated at FiO_2 100 per cent for two minutes to reduce hypoxaemia.

Routine use of hyperinflation is not recommended due to the risk of barotrauma from large tidal volumes and high peak pressures, as well as patient discomfort (Rose & Paulus, 2024). Hyperinflation should be delivered by the ventilator to control tidal volume and inspiration peak pressure.

Closed-suctioning technique is recommended for mechanically ventilated people, as it facilitates continuous ventilation and oxygenation during suctioning (Porritt, 2022a).

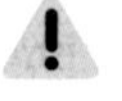
Safety

Ensuring adequate hydration and humidification is more successful in maintaining thin secretions than routine normal saline (NS) instillation (Porritt, 2022a). Routine instillation of sterile NS is no longer recommended for children or adults. This has been associated with adverse events, including excessive coughing; decreased oxygen saturation; bronchospasm; dislodgement of the bacterial biofilm colonising the endotracheal tube into the lower airway; pain, anxiety and dyspnoea; tachycardia; and increased intracranial pressure (Porritt, 2022b).

Open the sterile glove and suction catheter packages. For this procedure, you will need a face shield or goggles, a mask and a plastic apron. These must be applied prior to putting on your sterile gloves.

PERFORM ARTIFICIAL AIRWAY SUCTIONING

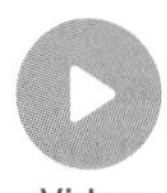

Video

Safety

Hand hygiene

Artificial airway suctioning is an invasive procedure and may lead to contamination of the lower airways (Porritt, 2022a; Rose & Paulus, 2024). Hand hygiene must occur on entering the person's bed area; prior to donning gloves to perform the suctioning procedure; on completion of the suctioning procedure following glove removal; and on leaving the person's bed area. Aseptic Non Touch Technique (ANTT) (see **Clinical Skill 7**) is recommended during open suctioning technique (Porritt, 2022a; Rose & Paulus, 2024).

Safety

The *Australian Guidelines for the Prevention and Control of Infection in Healthcare* (National Health and Medical Research Council [NHMRC], 2019) state all procedures generating or having potential to generate secretions or excretions require healthcare workers to wear either a face shield or a mask worn with protective goggles. See TABLE 62.4 for recommended PPE for closed-system suctioning and open suctioning. Refer to the facility's infection prevention and control guidelines.

TABLE 62.4 Recommended PPE for closed-system suctioning and open suctioning

PPE	CLOSED-SYSTEM SUCTIONING	OPEN SUCTIONING
Mask/goggles or face shield	Yes	Yes
Gown/apron	Yes	Yes
Gloves	Non-sterile	Sterile
Suction catheter	Closed-system catheter changed as per manufacturer's recommendation	Sterile suction catheter Discarded post-procedure
Field	Clean	Aseptic

SOURCE: NHMRC (2019). *AUSTRALIAN GUIDELINES FOR THE PREVENTION AND CONTROL OF INFECTION IN HEALTHCARE.* COMMONWEALTH OF AUSTRALIA. RETRIEVED FROM HTTP://WWW.NHMRC.GOV.AU.

Open-suction method

Turn on the suction device and connect it to the suction tubing. Set the regulator to the desired setting (see TABLE 62.3). Tape the disposable bag to the locker within easy reach for the disposal of used items.

Don gloves

Some facilities require you to wear a sterile glove during artificial airway suctioning to maintain suction catheter sterility and to protect you from bodily secretions. To do this, put the non-sterile glove on your non-dominant hand. Put the sterile glove on your dominant hand (see **Clinical Skill 8**). Maintain ANTT (with your designated suction hand) throughout the procedure.

Pick up the suction catheter

Pick the catheter up in your dominant hand, coil the distal length around your fingers and attach the proximal end of the adaptor. Use your non-dominant gloved hand to manipulate the tubing. Hold the distal end of the suction catheter with your dominant hand and dip it into sterile saline. Briefly apply suction by occluding the proximal port with the thumb of your non-dominant hand to test the equipment and lubricate the tip.

Remove the tracheostomy mask or humidification device if used, and place on a waterproof sheet.

Insert the catheter tip

As you insert the catheter tip, ask the person to take a couple of deep breaths. Talking with the person helps prepare them for the unpleasant sensations felt during suction.

Avoid contaminating the catheter tip by not touching the sides of the artificial airway tube. Using your dominant hand, gently and quickly insert the catheter to the required depth. Deep suctioning is to be avoided, as it is associated with airway mucosal damage and inflammation and may induce bronchial bleeding with subsequent risk of airway occlusion (Mbinji, 2022a).

Inserting the catheter at the end of inspiration generally causes an increase in cough strength, as the maximum tidal volume is achieved with the greatest elastic recoil, which is important for maximum cough generation. This increases secretion mobilisation and removal and reduces the risk of suction-induced hypoxia. Additionally, it is less distressing for the person to cough after taking a deep breath rather than at the end of expiration.

Apply suction and withdraw the catheter

Inform the person suction is about to occur and that it will make them cough. Occlude the suction port and apply continuous suction as you withdraw the catheter slowly (without rotation or twirling) over 10 to 15 seconds. Longer periods are associated with increased hypoxaemia and trauma. Intermittent suction increases mucosal damage. Multi-eyed catheters draw secretions from all sides without rotation.

Assess the secretions removed while suctioning.

Reconnect the tracheostomy mask, humidification or oxygen devices

Reapply the tracheostomy mask, the humidification device or oxygen if required within 10 seconds of completing suctioning. Assess the person's oxygen saturations post-procedure and consider increasing supplementary oxygen if saturations have decreased. Assess the person's vital signs. If the person is ventilated, assess the tidal volume and peak pressure post-procedure. Reassess the person's respiratory status to evaluate their response to suctioning.

?

If secretions remain, repeat the procedure until the airway is clear; however, ensure that the person has sufficient rest after each suction episode. If the facility's guidelines permit a second suctioning using the same catheter, remove thick secretions and clean the lumen of the catheter by suctioning some water until the catheter is clear. (Consult the facility's guidelines regarding catheter reuse.)

If a new sterile catheter and sterile glove are required, remove the suction catheter and the sterile glove. Secretions are cleared from suctioning tubing by suctioning water until tubing is clear.

Remove the non-sterile glove. Perform hand hygiene and don new gloves and repeat the suctioning procedure. The number of suction passes should be kept to a minimum. Follow the facility's guidelines regarding the maximum number of suctioning attempts.

Closed-suction method

The following equipment is required for the closed-suction method:

- in-line closed-suction system
- NS (10 to 20 mL) in a syringe
- Ambu bag and appropriately sized mask
- clean gloves and PPE.

Secure the connecting tube

Perform hand hygiene and put on PPE.

Secure the connecting tube to the closed-system suction port (follow the manufacturer's instructions) and ensure the sterility of the connection port. Determine the appropriate safe suction level. Align the catheter under the lavage port before applying suction (again, follow the manufacturer's instructions). Ensure the tip of the Y-adaptor touches a marked whole centimetre number (e.g. 18 cm) on the endotracheal tube. Add 5.5 cm to this whole number for the correct catheter length (e.g. 18 cm + 5.5 cm = 23.5 cm).

Set the suction regulator at the appropriate suction level while the thumb port of the catheter is depressed (or as per the manufacturer's instructions). This prepares for suctioning and limits the amount of negative pressure, thereby limiting damage to the tracheal epithelium. Adequate pressure is required to effectively remove secretions. Follow the manufacturer's directions for suction pressure levels with closed-suction systems.

Preoxygenate as per the facility's guidelines. Preoxygenation increases arterial oxygen levels in preparation for suctioning.

Advance the catheter

Advance the catheter until the measured number is aligned with the lavage port. The most efficient catheter advancement occurs when the bag covering the catheter bunches up behind your fingers (Dougherty, Lister & West-Oram, 2015).

Depress suction and hold

When the catheter is at the correct depth, apply suction then slowly withdraw the catheter (for 10 to 15 seconds). To prevent extubation, support the catheter at the artificial airway tube with your non-dominant hand while withdrawing the suction catheter. To minimise arterial oxygen desaturation and mucosal trauma, suctioning is limited to 15 seconds or less in adults, or 10 seconds or less in children (Porritt, 2022a; Rose & Paulus, 2024).

Cleanse the catheter

Withdraw the black tip of the catheter into the middle of the cleaning chamber and depress suction first, then gently squeeze the saline solution into the chamber. The catheter is to be flushed between each insertion of the catheter while watching the catheter window.

To prevent catheter movement between suctioning, lock the suction catheter when you have finished suctioning and cleaning it.

Reconfirm the security and position of the artificial airway

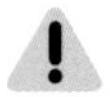

Safety

Ensure the artificial airway tube is secure to allow for immediate attention if needed. Report any change in the position of the tube immediately to a team leader.

Reassess respiratory status

After suctioning is completed, you need to monitor physiologic status, including vital signs, SpO_2, ICP (if monitoring is in situ) and the person's clinical appearance, including the colour of the skin and mucous membranes, diaphoresis and agitation (Rose & Paulus, 2024).

Post-assessment evaluates whether the person's condition has improved after the suctioning procedure. Report the following clinical manifestations to the team leader:

- diminished breath sounds
- increased peak airway pressures
- persistent coughing
- increased work of breathing
- inability to pass the suction catheter
- changes in quality or characteristics of secretions.

Suction the oropharynx and nasopharynx

Once the artificial airway is cleared of secretions, use another suction device to suction the oral and nasal pharynx (see **Clinical Skill 61**). Periodic suctioning of the upper airway prevents secretions pooling and potentially entering the lower airways and causing aspiration pneumonia. Upper-airway suctioning occurs after tracheal suctioning because the nose and mouth are not as clean as the trachea. Some facilities require a sterile catheter for each of these areas – check the facility's guidelines.

Provide oral care

Regular oral care (see **Clinical Skill 56**) provides comfort and reduces the incidence of hospital-acquired infections.

Remove gloves, perform hand hygiene and remove remaining PPE.

Post-procedure

Assist the person to a comfortable position. Replace the call bell and anything that was moved during the procedure so that it is within reach. If FiO_2 was increased, reassess the person and their SpO_2 after they have settled. If the person's levels are within their desired parameters, readjust the oxygen flow to the original flow rate.

CLEAN, REPLACE AND DISPOSE OF EQUIPMENT

For open suctioning, wrap the suction catheter around your gloved dominant hand and peel the glove off to envelop the catheter. Discard the glove, the catheter and the wrappings in the bag. Remove and dispose of waterproof sheets. Close the bag and place it in the contaminated waste bin.

Discard the remainder of the solution used for cleaning the suction catheter and tubing. Clean and replace the bowl as per the facility's guidelines. Remove the non-sterile glove and dispose of it in the contaminated waste bin.

As needed or as per facility guidelines, empty and rinse the suction collection container. Replace equipment to ensure an adequate supply when the person requires suctioning again. Change the closed-suction system every 24 to 72 hours, depending on the facility's guidelines.

DOCUMENTATION

Document the date and time; the initial assessment; the procedure; the amount, colour, consistency and odour of secretions, and any specimens taken; the person's response to suctioning and their respiratory and oxygenation status following the procedure; and any unexpected outcomes and related interventions necessary to correct these before, during and after suctioning.

CLINICAL SKILLS ASSESSMENT

Artificial airway suctioning

Demonstrates the ability to effectively and safely suction a person with an endotracheal tube or tracheostomy via the open- or closed-suctioning method. Incorporates the *National Safety and Quality Health Service Standards*: 2 Partnering with consumers, 3 Preventing and controlling healthcare-associated infections, 5 Comprehensive care, 6 Communicating for safety, and 8 Recognising and responding to acute deterioration (Australian Commission on Safety and Quality in Health Care [ACSQHC], 2021).

Performance criteria	1	2	3	4	5
(Numbers indicate NMBA *Registered Nurse Standards for Practice*)	**(Dependent)**	**(Marginal)**	**(Assisted)**	**(Supervised)**	**(Independent)**
1. Identifies indication – performs respiratory assessment (1.1, 3.3, 3.4)	☐	☐	☐	☐	☐
2. Evidence of therapeutic interaction with the person, e.g. gives the person a clear explanation of the need for the procedure, effects and procedural consequences (1.4, 1.5, 2.1, 2.2, 3.2)	☐	☐	☐	☐	☐
3. Demonstrates clinical reasoning abilities, e.g. assesses the person prior to the procedure, identifies indications, contraindications, and potential complications identified during and after suctioning (1.1, 1.2, 1.3, 1.5, 4.1, 4.2, 4.3, 5.1, 6.1)	☐	☐	☐	☐	☐
4. Gathers equipment (1.1, 5.5, 6.1): ■ tracheostomy emergency equipment ■ suctioning apparatus ■ a sterile bottle of water ■ gloves (sterile and non-sterile) ■ personal protective equipment (goggles, mask or face shield/apron/gloves as per facility infection and prevention control procedural guidelines) ■ waterproof sheet ■ waterproof disposal bag ■ Ambu bag and oxygen ■ stethoscope ■ a Yankauer suction catheter ■ oral care equipment	☐	☐	☐	☐	☐
5. Performs hand hygiene (1.1, 3.4, 6.1)	☐	☐	☐	☐	☐
6. Turns the suction device on and sets the regulator; checks pressure by suction tubing occlusion (1.1, 6.1)	☐	☐	☐	☐	☐
7. Identifies need to preoxygenate and, if appropriate, preoxygenates (4.1, 6.1)	☐	☐	☐	☐	☐
8. Open-suctioning method: attaches the catheter tip to the suction tubing and tests the equipment (6.1) Closed-suctioning method: secures tubing to the closed-suctioning equipment as per the manufacturer's instructions (6.1)	☐	☐	☐	☐	☐
9. Dons sterile gloves (where appropriate) and other PPE (1.1, 3.4, 6.1)	☐	☐	☐	☐	☐
10. Open-suctioning method: lubricates and inserts the catheter (6.1) Closed-suctioning method: advances closed-suction catheter to the required depth (6.1)	☐	☐	☐	☐	☐
11. Replaces the tracheal mask, humidification device or oxygen therapy as required and reassesses respiratory and oxygenation status (4.1, 4.2, 4.3, 6.1)	☐	☐	☐	☐	☐
12. Suctions the oropharyngeal and nasopharyngeal spaces (6.1)	☐	☐	☐	☐	☐
13. Assists the person to reposition, replaces the call bell and anything that was moved during the procedure so that it is within the person's reach (2.3, 4.1, 4.2, 4.3, 6.1)	☐	☐	☐	☐	☐

Performance criteria	1	2	3	4	5
(Numbers indicate NMBA *Registered Nurse Standards for Practice*)	**(Dependent)**	**(Marginal)**	**(Assisted)**	**(Supervised)**	**(Independent)**
14. Provides oral care (6.1)	☐	☐	☐	☐	☐
15. Cleans, replaces and disposes of equipment appropriately (3.6, 6.1)	☐	☐	☐	☐	☐
16. Documents relevant information and ensures that reporting and documentation are timely and accurate (1.1, 1.4, 1.6, 2.2, 2.7, 3.5, 3.7, 6.1, 6.2, 6.5, 7.3)	☐	☐	☐	☐	☐
17. Demonstrates the ability to link theory to practice (1.1, 3.3, 3.4, 3.5)	☐	☐	☐	☐	☐

Student:

Clinical facilitator: Date:

CHAPTER 63

TRACHEOSTOMY CARE

INDICATIONS

A tracheostomy is a surgical opening below a person's larynx into their trachea, usually into the second or third tracheal ring below the cricoid cartilage into which an indwelling tube is placed to overcome upper airway obstruction, facilitate mechanical ventilatory support, and enable the removal of tracheobronchial secretions.

A tracheostomy may be required temporarily or permanently due to:

- head and neck surgery
- maxillofacial trauma
- congenital anomaly, such as laryngeal hypoplasia or vascular web
- supraglottic or glottic pathologic condition, such as infection, neoplasm or bilateral vocal cord paralysis
- upper airway oedema from trauma, burns, infection or anaphylaxis (Joanna Briggs Institute, 2022; Matthew, 2022).

Advantages of tracheostomy over long-term endotracheal intubation for a person include:

- reduced laryngeal ulceration
- reduced respiratory resistance resulting in reduced work of breathing
- more easily tolerated
- improved ability to communicate (Joanna Briggs Institute, 2022; Sivapuram, 2022b).

Tracheostomy can be performed using a surgical technique, percutaneous dilatational technique or mini-tracheostomy tube (Joanna Briggs Institute, 2022; Matthew, 2022). In critical care areas in Australia and New Zealand, percutaneous dilatational technique is more commonly performed than surgical technique.

Contraindications to percutaneous dilatational technique include:

- uncorrected coagulopathy
- severe local sepsis
- high positive end-expiratory pressure as compared to fraction of inspired oxygen
- elevated intracranial pressure
- tracheal obstruction
- unusual neck anatomy
- need for emergency airway management (Matthew, 2022).

Mini-tracheostomies are small-bore, cuffless tubes inserted through the cricothyroid tissue into the trachea. Indications for a mini-tracheostomy tube include secretion retention, people with a high risk of postoperative pulmonary complications due to either an infective cough or because they are unable to perform effective chest physiotherapy (e.g. following lung or cardiac surgery), or an emergency when a person has a total airway obstruction (Matthew, 2022). Unlike other invasive ventilator systems, a mini-tracheostomy tube allows a person to speak.

Tracheostomy tubes (TTs) are cuffed or uncuffed. They vary in their composition, number of parts, shape and size. The type of TT is chosen to facilitate secretion clearance or communication, or to accommodate differing anatomy. The length and curve are important to avoid dislodgement during coughing or head turning. Previously, TTs were made from stainless steel, sterling silver or rubber. Increasingly, TTs are made from disposable non-reactive plastics.

A short-term TT is usually a single cuffed tube. A long-term TT has three parts: an inner cannula (a smooth tube with a locking device), an outer cannula (flange, cuff and pilot tube) and an obdurator (a round, smooth tip facilitates non-traumatic tube insertion) (Sivapuram, 2022b). Inner cannulae (reusable or disposable) reduce secretion accumulation in the TT.

The key nursing concept of tracheostomy management is to ensure the person's airway remains patent. A blocked or partially blocked tracheostomy tube results in severe respiratory distress (Sivapuram, 2022b). Additionally, nursing care of a person with a TT aims to prevent site infection and tube dislodgement or accidental decannulation, and to provide adequate humidification, appropriate cuff pressure management and suctioning to maintain airway patency.

Keeping the stoma site clean and dry reduces infections of the site and lower airway pneumonia by removing microorganisms before they migrate to the person's lower airways. Tracheostomy care facilitates healing, prevents peristomal skin excoriation and promotes comfort.

EVIDENCE OF THERAPEUTIC INTERACTION

Introduce yourself and inform the person of your designation. Clearly explain the suctioning procedure, including the need for suction, consequences of not suctioning when required, and effects of suctioning, and clarify any immediate concerns. Repeat this information prior to each suctioning procedure, as some people may not recall previous instructions. This helps reduce the person's anxiety and gains their cooperation, reducing the risk that they will touch or contaminate sterile items and minimising the risk of inadvertent tube dislodgement. Talk about the most comfortable position for the person to be in during the procedure and discuss procedural expectations. Explaining to the person how they can assist enables them to actively participate in their care. Answering questions honestly fosters trust.

Screen the bed area or close the door to provide privacy for the person. Tracheostomy care is a two-person procedure. One of these must be a registered nurse (RN).

Communication

People communicate in different ways, such as using gestures, facial expressions, body postures and vocalising. Most TTs are positioned below vocal cords, which impacts on the person's ability to produce a normal voice (Edwards, 2022). Inability to speak can evoke feelings of insecurity and panic, and at times frustration for the person, staff and family.

Refer a person with a new tracheostomy to a speech pathologist for assessment and provision of communication aids such as letter boards, pen and paper, magic slates or electronic devices. These aids require patience, coordination and endurance, which is often difficult for an acutely ill person with musculoskeletal weakness, coordination difficulties or slowed thought processing due to prolonged illness, especially in older adults (Matthew, 2022).

For people with established tracheostomy tubes, it is essential that communication methods are identified in discussion with the person and their family. These methods must be documented on the person's plan of care and verbally handed over to staff to ensure adequate communication and appropriate understanding of the person and their needs.

A speaking valve is a small plastic device with a silicone one-way valve. The valve opens on inspiration, allowing air to enter the TT, and closes on exhalation, directing air up the trachea, larynx, nose and mouth, as in normal breathing and normal speech. The person's tolerance of the speaking valve depends on the patency of the airway around and above the TT. To exhale sufficiently, the person must have sufficient airway patency around the TT, through the larynx and out of the nose and mouth (Rose & Paulus, 2024). If the person is unable to adequately exhale with the speaking valve in place, they may become distressed, which can lead to air trapping or lung barotrauma.

Whatever form of communication is used, it is important to provide the person time to express themselves.

DEMONSTRATE CLINICAL REASONING

Care for a person with a tracheostomy

Immediate postoperative and ongoing priorities of care for a person with a tracheostomy include ensuring TT is securely in place and the person's airway is patent. A person's comfort is imperative throughout the postoperative period. Pain should be proactively managed as per the facility's guidelines.

Tracheostomy emergencies

The three most common tracheostomy emergencies are haemorrhage, tube dislodgement and tube obstruction, which are summarised in TABLE 63.1. Percutaneous dilatational technique results in fewer wound infections, decreased bleeding and reduced mortality compared to surgical technique (Rose & Paulus, 2024; Sivapuram, 2022b).

TABLE 63.1 Common tracheostomy emergencies

EMERGENCY	DESCRIPTION

Haemorrhage	• A small amount of self-limiting bleeding is expected after the initial procedure and tracheostomy tube changes
	• Continued minimal or large amounts of bleeding may require exploration of the site to ligate a bleeding vessel
	• The surgeon needs to be contacted
	Tracheoinnominate fistula:
	• Occurs when the innominate artery becomes eroded through the trachea, causing massive haemorrhage. Generally, occurs three to four weeks after surgery due to one of the following predisposing factors:
	  • high cuff inflation pressures exceeding tracheal capillary perfusion pressure
	  • improper placement of the cannula tip (from direct weight or torque on the TT from the ventilator circuit)
	  • low tube placement
	  • hyperextension of the head
	  • radiotherapy or steroid use
	• Preventative measures include:
	  • maintaining cuff inflation pressure between 20 to 25 mmHg or 20 to 30 cm H_20
	  • removing added weight and traction from the ventilator circuit
	  • keeping the TT in a midline and neutral position

EMERGENCY	DESCRIPTION

Tube dislodgement and loss of airway	• Dislodgement of the TT during the first postoperative week is a medical emergency. The immature stoma quickly collapses if the tube is dislodged or inadvertently removed
	• Check tube security frequently and always before moving the person
	• A dislodged tube from a mature tracheostomy should be replaced with the same size tube, a tube one size smaller or an endotracheal tube through the stoma
	• In an emergency, a person with a dislodged TT that is unable to be reinserted should be intubated
	• *Decannulation* means the tube is completely dislodged
	Partial TT dislodgement:
	• Means the tube tip lies within a false passage anterior to the trachea. It is potentially more harmful than decannulation due to delayed diagnosis resulting in aspiration or decreasing gas exchange. Predisposing factors include:
	  • loose ties
	  • neck or airway oedema
	  • excessive coughing
	  • agitation or being under sedation
	  • morbid obesity
	  • TT too short for the tract
	  • technique used to place the TT
	  • downward traction caused by ventilator circuit weight
	• *Preventative measures include:*
	  • maintaining effective analgesia and sedation if required
	  • keeping tracheostomy ties secure and snug (no more than a single finger should fit under the ties)
	  • removing added weight and traction from the ventilator circuit
	  • keeping the TT in a midline and neutral position
	  • minimising transport of the person as much as possible

Tube obstruction	Acute obstruction is most likely caused by a mucous plug; it could also be caused by obstructing granuloma or tube insertion into a false track
	• Predisposing factors include:
	  • endoluminal mucous impaction caused by humidity deficiency
	  • tenacious secretions
	  • decreased neurological and muscular performance
	  • decreased active cough reflexes and efforts
	• Preventative strategies:
	  • change the inner cannula daily or more frequently if necessary
	  • perform tracheal suctioning to confirm TT placement
	  • stimulate production of secretions
	  • facilitate removal of secretions
	• An open tracheostomy requires added humidity to provide comfort, prevent mucous membranes drying, and prevent thickening of secretions
	• A progressive mobility program incorporating upper limb range of motion exercises helps mobilise secretions
	• Sitting the person in a chair helps maintain a functioning position – a more effective diaphragm promotes a more effective cough

SOURCES: EDWARDS, J. (2022). *TRACHEOSTOMY: DRESSING* [EVIDENCE SUMMARY]. ADELAIDE, SA: JOANNA BRIGGS INSTITUTE EBP DATABASE, JBI@OVID; MATHEW, S. (2022). *MINI-TRACHEOSTOMY: EFFECTIVENESS.* [EVIDENCE SUMMARY]. ADELAIDE, SA: JOANNA BRIGGS INSTITUTE; ROSE, L. & PAULUS, F. (2024). VENTILATION AND OXYGEN MANAGEMENT. IN L. AITKEN, A. MARSHALL & T. BUCKLEY (EDS), *ACCCN'S CRITICAL CARE NURSING* (5TH ED.), PP. 521–66. CHATSWOOD, NSW: MOSBY; SIVAPURAM, M. (2022B). *TRACHEOSTOMY: MANAGEMENT OF PATIENTS.* ADELAIDE, SA: JOANNA BRIGGS INSTITUTE.

TABLE 63.2 Immediate postoperative and long-term tracheostomy complications

IMMEDIATE POSTOPERATIVE COMPLICATIONS	LONG-TERM COMPLICATIONS
• Blocked or dislodged tube • Bleeding from the airway/TT • Pneumothorax • Subcutaneous and/or mediastinal emphysema • Respiratory and/or cardiovascular collapse • Aspiration	• Acute airway obstruction • Blocked or dislodged tube • Infection (localised to stoma or tracheobronchial) • Aspiration • Tracheal trauma • Stomal or tracheal tissue granuloma • Tracheal stenosis • Tracheomalacia • Tracheooesophageal fistula • Vocal cord injury • Swallowing difficulties • Scarring

SOURCES: EDWARDS, J. (2022). *TRACHEOSTOMY: DRESSING* [EVIDENCE SUMMARY]. ADELAIDE, SA: JOANNA BRIGGS INSTITUTE EBP DATABASE, JBI@OVID; MATHEW, S. (2022). *MINI-TRACHEOSTOMY: EFFECTIVENESS.* [EVIDENCE SUMMARY]. ADELAIDE, SA: JOANNA BRIGGS INSTITUTE; ROSE, L. & PAULUS, F. (2024). VENTILATION AND OXYGEN MANAGEMENT. IN L. AITKEN, A. MARSHALL & T. BUCKLEY (EDS), *ACCCN'S CRITICAL CARE NURSING* (5TH ED.), PP. 521–66. CHATSWOOD, NSW: MOSBY.

Preventative measures

Assessing the person frequently, early identification and prompt management of complications, regular tracheostomy care, maintaining the person's hydration and nutritional status, and inspired air humidification help prevent respiratory emergencies. See TABLE 63.2 for possible immediate and long-term postoperative complications.

Routine care

Immediate and routine care incorporates regular assessment of the person and airway management. To prevent postoperative infection, keep the incision clean and dry (Overall, 2023). Leave the tracheostomy to heal for five to seven days and assist the cutaneo-endotracheal tract to become stable and patent (Sivapuram, 2022b).

Stoma care includes routine site observations. Report and accurately document any assessment findings of redness, swelling, increased discomfort during care, odour and evidence of granulation tissue (Overall, 2023).

Clean the stoma daily using a sterile solution of 0.9 per cent normal saline (NS) to ensure the stoma and peristomal skin is clean and dry. This avoids irritation, maceration and skin breakdown from continued moisture, and removes dried secretions (Edwards, 2022; Overall, 2023; Sivapuram, 2022b). Keep the site dry using TT sponges or skin barrier dressings to prevent skin breakdown and infections. See TABLE 63.3 for an overview of tracheal stoma dressings.

Humidification

A tracheostomy bypasses the upper airway, preventing normal humidification and filtration of inhaled air. Unless air inhaled via the TT is humidified, the tracheal epithelium and bronchi become dry, which increases the risk of tube blockage. Tracheal humidification can be provided by a heated humidifier, a heat and moisture exchanger (HME) or a tracheostomy bib. See TABLE 63.4 for an overview of these humidification methods.

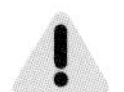
Safety

Without humidification, the person's mucus becomes thick and difficult to expectorate, increasing the risk of lower respiratory tract infections and airway obstruction from endoluminal mucous impaction (Overall, 2023; Sivapuram, 2022b). Secretions remaining tenacious with humidification may require saline nebulisers two-hourly to four-hourly (Sivapuram, 2022b).

Suctioning

If a person is unable to clear their secretions, perform suctioning to maintain a clear airway by removing secretions and preventing the formation of a mucous plug (Sivapuram, 2022b). The frequency of airway suctioning is determined by the person's individual need (see **Clinical Skill 62**).

TABLE 63.3 Tracheal stoma dressings

DRESSING TYPE	SUGGESTED USE
TT gauze sponges	Minimal to moderate secretions
Polyurethane foam (e.g. Lyofoam)	Copious secretions
Hydrocolloid (DuoDERM), which can be used as primary skin protection and then covered with a TT gauze sponge to absorb secretions	Potential or actual skin breakdown from copious secretions
Silicone foam (Mepilex) can be used as primary skin protection and then covered with a TT gauze sponge to absorb secretions	• Potential or actual skin breakdown from copious secretions • To cushion skin from the neck flange

SOURCE: ADAPTED FROM EDWARDS, J. (2022). *TRACHEOSTOMY: DRESSING* [EVIDENCE SUMMARY]. ADELAIDE, SA: JOANNA BRIGGS INSTITUTE EBP DATABASE, JBI@OVID.

TABLE 63.4 Humidification methods

HUMIDIFICATION METHODS	INDICATIONS AND NURSING CONSIDERATIONS
Heated humidification delivers gas heated to body temperature via a heated water bath prior to inspiration	• Oxygen delivery via tracheostomy mask • Mechanical ventilation • Respiratory infection with increased secretions • Management of thick secretions • Humidification temperature set at 37 °C delivers temperatures 36.5 to 37.5 °C at the tracheostomy site
HMEs absorb the person's expired air, heat and moisture via a hygroscopic paper surface, part of which is delivered during their next inspiration	• Recommended for all people with TT • HME with an oxygen port is suitable for low-flow oxygen administration • Fits directly onto TT • Changed daily or as needed if the filter appears excessively moist or blocked • Do not wet the HME filter prior to use
Tracheostomy bibs are made of a specialised foam that traps moisture from expired air moisture. The foam moistens and warms air to be inspired	• Suitable for people no longer requiring oxygen therapy • Bibs work in a similar way to HME devices • Reusable • Change daily or more frequently as required • Wash hands in warm water using a mild detergent/soap, rinse thoroughly and allow to air dry • Tracheostomy bibs should be discarded monthly or more frequently if discoloured or damaged

SOURCES: OVERALL, B. (2023). *TRACHEOSTOMY: STOMA CARE*. ADELAIDE, SA: JOANNA BRIGGS INSTITUTE; SIVAPURAM, M. (2022B). *TRACHEOSTOMY: MANAGEMENT OF PATIENTS*. ADELAIDE, SA: JOANNA BRIGGS INSTITUTE.

Suctioning indications include:

- audible, palpable or visible secretions (e.g. sputum, gastric or upper airway contents, or blood)
- coarse, reduced or absent breath sounds on auscultation
- reduced airflow
- increased spontaneous coughing
- rise in airway pressures
- suspected aspiration
- deterioration of peripheral oxygen saturations, increased respiratory rate, increased work of breathing
- increased heart rate and blood pressure
- restlessness/agitation or diaphoresis (Joanna Briggs Institute, 2022; Sivapuram, 2022b).

Periodically suctioning the upper airways removes oral and pooled secretions above the TT cuff, which reduces the risk of aspiration (Sivapuram, 2022b). People with a tracheostomy have altered upper airway function and increased oral care requirements.

Cuff inflation pressures

Cuff inflation techniques and cuff inflation pressure measurement are essential aspects of caring for a person with a cuffed TT. The cuff is an inflatable balloon surrounding the shaft near the tube's distal end. The cuff does not secure the tube in the trachea. Risks associated with cuff inflation pressures below 20 mmHg or above 25 mmHg include pharyngeal secretions or gastric content contaminating the airway and loss of tidal volume during mechanical ventilation. Risks associated with cuff inflation pressures above 25 mmHg include tracheal ischaemia leading to necrosis, tracheal stenosis, tracheo-oesophageal fistula and tracheomalacia (Edwards, 2022; Overall, 2022; Rose & Paulus, 2024).

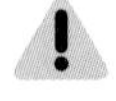
Safety

In Australia and New Zealand, cuff pressure measurement is the most frequently used method to monitor cuff inflation pressure and to ensure it remains between 20 and 25 mmHg (Overall, 2022; Rose & Paulus, 2019). Body position and head movement, tube position and airway pressures alter cuff inflation pressures. These are monitored once per shift and after TT manipulation (Overall, 2022).

Routine cuff deflation is unnecessary. It is indicated in order to evaluate cuff leakage, after cardiopulmonary arrest, and after surgery to re-evaluate cuff volume (Sivapuram, 2022b).

Other relevant issues

Altered body image is also an issue for people with a tracheostomy. The stoma is perceived as disfiguring and ugly. Fear and anxiety are common responses to the inability to speak or breathe. Ensure the person has their call bell within easy reach at all times.

It is important to assess nutritional and fluid status. The TT impairs swallowing, compromising the person's nutritional status. Ensure the person is adequately hydrated to facilitate the removal of respiratory secretions.

Assess the person

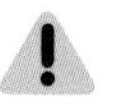
Safety

Prior to suctioning, consider the person's potential complications and contraindications.

LOOK at the person's colour, respiratory rate, depth and effort; for any accessory respiratory use; chest expansion – symmetrical or asymmetrical; and visible secretions in tube. Changes in vital signs.

LISTEN to the person's description of breathlessness, dyspnoea, anxiety, requests for suctioning or reports of pain; for air entry – good, fair or poor; any adventitious sounds; and airflow from tube.

FEEL for movement of expired air and cuff leakage.

Assess the person's respiratory status for ease of breathing, rate, rhythm and depth (see **Clinical Skill 19**).

Auscultate the lungs to assess bilateral breath sounds, which verifies tube placement. Assess for cuff leakage (e.g. an audible or auscultated respiratory leak over larynx, or the person's audible vocalisations).

Monitor the person's oxygen saturation before, during and after the procedure. Ensure their SpO_2 is 95 per cent or greater (Porritt, 2022b). Check that the pilot balloon (a tiny balloon near the inflation port of the cuff) is intact and inflated.

Assess the character and amount of the secretions at the stoma and any drainage on the tracheostomy dressing and ties. The stoma or incision is also assessed for tenderness, swelling and odour.

Assess the person's general condition (e.g. nutrition and hydration) and factors influencing tracheal care (e.g. infection and humidification), as well as their ability to learn and look after their tracheostomy.

Position the person

Depending on the person's condition, lay the person flat or in a semi-Fowler's position to make the tracheostomy site more accessible. A semi-Fowler's position facilitates oxygenation and ventilation; it also reduces stimulation of the gag reflex and the risk of aspiration.

Place a towel or absorbent pad on the person's chest to protect their clothing and bed linen.

PERFORM TRACHEOSTOMY CARE

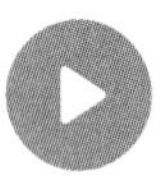
Video

Hand hygiene

Hand hygiene (see **Clinical Skill 5**) is a standard precaution to remove transient microorganisms from your hands, preventing cross-contamination. Put on PPE before you perform hand hygiene. Hand hygiene must occur on entering the person's bed area; prior to donning gloves to perform the tracheostomy care; on completion of tracheostomy following glove removal; and on leaving the person's bed area.

GATHER EQUIPMENT

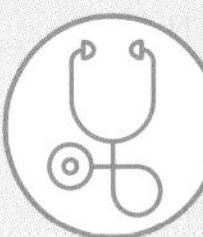

When caring for a person with a tracheostomy, check that the general and emergency equipment is available at the person's bedside and functioning (review the facility's policy for required emergency and general equipment). This facilitates prompt response and management of postoperative emergencies and complications, and must be readily accessible in case of emergency airway obstruction or accidental TT decannulation (Edwards, 2022).

Gather the following equipment to assist in efficient preparation:

Tracheostomy emergency equipment	Includes: • Spare tracheostomy tubes, one in the same size and one size smaller, both the same type as the one in place (with required introducer) • Tracheostomy dilator • Spare ties (cotton and Velcro) • Scissors (or chain cutters as applicable) • An oxygen source, a resuscitation bag and an appropriately sized mask • Functioning wall or portable suction • Appropriately sized suction catheters • A Yankauer suction catheter • 10 mL syringe (not required for cuffless tubes) • Water-based lubricant for tube changes (Edwards, 2022; Rose & Paulus, 2024; Sivapuram, 2022b)
A tracheostomy dressing or a basic dressing package	• If using a basic dressing pack, add a tracheostomy dressing, lint-free cotton-tip applicators, and a small brush or pipe cleaner for a TT with an inner cannula • Frayed edges are a potential infection source and shed lint may be inhaled (Edwards, 2022); if a commercial tracheostomy dressing is unavailable, fold lint-free gauze squares to the appropriate shape
0.9% normal saline (NS)	Used to clean the stoma
Cleaning solution	The inner cannula needs to be consistent with manufacturer's instructions (Joanna Briggs Institute, 2022); for example, Shiley™ TT – warm running water; Bivona® TT – mild liquid soap, tap water or boiled water
Sterile scissors	Used to cut the tracheostomy ties
Sterile gloves (two pairs) and clean gloves	• Sterile gloves are needed to protect the person and you from microorganisms • Non-sterile gloves are used while the ties are changed
Personal protective equipment (PPE)	Include a gown or apron, and face and eye protection if there is a risk of contact with blood or body fluids; for example, if the person has a good cough reflex or sneezes during the procedure
Tracheostomy ties (if not in the care kit)	Prepackaged twill tape or soft ribbon with Velcro fasteners
Tracheostomy suction supplies	See 'Gather equipment' in **Clinical Skill 62**
Heat moisture exchange device 'Swedish nose'	A filter/humidifier placed over the tracheostomy
Skin barrier film pad	Silicone foam (Mepilex) to provide primary skin protection
Dressing trolley	To place the items on to take to the person's bedside and to establish a critical aseptic field
Pulse oximeter	• Displays the pulse rate and the SpO_2 level (see **Clinical Skill 12**) • Is required to monitor oxygen saturation
Towels	To aid with positioning the person

Prepare the tracheostomy care kit

Use Aseptic Non Touch Technique (ANTT) to establish a critical aseptic field (see **Clinical Skill 7**). Place NS in one basin. Depending on the secretions around the stoma, open several sterile cotton-tip applicators. Open the tracheostomy dressing. Cut two 40 cm ties. Prepare the suctioning equipment. Put on gloves (according to the facility's guidelines).

Suction the tracheostomy tube

(See also **Clinical Skill 62**.) If the person is on oxygen, place the oxygen and humidification source near their stoma and ask them to breathe deeply. (See also **Clinical Skill 60**.)

Remove the inner cannula

After suctioning, remove the inner cannula if it is in situ. With gloved hands, hold the flange in one hand and the inner cannula in the other; gently twist (usually an anticlockwise turn) to unlock the inner cannula and gently remove it towards you in line with the TT.

Place the inner cannula in a kidney dish with the recommended cleaning solution.

Replace the inner cannula

Insert the spare inner cannula into the tracheostomy. Lock it into place by turning it clockwise.

Quinney and Dwyer (2021) recommend using two inner cannulae. When one is removed, it is replaced by the second immediately. The 'used' inner cannula is then cleaned as per the manufacturer's instructions and preserved for the next time the inner cannula is cleaned.

Remove the dressing

Gently loosen and remove the soiled dressing from around the stoma. Fold it into the palm of the glove, enfolding the dressing as the glove is removed. Discard the dressing, the glove and the tracheostomy suction tubing into the clinical waste bin.

Clean and dry the stoma

Gently clean the site using sterile cotton-tip applicators dipped in NS. Remove secretions from around and on the exposed outer cannula surfaces. Pass the swab beneath the TT flange. Dry it in the same manner. Avoid moving the TT (Edwards, 2022). Dry the peristomal skin using gauze squares. Observe the condition of the stoma and peristomal skin and report any abnormalities.

Redress the stoma site

Gently ease a segment of slit tracheostomy dressing under the flange on either side of the TT. Then remove the gloves and perform hand hygiene.

Change the tracheostomy ties

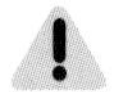
Safety

Perform hand hygiene/alcohol-based hand rub (ABHR) and use PPE, including non-sterile gloves and safety glasses. Before you begin the procedure, explain to the person what you are going to do.

Two nurses are required to change tracheostomy ties. The assistant holds the TT in position while the RN cuts the ties and removes and discards the soiled tapes (Edwards, 2022).

Do not change the ties during the initial 48 to 72 hours because of the risk of stoma closure if inadvertent decannulation occurs.

Even though cotton tape is inexpensive and readily available, it is easily soiled and traps moisture, causing skin irritation; Velcro ties are more commonly used. The procedures for changing both types of ties are discussed in the following sections.

Procedure for changing cotton ties

1. Prepare two equal lengths of tie long enough to go around the person's neck.
2. Lie the person down with their neck gently extended by a small rolled towel placed under their shoulders. Alternatively, the person may like to sit up in bed or in a chair.
3. Changing cotton ties is a two-person procedure. The first person holds the TT securely in place. The second person removes the existing cotton ties and then inserts a clean tie through the holes on either side of the flange.
4. Use double knots without any bows to tie both sides together. Well-secured tapes without any padding allow two fingers to slip between the tape and the person's neck. The ties should feel firm against your fingers to prevent accidental TT dislodgement. They should also be comfortable for the person, and not apply pressure on the jugular veins (Joanna Briggs Institute, 2022).
5. Remove and discard gloves and perform hand hygiene.
6. Replace the oxygen and humidification source.

Procedure for changing Velcro ties

1. Prior to each use, check the Velcro ties to ensure they are adherent; if not, discard and replace them.
2. Changing Velcro ties is a two-person procedure. The first person holds the TT securely in place. The second person:
   - removes the existing Velcro ties
   - inserts the clean Velcro ties through one side of the flange, passing the tie around the back of the person's neck and inserting the Velcro tie through the other side of the flange.
3. Adjust the ties so two fingers can slip between the tie and the person's neck. Observe the person's neck to ensure skin integrity.
4. Wash Velcro ties daily in warm, soapy water. Rinse and dry completely before reusing. Remove and discard gloves and perform hand hygiene.
5. Replace the oxygen and humidification source.

Check the cuff pressure

Check that the cuff pressure is between 20 and 25 mmHg using a cuff pressure manometer.

Provide oral hygiene

Providing oral hygiene for the person is both a hygiene and a comfort measure. See **Clinical Skill 56** for more on this procedure.

Post-procedure

Assist the person to a comfortable position, replacing the call bell and anything moved during the procedure so that it is within their reach.

Cleanse the inner cannula

Put on the second pair of sterile gloves. Gently but vigorously brush the inside and the outside of the cannula. Clean the inner cannula as per the manufacturer's instructions.

Run a gentle flow of tap water. Align the inner cannula to enable tap water to pour through the inner cannula for two to three minutes or until all secretions are removed. Mechanical force and friction remove dried secretions. Avoid hydrogen peroxide, Milton or hot water as these can shorten the inner cannula life.

Tap the inner cannula to remove excess NS and to prevent aspiration of the liquid. Dry the inner cannula with a hand towel. Visually check the inner cannula for remaining crusts and secretions and the outer cannula for excess secretions. If necessary, use a sterile suction tube to suction the cannula.

Store the dried inner cannula in a clean container ready for the next inner cannula change.

> Notify the RN or team leader if all secretions are unable to be cleaned from the inner cannula. Generally, the inner cannula is discarded if all secretions are unable to be removed. Indicator humification levels may need to be increased, or inner cannula may require an increase cleaning frequency.

CLEAN, REPLACE AND DISPOSE OF EQUIPMENT

All materials contaminated with tracheal secretions (e.g. gloves, gauze and cotton-tipped applicators) are to be discarded in the clinical waste bin. Bottles of NS can be reused within 24 hours if the time and date of opening are appropriately marked on the label. Solution is considered sterile for 24 hours after opening. At the next use, discard a few millilitres of solution to cleanse the bottle's lip before pouring it into a sterile basin.

DOCUMENTATION

The time, date and procedure are documented on the clinical notes. Document any secretions, including amount, colour, consistency and any odour noted. Record high or low cuff inflation pressure at each shift and inner cannula inspection and change on a tracheostomy care sheet. High or low cuff pressures must be reported to the shift coordinator. Also record the person's response to the procedure.

CLINICAL SKILLS ASSESSMENT

Tracheostomy care

Demonstrates the ability to effectively and safely care for a person with a tracheostomy tube in situ. Incorporates the *National Safety and Quality Health Service Standards*: 2 Partnering with Consumers, 3 Preventing and Controlling Healthcare-Associated Infection, 5 Comprehensive Care, 6 Communicating for Safety, and 8 Recognising and Responding to Acute Deterioration (Australian Commission on Safety and Quality in Health Care [ACSQHC], 2021).

Performance criteria	1	2	3	4	5
(Numbers indicate NMBA *Registered Nurse Standards for Practice*)	(Dependent)	(Marginal)	(Assisted)	(Supervised)	(Independent)
1. Identifies indication (1.1, 3.3, 3.4)	☐	☐	☐	☐	☐
2. Discusses the procedure with the person, e.g. gives the person a clear explanation of the need for the procedure, effects and procedural consequences (1.1, 1.2, 1.3, 1.5, 2.2, 2.3, 5.1, 6.1)	☐	☐	☐	☐	☐
3. Evidence of therapeutic interaction with the person, e.g. gives the person a clear explanation of the procedure (1.4, 1.5, 2.1, 2.2, 3.2)	☐	☐	☐	☐	☐
4. Demonstrates clinical reasoning, e.g. assesses and positions the person, assesses the person and appropriately repositions them (4.1, 4.2, 4.3, 6.1)	☐	☐	☐	☐	☐
5. Gathers equipment (1.1, 5.5, 6.1): ■ tracheostomy emergency equipment ■ tracheostomy dressing/basic dressing package ■ 0.9% normal saline ■ cleaning solution ■ sterile scissors ■ sterile gloves (two pairs) and clean gloves ■ personal protective equipment ■ tracheostomy ties and suction supplies ■ a 'Swedish nose' ■ skin barrier film pad ■ dressing trolley ■ pulse oximeter ■ towels	☐	☐	☐	☐	☐
6. Performs hand hygiene and dons gloves (1.1, 3.4, 6.1)	☐	☐	☐	☐	☐
7. Prepares equipment (1.1, 6.1)	☐	☐	☐	☐	☐
8. Suctions the tracheostomy tube (4.1, 4.2, 4.3, 6.1)	☐	☐	☐	☐	☐
9. Removes the old dressing (6.1)	☐	☐	☐	☐	☐
10. Cleanses the inner cannula and replaces it (6.1)	☐	☐	☐	☐	☐
11. Cleans and dries the stoma (6.1)	☐	☐	☐	☐	☐
12. Redresses the stoma site (6.1)	☐	☐	☐	☐	☐
13. Changes the tracheostomy ties (6.1)	☐	☐	☐	☐	☐
14. Measures the cuff inflation pressure (4.2, 6.1)	☐	☐	☐	☐	☐
15. Provides oral hygiene (6.1)	☐	☐	☐	☐	☐
16. Ensures that the person is comfortable post-procedure (2.3, 4.1, 4.2, 6.1)	☐	☐	☐	☐	☐
17. Cleans, replaces and disposes of equipment appropriately (3.6, 6.1)	☐	☐	☐	☐	☐
18. Documents relevant information (1.1, 1.4, 1.6, 2.2, 2.7, 3.5, 3.7, 6.1, 6.2, 6.5, 7.3)	☐	☐	☐	☐	☐
19. Demonstrates the ability to link theory to practice (1.1, 3.3, 3.4, 3.5)	☐	☐	☐	☐	☐

Student:

Clinical facilitator: Date:

CHAPTER 64

CHEST DRAINAGE SYSTEM ASSESSMENT AND MANAGEMENT

INDICATIONS

Chest or intrapleural drains are used to remove air, fluid, pus or blood collection from the pleural space into a collecting system to restore normal respiratory expansion and function (Wagner et al., 2019). The purpose of chest drainage systems is to maintain respiratory and haemodynamic stability by draining the pleural and mediastinal spaces of air (pneumothorax), blood (haemothorax), fluid (pleural effusion), or pus (empyaema) (Slade, 2023). Lungs collapse when the negative pressure in the pleural cavity is lost. If the lung is not reinflated and negative intrathoracic pressure restored within the pleural space, respiratory collapse and death will occur (Hawley, Gunn & Elliott, 2014). See TABLE 64.1 for an overview of clinical situations that may require chest drain insertion.

To avoid vital structures, chest drains are generally inserted under point-of-care ultrasound guidance or within the 'triangle of safety', the borders of which are midaxillary line (posterior limit), pectoral groove (anterior limit), and between the third and fifth intercostal space (McElnay & Lim, 2017).

Spontaneous pneumothoraxes and non-viscous effusions are drained with smaller-sized drains (8 to 18 Fr/Ch). These are better tolerated and are associated with less discomfort. However, traumatic pneumothoraxes, haemothoraxes and empyaemas need larger drains (24 to 32 Fr/Ch) (Slade, 2023).

After the chest tube is inserted, the tube should be connected to a pre-prepared chest drainage system and the position of the tube confirmed by X-ray.

TABLE 64.1 Causes of pneumothorax and haemothorax

EXTERNAL CAUSES	INTERNAL CAUSES
Thoracic surgery (e.g. open thoracic surgery)	Open communication between alveoli and pleural cavity (e.g. spontaneous pneumothorax or ruptured emphysematous bleb)
Penetrating chest trauma (e.g. knife or bullet)	Procedural rupture of visceral pleura (e.g. during lung tissue biopsy)
Unintentional catheter entry into intrapleural space during central line placement	Barotrauma (e.g. during mechanical ventilation positive end expiratory pressure)
Chest contusion	

SOURCES: SLADE, S. (2023). *CHEST DRAINS: INSERTION.* ADELAIDE, SA: JOANNA BRIGGS INSTITUTE EBP DATABASE, JBI@OVID. 2020; JBI1630; WAGNER, K. D., HARDIN-PIERCE, M. G., WELSH, D. & JOHNSON, K. (2019). *HIGH-ACUITY NURSING* (7TH ED.). UPPER SADDLE RIVER, NJ: PEARSON.

EVIDENCE OF THERAPEUTIC INTERACTION

Conditions affecting breathing and oxygenation produce anxiety because of the associated feelings of impending death. As a person's anxiety level increases, so does the body's need for oxygen, creating a vicious cycle. People with chest drains require reassurance and information about their condition and the chest drainage system, to help reduce anxiety.

Explain that nursing staff will be regularly assessing their status and the chest tube and drainage system, including the site, bubbling, drainage, swinging, and suction pressure (Slade, 2023). Ask them to report any shortness of breath or chest pain.

Remind them not to put the chest drainage system above their chest. Explain to the person that their chest drain is sutured in place, and that moving in bed or around the room should not cause it to be displaced. Remind them that although the tubing is flexible, they should not kink the tubing or lie on it, which obstructs the tube. Inform the person what to expect in regard to the amount of drainage. Most thoracic surgery produces sanguineous drainage in diminishing amounts for the initial 72 hours. The person should also be aware that fluctuation of the water level and intermittent bubbling is to be expected. Inform them of the importance of effective pain management and about the availability of prescribed analgesia and other pain management strategies.

DEMONSTRATE CLINICAL REASONING

There are a variety of systems available. The most common is a disposable, self-contained, three-chamber system that incorporates the collection or drainage chamber, the water-seal chamber and the suction chamber. These commercial systems have generally replaced the older three-bottle chest drainage systems. Chest drainage systems are closed to atmospheric pressure and are designed to allow air or fluid to be removed from the pleural cavity, while also preventing backflow of air or fluid into the pleural space. When the person exhales, the air or fluid in the intrapleural cavity is forced into and through the chest tube and tubing. Air bubbles out of the tubing and into the water-sealed chamber then up into the atmosphere. Fluid is collected in the drainage chamber.

A *dry chest drainage system* may be used in the facility. As the name implies, these do not require water in the suction chamber. Suction is regulated via a dial on the system or wall suction (Mbinji, 2022b). Consult the manufacturer's instruction to verify operation and checking of the system used at the facility.

A *flutter valve* (Heimlich valve or Pneumostat) is a small, one-way, portable valve system used to transport or for ambulant people (Deakin, 2019). Flutter valves allow air or fluid to drain and not to backflow into the pleural cavity. This valve is used for clinically stable people with a pneumothorax, in which case it is not connected to a drainage system. Alternatively, it can be attached to a closed drainage system to collect drainage from a small haemothorax (Deakin, 2019). Major advantages of the flutter valve for the person include its light weight, comfort, increased mobility, and reduced length of hospital stay (Deakin, 2019).

Safety considerations

Safety

All procedures associated with the chest drainage system (insertion, setting up or change) incorporate the principles of surgical Aseptic Non Touch Technique (ANTT): surgical hand scrub, gloves, gown, antiseptic preparation for the insertion site and adequate critical aseptic field. This avoids infection of the wound site or secondary empyaema (Slade, 2023).

Specific safety considerations when caring for a person with a chest drainage system include:

- Ensure the chest drainage unit and all tubing are below the person's chest level to facilitate drainage and never lift the chest drainage above the person's chest level. This prevents fluid flowing backwards into the pleural cavity.
- Tubing should have no kinks or obstructions inhibiting drainage.
- Ensure all connections between the chest tubes and the drainage unit are tight and secure.
- Tubing should be anchored to the person's skin to prevent drain pulling.
- Ensure the chest drainage unit is securely positioned on its stand or hanging on the bed.
- Ensure the water seal is maintained at 2 cm at all times (Mbinji, 2022b; Slade, 2023).
- Ensure that emergency bedside equipment is available (see 'Gather equipment').

Safety

If accidental drain disconnection occurs, options include immediate reconnection (connections are cleaned with alcohol and reconnected if uncontaminated); placing the tube in a 250 mL bottle of sterile saline or water, 2 to 4 cm below the surface; or leaving the tube open rather than clamping until another drainage system is prepared (Slade, 2023).

If the chest tube is accidentally removed, a sterile occlusive dressing is placed over the site and taped on three sides only to ensure that air can escape (Mbinji, 2022b). The team leader and medical staff must be notified immediately. Gather the equipment for intercostal catheter reinsertion and reconnection to the underwater seal drain (UWSD). Until another chest tube is inserted, administer oxygen, monitor the person's SpO_2 and assess for the development of a tension pneumothorax.

A tension pneumothorax is a medical emergency involving significant and progressive respiratory and haemodynamic compromise (Slade, 2023). If the lung is not reinflated, respiratory collapse and death will occur (Mbinji, 2022b). Clinical manifestations of a tension pneumothorax include hypotension, shock, distended neck veins, severe dyspnoea, tachypnoea, tachycardia, unilateral chest movement, absent breath sounds on the affected side, tracheal deviation to the unaffected side, and muffled heart sounds (Wagner et al., 2019).

Effective coughing and deep-breathing exercises

Effective coughing and deep-breathing exercises are difficult, if not impossible, to achieve if the person is experiencing pain. Inserting a chest drain causes tissue damage, activating nerve fibres surrounding the insertion site, and while the drain is in place the nerve fibres cannot heal. Chest tube-related pain is common and pain assessment needs to be conducted regularly with appropriate analgesia administered (Slade, 2023).

Inadequate pain control causes shallow respirations and may cause splinting. The person may also avoid coughing, resulting in atelectasis leading to chest infections. This requires a comprehensive pain management plan involving the person and the interdisciplinary team to manage all stages of the chest drainage process (insertion, management of the drain during drainage, and removal) (Slade, 2023). Appropriate pain management promotes the person's ability to mobilise and to participate in deep-breathing exercises and chest physiotherapy.

Assist the person into a semi-Fowler's position to aid removal of air, or a high Fowler's position to aid the removal of fluid. Change the person's position two-hourly to assist with comfort and to increase and change the intrapleural cavity area being drained.

GATHER EQUIPMENT

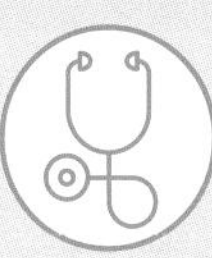

Gathering equipment is an organisational step that helps to create a positive environment for a successful interaction. It ensures that you have all needed material, boosts the person's confidence and trust in you, and increases your self-confidence. While gathering the equipment, you can mentally rehearse the procedure. Equipment includes the following items:

EQUIPMENT	EXPLANATION
Emergency bedside equipment	• A set of two padded clamps • A 250 mL bottle of sterile water or normal saline (NS) • Two suction outlets: one for the chest drain and one for airway management • A sterile occlusive dressing and tape (Slade, 2023) • Review the facility's guidelines for the bedside emergency equipment required
Sphygmomanometer, stethoscope, thermometer, pulse oximeter and watch with a second hand	Used for assessing vital signs and respiratory status

Assist the person to sit upright and splint their affected side or the sternum (if a mediastinal tube is in situ) with a folded towel or hand to decrease discomfort. An incentive spirometer is useful to assist the person in their deep-breathing exercises.

Coughing and deep respirations are necessary to force air and fluid out of the intrapleural cavity. These increase the rate at which the lungs re-expand and prevent respiratory complications associated with retained secretions. These exercises should be done hourly while the person is awake.

Encourage active or passive range of motion exercises on the arm of the affected side, as the person may limit their movement of that arm to reduce discomfort at the insertion site, resulting in joint discomfort and potential joint complications (Wagner et al., 2019). If the person is able, they should be encouraged to walk around. However, a chest drainage system requiring external suction restricts the person to the bedside (Mbinji, 2022b).

PERFORM AN ASSESSMENT OF A PERSON WITH A CHEST DRAINAGE SYSTEM

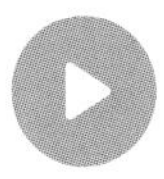
Video

Hand hygiene

Hand hygiene (see **Clinical Skill 5**) is an infection-control measure, removing transient microorganisms from your hands to prevent cross-contamination.

Assess the person and chest drain

At the beginning of your shift, assess the person and the chest drain and ensure all safety equipment is available and in working order. You will need to take a holistic approach when assessing a person with a chest drainage system, in addition to making specific assessment of the chest tube and drainage system. Clinical assessment takes into consideration the person's risk factors associated with chest drain insertion. Refer to the facility's guidelines regarding the frequency of ongoing assessments.

Assessing the person's status includes their respiratory status, chest movement and the quality of respirations and rate (see TABLE 64.2).

Clinical manifestations of extending haemothorax include diminished or absent breath sounds, dyspnoea and cyanosis.

Clinical manifestations of an extending pneumothorax include an increased area of absent breath sounds, hyper-resonance, subcutaneous emphysema and crepitus, tachycardia, increased respiratory distress, cyanosis, restlessness, sudden sharp focal chest pain and confusion.

Post-assessment

Assist the person to a comfortable position, replacing the call bell and anything that was moved during assessment so that it is within their reach. Perform hand hygiene.

CLEAN, REPLACE AND DISPOSE OF EQUIPMENT

Prompt replacement of equipment and leaving a clean and tidy workspace increases efficiency and demonstrates regard for fellow staff members.

DOCUMENTATION

Documenting care given to a person with a chest drain must include their vital signs, respiratory and oxygenation parameters, the appearance of the chest tube insertion site, excessive bleeding, the presence of subcutaneous emphysema, chest drainage anomalies such as excessive volume or change in drainage appearance, and the person's response to interventions. Many facilities provide specific documentation sheets for these assessments.

Document nursing interventions; for example, teaching, effectiveness of pain management, and effectiveness of coughing and deep-breathing exercises.

TABLE 64.2 Clinical assessment of a person with a chest drainage system

ASSESSEMENT	DESCRIPTION
Assessment of the person	• Vital signs (see **Clinical Skills 10 and 11**) • Respiratory status: breath sounds auscultation (see **Clinical Skill 19**), comparing the unaffected side with the affected side • Oxygenation status: assess the person's level of consciousness, pulse oximetry (see **Clinical Skill 12**), skin and mucous membrane colouring, respiratory effort and work of breathing • Pain assessment (see **Clinical Skill 13**)
Chest tube insertion site	• Occlusive dressing should be dry and intact; reinforce as necessary • Assess for fluid drainage, infection and subcutaneous air infiltration • If the dressing requires changing, assess the skin appearance at the tube insertion (ensure the chest drain is positioned well – not kinked and no tube eyelets visible) and suture (intact) sites • Assess the site for excessive bleeding • Palpate around the dressing site for subcutaneous emphysema – if the affected area is enlarging, mark the edge with a pen to evaluate the rate and extent of spread
Chest drainage system	Extension tubing: • To avoid unintentional disconnection, assess all tubing connections are secured (in a spiral wrapping method or goal post method; two strips of tape placed longitudinally down all connections and covered at either end with more tape, allowing connections to be visualised) • To avoid decreased drainage from dependent looping, loop extension tubing horizontally on the bed • A rolled towel under the person when side-lying (on side of chest drain) keeps weight off the tubing Drainage chamber: • Assess and document blood/fluid drainage volume in the drainage chamber • Mark the volume on the outside of the drainage chamber, with time and date of marking • Hourly document amount of fluid in the drainage chamber on the Fluid Balance Chart • Calculate and document total hourly output if there are multiple drains • Calculate and document cumulative total output • Assess appearance (e.g. sanguineous, serosanguineous, serous, purulent) • Drainage should not be frankly bloody for more than a few hours • Be alert for potential haemorrhage – reversal of drainage appearance (serous to serosanguineous to sanguineous) • Be aware of the expected volume of bleeding in the first 24 hours following surgery and report drainage above the anticipated volume • Excessive drainage more than 100 mL per hour needs to be reported to your team leader and the surgeon. The initial 24 hours can see up to 1000 mL of serosanguineous fluid • Report any sudden decrease or absence of drainage associated with respiratory distress • Blocked drains are a major concern following cardiac surgical procedures due to the risk of cardiac tamponade. Notify your team leader and the medical staff if a drain with ongoing loss suddenly stops draining • If clots are present – only milk or strip a tube if the obstruction is restricting drainage and then only the portion that is blocked. Milking chest drains in some facilities is only to be done with written orders from medical staff. Milking drains creates a high negative pressure that causes pain, tissue trauma and bleeding (Slade, 2023) Water-sealed chamber: • Check that the chamber is below chest level • Ensure the system is upright and the end of the tubing is below the waterline • Check the water level is at the appropriate level for the system – refill as necessary • Observe fluid level fluctuation – water should rise with inspiration and fall with expiration (oscillation or swing); this will diminish as pneumothorax resolves. Fluctuation stops when the lung is re-expanded, if tubing is obstructed or if there are loose connections. If the fluctuation stops and the lung is not re-expanded, check the tubing for air leaks or obstruction. There is no swing in the water-sealed chamber in mediastinal drains, which are inserted following some types of cardiac surgery • Observe for bubbling – should be intermittent if the person has a pneumothorax. Constant bubbling indicates a large air leak between the person and drain. Assess the person's condition and check the drain for disconnection, dislodgement or loose connection. Notify your team leader and medical staff immediately if the problem cannot be resolved. Some systems continually bubble when attached to a suction unit. Turn off the suction unit briefly to determine if there is bubbling
	Suction chamber: • Suction is not always required and may lead to tissue trauma and prolongation of an air leak in some people (Slade, 2023). If suction is required, medical staff must provide written orders. Some clinical areas may use an orange 'Chest Drain Orders' sticker, which is placed in the person's progress notes. When suction is used within the system, check that settings remain as ordered • Monitor the water level in the chamber to ensure it is at 20 cm H_2O or other prescribed level – refill as necessary • If external suction is used, check that the chamber bubbling is a gentle bubbling action – decrease external suction as necessary • High-volume, high-pressure suction units should be avoided, as these may lead to air stealing and hypoxaemia, perpetuation of persistent air leaks, and damage to lung tissue becoming trapped in the catheter (Slade, 2023)

CLINICAL SKILLS ASSESSMENT

Chest drainage system assessment and management

Demonstrates the ability to effectively and safely assess a person who has a chest drainage system. Incorporates the *National Safety and Quality Health Service Standards*: 2 Partnering with Consumers, 3 Preventing and Controlling Healthcare-Associated Infection, 5 Comprehensive Care, 6 Communicating for Safety, and 8 Recognising and Responding to Acute Deterioration (Australian Commission on Safety and Quality in Health Care [ACSQHC], 2021).

Performance criteria	1	2	3	4	5
(Numbers indicate NMBA *Registered Nurse Standards for Practice*)	**(Dependent)**	**(Marginal)**	**(Assisted)**	**(Supervised)**	**(Independent)**
1. Identifies indication (1.1, 3.3, 3.4)	☐	☐	☐	☐	☐
2. Discusses the assessment and special considerations (1.1, 1.2, 1.3, 1.5, 2.2, 2.3, 4.1, 4.2, 4.3, 5.1, 6.1, 6.5)	☐	☐	☐	☐	☐
3. Evidence of therapeutic interaction with the person, e.g. provides a clear explanation of the assessment, reassures the person (1.4, 1.5, 2.1, 2.2, 3.2)	☐	☐	☐	☐	☐
4. Demonstrates clinical reasoning, e.g. takes into consideration safety considerations, effective coughing and deep-breathing exercises (1.4, 1.5, 2.1, 2.2)	☐	☐	☐	☐	☐
5. Teaches and encourages coughing and deep-breathing exercises (3.2, 6.1)	☐	☐	☐	☐	☐
6. Gathers equipment (1.1, 5.5, 6.1): ■ emergency bedside equipment ■ sphygmomanometer ■ stethoscope ■ thermometer ■ pulse oximeter ■ watch with a second hand	☐	☐	☐	☐	☐
7. Performs hand hygiene (1.1, 3.4, 6.1)	☐	☐	☐	☐	☐
8. Assesses the person's respiratory and oxygenation status, vital signs and pain level as per the health facility's guidelines (1.4, 4.1, 4.2, 6.1)	☐	☐	☐	☐	☐
9. Assesses the chest drainage system as per the facility's guidelines (1.4, 4.1, 4.2, 6.1)	☐	☐	☐	☐	☐
10. Assists the person to reposition, replaces the call bell and anything moved during the procedure so that it is within the person's reach (2.3, 4.1, 4.2, 4.3, 6.1)	☐	☐	☐	☐	☐
11. Cleans, replaces and disposes of equipment appropriately (3.6, 6.1)	☐	☐	☐	☐	☐
12. Documents relevant information (1.1, 1.4, 1.6, 2.2, 2.7, 3.5, 3.7, 6.1, 6.2, 6.5, 7.3)	☐	☐	☐	☐	☐
13. Demonstrates the ability to link theory to practice (1.1, 3.3, 3.4, 3.5)	☐	☐	☐	☐	☐

Student:

Clinical facilitator: Date:

PART 11

REFERENCES

Aginga, C. (2021). *Skin assessment: Ethnic diversity* [Evidence summary]. Adelaide, SA: Joanna Briggs Institute.

Ahmed, E-I. & Eid, R. (2022). *Oropharyngeal suctioning: Safe and effective practice.* [Evidence summary]. Adelaide, SA: Joanna Briggs Institute.

Australian Commission on Safety and Quality in Health Care (ACSQHC) (2021). *National safety and quality health service standards* (3rd ed.). Sydney, NSW: ACSQHC.

Deakin, L. (2019). *Heimlich valves: Clinician information.* [Evidence summary]. Adelaide, SA: Joanna Briggs Institute.

Dougherty, L., Lister, S. & West-Oram, A. (eds) (2015). *The Royal Marsden manual of clinical nursing procedures* (9th ed.). Oxford, UK: Wiley-Blackwell.

Eastwood, G. M., O'Connell, B., Considine, J. & Greenslade, L. (2015). Oxygen therapy in clinical practice: Management or mismanagement. *Australian Critical Care, 28*(1), 41.

Edwards, D. (2022). *Tracheostomy: Dressing* [Evidence summary]. Adelaide, SA: Joanna Briggs Institute EBP Database, JBI@Ovid.

Fong, E. (2021a). *Chemotherapy: Adverse effects (pulmonary)* [Evidence summary]. Adelaide, SA: Joanna Briggs Institute.

Fong, E. (2021b). *Oxygen therapy: Hospital setting.* [Evidence summary]. Adelaide, SA: Joanna Briggs Institute.

Hawley, D., Gunn, S. & Elliott, R. (2014). *The clinical effectiveness of suction versus water seal for optimal management of pleural chest tubes in adult patients: A systematic review.* Adelaide, SA: Joanna Briggs Institute.

Joanna Briggs Institute (2020). *Long term oxygen therapy (LTOT)* [Recommended practice]. Joanna Briggs Institute EBP Database, JBI@Ovid. 2020; JBI6718.

Joanna Briggs Institute (2022). *Tracheostomy: Cleaning inner cannula* [Recommended practice]. Adelaide, SA: Joanna Briggs Institute.

Kydonaki, K. & Parke, R. (2024). Respiratory assessment and monitoring. In L. Aitken, A. Marshall & T. Buckley (eds), *ACCCN's critical care nursing* (5th ed.), pp. 439–76. Chatswood, NSW: Mosby.

Lister, S., Hofland, J. & Grafton, H. (eds) (2020). *The Royal Marsden manual of clinical nursing procedures* (10th ed.). Oxford, UK: Wiley-Blackwell.

Marieb, E. N. & Hoehn, K. (2019). *Human anatomy and physiology* (11th ed.). Glenview, IL: Pearson.

Mathew, S. (2022). *Mini-tracheostomy: Effectiveness.* [Evidence summary]. Adelaide, SA: Joanna Briggs Institute.

Mbinji, M. (2022a). *Artificial airway: Subglottic suctioning.* [Evidence summary]. Adelaide, SA: Joanna Briggs Institute.

Mbinji, M. (2022b). *Chest drains: Maintenance.* [Evidence summary]. Adelaide, SA: Joanna Briggs Institute.

McElnay, P. & Lim, E. (2017). Modern techniques to insert chest drains. *Thoracic Surgery Clinics, 27*(1), 29–34. https://doi.org/10.1016/j.thorsurg.2016.08.005

National Health and Medical Research Council (NHMRC) (2019). *Australian guidelines for the prevention and control of infection in healthcare.* Commonwealth of Australia. https://www.nhmrc.gov.au

Overall, B. (2022). *Tracheostomy (adult and pediatric): Cuff management* [Evidence summary]. Adelaide, SA: Joanna Briggs Institute.

Overall, B. (2023). *Tracheostomy: Stoma care.* [Evidence summary]. Adelaide, SA: Joanna Briggs Institute.

Porritt, K. (2022a). *Endotracheal suctioning (adult, pediatric and neonatal): Frequency and duration* [Evidence summary]. Adelaide, SA: Joanna Briggs Institute.

Porritt, K. (2022b). *Suctioning (endotracheal or tracheostomy): Installation of normal saline.* Adelaide, SA: Joanna Briggs Institute.

Quinney, L. & Dwyer, T. (2021). Oxygenation. In B. Kozier, G. L. Erb, A. Berman, S. Snyder, T. Levett-Jones, T. Dwyer, M. Hales, N. Harvey, L. Moxham, T. Park, B. Parker, K. Reid-Searl & D. Stanley, *Kozier & Erb's fundamentals of nursing* (3rd Australian ed.), vol. 3, pp. 1516–61. Frenchs Forest, NSW: Pearson.

Rose, L. & Paulus, F. (2024). Ventilation and oxygen management. In L. Aitken, A. Marshall & T. Buckley (eds), *ACCCN's critical care nursing* (5th ed.), pp. 521–66. Chatswood, NSW: Mosby.

Sivapuram, M. S. (2022a). *Acute medical patients: Oxygen therapy.* [Evidence summary]. Adelaide, SA: Joanna Briggs Institute.

Sivapuram, M. S. (2022b). *Tracheostomy: Management of patients.* [Evidence summary]. Adelaide, SA: Joanna Briggs Institute.

Slade, S. (2023). *Chest drains: Insertion.* [Evidence summary]. Adelaide, SA: Joanna Briggs Institute.

Swe, K. K. (2021). *Acute myocardial infarction: Oxygen inhalation.* [Evidence summary]. Adelaide, SA: Joanna Briggs Institute.

Therapeutic Goods Administration (2017). *Poisons Standard 2017.* Australian Government Department of Health. https://www.legislation.gov.au/Details/F2017L01285

Wagner, K. D., Hardin-Pierce, M. G., Welsh, D. & Johnson, K. (2019). *High-acuity nursing* (7th ed.). Upper Saddle River, NJ: Pearson.

PART 12

TRANSFUSION AND BLOOD PRODUCTS

65 BLOOD TRANSFUSION

66 VENIPUNCTURE

Note: These notes are summaries of the most important points in the assessments/procedures and are not exhaustive on the subject. References of the materials used to compile the information have been supplied. The student is expected to have learnt the material surrounding each skill as presented in the references. No single reference is complete on each subject.

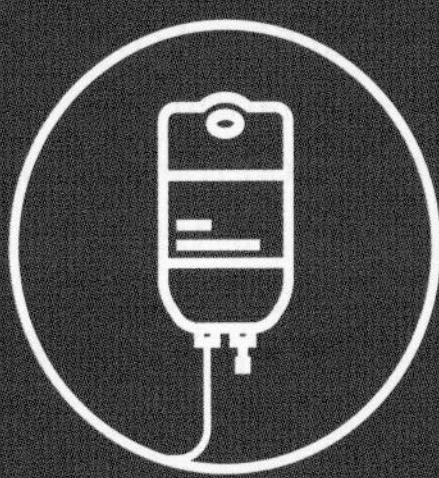

CHAPTER 65

BLOOD TRANSFUSION

INDICATIONS

Blood components (e.g. red blood cells, platelets, plasma and globulins) have complex functions, and administering them replaces fluids and restores other body functions (e.g. clotting, oxygen carrying capacity). Significant loss of whole blood or loss of one or more of the components has far-reaching consequences (e.g. reduced tissue oxygenation, clotting difficulties, immunological deficits). Therefore, the indications for blood product transfusion include:

- blood loss (e.g. from trauma, surgery, haemorrhage)
- severe anaemia
- replacement of fluid and protein
- restoration of oncotic pressure
- replacement of essential clotting factors.

Verify the blood product order

The physician orders the type of blood product and the amount to be infused. This is a legal prescription. The person's written consent is required for the transfusion and must be verified prior to initiating the transfusion.

Blood grouping and blood cross-matching

The recipient's blood is grouped and cross-matched with the donor blood before starting the transfusion. Because blood is living tissue, a blood transfusion is actually transplantation. There is a possibility of fatal transfusion/transplant reactions, and that is why rigorous procedures for identifying the person and the blood product are carried out as preventative measures.

Blood is obtained from volunteers in Australia and New Zealand. Blood can be collected as whole blood or in a process of apheresis, where blood is drawn from a volunteer, immediately separated into platelets or plasma (whichever is required) and the remainder of the blood plus some normal saline are returned to the volunteer (Australian Red Cross Lifeblood [ARCL], 2022).

Human blood is grouped into four classifications based on immune reactivity: A, B, O and AB. It is tested twice for groupings and the rhesus (Rh) factor (either positive or negative) is also determined. Eighty-five per cent of the population has Rh antibodies on the surface of the red blood cells (RBCs), which indicates the blood is Rh positive. Generally speaking, the blood of any one group is incompatible with the blood of another group. Mismatched blood, either in grouping or in Rh factor, causes haemolytic reactions. In emergency situations, however, type O negative RBCs (but not plasma) can be used for people with other types of blood. O negative RBCs have no surface antigens and are negative to the Rh factor and react minimally with the other blood types and Rh-positive antibodies.

As well as compatibility testing, blood in Australia and New Zealand is tested for various viral infections, including hepatitis and human immunodeficiency viruses (HIV). The ARC provides blood that is among the safest in the world (ARCL, 2022). Some people prefer to use autologous blood transfusions where their own blood is collected some time previous to the planned surgery and given back to them during/after surgery as needed.

NB: This is a brief summary of the available information on blood transfusion. Please read more widely in your medical surgical text or on the numerous online resources, such as:

- Australian Red Cross Lifeblood: https://www.lifeblood.com.au/health-professionals/testing/donation
- Blood transfusion administration and checklist: https://transfusion.com.au/transfusion_practice/administration
- NZ Blood: https://www.nzblood.co.nz/about-blood.

Some interesting facts about blood components and blood transfusions are available online at the BloodSafe website: http://www.bloodsafelearning.org.au.

EVIDENCE OF THERAPEUTIC INTERACTION

Explain the entire procedure to the person and reiterate its benefits to gain their cooperation. Alert the person to report back pain, fever and chills, itching or alterations in respiratory status, as these indicate a reaction to the blood. Ask them to report any alterations (sensations, feelings) felt during the transfusion. Prompt reporting of symptoms will lead to the earliest possible treatment and minimisation of harm.

DEMONSTRATE CLINICAL REASONING

Blood products

Blood products include: whole blood, packed red cells, plasma, platelets, serum albumin and cryoprecipitate. Only the components of blood are used. Whole blood is no longer available from the Australian Red Cross Blood Service or the New Zealand Blood Service (NZBS). It is now used to obtain its components (red blood cells, plasma, platelets, clotting factors) and other fractions of blood. The use of blood component transfusion for many people is questionable. The Patient Blood Management protocol has reduced the number of blood component transfusions undertaken in hospitals. This protocol includes treatment of anaemia (e.g. prior to surgery, for iron deficient anaemia), minimising blood loss and bleeding during surgeries, optimisation of coagulation, and employing true person-centred decision making (Ozawa et al., 2023).

Packed red cells

Packed red cells (RBC) are created by removing the plasma from whole blood. They are used for anyone requiring increased oxygen-carrying capacity without excess fluid (e.g. following surgery with blood loss, anaemia). RBCs are leucodepleted (the white cell components are removed) as the white cells serve no purpose and can contribute to adverse reactions (Australian and New Zealand Society of Blood Transfusion [ANZSBT] & Australian College of Nursing [ACN], 2020). They can be safely stored at an optimum temperature (–2 to –60 °C) for up to 42 days (ARCL, 2021d). They are generally infused at a rate of one unit over 60 to 180 minutes, but must be infused within four hours after removal from the controlled temperature refrigerator.

Plasma

Plasma is the liquid portion of blood. It is used to restore lost fluid and protein in the intravascular compartment. Plasma, taken from fresh whole blood, is usually frozen to preserve the clotting factors. However, rewarming (even using a blood warmer) can degrade protein and the clotting factors, so frozen plasma is used quickly after thawing to maintain its coagulation and other plasma effects (Heger, Pock & Romisch, 2017). It is usually infused over 30 minutes per unit. Plasma does not need to be typed and cross-matched as it contains no RBCs, but it should be of the same blood type as it may contain anti-A or anti-B antibodies (NZBS, 2016).

Platelets

Platelets are separated out of the plasma and used to assist people with clotting abnormalities and tissue repair (National Blood Authority Australia, n.d.). They are leucodepleted and irradiated to inactivate lymphocytes, which left, could precipitate a nearly always fatal graft versus host disease. Since the plastics used in the container bag affect platelets by causing them to clump, the container is to be gently rocked during administration to prevent this. Platelets are administered over 15 to 30 minutes per pack (ANZSBT & ACN, 2020); in New Zealand, it is 30 to 60 minutes per standard equivalent dose (NZBS, 2016). Platelets must not be transfused through a blood administration set that has been used for red cells, as red cell debris in the inline filter may trap infusing platelets.

Serum albumin

Serum albumin is a large-molecule blood protein used to increase oncotic pressure in the intravascular space, causing fluid shift from the interstitial to the intravascular space. This assists in correcting hypovolaemia. Few incompatibilities have been noted; therefore, infusion compatibility testing is not usually required. Follow facility protocols for infusion rates.

Cryoprecipitate

Cryoprecipitate is a solution precipitated from plasma containing Factor VIII, and other clotting factors haemophiliacs are missing. It is available in all blood types. Small amounts (10 to 15 mL) are usually administered over 30 to 60 minutes.

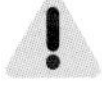
Safety

Infusion times are dependent on the recipient (e.g. a child, someone with heart or renal failure would have a slower rate to prevent fluid overload) and the situation (e.g. someone with acute bleeding or hypovolaemic shock would be transfused rapidly, or with a major haemorrhage, as fast as the person and the intravenous [IV] access could tolerate).

Caution

Safety

Medication is not administered with the blood transfusion (ANZSBT & ACN, 2020). IV fluids other than normal saline (NS) are not used with blood components (with rare exceptions [e.g. ABO-compatible plasma, 4% albumin or other suitable plasma expanders] – as ordered by the physician (ARCL, 2020b).

ELDER CARE

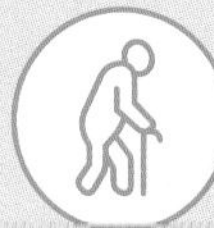

Sharp et al. (2021) demonstrated the safety of home-based blood administration and found it reduced the burden and cost of hospital administration for both the person and the healthcare system. The practice of visiting registered nurses (RNs) administering blood in homes or residential facilities will increase because the incidence of developing haematological disorders (e.g. anaemia, haematological malignancies) increases with age. The risk of adverse reactions to transfused blood components is unaffected by age or gender (Sharp et al., 2021).

THE PERSON LIVING WITH SEVERE OBESITY

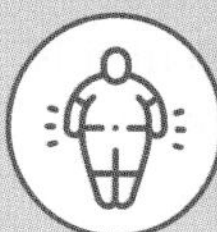

Venipuncture attempts may be difficult due to the extra tissue, and the severely obese person may need to have a peripherally inserted central catheter line inserted (which can remain in situ for several weeks) for the duration of their need for intravenous access. (See **Clinical Skills 15 and 23** for a brief explanation of issues for people living with severe obesity.)

GATHER EQUIPMENT

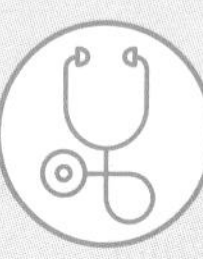

Gathering equipment is an organisational step that helps to create a positive environment for a successful interaction. While gathering the equipment, you can mentally rehearse the procedure. Equipment may include the following items:

EQUIPMENT	EXPLANATION
Blood order sheet	• Part of the identification of the person • To verify the order • Taken by an RN to the blood bank refrigerator to cross-check with the blood product being retrieved
Consent form	• Check that the person has signed it • The doctor will have explained the reason for the blood component, what to expect, any common adverse reactions plus any rare but serious reactions, and any alternative to the transfusion
Equipment to initiate an IV of NS	This equipment is assembled if an IV infusion is not established (see **Clinical Skill 31**)
Blood transfusion-giving set	• A blood transfusion-giving set with a 170 to 200 micron filter (ARCBS, 2016) is needed • A straight set that is similar to a normal IV giving set but has a filter • A double spike set with a filter (one spike for the blood bag, one for a NS bag) is often used so that the NS infusion is not discontinued during blood infusion and is available to keep vein open (KVO) between units (ANZSBT & ACN, 2020) • Some giving sets have 15 drops per mL drip rate (to accommodate the viscosity of RBCs), so take care when calculating the drip rate
Infusion pump	Must be compatible with blood and with drops per mL to ensure the ordered rate of administration
Blood warmer	• To warm the refrigerated blood components if large quantities of blood are required • Cold blood contributes to hypothermia (Lotterman & Sharma, 2023)
Clean gloves	For your protection

ADMINISTER A BLOOD TRANSFUSION

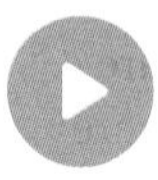

Video

An IV infusion of NS is required to begin a transfusion. An assessment of the person and verification of their identity and consent are also completed prior to administering blood.

Hand hygiene

Hand hygiene (see **Clinical Skill 5**) is essential since intravenous access is an invasive procedure. Hand hygiene removes transient microorganisms from your hands, preventing cross-contamination.

Establish an intravenous infusion with normal saline

A specially trained RN or medical staff member establishes IV access (see **Clinical Skill 31**). NS is the only IV solution used during a blood transfusion. It is isotonic and therefore does not cause RBC lysis or clumping (ANZSBT & ACN, 2020). An 18 to 20 gauge cannula or needle is used to establish the IV so that no damage occurs to blood cells from being forced to flow through small-bore devices. The tubing and the blood filter are primed with NS. If a pump is used for the infusion, it must be one that does not damage the RBCs.

Assessment

Baseline assessment

Establish a baseline (15 minutes before the transfusion) prior to starting so that any changes during or after the transfusion can be monitored.

LOOK – take the person's blood pressure, temperature, pulse, respiratory rate, oxygen saturation and document. A temperature of 38.8 °C or greater must be reported to the physician before starting the transfusion. Observe for pre-existing rashes. Assess the IV site. Other baseline data relating to the person's pathology is then noted (e.g. haemoglobin, haematocrit). Confirm the person's written consent for the transfusion.

LISTEN to breath sounds and to their comments when you ask the person about known allergies or any reactions to previous blood products.

Ask the person to empty their bladder. In case of a reaction, a urine sample produced during the transfusion will be required. Transfusion reactions can cause kidney dysfunction and haemoglobinuria.

Verification

Safety

The blood product must be initiated within 30 minutes of arrival on the ward (ANZSBT & ACN, 2020); if not, it must be returned to the blood bank or a blood-specific refrigerator for storage at the optimum temperature. This minimises the risk of bacterial contamination and lysis of RBCs. Blood components are removed from storage and administered one unit at a time.

An RN brings the blood product to the ward and, with a second RN (i.e. two licensed healthcare professionals), checks the person's identification, the blood order sheet and the information on the blood product to ensure they are all the same. The person's consent to the transfusion is rechecked. Do *not* spike the blood/component unit until verification is complete.

The minimum verification is:

- the person's name (ask them to state and spell their name) and date of birth
- their identification/medical record number (check against the armband)
- their blood group and Rh type and those of the blood unit
- the original prescription (i.e. the type of blood component/number of units)
- the expiration date and time of the unit of blood
- the unit of blood's ID number (there will be a removable duplicate sticker or bar code for eMedical record to use in documentation).

The policies of some facilities may be broader. If there are any discrepancies, the blood is not administered.

Administer the transfusion

Initiate the blood transfusion

The blood product is administered by one of the RNs who identified the blood and the person. Assess patency of the IV cannula.

1. Check that the pack has not been compromised, there are no clots, discolouration or turbidity (ARCBS, 2016).
2. Gently invert the blood bag several times to ensure the components are mixed.
3. Perform hand hygiene. Put on gloves.

Use the following steps when you are required to complete this procedure using a double-input blood transfusion set:

1. Close the three clamps (on both input-port [short] tubing and on the recipient end [long] tubing of the blood-giving set).
2. Expose the port of the saline bag, remove the cap from the spike, spike the port and hang it. Expose the port of the blood bag, remove the cap from the spike and spike the port with the other arm of the blood-giving set. (Check the manufacturer's direction, some blood-giving sets have designated saline arms [with a one-way valve, to prevent backflow of blood into the NS bag] and blood arms). Hang the blood.
3. Unclamp the saline arm and fill the filter to prevent air from entering the system and promote a smooth flow of blood. Prime the remainder of the tubing (to the person) of the blood-giving set with the saline (so you can see and eliminate any air in the tubing). Clamp then attach the saline-filled line to the existing cannula. Unclamp the saline-filled line to establish patency of the line and the flow (at a KVO rate).
4. Clamp the saline arm (above the filter) so blood is not drawn into the saline bag. Unclamp the blood arm tubing and let gravity pull blood into the filter. Blood is usually infused by itself (i.e. the NS is off during the transfusion).
5. If large volumes of blood are to be infused, a blood-warming device may be used to prevent hypothermia.

Use the following steps when you are required to complete this procedure using a single-input blood transfusion set (used when no extra fluid is needed, less expensive):

1. Close the clamp on both the short input port tubing and the long recipient tubing.
2. Expose the port of the blood bag, remove the cap from the spike and spike the port. Hang the blood.
3. Unclamp the input port tubing and fill the filter to prevent air from entering the system and promote a smooth flow of blood. You may need to squeeze the filter very gently to start the blood flow.
4. Prime the remainder of the tubing (to the person) with the blood (eliminate any air in the tubing). Clamp.

5. Attach the blood-filled line to the cannula, unclamp and set the rate.
6. If large volumes of blood are to be infused, a blood-warming device may be used to prevent hypothermia.

However, this method does not allow for an NS flush to empty the line of blood when the bag is empty. With this method, an NS bag and giving set at the bedside are advised in case of a reaction to KVO for any emergent medication administration.

Begin the blood infusion slowly

Safety

Transfusion reactions often occur within the first 15 minutes of initiation of the blood transfusion. Begin the infusion slowly at a rate of 2 mL/minute for the first 15 minutes (Lotterman & Sharma, 2023) to reduce the amount of donor RBCs in the system. Less stimulus to react against reduces the severity of any reaction. After the initial slow start, set the flow to the rate ordered. Remain with the person for the initial 15- to 30-minute period to observe for possible reactions. Blood components are given within different timeframes for each, as noted above. The RBCs may be given faster in someone with acute or massive bleeding. Rapid transfusion increases the risk of a reaction and circulatory overload. A transfusion time of longer than four hours increases bacterial growth and subsequent septic reaction.

Monitor the person

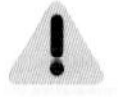

Safety

During the transfusion, take vital signs (temperature, pulse and respiration rate, blood pressure, O_2 saturation and listen to breath sounds) 15 minutes after initiation, and stay with the person for at least the first 30 minutes of the transfusion (ARCL, 2020b).

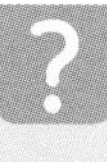

If a second (or more) pack of blood is required, the person is closely monitored (q15min) for the first 30 minutes of each pack.

The vital signs are taken frequently (every 30 to 60 minutes) throughout and following the transfusion, depending on hospital policy. Many complications can occur during or following a blood transfusion. Serious and life-threatening reactions can occur unpredictably and progress rapidly (see TABLE 65.1). Close observation throughout the transfusion is mandatory.

TABLE 65.1 Transfusion reactions

MILD TRANSFUSION REACTIONS			
Transfusion reaction	**Cause**	**Signs/symptoms**	**Nursing care**
Mild febrile reaction	Immune response to white cell fragment/antigens	• Mild fever <1.5 °C over baseline • Headache • Tachycardia • Normotensive	• *Standard transfusion reaction care (see below) • Give antipyretics as ordered • Reassure • Cautiously restart the transfusion (as ordered)
Mild allergic (urticarial) reaction	Immune response to plasma proteins in donor blood	• Urticaria over <2/3 of the body • Pruritus • Headache • Normotensive	• *Standard transfusion reaction care • Give antihistamines as ordered • Reassure • Cautiously restart the transfusion (as ordered)
MODERATE TO SEVERE TO LIFE-THREATENING TRANSFUSION REACTIONS			
Transfusion reaction	**Cause**	**Signs/symptoms**	**Nursing care**
Acute haemolytic reaction (occurs within first few minutes or as little as 10 mL of infused blood)	ABO incompatibility (most often due to checking error in the lab or at the bedside)	• Fever (>39 °C) chills/rigor • Haemoglobinuria • Tachycardia • Constricting chest or lumbar pain • Hypotension • Uncontrollable bleeding • Heat along infusing vein • Hyperbilirubinaemia	• *Standard transfusion reaction care • Keep the vein open (do not flush the blood tubing – use a new NS bag and giving set so no more blood is infused) • Collect a urine sample for testing • Supportive care as needed (antipyretics, O_2, may need transfer to ICU) • Notify blood bank • Return remaining blood and tubing to the blood bank in a sealed and labelled biohazard bag
Severe allergic/ anaphylactic reaction (occurs within seconds to minutes of start of transfusion)	Severe immune response to plasma proteins in the donor blood	• Dyspnoea, bronchospasm, wheezing, angio-oedema • Hypotension • Tachycardia • Flushing, facial oedema • Anxiety • Nausea and vomiting • Widespread rash	• *Standard transfusion reaction care • Keep the vein open (as above) • Supportive care as needed (antihistamines, adrenaline, corticosteroids as ordered, O_2, elevate head of bed, may need transfer to intensive care unit [ICU]) • Notify blood bank • Return remaining blood and tubing to the blood bank (as above)

MODERATE TO SEVERE TO LIFE-THREATENING TRANSFUSION REACTIONS			
Transfusion reaction	**Cause**	**Signs/symptoms**	**Nursing care**
Bacterial contamination (starts within 24 hours of initiation of a transfusion) Septic shock	Bacterial contamination of the blood component (rare – plasma most affected, as it is kept at 22 °C)	• High fever • Chills/rigors • Vomiting • Abdominal cramps • Diarrhoea • (Symptoms dependent on contaminant)	• *Standard transfusion reaction care • Keep the vein open (as above) • Supportive care as needed (antipyretics, O_2, may need transfer to ICU) • Notify blood bank • Return remaining blood and tubing to the blood bank (as above)
Transfusion associated cardiac overload (occurs within six hours of start of blood transfusion)	Frailty, very young or old, medical problems – cardiac or renal	• Dyspnoea • Tachycardia • Hypertension • Decreased O_2 saturation • Cough	• *Standard transfusion reaction care • Keep the vein open (as above) • Supportive care as needed (diuretics, O_2, may need transfer to ICU)
Transfusion-associated acute lung injury (occurs from two to six hours from start of blood transfusion)	Donor antibodies react with recipient's neurophils to damage lung epithelium	• Severe dyspnoea • Tachycardia • Hypotension • Decreased O_2 saturation • Cough – may have frothy blood-tinged sputum • Mild fever	• *Standard transfusion reaction care • Keep the vein open (as above) • Supportive care as needed (O_2, elevate head of bed, may need ventilatory support – transfer to ICU)

* Standard transfusion reaction care: Stop the transfusion immediately; report to medical officer; recheck all identifying documentation of blood and person; monitor closely – q15min (temperature, pulse and respiration [TPR], blood pressure [BP], O_2 saturation, symptoms); follow the facility's Adult Deterioration Detection System [ADDS] protocol; remain with the person and reassure them; document.

SOURCES: AUSTRALIAN RED CROSS LIFEBLOOD (2020A). *CLASSIFICATION & INCIDENCE OF ADVERSE EFFECTS*. RETRIEVED FROM HTTPS://TRANSFUSION.COM.AU/ADVERSE_TRANSFUSION_REACTIONS, ACCESSED 10 AUGUST 2020; JOINT UNITED KINGDOM (UK) BLOOD TRANSFUSION AND TISSUE TRANSPLANTATION SERVICES PROFESSIONAL ADVISORY COMMITTEE (2013 – UPDATED MAY 2020). *GUIDELINES FOR THE BLOOD TRANSFUSION SERVICES IN THE UK*. RETRIEVED FROM HTTPS://WWW.TRANSFUSIONGUIDELINES.ORG/RED-BOOK, ACCESSED 10 AUGUST 2020.

Complete the transfusion

When the blood unit is empty (assuming no adverse reactions), open the clamp on the saline solution and flush the lines with saline. This ensures the person receives the entire amount of blood. Perform hand hygiene, put gloves on and disconnect the blood unit and the blood administration set from the IV tubing. Determine if the person requires either further blood products or intravenous solutions. If not, discontinue the IV. If further units of blood are required, a fresh transfusion-giving set is required every 12 hours (ANZSBT & ACN, 2020).

Continue to monitor the person

Monitor the person for altered vital signs or the appearance of symptoms hourly for four hours, then every four hours for the next 24 hours in case a delayed reaction occurs. If symptoms do occur, notify the physician. Check the medication chart for any medications to be given in between units (e.g. frusemide).

CLEAN, REPLACE AND DISPOSE OF EQUIPMENT

Perform hand hygiene and put on gloves. Some facilities require the completed blood unit be kept for 24 hours in case a delayed reaction occurs. If so, place the empty blood unit (minus the insertion spike(s) from the administration set, which is cut off and goes in the sharps container) in a biohazard bag, seal, label and store as directed. Remove gloves and perform hand hygiene. After 24 hours, dispose of the blood unit in a contaminated waste unit.

DOCUMENTATION

Many facilities have specific documentation forms/electronic forms for blood transfusions, with spaces for various observations. If not, modify the vital signs sheet to use during the transfusion.

Document the following in the notes:

- date and time (each) transfusion was commenced and completed
- type of blood component used, number of units and the sequence number of each unit (if more than one)
- batch number – blood units have a peel-off identification tab or bar code with the unit ID number, group and Rh factor, so that errors in transcription are avoided. Remove this tab and place it in the person's progress notes at commencement of the (each) transfusion (or read the bar code into the e-medical record). Note the time when each unit was completed
- incidence and management of any adverse events
- signature of the person administering and the person checking the blood units (ARCL, 2021c).

All transfusion documentation is to be carefully completed in the person's medical record file.

CLINICAL SKILLS ASSESSMENT

Blood transfusion

Demonstrates the ability to effectively and safely administer a blood transfusion. Incorporates the *National Safety and Quality Health Service Standards*: 2 Partnering with consumers, 3 Preventing and controlling healthcare-associated infections, 4 Medication safety, 5 Comprehensive care, 6 Communicating for safety, 7 Blood management, and 8 Recognising and responding to acute deterioration (Australian Commission on Safety and Quality in Health Care [ACSQHC], 2021).

Performance criteria	1	2	3	4	5
(Numbers indicate NMBA *Registered Nurse Standards for Practice*)	(Dependent)	(Marginal)	(Assisted)	(Supervised)	(Independent)
1. Identifies indication (1.1, 3.3, 3.4)	☐	☐	☐	☐	☐
2. Verifies the validity of the blood product order (1.4, 3.4, 6.2, 6.5)	☐	☐	☐	☐	☐
3. Displays knowledge of blood groups and blood matching (1.1, 3.4)	☐	☐	☐	☐	☐
4. Evidence of therapeutic interaction with the person, e.g. gives the person a clear explanation of the procedure (1.4, 1.5, 2.1, 2.2, 3.2)	☐	☐	☐	☐	☐
5. Demonstrates clinical reasoning; displays knowledge of blood products (1.1, 1.2, 1.3, 1.5, 3.4, 4.1, 4.2, 4.3, 5.1, 6.1)	☐	☐	☐	☐	☐
6. Gathers equipment (1.1, 5.5, 6.1): ■ blood order sheet ■ consent form ■ equipment to initiate an IV of normal saline ■ blood transfusion-giving set ■ infusion pump ■ blood warmer ■ clean gloves	☐	☐	☐	☐	☐
7. Performs hand hygiene (1.1, 3.4, 6.1)	☐	☐	☐	☐	☐
8. Establishes an intravenous infusion with normal saline (1.4, 4.1, 4.2, 4.3, 6.1)	☐	☐	☐	☐	☐
9. Records vital signs (4.1, 4.2, 4.3, 6.1)	☐	☐	☐	☐	☐
10. Identifies the person and the blood product according to policy (1.1, 6.1)	☐	☐	☐	☐	☐
11. Initiates the blood transfusion (1.1, 6.1)	☐	☐	☐	☐	☐
12. Begins the blood infusion slowly (1.1, 6.1)	☐	☐	☐	☐	☐
13. Monitors the person (1.1, 4.1, 4.2, 4.3, 6.1)	☐	☐	☐	☐	☐
14. Completes the transfusion (1.1, 6.1)	☐	☐	☐	☐	☐
15. Continues to monitor the person (1.1, 4.1, 4.2, 4.3, 6.1)	☐	☐	☐	☐	☐
16. Cleans, replaces and disposes of equipment appropriately (3.6, 6.1)	☐	☐	☐	☐	☐
17. Documents relevant information (1.1, 1.4, 1.6, 2.2, 2.7, 3.5, 3.7, 6.1, 6.2, 6.5, 7.3)	☐	☐	☐	☐	☐
18. Demonstrates the ability to link theory to practice (1.1, 3.3, 3.4, 3.5)	☐	☐	☐	☐	☐

Student:

Clinical facilitator: Date:

CHAPTER 66

VENIPUNCTURE

INDICATIONS

Venipuncture is an advanced skill to access the venous system via a needle to obtain blood for diagnostic purposes or to monitor response to treatment. Blood tests provide valuable information about a person's nutritional, haematological, metabolic, immune and biochemical status. Testing blood composition (detecting analytes [e.g. medications, ethanol], hormones, nutrients and metabolites [e.g. glucose]), oxygen levels and pulse rate using a hydrogel-coated chemical biosensor that identifies the person by fingerprint, collects molecules on the skin that are released through sweat, analyses the molecules and encrypts the information has been developed (Lin et al., 2022). This will reduce the need for many venipunctures when it becomes widely available. However, conventional venipuncture remains the current practice.

Blood tests are ordered by the medical staff. Venipuncture is an invasive procedure and requires consent; in this instance, the person's cooperation with a procedure is an implied consent and written consent is not needed.

Most facilities require nurses to undertake advanced training to qualify them to establish an intravenous (IV) access device.

There are needleless blood-drawing devices in development. One is a device that sits on the skin and, when activated, punctures the skin with 30 microneedles that pull capillary blood into the receptacle over approximately two minutes (Hein, 2017). Another device uses an existing IV line by inserting a small cannula downstream from the tip to draw blood. For haematology, it reduces pain, eliminates 'missed' attempts and needlestick injuries (Pendleton & LeFaye, 2022). The Australian states are inconsistent in their policies regarding peripherally inserted venous cannulas (PIVCs) to sample blood (Davies et al., 2020). Please refer to the facility's protocols.

EVIDENCE OF THERAPEUTIC INTERACTION

Clearly explain the procedure to allay fears and anxiety. Many people have a deep-seated fear of needles. Anxiety about the procedure may result in vasoconstriction (Shah et al., 2020). Emphasising the necessity and the benefits helps the person to accept the unpleasant procedure and provide tacit consent. Do not be dishonest about the discomfort; give reassurance and emphasise that it will be completed quickly.

Ask about allergies/sensitivities to latex, antiseptics and adhesives. Ask about a history of fainting when blood is drawn – the person may be more comfortable and safer lying down.

DEMONSTRATE CLINICAL REASONING

Safety considerations are an important aspect of any clinical procedure, but especially so of invasive procedures. Preparing the environment for privacy and your convenience, assessing the site and assembling the equipment precede accessing the vein.

Safety considerations

Safety

The venous system is a closed sterile system that venipuncture breaches, providing an entry point for microorganisms. Aseptic Non Touch Technique (ANTT) is essential for venipuncture (see **Clinical Skill 7**).

Maintain standard precautions when undertaking venipuncture, since blood easily contaminates your skin. Various vacuum systems are used to reduce the risk of needle-stick injuries to healthcare workers. These provide a safer method for collecting blood samples and are preferable to using a needle and syringe. Familiarise yourself with the integrated safety devices available at the facility where you are working. Vein visualisation instruments for locating veins not visible to the naked eye are available (e.g. near-infrared spectography, ultrasound) (Kaganovskaya, Capitulo & Wuerz, 2023). Use these if they are available.

Ask the person to state their full name and date of birth. Check their identification band or scan the bar code against the request form to ensure the specimen is obtained from the correct person. Label the blood draw tubes at this point so there is no mix-up with the identification of the sample.

Knowledge of the person's medical history, current and recent medications and diagnosis is essential. If there are bleeding disorders (e.g. pancytopenia, thrombocytopenic purpura) or a recent history of steroid or anticoagulant use, including aspirin, pressure needs to be applied to the puncture site for longer.

Determine any preparation required (e.g. fasting) and that it has been done or if there is a specific time requested. If a topical anaesthetic is to be used (e.g. EMLA cream [Eutetic Mixture of Local Anaesthetics]), it must be in contact with intact skin for an hour prior to the procedure for good effect (Babamohamadi et al., 2022).

The medical staff complete laboratory requisitions for all blood tests. The healthcare professional collecting the specimen provides their name, signature and the time and date of collection.

Prepare the environment

Provide privacy for the person by closing the curtains or the door to their room. Provide good illumination for the procedure. Raise or lower the bed to a comfortable working position to reduce strain on your back muscles and to improve access to the venipuncture site.

Assess the site

Visually inspect the veins on both arms. Veins adjacent to an infection, bruising or phlebitis are not considered because of the risk of causing more local tissue damage or systemic infection (Sivapuram, 2019). Avoid areas of previous venipuncture to reduce the build-up of scar tissue, which makes accessing the vein difficult and painful. When choosing the arm to be used for venous access, be aware of such conditions as lymphoedema, a mastectomy or axillary node dissection on that side, an established intravenous access, an arteriovenous shunt, or a haematoma at the potential site that precludes use of that arm for venous access. Age, weight and preference of the person also influence the choice of site.

The vein chosen for access is often in the antecubital fossa – the median cubital vein is the usual choice in order to avoid haematoma formation, nerve injury and chronic persistent pain (Sivapuram, 2019). However, be aware that others may be more suitable, such as the basilic and cephalic veins. The median cubital, basilic and cephalic veins are straight and strong, and suitable for large-gauge venipuncture. They are superficial and accessible. The basilic and cephalic veins require stabilisation as they tend to roll.

LOOK for an unused vein, easily detected by inspection and palpation, that is patent and healthy (Brown, 2020).

LISTEN to the person's comments about potential problems (as above).

FEEL for a soft, bouncy vein that refills when depressed.

Consult an anatomy and physiology text for more information on the veins of the arm.

?

If the veins in the arms are unsuitable or inaccessible, access the superficial veins in the back of the hand or wrist for venipuncture. Do not use the veins in the underside of the wrist (Strasinger & DiLorenzo, 2019).

To engorge veins, warm the limb and keep it dependent for a few minutes. This increases blood volume in the venous system and makes access easier.

Provide comfort

Venipuncture can be distressing and painful, though usually for only a short time. EMLA cream is effective, but requires skin contact for an hour (Babamohamadi et al., 2022). Zempsky, Schmitz and Meyer (2016) demonstrated that lidocaine powder applied to the skin at the site one to three minutes prior to venipuncture reduced pain in both adults and children. A spray-coolant may be used. Follow the protocol at the facility.

ELDER CARE

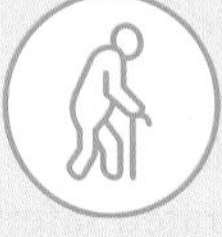

Physiological changes to skin (e.g. loss of elasticity, moisture and support structures), reduced muscle size, altered peripheral vascular competency (decreasing circulation) and a propensity to cold and chills (causing vasoconstriction) all impact on venipuncture in elderly adults. Hearing loss, reduced eyesight and, for some, confusion and dementia, increase the stress of this procedure. Use excellent communication skills, respect, calmness, kindness and reassurance to decrease the negative impact and increase comfort (Brown, 2020).

The near-infrared visualisation device is useful in this demographic group (Kaganovskaya, Capitulo & Wuerz, 2023). Use warm towels on the arm and place the arm in a dependent position (below the heart) for several minutes to increase vasodilatation. Place the tourniquet over a sleeve or towel to prevent skin damage. Take care with the angle of the needle, as vessels may be shallower in an elderly person. Older people often have very prominent veins that rise above the surface of their hand or arm. You will need to adjust the angle of entry (flatter) to avoid puncturing the opposite wall of the vein. Skin and vein walls are more fragile, use gentleness when accessing the vein. The veins may roll more easily and need to be stabilised with your thumb below the intended venipuncture site.

THE PERSON LIVING WITH SEVERE OBESITY

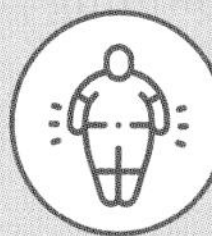

You may find the veins in someone who is severely obese buried very deep and very difficult to locate or access. Kaganovskaya, Capitulo and Wuerz (2023) found vein visualisation technology devices that use near-infrared light or ultrasound to assist location of peripheral veins to be useful. However, these may not be available to assist you. If you do not access the vein on the first attempt, ask an experienced phlebotomist or a more experienced nurse (preferably from the IV team) to access the vein.

GATHER EQUIPMENT

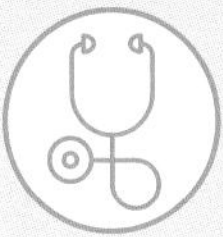

Gathering equipment is an organisational step that helps to create a positive environment for a successful interaction. It ensures that you have all needed material, boosts the person's confidence and trust in you, and increases your self-confidence. While gathering the equipment, you can mentally rehearse the procedure. Equipment may include the following items:

EQUIPMENT	EXPLANATION
Absorbent pad	To protect bed linen
Clean gloves	To uphold standard precautions
Tourniquet	Impedes venous return, engorging the veins and facilitating access (single-use, latex-free, as available)
EMLA cream, Lidocaine powder or a spray coolant	To numb the skin momentarily during venipuncture (use according to the facility's procedure)
Alcowipes	• Used to cleanse the skin prior to inserting the needle because alcohol destroys microorganisms on the skin • Use an alcohol-based solution such as chlorhexidine 0.5 per cent in 70 per cent alcohol to remove the risk presented by the person's skin flora • Rub firmly for 30 seconds. Allow the area to dry, facilitating disinfection and preventing a stinging pain on needle insertion (Marcelino & Shepard, 2023) • Chlorhexidine gluconate is a topical antiseptic that remains on the skin to reduce the incidence of skin contaminants (Marcelino & Shepard, 2023)
Butterfly needle and cannula extender	• To access the vein • Available with a Vacutainer attachment • A needle (21 to 23 gauge) and a 5 to 10 mL syringe can be used to draw the blood from the venous system • A 20 to 22 gauge needle enables the blood to be withdrawn at a reasonable speed without undue discomfort to the person and prevents cellular components of the blood (red blood cells) from being crushed (haemolysis), which occurs if pulled through a smaller needle, or sheared if pulled through a larger one (Ally, 2019) • Most haematological tests require 5 to 10 mL of blood
Vacutainer	• Specialist equipment used for accessing a vein • Consists of a plastic holder with a double-sided needle screwed in and a stoppered vacuum test tube

Appropriate test tubes and indelible pen	• To collect blood for different tests
	• The stoppers are colour-coded to indicate the types of diagnostic studies
	• A chart with a list of the various tests and the appropriate test tube will be available
	• Some tubes contain preservatives, others contain anticoagulants or coagulants, and some contain nothing
	• Collect the blood samples in the following order to minimise the risk of transferring additives from one tube to another:
	  ◦ blood culture tube
	  ◦ glass or non-additive tubes; coagulation occurs in this tube
	  ◦ serum tubes with or without clot activator or gel separator
	  ◦ additive tubes such as gel separator
	  ◦ tubes that contain clot activator or heparin
	  ◦ heparin tubes
	  ◦ EDTA tubes (an anticoagulant used for preserving the blood)
	  ◦ other tubes, e.g. trace elements (Sivapuram, 2019)
	Use the person's individual identification stickers. If you need to write on the label, an indelible pen is used to ensure the label remains readable if it becomes damp

Sharps container	Used to receive needles following use and reduce the incidence of needle-stick injuries
Gauze dressing, low-lint swabs and a Band-Aid or an adhesive pressure pad	Used to apply pressure to the puncture site for a short while (20 minutes to an hour, depending on the person) to allow the puncture site to close

PART 12

PERFORM A VENIPUNCTURE

Video

After the arm has been assessed, the tourniquet is applied to distend the veins. A vein is located, the area cleansed and the butterfly needle inserted to draw the required amount of blood.

Hand hygiene

Hand hygiene (see **Clinical Skill 5**) removes transient microorganisms from your hands. This is an infection-control measure that prevents cross-contamination.

Assemble the equipment

Assemble the Vacutainer system or the syringe and needle in a convenient position. If using the syringe, loosen the plunger in the cylinder. Position the chosen arm by extending it to form a straight line from the shoulder to the wrist and well below the heart. Cover a small pillow or towel with the waterproof sheet and place it under the upper arm to stabilise the arm. The person may sit or lie down. Some people feel very faint when blood is being taken and may need to lie down. Perform hand hygiene.

Apply the tourniquet

Apply the tourniquet about 10 to 15 cm above the intended puncture site. It should be tight enough to impede venous flow, but not tight enough to impede arterial flow.

For a latex tourniquet, lie it flat against the skin and bring the ends together, with one lying on top of the other. Hold the bottom end in position. Lift, stretch and tighten the tourniquet with your other hand and, using two fingers, tuck the top tail under the bottom length, with both tails pointing away from the proposed puncture site so they don't contaminate it.

For a cloth tourniquet, lie it flat against the skin and clip the ends together. Place the clip on the outside of the arm so it does not interfere with the venipuncture site. Tighten the strap.

Check the distal pulse to make sure you have not occluded an artery. If you are unable to locate a pulse, release the tourniquet and reapply more loosely. Leave the tourniquet in place for one minute only, as prolonged tourniquet application may cause stasis, localised acidaemia, haemoconcentration (Strasinger & DiLorenzo, 2019) and haemolysis (Ally, 2019; Slade, 2019), and be very painful. If you are unable to find and access the vein within a minute, release the tourniquet, wait two minutes, and reapply it.

Locate the vein

Visually locate the vein. Palpate to determine the location and condition of the vein, and to distinguish veins from arteries and tendons or to detect deeper veins. Use the index and middle fingers of your non-dominant hand to palpate, because it increases the sensitivity and accuracy of vein location.

Ask the person to make a fist to increase the dilatation of the vein. If this is done quickly, or the fist is pumped, haemoconcentration and inaccurate results occur (Strasinger & DiLorenzo, 2019). Massaging the arm towards the tourniquet is both comforting and increases vasodilatation (Yasuda et al., 2019). The vein should feel round and firm and spring back when compressed.

> ? If the veins are difficult to locate, use additional assistive technologies such as a vein visualisation device or ultrasound. Ask for assistance from someone experienced in their use.

Release the tourniquet and relax the hand. Allow two minutes (in which you cleanse and dry the area) before reapplying the tourniquet. If you are using a cooling spray or Lidocaine spray to reduce the pain of venipuncture, this is when it is applied as the effect is immediate (it rapidly and temporarily lowers skin temperature resulting in decreased pain sensitivity and topical anaesthesia) (Khosravi Pour et al., 2023). Perform hand hygiene.

Cleanse the area

Put on clean gloves to protect both you and the person as part of standard precautions. Use the alcowipe to clean the area using circular strokes outwards from the intended puncture point for 5 to 7 cm to avoid bringing microorganisms into the cleaner area. Clean for 30 seconds and allow the area to dry for at least 30 seconds (Marcelino & Shepard, 2023). These authors recommend following with 2% chlorhexidine gluconate/70% alcohol swabs rubbed vigorously for five seconds and allowed to dry. Cleansing with chlorhexidine offers superior clinical protection, probably because of a more rapid action, a shorter drying time (it is combined with 70% alcohol), its persistent activity and thus longer residual effect at the site of skin puncture (O'Grady, 2023). If using the chlorhexidine gluconate/alcohol swab, rub vigorously for five seconds and allow to dry for at least five seconds (Marcelino & Shepard, 2023).

Access the vein and draw blood

Reapply the tourniquet. Ask the person to make and hold a fist (Canberra Hospital and Health Services, 2021). If you need to repalpate the site to find the vein, the area will have to be cleaned again. Uncap the needle.

With the Vacutainer (or the butterfly, or needle and syringe) in your dominant hand, stabilise the vein by stretching the skin taut below the intended puncture point using your non-dominant hand (Canberra Hospital and Health Services, 2021). Keep the needle parallel to the vein and above it. Insert the needle at 15 to 30 degrees elevation to avoid going through the other side of the vein. The angle is dependent on the size or depth of the vein. Keep the bevel of the needle upward to also prevent going through the opposite wall of the vein. Advance the needle through the skin and subcutaneous tissue and gently but firmly through the vein wall. You may feel the difference in pressure as the needle advances from the tissue through the vein wall (most commonly felt in adults, less often in children or in the frail elderly).

Blood appears in the hub of the needle or out of the tubing of the butterfly needle but not in the Vacutainer needle device. Reduce the angle of descent when this flashback is seen or when puncture of the vein wall is felt. Release the tourniquet at this point (see below).

If using a needle and syringe, ensuring you have pulled slightly back on the plunger before venipuncture means a flashback of blood is seen in the barrel on successful entry into the vein. If there is no flashback, withdraw the needle slightly as it may be in contact with a valve.

Once there is a flashback, pull back slowly and steadily on the plunger until the amount of blood required is obtained. Forceful withdrawal of blood causes haemolysis (Ally, 2019).

Safety

If using the Vacutainer, firmly anchor the needle with the non-dominant hand to avoid dislodging it. Push a test tube onto the back part of the Vacutainer needle using your dominant hand. The vacuum in the test tube will pull the required amount of blood into it. If no blood appears in the container (because the vein was missed), do not use that container again as the vacuum will have been broken. If the attempt was unsuccessful, release the tourniquet, wait a few minutes and try again. Most facilities have a policy allowing only two unsuccessful attempts (to protect the person).

Release the tourniquet

Release the tourniquet as soon as the vein is entered and a good flow established to increase comfort, to restore circulation and to avoid inaccurate results caused by haemolysis, haemoconcentration or haemostasis (e.g. blood for calcium levels) (Ally, 2019) you must release the tourniquet within two minutes (Canberra Hospital and Health Services, 2021).

Withdraw the needle from the vein

Safety

Support the insertion site with gauze. Withdraw the needle at the same angle at which it was inserted to avoid tearing the vein. Do not apply pressure to the puncture site until after the needle is fully removed to decrease pain on removal, and to prevent damage to the intima of the vein and haematoma formation. Then apply pressure with the gauze for two to five minutes to assist clotting and to prevent bleeding and ecchymosis (ask the person to do this if they are able).

Post-procedure

Activate the needle safety cover or place the needle unit in the sharps container.

If the syringe and needle were used, clean (with alcowipe and let dry) the required test tube top and fill it using the same needle used to access blood. Again, the vacuum pulls the required amount of blood into the tube. Do not force the blood into the tube or underfill the test tube, as this will cause haemolysis (Ally, 2019). Wipe the top of the test tube with an alcowipe to remove any traces of blood.

If needed, gently rock the test tube six to 10 times to thoroughly mix the blood with any additives.

Remove and discard the gloves. Affix the adhesive, printed label to the test tube with the person's information (or use the indelible pen to fill in the label). Place the test tubes in a biohazard bag and send them and the laboratory requisition to the lab. Perform hand hygiene.

Check the site for haematoma formation, and place a Band-Aid (check for allergies to Band-Aids/tape) or pressure pad over the insertion site and the gauze to continue the pressure required to minimise bleeding. If the person has fragile skin, do not use a Band-Aid or tape; rather, apply pressure to the puncture site until bleeding has ceased. The person is advised to minimise activity with the involved arm and to maintain pressure on the site for five minutes. Observe the site for haematoma formation. Ask the person to leave the dressing on for half an hour.

CLEAN, REPLACE AND DISPOSE OF EQUIPMENT

Place needles (uncapped) in the sharps container for safety. The Vacutainer holder is single-use and is discarded with the attached needle into the sharps container. A single-use tourniquet is discarded in the contaminated waste bin. A reusable tourniquet must be decontaminated (follow manufacturer's instructions) before being returned to storage (Salgueiro-Oliveira et al., 2019). Wrap any gauze, alcowipes, used gloves and any other equipment contaminated with blood in the waterproof sheet and discard in the contaminated waste bin. Perform hand hygiene. For efficiency and collegial relationships, restock the tray as necessary with any equipment used.

DOCUMENTATION

Documentation of blood taken usually consists of a brief notation in the eHealth record or progress notes, including time, date, type of tests and the person's response. Document and report any abnormal test results to medical staff.

With thanks to Cindy Proctor, Certified Phlebotomist, for reviewing the material.

CLINICAL SKILLS ASSESSMENT

Venipuncture

Demonstrates the ability to effectively and safely obtain a blood sample from a vein. Incorporates the *National Safety and Quality Health Service Standards*: 2 Partnering with consumers, 3 Preventing and controlling healthcare-associated infections, 5 Comprehensive care, and 6 Communicating for safety (Australian Commission on Safety and Quality in Health Care [ACSQHC], 2021).

Performance criteria	1	2	3	4	5
(Numbers indicate NMBA *Registered Nurse Standards for Practice*)	(Dependent)	(Marginal)	(Assisted)	(Supervised)	(Independent)
1. Identifies indication (1.1, 3.3, 3.4)	☐	☐	☐	☐	☐
2. Outlines safety considerations (4.1, 4.2, 4.3, 6.1)	☐	☐	☐	☐	☐
3. Evidence of therapeutic interaction with the person, e.g. gives the person a clear explanation of the procedure (1.4, 1.5, 2.1, 2.2, 3.2)	☐	☐	☐	☐	☐
4. Demonstrates clinical reasoning; assesses arm, selects the site and assembles equipment (1.1, 1.2, 1.3, 1.5, 4.1, 4.2, 4.3, 5.1, 5.5, 6.1	☐	☐	☐	☐	☐
5. Gathers equipment (1.1, 5.5, 6.1): ■ absorbent pad ■ sharps container ■ clean gloves ■ tourniquet ■ Vacutainer and access device or syringe and needle and appropriate test tubes ■ alcowipes ■ cotton balls ■ Band-Aids	☐	☐	☐	☐	☐
6. Performs hand hygiene (1.1, 3.4, 6.1)	☐	☐	☐	☐	☐
7. Applies the tourniquet (6.1)	☐	☐	☐	☐	☐
8. Locates the vein and cleanses the area (1.1, 4.1, 4.2, 4.3, 6.1)	☐	☐	☐	☐	☐
9. Dons gloves (1.1, 3.4, 6.1)	☐	☐	☐	☐	☐
10. Accesses the vein (1.1, 6.1)	☐	☐	☐	☐	☐
11. Draws blood (6.1)	☐	☐	☐	☐	☐
12. Releases the tourniquet (1.1, 6.1)	☐	☐	☐	☐	☐
13. Withdraws the needle, applies pressure to the insertion site (1.1, 6.1)	☐	☐	☐	☐	☐
14. Cleans, replaces and disposes of equipment appropriately (3.6, 6.1)	☐	☐	☐	☐	☐
15. Documents relevant information (1.1, 1.4, 1.6, 2.2, 2.7, 3.5, 3.7, 6.1, 6.2, 6.5, 7.3)	☐	☐	☐	☐	☐
16. Demonstrates the ability to link theory to practice (1.1, 3.3, 3.4, 3.5)	☐	☐	☐	☐	☐

Student:

Clinical facilitator: Date:

REFERENCES

Ally, A. (2019). Avoiding hemolysis in blood sample collection and processing. *Fisher Clinical Services.* https://www.fisherclinicalservices.com/en/learning-center/insights-blog-overview/avoiding-hemolysis-in-blood-sample-collection-and-processing.html

Australian Commission on Safety and Quality in Health Care (ACSQHC) (2021). *National safety and quality health service standards* (3rd ed.). Sydney, NSW: ACSQHC.

Australian and New Zealand Society of Blood Transfusion (ANZSBT) & Australian College of Nursing (ACN) (2020). *Guidelines for the administration of blood products* (3rd ed.). https://anzsbt.org.au/wp-content/uploads/2020/03/ANZSBT-Administration-Guidelines-Revised-3rd-edition-Publication-Version-FINAL-20191002.pdf

Australian Red Cross Blood Service (ARCBS) (2016). *Appropriate transfusion practice.* https://www.transfusion.com.au/transfusion_practice/administration

Australian Red Cross Lifeblood (ARCL) (2020a). *Classification & incidence of adverse effects.* https://transfusion.com.au/adverse_transfusion_reactions

Australian Red Cross Lifeblood (ARCL) (2020b). *Preparing to administer a blood component including equipment.* https://transfusion.com.au/transfusion_practice/administration

Australian Red Cross Lifeblood (ARCL) (2021a). *Donation testing.* https://www.lifeblood.com.au/health-professionals/testing/donation

Australian Red Cross Lifeblood (ARCL) (2021b). *Administration: Equipment required.* https://www.lifeblood.com.au/health-professionals/clinical-practice/transfusion-process/administration

Australian Red Cross Lifeblood (ARCL) (2021c). *Documentation and traceability.* https://www.lifeblood.com.au/health-professionals/clinical-practice/transfusion-process/documentation-traceability

Australian Red Cross Lifeblood (ARCL) (2021d). *Storage and handling.* https://www.lifeblood.com.au/health-professionals/products/storage-and-handling.

Australian Red Cross Lifeblood (ARCL) (2022). *Platelets.* https://www.lifeblood.com.au/health-professionals/products/blood-components/platelets

Babamohamadi, H., Ameri, Z., Asadi, I. & Asgari, M. (2022). Comparison of the effect of EMLA™ cream and the valsalva maneuver on pain severity during vascular needle insertion in hemodialysis patients: A controlled, randomized, clinical trial. *Evidence-Based Complementary and Alternative Medicine,* Article ID 8383021. https://doi.org/10.1155/2022/8383021

BloodSafe eLearning Australia (2015). *Clinical decision making.* Transfusion Practice Course. https://learn.bloodsafelearning.org.au/mod/elmo/view.php?id=2

Brown, K. (2020). *Phlebotomy Ps and Qs: Problems and quandaries in specimen collection.* California Association for Medical Technology Workshop, North Hollywood, CA, 15 March 2020. https://camlt.org/wp-content/uploads/2020/02/Phlebot-Ps-and-Qs-CAMLT-2020.pdf

Canberra Hospital and Health Services (2021). *Clinical procedure: Venepuncture blood specimen collection.* https://www.health.act.gov.au

Davies, H., Coventry, L., Jacob, A., Stoneman, L. & Jacob, E. (2020). Blood sampling through peripheral intravenous cannulas: A look at current practice in Australia. *Collegian, 27*(2), 219–25. https://doi.org/10.1016/j.colegn.2019.07.010

Heger, A., Pock, K. & Romisch, J. (2017). Thawing of pooled, solvent/detergent-treated plasma octaplasLG®: Validation studies using different thawing devices. *Transfusion Medicine and Hemotherapy, 44,* 94–8. https://doi.org/10.1159/000460302

Hein, I. (2017). Needleless, pain-free blood draw device coming to market. *Medscape Nurses, from Consumer Technology Association, 2017 Digital Health Summit,* 6 January.

Joint United Kingdom (UK) Blood Transfusion and Tissue Transplantation Services Professional Advisory Committee (2013, updated May 2020). *Guidelines for the blood transfusion services in the UK.* https://www.transfusionguidelines.org/red-book

Kaganovskaya, M., Capitulo, K. & Wuerz, L. (2023). Current and emerging vein identification technology for phlebotomy and peripheral I.V. Cannulation. *Nursing, 53*(2), 39–45. https://www.researchgate.net/profile/KathleenCapitulo/publication/368536759_20 23Current_and_emerging_vein_identification13/links/63ed5ed72958d64a5cd0a6 50/2023-Current-and-emerging-vein-identification13.pdf

Khosravi Pour, A., Hejazi, S., Kameli, A., Azizi, T., Armat, M. & Eshgh, M. (2023). Cooling spray or lidocaine spray and needle insertion pain in hemodialysis patients: An open-label cross-over randomized clinical trial. *BioMedicalCentral Anesthesiology, 23*(69). https://doi.org/10.1186/s12871-023-02028-w

Lin, S., Zhu, J., Yu, W., Wang, B., Sabet, K., Zhao, Y., Cheng, X., Hojaiji, H., Lin, Tan, J., Milla, C., Davis, R. & Emaminejad, S. (2022). A touch-based multimodal and cryptographic bio-human–machine interface. *Proceedings of the National Academy of Sciences (PNAS), 119*(15), e2201937119. https://doi.org/10.1073/pnas.2201937119

Lotterman, S. & Sharma, S. (2023). Blood transfusion. In *StatPearls [Internet].* Treasure Island (FL): StatPearls Publishing. https://www.ncbi.nlm.nih.gov/books/NBK499824

Marcelino, C. & Shepard, J. (2023). A quality improvement initiative on reducing blood culture contamination in the emergency department. *Journal of Emergency Nursing, 49*(2), 162–71. https://doi.org/10.1016/j.jen.2022.11.005

National Blood Authority Australia (n.d.). *Overview: About blood.* National Blood Authority Australia. https://www.blood.gov.au/about-blood

New Zealand Blood Service (NZBS) (2016). *A guide to the clinical use of blood components, blood products and blood transfusion procedures in New Zealand.* Auckland, NZ: New Zealand Blood Service.

O'Grady, N. (2023). Prevention of central line–associated bloodstream infections. *New England Journal of Medicine, 389,* 1121–31. https://doi.org/10.1056/NEJMra2213296

Ozawa, S., Ozawa-Morriello, J., Rock, R., Sromoski, M., Walbolt, S., Hall, T. & Pearse, B. (2023). Patient blood management as an emerging concept in quality: The role of nurses. *Journal of Nursing Care Quality, 10,* 1097. https://doi.org/10.1097/NCQ.0000000000000734

Pendleton, B. & LaFaye, R. (2022). Multicenter study of needle-free blood collection system for reducing specimen error and intravenous catheter replacement. *Journal for Healthcare Quality, 44*(2), e24–e30. https://doi.org/10.1097/JHQ.0000000000000331

Salgueiro-Oliveira, A. S., Costa, P. J., Braga, L. M., Graveto, J. M., Oliveira, V. S. & Parreira, P. M. (2019). Health professionals' practices related with tourniquet use during peripheral venipuncture: A scoping review. *Revista Latino-Americana de Enfermagem, 27,* e3125. https://doi.org/10.1590/1518-8345.2743-3125

Shah, P., Khaleel, M., Thuptimdang, W., Sunwoo, J., Veluswamy, S., Chalacheva, P., Kato, R. M., Detterich, J., Wood, J. C., Zeltzer, L., Sposto, R., Khoo, M. & Coates, T. D. (2020). Mental stress causes vasoconstriction in subjects with sickle cell disease and in normal controls. *Haematologica, 105*(1), 83–90. https://doi.org/10.3324/haematol.2018.211391

Sharp, R., Turner, L., Altschwager, J., Corsini, N. & Esterman, A. (2021). Adverse events associated with home blood transfusion: A retrospective cohort study. *Journal of Clinical Nursing, 30,* 1751–9. https://doi.org/10.1111/jocn.15734

Sivapuram, M. S. (2019). *Venipuncture (adults): Risks of blood specimen collection* [Evidence summary]. Joanna Briggs Institute EBP Database, JBI@Ovid. 2019; JBI145.

Slade, S. (2019) *Blood specimen collection: Hemolysis prevention* [Evidence summary]. Joanna Briggs Institute EBP Database, JBI@Ovid. 2019; JBI1657.

Strasinger, S. & DiLorenzo, M. (2019). *The phlebotomy textbook* (4th ed.). Philadelphia, PA: Davis.

Yasuda, K., Sato, S., Okada, K. & Yano, R. (2019). The venodilation effects of tapping versus massaging for venipuncture. *Japanese Journal of Nursing Sciences, 16,* 491–9. https://doi.org/10.1111/jjns.12261

Zempsky, W., Schmitz, M. & Meyer, J. (2016). Safety and efficacy of needle-free powder lidocaine delivery system in adult patients undergoing venipuncture or peripheral venous cannulation: A randomized, double blind, placebo-controlled trial. *Clinical Journal of Pain, 32*(3), 211–17. https://doi.org/10.1097/AJP.0000000000000257

PART 13

WOUND MANAGEMENT

67 DRY DRESSING TECHNIQUE

68 COMPLEX WOUNDS: DRAIN CARE AND SUTURE, STAPLE OR CLIP REMOVAL

69 COMPLEX WOUNDS: WOUND IRRIGATION

70 COMPLEX WOUNDS: FILLING A WOUND; NEGATIVE PRESSURE WOUND THERAPY

Note: These notes are summaries of the most important points in the assessments/procedures and are not exhaustive on the subject. References of the materials used to compile the information have been supplied. The student is expected to have learnt the material surrounding each skill as presented in the references. No single reference is complete on each subject.

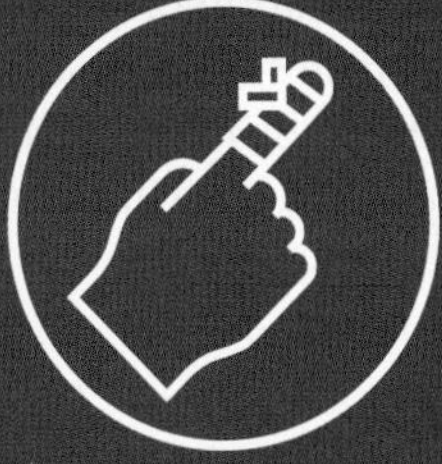

CHAPTER 67

DRY DRESSING TECHNIQUE

INDICATIONS

The purpose of wound care is to assist the physiological processes of healing effectively and in the shortest time possible. Dry dressings are used most commonly for uncomplicated postoperative incisions and for abrasions. The wound will have little or no drainage and is expected to heal without incident (e.g. simple cuts, scrapes, lacerations, skin tears and surgical incisions). The dressing is protective, reduces the introduction of microorganisms, reduces discomfort or accidental trauma to the site and speeds healing by keeping the wound surface moist. However, Dias et al. (2023) found no conclusive evidence that dressings over surgical incisions healing by primary intention prevented surgical site infections, improved scarring, reduced pain, eased removal or were more acceptable to the person. Undisturbed wound healing is optimum (depending on the person [e.g. their comorbidities, age, high body mass index (BMI)]), with dressing changes only recommended for saturation of the wound dressing material, excessive bleeding, suspected local/systemic infection (e.g. local wound pain, redness, swelling) and potential dehiscence (Morgan-Jones et al., 2019). Unfortunately, this consortium of surgeons noted that 'dressing change "ritualism" has been identified as a wider issue in wound care, and this particularly applies to post-surgical incision wounds, where pre-set schedules may be in place regardless of individual clinical need' (p. 4). Most people would prefer, at least initially, to have a dressing over their incision site to protect it from irritation or trauma, and for some, to hide the incision. Wounds should be assessed to observe the need for cleansing and replacing the dressing. Note that some agencies consider the dressing of a clean surgical incision, once it is re-epithialialised, to warrant a clean approach rather than an aseptic dressing technique. Showering and a simple wound covering generally suffice (Schellack, 2020). Check the policies of the facility. Both clean and aseptic methods of cleansing a wound are presented in this Clinical Skill.

EVIDENCE OF THERAPEUTIC INTERACTION

Explain the procedure, the reason for assuming a particular position and your expectations of the person. This helps ensure their cooperation, reduces the risk that they will touch either the wound or something sterile, and reduces the necessity of talking during the procedure. These actions will reduce contamination of the wound and of sterile items. You will be able to gain their consent and reduce any anxiety they may have.

DEMONSTRATE CLINICAL REASONING

Preparation of the environment, attention to the person's comfort and positioning all make changing the dressing simpler, safer and easier. A brief health assessment will help you make decisions on care.

Prepare the environment

Provide privacy to minimise embarrassment. Restrict airflow (i.e. close windows and curtains and shut off fans) so that airborne microorganisms are less likely to contaminate the wound. Adjust lighting to assist with assessment and treatment. Place a waterproof disposal bag with a cuff near the person's bedside or clip it onto the side of the dressing trolley to receive contaminated articles and to prevent transmission of microorganisms (the plastic package of the dressing pack is often used). The bag should be placed between the wound and the sterile field so that contaminated material is not carried over it. A folded cuff on the bag ensures that the bag's outer surface is not contaminated. A bulldog clip is used in preference to tape as the accumulation of adhesive on the trolley over time provides a harbour for microorganisms.

ELDER CARE

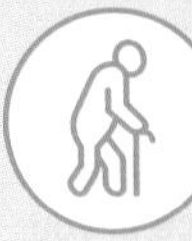

Take care not to expose any more of the person's body than necessary, as usually elderly people feel the cold more than younger people due to vasoconstriction in their limbs. Assess the elderly person's skin texture and integrity prior to using adhesive or even paper tape. Fragile elderly skin tears easily. Sinha, Free and Ladlow (2022) recommend NOT using any adhesive on the forearms/hands of people with fragile skin (may cause skin tears), but using a foam dressing covered with silicone and using a remover wipe to remove the dressing. Use a gauze (e.g. Tubigrip netting) or elastic bandage around the limb to secure the dressing. Use tape on the dressing material only.

THE PERSON LIVING WITH SEVERE OBESITY

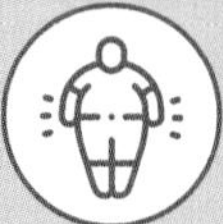

Adipose tissues have poor blood supply and inadequate tissue oxygenation, which alters wound healing. The severely obese person has a raised core body temperature (due to the insulating effect of adipose tissue), resulting in increased perspiration, moist skin (especially in folds – axilla, under breasts, under abdominal 'apron', perineum) that can frequently result in bacterial or fungal growth (Earlam & Woods, 2020) and delay healing. The moist skin also reduces the adhesion of dressings/tape. You may need to reinforce or replace tape between dressings.

Position the person

Position the person comfortably to reduce movement during the procedure, which can contaminate sterile items. When positioning, consider the time the person will need to stay still and the area to be exposed. Attend to your own comfort when doing the procedure to prevent wound contamination and self-injury from assuming an awkward position. Raise the bed to a comfortable height for you (about waist level). Most people find that working with their dominant hand positioned closest to the bottom of the bed allows for the greatest manoeuvrability.

Offer a bedpan, urinal or assistance to the toilet prior to the procedure, which will reduce unnecessary interruptions and increase their comfort. Give analgesia 20 to 30 minutes before the procedure (as necessary) to reduce discomfort, increase cooperation and aid relaxation. Time the dressing change in consultation with the person, to coincide with the timing of doctors' rounds (so they can assess the wound without removing the dressing twice), and so that rest periods or mealtimes are not disrupted. Some surgeons do not permit nursing staff to change the first dressing at 24 to 48 hours post-operation, and change it themselves. Check the facility's procedure.

Brief health assessment

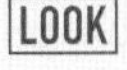

at information in the person's health record for any comorbidities, their nutritional and hydration status, if there are signs of systemic infection, the cause of the wound (e.g. clean surgical incision, traumatic wound). This information will help you to make appropriate decisions about their care (Annesley, 2019). Take the vital signs to check that all are within normal range for the person (especially temperature).

PERFORM DRY DRESSING TECHNIQUE

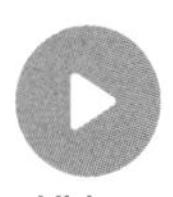

Video

Hand hygiene

Put on a plastic apron, mask and eye protection (as required) prior to hand hygiene so you don't contaminate clean hands by touching your face, hair or uniform. Perform hand hygiene (see **Clinical Skill 5**) and put on clean gloves (see **Clinical Skill 6**). Hand washing is the most significant factor in reducing wound infections (Smith, 2020).

Aseptic technique for cleaning a wound

Remove the soiled dressing

Remove the tape carefully. Hold the skin around the tape and pull the tape towards the wound to reduce stress on the fresh incision. Use short gentle pulls parallel to the skin to minimise pain. A non-irritating solvent can be used to remove adhesive painlessly (use the facility's protocol).

?

If the dressing adheres to the wound, moisten it with sterile NS and leave it for a few minutes. This loosens the dried drainage so that new granulating tissue is not pulled off the healing wound.

Next, remove the dressing with the soiled surface away from the person to reduce possible distress. Assess it for drainage, noting amount, colour, consistency and odour. Assess the undressed wound (see below). Carefully place the dressing (usually folded over itself) in the disposal bag without contaminating the outside of the bag. Blood and fluid on the skin around, but not close to, the wound should be removed with a warm washcloth. Remove your gloves and place in the disposal bag.

PART 13

GATHER EQUIPMENT

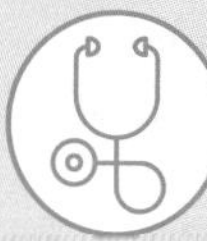

Gather and prepare the equipment for the procedure before proceeding to the bedside. This ensures that you have all items and allows you to mentally rehearse the steps in the procedure. It prevents the need for assistance to obtain forgotten items, since leaving an aseptic set-up risks contamination. Being organised enhances your self-confidence and promotes the individual's confidence in you.

EQUIPMENT	EXPLANATION
Dressing trolley (dedicated to aseptic uses)	• To transport materials to and from the bedside • Must be cleaned with antiseptic or detergent wipes before placing equipment onto it (Denton & Hallam, 2020a)
Dressing packs	• Sterile pack sealed in a (usually) plastic bag. Check the expiry date and for intactness (Denton & Hallam, 2020b) • Usually commercially supplied. Each contains a waterproof wrapper that becomes the critical aseptic field when the pack is unwrapped. There is a receptacle with gauze squares that is used as a solution bowl • There are usually sufficient supplies in this for a minimally draining wound. If the wound drainage is more than a small amount, additional supplies of sterile gauze squares for cleansing and drying are added • Usually contains three forceps in the pack (ask if you are unsure, so you can obtain an extra forceps if needed) • Sits on the top of the trolley; the remainder of the equipment is placed on the lower shelf
Waterproof bag	• To contain all used and contaminated material to prevent transmission of microorganisms (often the packaging from the dressing pack is sufficient) • Is clipped to the trolley with a bulldog clip (or similar)
Sterile solution	• Usually normal saline (NS) is used to cleanse the wound • The small amount needed is supplied in plastic ampoules of 10 mL and 20 mL • Warmed solutions reduce stress reactions in most people and reduce disruption of the healing process
Wound ruler	May be needed to assess the wound, although often not necessary in a simple non-infected incision
Dressings Watch for new materials (e.g. bamboo viscose and polysaccharide chitosan fabrics) that are biocompatible, with good absorbency, mechanical integrity, reduced wound adhesion and good healing properties (Shyna et al., 2020)	• To protect the wound • Non-adherent dressings with a hypo-allergenic covering are frequently used; these promote absorption while minimising wound adherence to the dressing by dried exudate (e.g. Telfa, Primapore, Melolin). Melolin is generally obtained from the central sterile services department (CSSD) in sterile packs that have been cut to size. Use of a non-adherent dressing prevents trauma to the wound during removal (Williams, 2020) • Moisture-retentive dressings have demonstrated superiority to simple dry dressings in assisting with wound healing. The natural moisture produced by the wound has proteins and cytokines that facilitate the formation of granulation tissue and healing (Sinha, Free & Ladlow, 2022) • Gauze dressings are also absorbent but adhere to a draining wound and cause trauma, disruption of granulation and pain when removed. They may be used over the top of the non-adherent dressing for extra bulk. There is no clear evidence that one dressing type is better than another in reducing the risk of surgical site infection (Williams, 2020) • Follow the facility's dressing protocol
Tape	• To secure the dressing to dry intact skin. Many dressings are 'island' types with the dressing material surrounded by adhesive (e.g. Primapore), making the use of tape unnecessary • Micropore or a paper tape are very effective at adhering to intact skin and are easier and less painful to remove than adhesive tapes. Preferred because many people are allergic or sensitive to adhesive tape
Gloves (clean)	• To remove the soiled dressing to minimise contamination • Some agencies also ask you to use sterile gloves during the actual dressing procedure; others rely on your use of Aseptic Non Touch Technique (ANTT) (see **Clinical Skill 7**) for the dressing procedure
Masks	Required by some agencies to prevent droplet spray from your respiratory tract from contaminating the wound
Apron	To prevent contamination to the site and protect your uniform
Goggles	Required if splashing is anticipated (unlikely for a dry dressing))

Some practitioners advocate leaving the final inner dressing in place until the critical aseptic field is established, then removing the dressing with an extra forceps, and disposing of the dressing and forceps in the waterproof bag. This reduces the chance of wound contamination (either by the person or from the environment) while you perform hand hygiene and set up the sterile field.

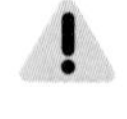
Safety

Follow the procedure for an aseptic or clinical hand wash (see **Clinical Skill 5**).

Establish a critical aseptic field

Open the dressing pack and tip the wrapped tray onto the top of the freshly cleaned trolley (use the package as your receptacle for contaminated items by cuffing it and clipping it to the edge of the trolley nearest to the person). Carefully manipulate the wrapped tray so the first fold is opened away from you. Take care to touch only the outside of the wrapper – the inside will become your critical field. Open the side flaps with the hand on that side (right hand, right fold of the wrap) so your hands are not moving across your critical field. Finally, open the wrapper flap closest to you. Adjust the position of the wrapper/tray by grasping the underside of the wrapper. Add all items necessary for the dressing using ANTT (see **Clinical Skill 7**). Add the solution. Perform hand hygiene

Put on sterile gloves (as per agency policy) (see **Clinical Skill 9** for open gloving method). Place the sterile drape beside the wound to extend the critical aseptic field and to help prevent contamination of equipment. Discard the cotton balls (if supplied), as these leave lint in the wound and along the incision line. Arrange the sterile items for convenience. Pour cleansing solution into one of the tray's pots. Soak half of the gauze squares with the cleansing solution.

Use the extra forceps to remove and discard the inner dressing if this has not been done.

Assess the wound

LOOK at the incision. There should be only minimal oedema, the incision line plus 1 to 2 cm of skin on either side may be pink to red, and warm. Are the edges well approximated? No gaping of the incision? Are the sutures/staples intact? Is there any sign of infection (erythema, purulent drainage, swelling) or haematoma?

Is there a drain present? Note location, type. Assess the drain incision as above. Measure the wound if indicated.

Assess the skin that was under the adhesive tape. Look for mechanical damage (skin tears, blisters, skin stripping); dermatitis (irritation, inflammation); maceration (wrinkled, moist skin from moisture trapped under the tape) and folliculitis (inflammation of hair follicles) (Fumarola et al., 2020).

LISTEN to any reports of incisional pain or pain in the immediate area.

FEEL (with sterile gloves on) the edges of the incision for oedema or induration. Be very gentle. There should be only minimal oedema, and feel firmer than the adjacent skin (i.e. induration).

SMELL any drainage (many infecting bacteria produce a distinctive odour).

Standardised systems for the assessment and documentation of wounds enable early identification of problems and early intervention to minimise harm (Boga, 2019).

Clean the wound

Squeeze excess solution out of the gauze squares with the sterile forceps so that there is no dripping solution to soil the linen. Place these in a dry 'pot' in the tray. Keep the forceps tip lower than the handles to prevent contamination by fluid travelling up and then down the handle. Use one gauze square for each stroke; cleanse the wound and surrounding skin until no trace of discharge is visible. Use the following principles (also see FIGURE 67.1):

1. Clean from the top of the incision to the bottom, since gravity pulls drainage to the bottom of the wound.
2. The incision is considered the least contaminated area and all strokes move outwards from the incision to prevent bringing microorganisms from the skin in towards it (Lalonde, Joukhadar & Janis, 2019).
3. Any area that looks infected is cleansed last.

Discard each swab into the waterproof bag. Using the same principles, dry the cleansed area with the dry gauze squares to promote comfort and to assist the tape to adhere.

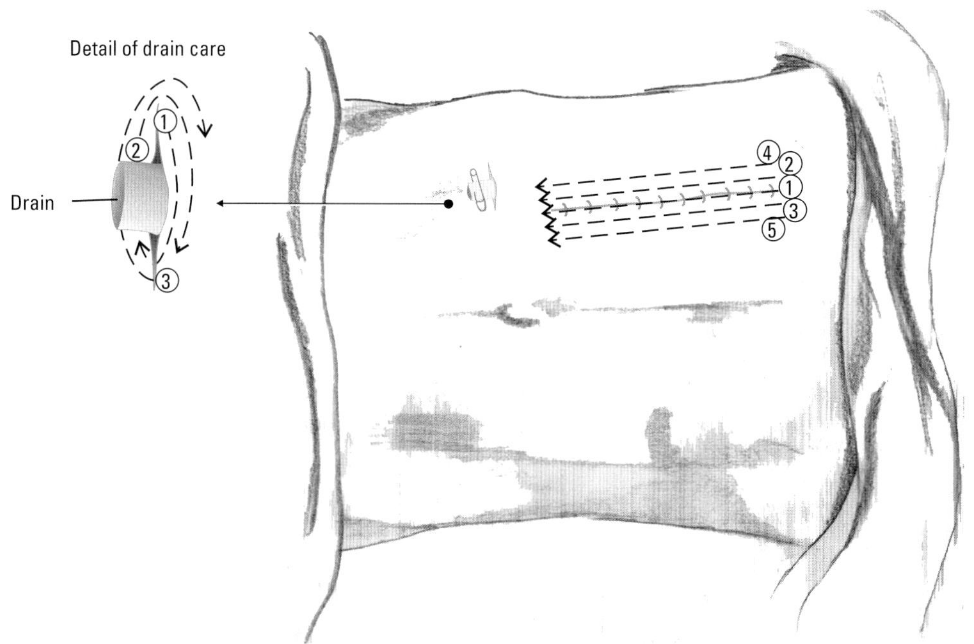

FIGURE 67.1 Direction of swab movement in an uncomplicated wound

Apply a dry dressing

Apply dressings to the incision or wound in layers to ensure optimal absorption. Use ANTT. The initial layer is usually Melolin, followed by gauze squares. If more drainage is expected, a thicker pad (e.g. Combine) is often applied. The incision may need more padding at the lower end to absorb extra drainage brought by gravity. Using a sterile dressing on a clean wound for longer than 48 hours is costly, prolongs hospitalisation and provides no benefits to the individual; however, a clean, protective dressing may increase comfort.

Remove your gloves and perform hand hygiene. Secure the dressing.

Clean method of cleansing a wound

Assess the wound

Perform hand hygiene and don clean gloves. Assess the person (e.g. severe obesity, comorbidities, diabetes) and the wound before determining that a clean method of wound care is appropriate. Remove the dressing to visually assess the wound (as with ANTT for cleaning a wound).

Showering the wound

Once the skin of a clean surgical incision is sealed (24 to 48 hours post-incision), showering the wound during personal hygiene is an acceptable alternative to using ANTT for cleaning the wound. The irrigating effect of the water dislodges contaminating debris and reduces bacterial contamination.

Shared bathrooms must be cleaned well between showers to reduce the risk of cross-contamination. Tap water suitable for drinking is as effective as sterile normal saline for preventing infections in open lacerations (Schellack, 2020), and can be safely used for clean surgical wounds. Teach the person to use only running water on the wound – no soap, lotion, antiseptic or bath gel, no face washer or similar – and to report any signs of infection or delayed healing to you.

If a dressing is applied to protect the wound, clean technique is to be used. Clean gloves are worn and the (usually) Primapore dressing is placed over the incision (dry skin), followed by gauze squares and tape if required to provide mechanical protection.

Remove your gloves and perform hand hygiene.

Secure the dressing

Secure the dressing with the selected tape (if not an 'island' dressing). Place the tape at the centre of the dressing and smooth evenly outwards, away from the midline. This reduces pulling and wrinkling of the skin from excessive tension. Apply tape strips at the ends of the dressing so that it cannot be folded back to expose the wound. Space the tape strips evenly across the middle of the dressing so that the dressing does not gape. If possible, place the tape in the opposite direction from a body action (i.e. in the same direction as a body crease or joint – not lengthwise over it) to help the dressing remain secure despite movement. Tape should extend 5 to 8 cm beyond the edge of the dressing so that it will securely adhere to the skin. Create a small tab by folding under the last 0.5 cm to make removal easier. Assist the person to a position of comfort that does not stress the incision or wound.

Remove your gloves and perform hand hygiene.

CLEAN, REPLACE AND DISPOSE OF EQUIPMENT

Perform hand hygiene and don clean gloves. Seal contaminated material in the disposal bag and then wrap it in the disposable wrapper that has formed the sterile field. Place the bundle on the bottom shelf of the trolley and then into the contaminated waste bin in the dirty utility room. Wipe down the trolley and the bulldog clip with the recommended solution. If gross contamination has occurred, use soap and water, then the solution. Return the trolley to its position in the clean service area of the unit. Shelve solutions to be reused in front of unopened solutions so that they can be used quickly and to avoid waste. Wash and dry any non-disposable equipment used (e.g. forceps) and return to the CSSD for sterilisation. Remove your gloves and perform hand hygiene.

DOCUMENTATION

Relevant information to be documented in the healthcare record includes the date and time, your assessment of the wound and drainage, the type of dressing applied and the person's response to the procedure (Do, Edwards & Finlayson, 2021).

CLINICAL SKILLS ASSESSMENT

Dry dressing technique

Demonstrates the ability to effectively and safely perform dry dressing technique. Incorporates the *National Safety and Quality Health Service Standards*: 2 Partnering with consumers, 3 Preventing and controlling healthcare-associated infections, 5 Comprehensive care, 6 Communicating for safety, and 8 Recognising and responding to acute deterioration (Australian Commission on Safety and Quality in Health Care [ACSQHC], 2021).

Performance criteria	1	2	3	4	5
(Numbers indicate NMBA *Registered Nurse Standards for Practice*)	(Dependent)	(Marginal)	(Assisted)	(Supervised)	(Independent)
1. Identifies indication (1.1, 3.3, 3.4)	☐	☐	☐	☐	☐
2. Evidence of therapeutic interaction with the person, e.g. gives the person an explanation of the procedure (1.4, 1.5, 2.1, 2.2, 3.2)	☐	☐	☐	☐	☐
3. Demonstrates clinical reasoning abilities, e.g. positions the person comfortably, administers analgesia if required, prepares the environment (1.1, 1.2, 1.3, 1.5, 4.1, 4.2, 4.3, 5.1, 6.1)	☐	☐	☐	☐	☐
4. Gathers equipment (1.1, 5.5, 6.1): ■ dressing trolley ■ dressing pack ■ waterproof bag ■ sterile solution ■ wound ruler ■ dressing ■ tape ■ gloves, apron, eye protection	☐	☐	☐	☐	☐
5. Performs hand hygiene and puts appropriate personal protective equipment on (1.1, 3.4, 6.1)	☐	☐	☐	☐	☐
6. Removes the soiled dressing (1.1, 6.1)	☐	☐	☐	☐	☐
7. Establishes the critical aseptic field (1.1, 3.4, 6.1)	☐	☐	☐	☐	☐
8. Cleans and assesses the wound (1.1, 3.4, 4.1, 4.2, 4.3, 6.1)	☐	☐	☐	☐	☐
9. Applies a dry dressing (1.1, 6.1)	☐	☐	☐	☐	☐
10. Secures the dressing (1.1, 6.1)	☐	☐	☐	☐	☐
11. Cleans, replaces and disposes of equipment appropriately (3.6, 6.1)	☐	☐	☐	☐	☐
12. Documents relevant information (1.1, 1.4, 1.6, 2.2, 2.7, 3.5, 3.7, 6.1, 6.2, 6.5, 7.2)	☐	☐	☐	☐	☐
13. Demonstrates the ability to link theory to practice (1.1, 3.3, 3.4, 3.5)	☐	☐	☐	☐	☐

Student:

Clinical facilitator: Date:

CHAPTER 68

COMPLEX WOUNDS: DRAIN CARE AND SUTURE, STAPLE OR CLIP REMOVAL

INDICATIONS: DRAIN REMOVAL

Wound drainage systems remove collections of fluid from around surgical incisions or wounds, to reduce:

- dead space (air) and to promote tissue approximation (bringing edges together)
- tension placed on the wound by accumulated fluid (blood, serum, pus), which prevents healing
- medium for growth of microorganisms, to prevent infection
- discomfort and pain from the pressure of fluid accumulation
- and to alert the care team to leaks in an anastomosis (Gibson & Lillie, 2019).

Drains are common accompaniments to large incisions, and the sites are usually situated a short distance from the incision and are assessed and dressed separately to the incision to reduce the risk of infection (Ramesh, 2020).

Know the type of drain in situ to facilitate its removal and to determine the equipment needed. The drain may or may not be sutured in place – ascertain this information from the theatre count sheet. There are two basic types of surgical drains:

- *Closed, active, evacuator or negative pressure drains* – use a vacuum to exert a low negative pressure on the site to remove exudates into a collection bottle.
- *Open or gravity drains* – deliver the exudates, using capillary action and slight pressure differences, to the surface where it is either collected in a container or soaked into the dressings. This type of drain has a safety pin through it, close to the skin, to prevent the drain from slipping into the wound.

Drains are monitored q8h, at a minimum, for dislodgement, patency, amount and type of drainage, signs of infection, integrity of the surrounding skin and, in the case of closed drains, the pressure being exerted. Record these observations in the eHealth record or nursing notes, and the volume on the intake/output sheet.

A drain is removed when it is no longer needed; that is, when there is no further drainage or the drainage is minimal (less than 30 mL/24 hours) (Ramesh, 2020). If left too long, the drain itself becomes a track for microorganisms to enter the wound. Kushner et al. (2021) found early removal irrespective of the amount of drainage does not increase the prevalence of infection or morbidity.

Drains are being used less frequently for most surgical procedures because their use can result in negative outcomes such as surgical site infections and increased length of hospital stay (Poeran et al., 2019). Although there are other types of drains (chest, hepatobiliary), their removal is reserved for the physician, and this skill focuses on surgical site drain removal.

Verify the order for drain removal

The doctor orders removal of a drain, usually on the second day post-operation. Some physicians order gravity drains (e.g. the Penrose drain) to be shortened for a couple of days before they are removed (discussed below). The orders include whether the incision dressing is to be changed or left intact, and whether suction is to be left on or not (e.g. orthopaedic drains are generally removed with the suction left on).

INDICATIONS: SUTURE, STAPLE OR CLIP REMOVAL

The edges of a wound need to be kept together (i.e. approximated) by some mechanical means until healing is sufficient that support is no longer necessary. This could be steri-strips if there is little tension on the incision line (usually superficial incisions). More recently, a synthetic topical glue has been introduced that keeps superficial wound edges approximated; provides a waterproof barrier for the wound; is non-invasive; is simple, fast and painless to apply; and sloughs off after a week or so (Jain & Wairkar, 2019). A zipper type skin closure system (adhesive bandage with an embedded mesh to strengthen it and provision to adjust the incisional closure to approximate edges) eliminates the need for sutures, staples or clips and is used as the primary closure (Alnachoukati, Emerson & Muraguri, 2019; Sadik et al., 2018). It is not removed for several days.

Currently, either sutures or skin clips or staples are still used to support larger incisions while the wound edges heal. Both methods are traumatic to already damaged tissues,

invasive, provide a focus for inflammation and a point of entry for infection. Cochetti et al. (2020) found no conclusive evidence of the superiority of either sutures or staples in reducing wound infection or postoperative events (e.g. dehiscence). Sutures were minimally better at decreasing postoperative infection and pain. Both are removed when the need to mechanically support the incision has passed.

The average time for removal of sutures, clips or staples is five to 14 days after injury (Tan, 2020); however, the timing of suture removal is dependent on the type and depth of the incision and where it is located on the body. For example, facial incisions are removed after four to five days; chest, lower limb and abdominal sutures after eight to 10 days; and feet and palms of the hands up to 14 days (Tan, 2020). Sutures/staples left after eight days will leave scars on each side of the incision due to epithelialisation of the suture hole (Tan, 2020). Deeper retention sutures remain in the tissues and are reabsorbed by the body over a short period of time.

Verify the order for suture, staple or clip removal

A doctor's order is required to remove the sutures, clips or staples. Often, the order will be to initially remove each alternate suture, clip or staple and the remainder on the next day. You must assess the incision (e.g. blood supply, infection) and individual sutures, clips or staples prior to removing them. Consider the factors that may delay wound healing before removal, including:

- age and frailty
- diseases and disorders (e.g. anaemia, autoimmune disorders, diabetes)
- previous surgery in the same area or using same suture line (e.g. caesarean section)
- drug usage (e.g. alcohol, nicotine, steroids, anti-inflammatories, cytotoxics)
- nutritional state (e.g. anaemia, malnutrition [undernutrition and obesity], dehydration, mineral, protein and/or vitamin deficiency).

EVIDENCE OF THERAPEUTIC INTERACTION

Explain the procedure and talk about the sensations the person can expect. This provides them with information that reduces anxiety and promotes cooperation and relaxation, which increase the person's ability to tolerate a stressful procedure.

DEMONSTRATE CLINICAL REASONING

Provide comfort measures

Privacy guards the person's dignity and reduces embarrassment at the exposure of (usually) private areas of the body. Offer the bedpan, urinal or the toilet before beginning the procedure for comfort and to prevent interruptions. Offer analgesia a half-hour before the procedure so that it has time to take effect and minimise discomfort. There can be considerable discomfort during closed drain (suction on) removal, and moderate discomfort during most drain removals and suture/staple/clip removal as you manipulate an incision. Alnachoukati, Emerson and Muraguri (2019) found staples to be more painful to remove than sutures, so consider analgesia carefully before removing staples or clips. Le May et al. (2021) demonstrated the effectiveness of virtual reality as a distraction in decreasing the pain during these medical procedures.

Position the person

Expose the drain or incision area. The position should be comfortable to facilitate relaxation and stillness during the procedure to reduce the possibility of contamination of the drain or incision site. Make sure you are also well positioned so you do not become fatigued.

ELDER CARE

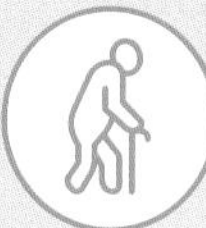

Elderly people often possess many of the factors that delay wound healing (e.g. frailty, comorbidities, dehydration, malnutrition, reduced circulation and polypharmacy), as well as possessing fragile skin and reduced subcutaneous tissues. This makes excellent assessment skills vital, so sutures/clips/staples are removed as soon as incisional healing permits to reduce the incidence of infection.

THE PERSON LIVING WITH SEVERE OBESITY

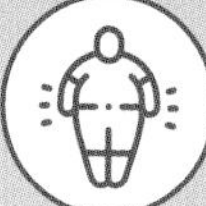

Assess well. Dehiscence is a very real possibility due to the pressure of excess tissue on the suture line and the poor healing ability of the severely obese individual. However, infection in the suture/staple insertion sites is also possible. Use caution as you remove every **<u>second</u>** suture/staple, and be prepared to support the incision line with butterfly tapes. If one area gapes, do not remove any more of the sutures/staples. (See **Clinical Skills 15 and 23** for a brief explanation of issues for people living with severe obesity.)

PART 13

GATHER EQUIPMENT

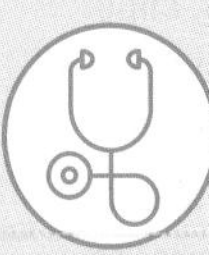

Gathering equipment is a time-management strategy, it creates a positive environment, promotes efficiency, boosts the person's confidence and trust in you and increases your self-confidence. It also provides an opportunity to mentally rehearse the procedure. Equipment will include the following:

EQUIPMENT	EXPLANATION
Dressing pack and normal saline (NS) or recommended solutions	To establish a sterile field and to cleanse the drain site
Appropriate dressing	To cover the drain site
Sterile safety pin	Used if the drain is to be shortened
Sterile scissors or sterile stitch cutters	To cut any retaining stitch in the drain and cut off excess drain material when shortening a gravity drain (straight scissors are preferred for drain shortening) Sterile scissors or stitch cutters are used to cut sutures. Tan (2020) recommends an 'iris scissor' as it is finer and less traumatic
Sterile clip or staple remover	For removal of staples, clips
Clean gloves	Worn to remove the soiled dressing from the drain site
Sterile gloves	Worn to manipulate the sterile items (e.g. scissors during suture removal and the drain removal)
Sharps container	For safe disposal if a stitch cutter is used
Waterproof pad	Protects the bed linen and the person during the procedure
Apron, face mask and goggles	To protect your uniform, skin and mucous membranes from body fluid splashes
Appropriate dressing	To cover the incision site after removing sutures/clips/staples

DRAIN CARE

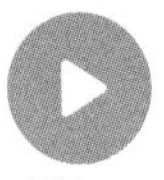

Video

Drain removal is ordered by the surgeon (or it is in the surgeon's protocol – check with the facility).

An important aspect of drain care is maintenance of the negative pressure in vacuum drains. This means checking the apparatus several times each shift and re-establishing the vacuum as necessary (each drain type will have a method of doing this, usually involving a very quick procedure [often just squeezing the reservoir]). Become familiar with the types of vacuum drains used at the facility and how to re-establish suction.

Determine if the drain is sutured in or not. This information should be on the theatre report or the nursing care plan.

When an unsutured drain is in situ, discuss the possibility of its spontaneous removal (e.g. during dressing changes, or the person may accidentally pull the drain out during movement). Reassure the person that this can occur and will be dealt with. Ask the person to take care when moving to reduce this possibility.

Drain removal is usually a simple aseptic procedure. Drains should be 'milked' prior to removal (Ramesh, 2020). Drain care (changing the dressing, removal) is a separate aseptic procedure from caring for the incision.

Hand hygiene

Hand hygiene (see **Clinical Skill 5**) removes transient microorganisms from your hands and is crucial to reduce wound contamination. Don a clean pair of gloves and other personal protective equipment as required.

Release the suction

Release the suction from the drain tubing (evacuator drains) by releasing the inlet clamp on the reservoir. This will minimise discomfort during removal. Orthopaedic drains are usually removed with the suction on so that all clots and any remaining fluid are removed with the drain. As this often causes more discomfort for the person, analgesia before the procedure is imperative.

'Milk' the drainage tube. With clean hands and gloves, hold the drain near its exit point and, with your dominant hand, gently squeeze the tube from the exit point towards the reservoir or end of the drain without releasing pressure on the tubing, pushing any discharge out of the tubing. Using an alcohol swab to do this eases the process by decreasing friction between your gloved fingers and the tube (Öztaş, Dursun & Öztaş, 2020).

Remove gloves and perform hand hygiene.

Set up the dressing tray

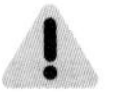

Safety

Set up the dressing tray using the principles of Aseptic Non Touch Technique (ANTT) (see **Clinical Skill 7**). The critical aseptic field provides a place to put the sterile scissors and/or stitch cutter (if needed) for later use. Place an absorbent pad between the drain site and the dressing trolley to prevent soiling of the bed linen.

Remove the drain dressing

Carefully remove the dressing to expose the drain. Use either clean gloves or forceps to remove the old dressing to prevent contaminating your hands. Aseptic/clinical hand washing (see **Clinical Skill 5**) is required because there is an open wound. Put on sterile gloves to ensure asepsis and to prevent transfer of microorganisms.

LOOK at the drainage – note colour, consistency and amount; and at the insertion site for erythema. Visually check if the drain is sutured in. Note if there is drainage or discharge from the insertion site.

FEEL the insertion site for induration (when you are removing or shortening the drain).

LISTEN to the person for reports of pain at the drain site.

SMELL for malodorous discharge.

Shorten the drain

Safety

If drain shortening is ordered (for gravity drains), use ANTT to cut and remove any retaining suture. Carefully pull out the drain to the length ordered by the surgeon (e.g. 5 cm). Insert a new sterile safety pin close to the skin, taking care not to puncture either yourself or the person. Use the sterile scissors to cut the drain between the two safety pins, then dispose of the cut drain end and safety pin in the rubbish bag. The pin reduces the risk of the drain going into the cavity.

Cleanse the drain site

Use NS or the recommended antiseptic solution and aseptic technique to prevent the transfer of microorganisms. One swab is used for each wipe. Start at the drain site and wipe in a circular pattern, spiralling outward for approximately 2 cm.

Cut the retaining suture

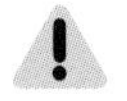

Safety

If applicable, using the sterile scissors or a stitch cutter, cut the retaining suture close to the skin. With sterile forceps, grasp the long tail of the cut suture (to prevent contaminated suture material being pulled through the skin) pull it steadily out, then remove the suture before pulling out the drain.

Remove the drain

Support the skin with a gauze square and gently remove the drain using a continuous, steady, slow motion. Distract the person while drawing out the drain to minimise discomfort. Prompting the person to breathe deeply is usually an effective distraction. Examine the drain end for intactness. Preserve it to be checked by a registered nurse (RN). Some facilities require that both observing nurses sign the theatre sheet verifying that the drain was intact when removed.

Clean the drain site

After the removal or shortening, often blood and drainage will be left on the surface. Clean it off using NS and ANTT.

Dress the drain site

When applying a new dressing to the drain/drain site, ensure that the drain is not folded onto itself, as this would cause a block in the drainage, increasing postoperative pain and chances of inflammation and infection.

Apply a dry sterile dressing (usually non-stick, such as Melolin) (see **Clinical Skill 67**) after drain removal to minimise the risk of infection. If the drain puncture site gapes, approximate the edges with a steri-strip. After shortening a drain, apply a dry sterile dressing with extra gauze under the drain and a thick dressing such as Combine to soak up any drainage. A stoma base and bag may be used over the drain if sufficient drainage is anticipated (see **Clinical Skill 72**). Maintain asepsis throughout the procedure to minimise the risk of contamination and subsequent infection. Remove your gloves and perform hand hygiene.

REMOVE A SUTURE, STAPLE OR CLIP

Sutures, staples and clips need to be removed after epithelialisation but before they become a focus of infection. Preparation of the equipment and assessment of the incision are important to efficient and safe removal of sutures, staples or clips.

Hand hygiene

Perform hand hygiene to remove microorganisms and to prevent cross-contamination (see **Clinical Skill 5**) of the wound if there are exposed tissues (e.g. dehiscence). Put on clean gloves. Use a plastic apron as required to protect your clothing and any other personal protective equipment needed.

Preparation

Set up the dressing tray

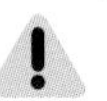

Safety

Use the ANTT principles to facilitate aseptic removal of the sutures, staples or clips (see **Clinical Skill 7**). Pour NS or ordered solutions. Put the sterile scissors, stitch cutter or clip remover on the critical aseptic field for later use. Arrange the tray. Place an absorbent pad between the incision site and the dressing trolley to prevent soiling of bed linen. Place a gauze square on the pad to drop the removed sutures, staples or clips onto.

Remove the dressing

Use either clean gloves or extra forceps to remove the old dressing to prevent contamination of your hands.

LOOK at the old dressing (check for amount, type and freshness of drainage) and discard it into the rubbish bag. Examine the incision (redness, approximation, discharge, or any gaping to determine the amount of healing) and the number of sutures/staples/clips and the type of suturing used. (See **Clinical Skill 67** for assessment of an incision.)

LISTEN to the person's reports of any discomfort from the incision or surrounding area.

Remove the gloves.

Put on sterile gloves

Perform clinical/aseptic hand hygiene and put on sterile gloves to ensure asepsis and to prevent the transfer of microorganisms.

Remove the sutures, staples or clips

Safety

This Clinical Skill discusses the removal of plain interrupted skin sutures only. Consult a nursing foundations text for removal of mattress interrupted sutures or any continuous sutures. Consult the facility and a senior nurse if retention sutures are to be removed. Usually, half of the alternate sutures are removed on one day and the remainder the next day. This supports the healing incision for an extra day.

The sutures, staples or clips are to be removed prior to cleansing the incision, unless there is gross contamination of the incision/sutures with drainage and blood. This is because dry suture material carries less contamination through the skin layers when being removed.

To remove sutures

1. Using one forceps in your non-dominant hand, grasp the knot.
2. Gently put tension on the knot until the suture comes away from the skin.
3. Slip the stitch cutter or suture scissors under the suture with the bowl of the crescent-shaped cutting edge up – at the end opposite to the knot or directly under the knot. This reduces the chance of infection by ensuring the least amount of contaminated suture material is pulled through the suture track and across the skin layers (Tan, 2020).
4. Slice or clip the suture as close to the skin as possible without endangering the person.
5. Steadily draw on the knot to pull the suture through the incision.
6. Some facilities require a more senior nurse to view the removed sutures. If so, discard the suture onto a gauze square. If this is not required, discard the suture into the rubbish bag. If the suture sticks to the forceps, wipe it off with a sterile gauze.
7. Remove every second suture, continuously inspecting the incision line for approximation. If there is no gaping, and the doctor has ordered the removal of all sutures, remove the remaining sutures.
8. Count the number of sutures you remove. Place the used stitch cutter in the sharps container.

To remove clips or staples

1. Gently insert the curved tip of the clip/staple remover under a clip/staple.
2. With the bowl of the curve facing up, gently but firmly squeeze the handle of the clip/staple remover. Do not pull upwards during the squeezing action. The squeeze bends the clip/staple in half and forces the edges of the clip/staple out of the skin.
3. When you can see both clip/staple ends, lift the clip/staple off the skin and discard it onto the gauze square. You may need to very carefully rock your hand from side to side to loosen the clip/staple ends from the skin (take care – this is painful).
4. Remove every second clip/staple and inspect the incision line.
5. If all clips/staples are to be removed and the incision line is intact, remove the remaining clips/staples.
6. Apply steri-strips along the entire incision line to provide support for an extra day or two (Tan, 2020).
7. Count the number of clips/staples you remove. Some facilities require a more senior nurse to view the removed clips/staples.

> ?
> Sometimes, wounds dehisce (gape) when a suture, clip or staple is removed. If so, leave the remaining sutures, clips or staples in place for an extra day or two. Apply a steri-strip to the incision at the point where the sutures, clips or staples came out to reapproximate the gaping wound edges and to support the open area of the wound. Inform the medical officer.

Clean the incision

Clean off any blood or fluid left on the surface by the removal of the sutures, clips or staples using gauze squares. Apply a dry sterile dressing (usually non-stick such as Melolin) to protect the wound (see **Clinical Skill 67**). Maintain asepsis throughout the procedure to minimise the risk of contamination and subsequent infection.

Remove your gloves and perform hand hygiene.

Post-procedure

Leave the person positioned comfortably with the call bell and their personal belongings within easy reach.

Following suture/staple/clip removal, teach the person to move the body part gently and only to the point of pain to reduce stress on the fresh incision line (Lalonde, Joukhadar & Janis, 2019). They should report any gaping of the incision line or drainage.

Remove a drain dressing after 24 hours. The site can be showered after 48 hours (Ramesh, 2020).

CLEAN, REPLACE AND DISPOSE OF EQUIPMENT

Wear clean gloves to protect yourself from contamination. Clean the scissors or clip/staple remover and send them to the central sterile services department (CSSD) for sterilisation. Discard disposables in the appropriate waste bin. Show the drain or the staples, clips or sutures to an RN as witness of their removal. Discard the staples or clips and the stitch cutter (if used) into a sharps container.

DOCUMENTATION

Drain removal

Measure or estimate, and record drainage on the fluid balance sheet and the drainage sheet to maintain an accurate record of the amount. Document the removal of the drain in the clinical notes or eHealth record, the care plan, the wound condition chart, the theatre count sheet (along with the signature of the witness), the fluid balance sheet and the wound drainage chart. Some facilities require the doctor's order sheet also to be signed.

Clinical notes should include the date and time of removal, witness and signature, amount and type of drainage (colour, consistency, clots or any odour), the condition of the skin around the drain incision, and the person's reaction to the procedure. Similar information is to be recorded for a drain shortening, including the length of drain removed.

Sutures, staples or clips removal

Document the condition of the incision line, and note any dehiscence, gaping, exudate or erythema. Also note the number and/or proportion of the sutures, or how many clips or staples were removed (e.g. eight alternate sutures removed). Also note the dressing that was applied afterwards.

PART 13

CLINICAL SKILLS ASSESSMENT

Complex wounds: drain care and removal and suture, staple or clip removal

Demonstrates the ability to safely remove sutures, staples and clips, or remove a drain. Incorporates the *National Safety and Quality Health Service Standards*: 2 Partnering with consumers, 3 Preventing and controlling healthcare-associated infections, 5 Comprehensive care, and 6 Communicating for safety (Australian Commission on Safety and Quality in Health Care [ACSQHC], 2021).

Performance criteria	1	2	3	4	5
(Numbers indicate NMBA *Registered Nurse Standards for Practice*)	(Dependent)	(Marginal)	(Assisted)	(Supervised)	(Independent)
1. Identifies indication for wound drainage system and drain removal (1.1, 3.3, 3.4, 6.2)	☐	☐	☐	☐	☐
2. Identifies indication for removal of the sutures, clips or staples (1.1, 3.3, 3.4, 6.2)	☐	☐	☐	☐	☐
3. Verifies written order to remove the drain or sutures, clips or staples (1.4, 3.4, 6.1, 6.2, 6.5)	☐	☐	☐	☐	☐
4. Evidence of therapeutic interactions with the person, e.g. gives the person a clear explanation of the procedure (1.4, 1.5, 2.1, 2.2, 3.2)	☐	☐	☐	☐	☐
5. Demonstrates clinical reasoning, e.g. provides privacy, pain relief and other comfort measures, positions the person (1.1, 1.2, 1.3, 4.2, 6.1)	☐	☐	☐	☐	☐
6. Gathers equipment (1.1, 5.5, 6.1): ■ dressing pack and recommended solutions ■ appropriate dressing ■ sterile safety pin ■ sterile scissors or stitch cutters, a clip or staple remover ■ clean gloves and sterile gloves ■ sharps container ■ waterproof pad ■ apron, face mask and goggles ■ appropriate dressing	☐	☐	☐	☐	☐
7. Performs hand hygiene (1.1, 3.4, 6.1)	☐	☐	☐	☐	☐
8a. Releases suction on the drain in preparation for removal (1.1, 6.1)	☐	☐	☐	☐	☐
8b. Sets up the dressing tray for drain removal (1.1, 6.1)	☐	☐	☐	☐	☐
8c. Removes the wound dressings and drain (1.1, 6.1)	☐	☐	☐	☐	☐
8d. Dons gloves (1.1, 3.4, 6.1)	☐	☐	☐	☐	☐
8e. Cleans around the drain with antiseptic solution (1.1, 6.1)	☐	☐	☐	☐	☐
8f. Cuts the suture and removes or shortens the drain (1.1, 6.1)	☐	☐	☐	☐	☐
9a. Sets up the dressing tray for removal of the sutures, clips or staples (1.1, 6.1)	☐	☐	☐	☐	☐
9b. Removes wound dressings (1.1, 6.1)	☐	☐	☐	☐	☐
9c. Assesses the suture line (1.1, 3.4, 4.2, 6.1)	☐	☐	☐	☐	☐
9d. Using aseptic technique, removes the suture/clip (1.1, 6.1)	☐	☐	☐	☐	☐
10. Cleanses and dresses the wound (1.1, 6.1)	☐	☐	☐	☐	☐
11. Cleans, replaces and disposes of equipment appropriately (3.6, 6.1)	☐	☐	☐	☐	☐
12. Documents relevant information (1.1, 1.4, 1.6, 2.2, 2.7, 3.5, 3.7, 6.1, 6.2, 6.5, 7.3)	☐	☐	☐	☐	☐
13. Demonstrates the ability to link theory to practice (1.1, 3.3, 3.4, 3.5)	☐	☐	☐	☐	☐

Student:

Clinical facilitator: Date:

CHAPTER 69

COMPLEX WOUNDS: WOUND IRRIGATION

INDICATIONS

Wound irrigations are performed to cleanse a wound of drainage and debris without disturbing new, granulating tissue. Irrigating wounds hydrates the healing tissue and improves visualisation of the base of the wound. Wounds that require irrigation are draining or producing debris (slough) or have an area of eschar. These wounds heal by secondary intention.

Biofilm is a proliferation of microbes that form a layer over the wound bed and become difficult to remove and to treat. Biofilms are characterised by a chronic inflammatory response with recurrent acute episodes resistant to both antimicrobial agents and to host defences (Bahamondez-Canas, Heersema & Smyth, 2019, p. 2). The inflammatory response delays cell proliferation plus the high levels of inflammatory mediators disrupts the normal process of proliferation and epithelialisation (Gajula, Munnamgi & Basu, 2020).

Irrigation promotes healing by removing debris, decreasing the microbial (fungal and bacterial) load in the wound, and loosening and removing eschar or necrotic tissue (International Wound Infection Institute [IWII], 2016). However, Rajhathy et al. (2023) warn that current wound care practices are based on expert opinion, not on solid research. These authors found little difference in surgical site infections between using wound irrigation and swabbing the wound with gauze.

Negative Pressure Wound Therapy (NPWT) with instillation is used in healing open wounds (those healing by secondary intention). The wound is filled with a solution, which is allowed to soak, then it is removed by extraction. This therapy is reported to decrease bacterial spread and contamination of the wound, increases circulation to the wound bed and encourages granulation tissue in a moist environment (McCaughan et al., 2020). Orlov and Gefen (2023) add that NPWT increases cell proliferation, clears wound infections earlier, decreases hospital stays and expedites wound closure. NPWT is commonly used and is being more thoroughly researched (Gabriel et al., 2021). (See the discussion in **Clinical Skill 70**.) Chronic wounds are those that do not progress through timely healing, and include pressure ulcers, diabetic foot ulcers and leg ulcers (Wounds Australia, 2016). Wound irrigation is one of the treatments used on chronic ulcers as part of the regimen to facilitate wound healing (Falcone et al., 2021). Please consult **Clinical Skill 59** as well as medical-surgical texts and specialist literature for discussion on chronic wounds and their treatment.

EVIDENCE OF THERAPEUTIC INTERACTION

Explain the procedure, the positioning and the expectations required of the person to ensure their cooperation, to reduce the risk of their touching something sterile and contaminating it, and to reduce the necessity of talking during the procedure. Tell the person about their wound (ask first to determine their readiness to learn) and its progress to empower them in their healthcare decisions and improve their self-management practices after discharge (Tobiano et al., 2022). Discuss the reason for the swab for culture and sensitivity (C&S) (see below) if one is needed, and let them know that there will be some discomfort during collection.

Wounds impact people psychologically as well as physically. Pain, altered body image, altered function, fear of disfigurement, or of the future, and perhaps grief affect those with chronic or large wounds. People with dark skin (Grabowski, Pacana & Chen, 2020) and Asian people are more prone to keloid formation (with resulting body image/psychological effects) following trauma or surgery (Ojeh et al., 2020). Listen carefully and be aware of their psychological wellbeing (Annesley, 2019).

DEMONSTRATE CLINICAL REASONING

Comfort

Offering a bedpan, urinal or assisting to the toilet prior to the procedure reduces unnecessary interruptions and increases comfort. A number of factors may cause pain during wound care, such as the disease process, the wound care procedure or product, skin problems, social or emotional issues or professional issues. Analgesia given 20 to 30 minutes prior to the procedure (as necessary and ordered) helps reduce discomfort, increases cooperation and helps relax the person. Record pain scores and vital signs for later comparison.

Prepare the environment

Provide privacy to minimise embarrassment. Restrict airflow by closing windows and curtains and shutting off fans, so that airborne microorganisms are less likely to contaminate the wound. Provide adequate lighting to assist in assessment and treatment. Clip a cuffed waterproof disposal bag near the bedside to receive contaminated articles to prevent transmission of microorganisms. The folded cuff on the bag ensures that the bag's outer surface is not contaminated.

Position the person

A comfortable position during the procedure reduces movement, which can contaminate sterile items. Consider the position in relation to the time the person needs to remain still and the body part being exposed to make irrigation accessible. Position them so that the irrigating solution flows through the wound from the cleanest area to the dirtiest area and out into the second basin. Place a protective pad under the person. Ensure you can comfortably access the wound site to eliminate contamination or self-injury from using an awkward position for the treatment.

ELDER CARE

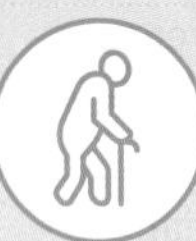

Elderly people both develop chronic wounds more readily (due to dry, thin, fragile skin, and little subcutaneous tissue increasing effects of pressure) and heal more slowly (from a combination of chronic diseases, decreased circulation, malnutrition and dehydration) than do younger people. The elderly and those who are immune compromised may not present with the classic signs of a wound infection but may lose their appetite, be drowsy, nauseous, restless or confused.

They may have difficulty in maintaining the required position for irrigating the wound without assistance from another nurse. Take care when bandaging that only paper tape, gauze netting or crepe bandaging is used to secure the dressing to preserve fragile skin. A consultation with a nutritionist may assist with the healing of the wound (Vranešić Bender & Krznarić, 2020).

THE PERSON LIVING WITH SEVERE OBESITY

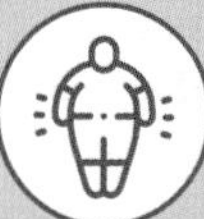

Severely obese people also develop chronic wounds more frequently than others (excess weight increasing pressure on bony prominences, limited mobility, reduced circulation, moist skin, friction when being moved) and healing is also impaired (again, nutrition is a big factor, as is infection following surgery, decreased vascularisation of adipose tissue) (Sen, 2019). Often, access to the wound of a severely obese person is difficult and a second nurse will be needed to support the person in the position required. These people also need excellent nutritional support.

GATHER EQUIPMENT

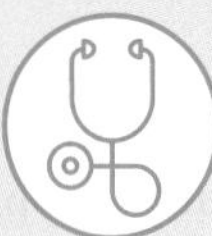

Gathering equipment for use during the procedure is a time-management strategy. Having all the necessary items available prevents having to seek assistance, since leaving a sterile set-up to obtain forgotten items risks contamination. Being organised increases your self-confidence and promotes the individual's confidence in you. Perform hand hygiene. Equipment will include the following:

EQUIPMENT	EXPLANATION
Dressing trolley	• To transport materials to and from the bedside • Must be cleaned before placing equipment onto it
Dressing pack	• Usually commercially supplied and contains a waterproof wrapper that becomes a critical aseptic field when the pack is unwrapped • A receptacle in the pack is used as a solution bowl • It contains gauze squares, a drape and some forceps
Sterile drape	To establish a critical aseptic field
Sterile solution	• To cleanse the wound – usually normal saline (NS) as it is isotonic and non-cytotoxic, or tap water in a clean vessel (Annesley, 2019) • Amount needed is dependent on amount of debris and bacterial load; 50 to 100 mL of NS or tap water per square centimetre is suggested (Lewis & Pay, 2023). As the amount is variable, check with the nursing care plan for previous care

EQUIPMENT	EXPLANATION
	• Warm solutions to near body heat to reduce discomfort and to prevent disruption of granulation (Royal Children's Hospital Melbourne [RCHM], 2023). Cold solutions slow healing. Warm the container in a warm bath • Infected wounds require a different solution. There is a great array of solutions available (e.g. chlorhexidine or Betadine solutions) • Antiseptic or antibiotic solutions tend to damage the granulating tissue and can contribute to development of antibiotic-resistant organisms (Annesley, 2019). They also prevent a culture swab from being accurate, as the swab is obtained following cleansing and debridement of the wound to ensure the microbes are recovered at or below the wound surface (Haalboom et al., 2019) • Antimicrobial and surfactant solutions dislodge biofilm to decrease chances of infection (IWII, 2016). New cleansing solutions for chronic and infected wounds (e.g. polyhexanide and betaine) are proving effective for treating colonised or infected wounds by disrupting biofilm and providing antimicrobial action
Wound ruler	To assess the wound, providing accuracy and consistency
Irrigating syringe	• A 30 to 50 mL syringe with a longer tip (or a 35 mL syringe with a 19-gauge catheter) that delivers a steady pressure (4 to 15 psi) of solution into the wound, dislodging debris without damaging granulating tissue or driving debris deeper (Lewis & Pay, 2023) • A pressure of 7 psi is safe and effective for wound irrigation and reduces the bacterial load by 80 per cent (Bonham, 2016; Lockwood, 2023). Squeezing the NS in a plastic ampoule/container into the wound does not generate enough pressure to dislodge debris and bacteria (Gabriel, 2021) • Commercial irrigation systems with shields that prevent splashback and flexible nozzle extensions are available but are used only for large wounds because of the cost
Two basins	One holds the sterile solution or tap water so it can be drawn into the syringe with minimal risk of contamination. A second is needed to collect the irrigant as it flows from the wound
Waterproof pad	A protective pad prevents soiling of the person's gown and bed linen and reduces your workload
Dressings	• Protect the wound (see **Clinical Skill 67**) • Optimal wound coverage requires moist dressings, which support autolytic debridement, absorb exudate, and protect surrounding normal skin (Daley, 2017)
Tape	Secures the dressing to dry intact skin (see **Clinical Skill 67**)
Clean gloves	To remove the soiled dressing to minimise contamination
Sterile gloves	To protect you and to reduce contamination
Apron, face mask and goggles	• To protect your uniform, skin and mucous membranes from body fluid splashes • Mask prevents droplets from your respiratory tract contaminating the wound and protects you from the aerosolised irrigating solution containing bacteria
Waterproof bag and bulldog clip	To contain contaminated material, preventing transmission of microorganisms
Sterile disposable containers, sterile cotton swabs Biohazard bag	• The swabs and a collection tube come in a sterile package to collect specimens for C&S, as required • Prepare a label with the person's information, site of the specimen swab, time and the test ordered • Some C&S tests require a specific medium for culturing (anaerobic, liquid or gel). Consider this when choosing an appropriate container for transport to the laboratory

PERFORM IRRIGATION OF A WOUND

Irrigating a wound must be done gently to minimise the risk of traumatising new tissue or of driving debris deeper into the wound. Follow the protocols of the facility.

Use personal protective equipment

Safety

Put on a plastic apron, a mask and eye protection prior to hand hygiene so that touching your face, hair or uniform does not contaminate your hands and any splash-back does not contaminate you or your uniform (Gabriel, 2021).

Hand hygiene

Perform hand hygiene to remove microorganisms and to prevent cross-contamination (see **Clinical Skill 5**).

Fry (2019) and Boyce (2023) found alcohol-based hand rub (ABHR) to be as effective as traditional aqueous hand washing in preventing surgical site infections.

Remove the soiled dressing

Remove the tape carefully by holding the skin around it and pulling it towards the wound so that stress is not applied to the open wound. Use short pulls parallel to the skin to minimise pain. Use clean gloves. If the old dressing adheres to the wound, moisten it with sterile NS and give it a few minutes to loosen so that new granulating tissue is not pulled off the healing wound. Then remove the dressing with the soiled surface away from the person to reduce possible distress. Assess the dressing (see below). Carefully place the dressing and the gloves in the disposal bag without contaminating the outside of the bag. Perform hand hygiene (see **Clinical Skill 5**).

Establish a critical aseptic field

Safety

Add all items necessary for the irrigation (see **Clinical Skill 7**), including the sterile pack (swab and container in a sterile bag) for collecting a specimen for culture and sensitivity if ordered. Add the solution. Place a sterile drape beside the wound to extend the sterile field and to help prevent contamination of equipment. Put on sterile gloves. Arrange the sterile items for convenience. Position one of the basins beneath the wound to catch the irrigating solution.

Assess the wound

Know the type of wound, its aetiology (original mechanism of injury), duration and the location of the wound. Find out about any systemic conditions that would affect wound repair (e.g. diabetes, severe obesity).

LOOK at:
- *wound dimensions* – length, width, depth; use a wound ruler and probe if necessary to determine undermined edges, sinuses
- *exudate* – type (e.g. purulent, serous, serosanguineous), amount, colour, consistency, odour
- *appearance of the wound bed* – granulating, sloughing, necrotic, foreign material, visible structures (e.g. tendons, bones), fistula formation
- *appearance of the wound edge* – raised, level, colour, tunnelled, rolled, undermined
- *integrity and characteristics of the surrounding skin* – healthy, erythematous, macerated, desiccated, alteration in pigmentation, dermatitis
- *phase of wound healing* – haemostasis, inflammation, reconstruction, maturation
- *signs of inflammation and infection* – purulent discharge, malodorous, erythematous, oedematous.

LISTEN to reports of wound pain (during dressing change? chronic? continuous?), its characteristics (location, intensity, duration, radiation, descriptive characteristics).

FEEL with sterile gloves the edges of the wound and peri-wound skin for oedema, induration and heat.

SMELL the discharge – many bacteria produce distinctive odours.

Adapted from: Nagle, Waheed & Wilbraham (2020).

Irrigate the wound

Irrigate a wound with a wide opening

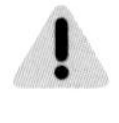
Safety

1. Using Aseptic Non Touch Technique (ANTT) (see **Clinical Skill 7**), clean the wound edges outward for approximately 5 cm (Lewis & Pay, 2023). See **Clinical Skill 67**.
2. Fill the syringe with warmed irrigating solution.
3. Hold the syringe tip 2.5 cm above the wound edge to prevent contamination of the tip (which would necessitate using another syringe).
4. Applying continuous pressure, flush the wound to remove debris and clean the wound.
5. Repeat the above steps until the irrigating solution draining into the basin is clear. This indicates the wound is clean.
6. Dry the peri-wound area using non-lint gauze squares to prevent skin maceration and to increase comfort.

Irrigate a deep or irregular wound or one with a small opening

1. Using ANTT, clean the wound edges outward for approximately 5 cm (Lewis & Pay, 2023). See **Clinical Skill 67**.
2. Fill the irrigating syringe.
3. Attach a small, soft catheter to permit direct flow into hidden areas of the wound.
4. Insert the moistened tip of the catheter into the wound until it touches a surface, then pull back about 1 to 2 cm to remove the tip from the fragile tissue.
5. Using slow, continuous pressure and rotating the tip of the catheter, flush the wound to reach every surface for cleansing.
6. Pinch off the catheter just below the syringe, keep the catheter tip in the wound and refill the syringe to avoid contamination of the solution.
7. Repeat steps 2 to 5 until the return flow is clear. The wound will take longer to empty because of the small opening.
8. Dry the wound using non-lint gauze squares to prevent skin maceration and to increase comfort.

Irrigation during a shower

For many wounds (e.g. lanced abscesses, chronic ulcers, shallow wounds), irrigation is done during the person's daily shower. Tap water has been demonstrated to be safe and effective for many types of 'clean' wounds (Holman, 2023) and reduces infection rates when compared to NS in acute wounds, although there was no difference in chronic wound healing rates (Lewis & Pay, 2023). The person must be immune competent if this method is used (Rajhathy et al., 2023).

Run the water for 15 seconds before applying it to the wound. Using a hand-held shower nozzle and gentle water pressure (cover nozzle with a clean face washer if necessary), direct warm tap water into the wound opening from approximately 30 cm away. Teaching the person to care for themselves helps them to return to the community at the earliest possible time.

?

If an acute wound shows signs of infection (e.g. malodorous, purulent drainage; inflammation in or around the wound; an increase in amount of drainage; or the person is febrile; or a chronic wound shows signs of spreading or of systemic infection [IWII, 2016]), a wound swab for C&S is taken. Obtain a specimen (see 'Obtain a specimen for culture and sensitivity') following wound cleansing so that infective material rather than colonising bacteria is obtained (Haalboom et al., 2019).

OBTAIN A SPECIMEN FOR CULTURE AND SENSITIVITY

Culture and sensitivity (C&S) is a laboratory test on wound material to diagnose an infection, including the responsible microorganism, the number of organisms present, and the effective antimicrobial agent. There are three methods of obtaining the wound material:

- a biopsy, which is invasive, painful, expensive and requires a physician to perform
- a needle aspiration of wound bed exudate, which can also be painful and requires skill and experience to undertake
- and a wound swab, which is non-invasive, relatively pain-free and practical as it is undertaken by the staff nurse.

Position the person for comfort and privacy, perform hand hygiene and use ANTT. Irrigate to clean and debride the wound with warm NS (no antimicrobial or antiseptic solutions). Remove the container and swabs from the bag (usually supplied as a unit in a sterile plastic bag) and take out the swabs. Moisten the swab tip with sterile NS. Be careful not to touch the sides of the wound or the surrounding skin. Firmly place the swab in the centre of the base of the wound where it is cleanest (do not collect necrotic material or dry crusted debris) or the leading edge of the infection (James, 2018). Rotate the swab several times over at least 1 cm^2 area of viable tissue in the wound base in a zigzag fashion, using enough pressure to express fluid from within the wound tissue (Haalboom et al., 2019). Again, being careful not to touch the wound sides or skin, withdraw the swab and carefully place it into the plastic tube. Seal it in with the cap and squeeze the opposite end to release the medium (if any) into the tube. Put the tube off the sterile field. Later, use the label to identify the person, time, date, clinical symptoms that prompted the C&S and any other pertinent information (e.g. post-operation day, diabetes). Note the anatomical position of the wound and any current or recent antibiotic cover (James, 2018). Place the swab in a biohazard bag. Take the swab to the laboratory immediately.

> ? If the wound has a sinus/pocket, use a separate swab and container. Label the container with 'from sinus' or something similar as well as the information discussed above.

Apply a sterile dressing

A protective dressing is applied to create a moist healing environment (enabling migration of tissue-repairing cells and spread of immune and growth factors), protect the wound, reduce the introduction of microorganisms, contain drainage, prevent odour, reduce movement, reduce accidental trauma to the site, provide comfort and decrease distress by covering the wound (Parker, 2019). There are various wound-management protocols used from here. Products are available to debride the wound, to maintain moisture and to remove exudate. Impregnated or plain gauze, hydrocolloids, hydrogels, alginate or bead dressings are variously available. Follow the facility's protocol.

Apply dressings to the wound in layers to ensure optimal absorption. Use aseptic technique (see **Clinical Skill 7**). Remove and discard gloves at this point.

Secure the dressing

Use the selected tape to secure the dressing comfortably (see **Clinical Skill 67**). Remove protective clothing and goggles. Perform hand hygiene. Reposition the person comfortably.

CLEAN, REPLACE AND DISPOSE OF EQUIPMENT

Wear clean gloves to protect yourself from contamination. Seal contaminated material in the disposable bag and then wrap it in the (disposable) wrapper that formed the sterile field. Place this material in the contaminated waste bin. Empty the basins into the hopper and wipe down with the recommended disinfectant solution. If gross contamination has occurred, use soap and water. Wash the basins and send to the central sterile services department (CSSD) for sterilisation. Label solutions to be reused with the date and time opened and shelve them in front of unopened solutions so that they can be used quickly, avoiding waste.

Remove your gloves and perform hand hygiene.

DOCUMENTATION

Note relevant information, including date and time, appearance of the wound and drainage, type of dressing applied and the person's response to the procedure. Record the C&S specimen and the time it was sent/taken to the laboratory. Note any sharp alteration in comfort level or fresh bleeding and report these to the shift coordinator. This validates the care given and provides a progress report of the person's condition.

CLINICAL SKILLS ASSESSMENT

Complex wounds: wound irrigation

Demonstrates the ability to effectively and safely irrigate a wound. Incorporates the *National Safety and Quality Health Service Standards*: 2 Partnering with consumers, 3 Preventing and controlling healthcare-associated infections, 5 Comprehensive care, 6 Communicating for safety, and 8 Recognising and responding to acute deterioration (Australian Commission on Safety and Quality in Health Care [ACSQHC], 2021).

Performance criteria	1	2	3	4	5
(Numbers indicate NMBA *Registered Nurse Standards for Practice*)	(Dependent)	(Marginal)	(Assisted)	(Supervised)	(Independent)
1. Identifies indication (1.1, 3.3, 3.4)	☐	☐	☐	☐	☐
2. Evidence of therapeutic interaction with the person, e.g. gives the person a clear explanation of the procedure (1.4, 1.5, 2.1, 2.2, 3.2)	☐	☐	☐	☐	☐
3. Demonstrates clinical reasoning, e.g. administers analgesia if required, prepares the environment and positions the person comfortably (1.1, 1.2, 1.3, 1.5, 4.1, 4.2, 4.3, 5.1, 6.1)	☐	☐	☐	☐	☐
4. Gathers equipment (1.1, 5.5, 6.1): ■ dressing trolley ■ dressing pack ■ sterile drape ■ sterile solution ■ wound ruler ■ irrigating syringe ■ two basins ■ waterproof pad ■ dressings and tape ■ clean gloves and sterile gloves ■ apron, face mask and goggles ■ waterproof bag and bulldog clip ■ sterile disposable containers	☐	☐	☐	☐	☐
5. Dons appropriate protective apparel (1.1, 3.4, 6.1)	☐	☐	☐	☐	☐
6. Performs hand hygiene (1.1, 3.4, 6.1)	☐	☐	☐	☐	☐
7. Removes the soiled dressing (1.1, 6.1)	☐	☐	☐	☐	☐
8. Establishes the critical aseptic field (1.1, 3.4, 6.1)	☐	☐	☐	☐	☐
9. Assesses the wound and irrigates it (1.1, 3.4, 4.3, 6.1)	☐	☐	☐	☐	☐
10. Obtains a specimen for culture and sensitivity, if ordered (1.1, 3.4, 4.3, 6.1, 6.2)	☐	☐	☐	☐	☐
11. Applies and secures the dressing (1.1, 6.1)	☐	☐	☐	☐	☐
12. Cleans, replaces and disposes of equipment appropriately (3.6, 6.1)	☐	☐	☐	☐	☐
13. Documents relevant information (1.1, 1.4, 1.6, 2.2, 2.7, 3.5, 3.7, 6.1, 6.2, 6.5, 7.3)	☐	☐	☐	☐	☐
14. Demonstrates the ability to link theory to practice (1.1, 3.3, 3.4, 3.5)	☐	☐	☐	☐	☐

Student:

Clinical facilitator: Date:

CHAPTER 70

COMPLEX WOUNDS: FILLING A WOUND; NEGATIVE PRESSURE WOUND THERAPY

INDICATIONS

Chronic wounds are those that do not progress through the normal stages of healing and are open for more than a month (Sen, 2019; Sussman, 2023). Chronic wounds usually occur in people with other major health concerns (e.g. advanced age [Gupta et al., 2019], obesity, malnutrition, comorbidities [e.g. diabetes, immunosuppression] and psychosocial stress [Sen, 2019]). Chronic wounds include pressure ulcers, diabetic foot ulcers, ischaemic ulcers and venous (leg) ulcers as well as surgical site infections (Wound Care Centers, 2020). Wound filling is used as part of the regimen to facilitate healing of chronic wounds. Please consult **Clinical Skill 59** plus fundamentals of nursing and medical-surgical texts and specialist literature for a more specific discussion of chronic wounds, filling materials and the extended treatment required for someone with a chronic wound.

Wound filling (Dieter, 2023) or, as previously known, packing, is indicated for stage 3 or 4 wounds, which are generally deep and narrow. For large ulcers with significant tissue deficit, the wound opening will decrease in size at a faster rate than the reduction in wound depth and size of wound tunnelling/undermining, causing premature closure with a dead space that invites infection (Dieter, 2023). Dieter (2023) preferred the term 'filling' as 'packing' indicates cramming or stuffing the material into the wound. Filling absorbs exudate, provides a moist environment and prevents premature closure of the top of the wound before granulation is complete at the base of the wound. This may be called wet-to-moist dressing. There are many filling/dressing materials that are effective.

Over-packing a wound causes excessive pressure on the tissue, causing pain, impaired blood flow, and potentially tissue damage and delayed healing. Under-filling or the filling material not touching the base and the sides of the cavity encourages undermining, sinus tract or tunnelling and there is a risk of the edges rolling and abscess formation (Dieter, 2023). Take care not to stuff the cavity, but to make sure the filling material touches all sides.

Ideally, the wound care packing/dressing will:

- be non-adherent to granulating tissue
- allow for oxygenation of the wound bed
- provide a moist environment for cell proliferation and migration of immune and growth factors
- be antibacterial
- need changing infrequently
- be cost-effective
- absorb exudate
- provide a physical barrier (Aljghami, Sundas & Amini-Nik, 2019).

New materials for filling and dressing wounds are being developed and trialled (e.g. wound dressings that change colour within four hours if the wound becomes infected, dressings specific to the person with diabetes) (Aljghami, Sundas & Amini-Nik, 2019). The physician orders the type of filling, although they are often guided by nursing staff. The type of dressing material to be used is specified in the physician's order and is recorded on the wound chart; and if the dressing material will be gauze ribbon (although no longer recommended), the solution to be used will be specified and recorded as well. (Note: do not insert dry gauze.) Check the chart to establish the materials required.

EVIDENCE OF THERAPEUTIC INTERACTION

Help the person understand the healing process. Determine their knowledge level and explain from there. Talk to them to relieve some anxiety associated with the procedure. Helping the person take control of the pain (e.g. offering analgesia, using relaxation exercises, guided imagery) and informing them of the timing of the procedure (when it will be done, stopping if pain becomes great) maintains autonomy and self-concept.

Conversing with the person during the procedure is a distraction for them and helps them to manage the discomfort. Take care to keep your voice and facial expression neutral when removing the dressing/filling, especially if it is malodorous.

DEMONSTRATE CLINICAL REASONING

Provide for comfort

Assess the person's pain level and administer analgesia so that peak performance of the medication occurs during the procedure. The pain of wound care is often underestimated, and people suffer needlessly because of it.

The procedure can take 15 to 20 minutes. Position the person to achieve efficient access to the wound and to maintain their comfort so that they are less likely to move and possibly contaminate sterile items. Consider your own comfort as well. Elevate the bed to a comfortable working height and position the person to reduce your muscle strain and to minimise possible wound contamination from inadequate exposure.

Close the door or curtains and hang 'Do not disturb' signs to assure privacy. Drape the person with a bath blanket to reduce exposure and to provide warmth. Providing privacy increases trust and reduces embarrassment.

Preparation

Consult the healthcare record and other healthcare personnel for relevant information about the wound and the person. Prior knowledge facilitates the procedure and alerts you to special requirements (e.g. the need for assistance). Consider the person's age, weight and ability to assist you (e.g. dementia, confusion). You may need assistance to help minimise movement. The healthcare record will tell you the size and location of the wound, which dressing and filling material to use, and the amount of filling (and solution) you will need.

ELDER CARE

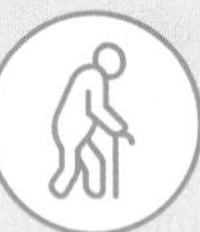

Elderly people develop chronic wounds more readily (due to dry, thin, fragile skin, and little subcutaneous tissue increasing effects of pressure) and heal more slowly (from a combination of chronic diseases, decreased circulation, malnutrition and dehydration) than do younger people. They may have difficulty in maintaining the required position for irrigating and filling the wound without assistance from another nurse. This procedure can take 20 minutes or more. Take care when bandaging that only paper tape, gauze netting or crepe bandaging is used to secure the dressing to preserve fragile skin. A consultation with a nutritionist may assist with the healing of the wound (Vranešić Bender & Krznarić, 2020).

THE PERSON LIVING WITH SEVERE OBESITY

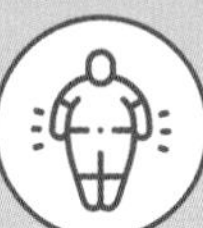

Severely obese people also develop chronic wounds more frequently than others (excess weight increasing pressure on bony prominences, limited mobility, reduced circulation, moist skin, friction when being moved), plus they are more prone to dehiscence following surgery, and their healing is also impaired (again, nutrition is a big factor, as is infection following dehiscence and surgery, decreased vascularisation of adipose tissue) (Sen, 2019). Often, access to the wound of a severely obese person is difficult and a second nurse will be needed to support the person in the position required. These people also need excellent nutritional support.

GATHER EQUIPMENT

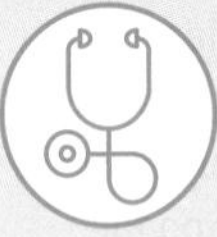

Appropriate wound dressing selection is guided by an understanding of wound dressing properties and an ability to match the level of drainage and depth of a wound (Royal Children's Hospital Melbourne [RCHM], 2023). The size and nature of the wound determines the equipment needed. Gather it all before the procedure to manage your time and increase your confidence. A mental rehearsal boosts confidence and ensures that no equipment is forgotten. The following list suggests equipment and materials generally used for filling a wound:

EQUIPMENT	EXPLANATION
Dressing trolley	• To transport materials to and from the bedside • Must be cleaned before placing equipment onto it
Dressing set or irrigation tray	To cleanse the wound
Waterproof bag	• Receives used materials so they will not cross the sterile field • Is cuffed and clipped to the trolley with a bulldog clip (or similar)
Clean gloves	To remove the dressing and the old filling before the wound is cleansed
Sterile gloves	To prevent wound contamination with microorganisms from your hands
Sterile lint-free gauze squares	For cleansing the wound if it is not irrigated (as per facility policy)
Normal saline (NS) (or other cleansing solutions as ordered)	• To cleanse or irrigate the wound • NS is the preferred solution since it is isotonic, although it has no antiseptic properties
Probe and forceps	• To estimate the wound contour • Extra sterile forceps are used with the probe to assist in inserting filling material into the entire wound

EQUIPMENT	EXPLANATION
Sterile scissors	• You cut the required amount of packing material (e.g. ribbon gauze or rope) from the package supplied • Often, you need less material than is supplied, and excess filling material that sits on intact skin eventually macerates the skin
Filling material: hydrogel, hydrocolloid alginate and gauze ribbon	• *Hydrogel* is an absorptive paste or gel used to debride the wound and to provide a moist healing environment. It is supplied in sheets or as a viscous gel that is squeezed into the wound and conforms to the shape of the cavity. It is not recommended for areas that are difficult to clean (e.g. undermined or tunnelled areas) because of the possibility of leaving contaminated material in the wound. Generally changed daily. Needs a secondary dressing
	• *Hydrocolloid alginate* rope is used for filling. It is composed of material extracted from seaweed, which expands as exudate is absorbed, forming a gel layer next to the wound surface. This material absorbs exudate, conforms to irregular spaces, eliminates dead space, promotes autolytic debridement and maintains a moist environment (Schluer, 2021). It is more cost-effective than gauze, as it remains in place for three to five days • *Gauze* ribbon or woven gauze (not recommended) is a narrow ribbon of gauze material or squares of woven gauze fluffed out, wetted with a solution and inserted into the wound. It is changed at least daily. Should no longer be used (Cutting, White & Legerstee, 2017)
Moisture-retentive dressings and occlusive dressings	Frequently used. Familiarise yourself with those used in the facility in which you are working (e.g. transparent film, silicone-based dressings)
Sterile dressing	• To cover the wound • Is often non-adherent to avoid fibres being left in the wound bed and delaying healing (e.g. Telfa) or hydrocolloid to protect the wound and keep it moist, resulting in a well-hydrated wound bed, which promotes rapid healing
Tape or tubular mesh	To secure the dressing. Ensure it is the gentlest tape available (e.g. for anyone at risk of skin damage from tape [Fumerola et al., 2020])
Apron, goggles and mask	To protect you from sprays of body fluids and infectious material and to reduce the transmission of microorganisms

FILL A WOUND

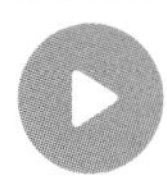
Video

Filling a wound is a skill that requires concentration, practice and patience. Use Aseptic Non Touch Technique (ANTT) (see **Clinical Skill 7**).

This method of wound management is being superseded for many types of uncomplicated wounds (e.g. chronic, pressure, diabetic and neuropathic wounds) by Negative Pressure Wound Therapy (NPWT), which stimulates granulation tissue, increases local blood flow to the wound bed, reduces wound odour, provides a moist environment and manages exudate (McCaughan et al., 2020). Further research to support these claims is needed beyond anecdotal evidence (McCaughan et al., 2020). See the section on NPWT below.

Use personal protective equipment

Put on an apron, goggles and/or a mask as needed before you wash your hands to prevent contamination of clean hands. Clip the waterproof bag to the side of the trolley.

Hand hygiene

Hand hygiene (see **Clinical Skill 5**) is an infection-control measure preventing cross-contamination. Don clean gloves to protect yourself from pathogenic microorganisms.

Remove the dressing

Loosen all the tapes (pull adhesive tapes parallel to the skin and towards the wound), grasp the old dressing and the end of the filling if rope or ribbon is used, and gently ease the dressing and filling out and off the person. Assess the amount and type of drainage. Take note of the old dressing and filling to determine the amount of new filling and dressing material needed. If that dressing and filling adequately contained the wound drainage, or debrided the wound, use it as a guide. If not, decide whether more or fewer materials are required to improve the function.

> ?
>
> **If the filling is dry and sticking to the wound, moisten it with sterile NS, wait a few moments and remove it – this protects granulating tissue. Wet-to-dry filling/dressings are considered sub-optimal care, as wound pain is two to three times higher during dressing changes when compared to advanced wound care products (Sahnan et al., 2017). They delay wound healing and increase the incidence of wound infection. Despite decades of research demonstrating the problems associated with wet-to-dry gauze dressings, their use is still common.**

Observe the filling for amount of exudate, colour, odour and consistency before disposing of it, and placing the filling and the gloves in the waterproof rubbish bag. Perform hand hygiene for a sterile procedure.

Establish a critical aseptic field

Use ANTT principles (see **Clinical Skill 7**). Put on sterile gloves and prepare all the material. For example, cut off the required length of ribbon or rope (sterile scissors), wet the ribbon with ordered solution and squeeze out the excess so the filling is damp – not sopping.

Cleanse the wound

Irrigate or use forceps and gauze squares (as per wound assessment and/or facility policy) to clean the wound and dry well (see **Clinical Skill 67**).

Assess the wound and wound margins

Monitor the healing of the wound and the condition of the surrounding skin. Use the probe in deep wounds and in undermined edges to ascertain the extent of the wound. Any deep cavity or tunnel (12 to 15 cm) should be attended by a physician, nurse practitioner or wound clinician.

LOOK at the granulation tissue – is it healthy pink to ruddy red? Friable? Discoloured? Bleeding? Be able to describe it. Look at the wound edges and periwound skin, considering colour, exudate, inflammation and irritation (see below).

LISTEN to the person's reports of pain – is the wound pain localised to the wound and immediate area? Is it more intense during dressing changes? Or does the pain not abate between dressings?

FEEL the wound edges for induration.

SMELL the wound to determine if the exudate is malodorous.

Assess the skin under the removed adhesive tape for mechanical injury (blisters, skin tears or skin stripping), maceration (damp, discoloured skin with wrinkles), folliculitis (inflamed hair follicles) or dermatitis (reddened irritated, inflamed skin). If these are present, document and report it. Determine what to use to secure the dressing (e.g. tubular net, crepe bandages, elastic bandages, stoma wafers). You may need to consult with a wound care specialist nurse.

Fill/pack the wound

Use the recommended filling material:

Safety

- Squeeze *hydrogel* into the base of the wound, using less than would be required to fill the cavity since it will expand with exudate.
- Fill the *hydrocolloid rope* loosely into the wound as it, too, expands with exudate.
- Dampen gauze ribbon or *lint-free gauze* with the solution and fill more closely, but not crammed, into the cavity (again – not recommended, but may be ordered).

Safety

Wherever possible, use a single piece (ribbon, rope, sheet, wafer) of filling to avoid a second piece being inadvertently left in the wound to become a focus of infection.

Sterile gloves as well as forceps are needed to handle the filling material. Use the probe to gently push the rope into the base of the cavity. *Do not use force* or pack the material in tightly, which would damage the new granulation in the wound. Take great care not to contaminate the probe or rope on the edges or base of the wound. One method is to wind a short length of the rope onto the forceps and use the probe to slide the material off the forceps into place. There are other methods of accomplishing this – practice and manual dexterity are required. Keep track of the amount of filling material you use. A very small 'tail' of the filling material can be left on top of the first dressing layer to facilitate removal next time. Do not leave damp filling material resting on the intact skin of the wound edge because it could macerate or erode the edge (Ayello & Sibbald, 2022).

Apply a dry dressing

Many newer dressings reduce healing time, pain, airborne contamination during dressing changes and the costs involved (Schluer, 2021). An appropriate moist wound environment maximises the biological processes required for wound healing (Gupta et al., 2019). Dressings are usually limited to those available at the facility.

Apply dressings in layers to ensure optimal absorption. Use ANTT principles. The initial layer is usually a non-stick, moisture-proof dressing, ideally with a fluid-lock technology (Ayello & Sibbald, 2022), followed by gauze squares. If more drainage is expected, a thicker pad (e.g. Combine) is applied. The wound may need more padding at the lower end to absorb extra drainage brought by gravity. Remove and discard your gloves at this point. Perform hand hygiene.

Secure the dressing

Use the selected tape to comfortably secure the dressing (see **Clinical Skill 67**). Tubular mesh may be useful, depending on the location of the wound.

Perform hand hygiene.

Closer to discharge, the individual and their support person are taught the dressing technique, using coaching and return demonstration (see **Clinical Skill 27**) to prepare them to care for the wound themselves. This may not be feasible, depending on the location of the wound, its severity and the individual's desire and ability to undertake this aspect of self-care.

Post-procedure

Assist the person to a comfortable position that does not stress the wound. Return the bed to a lower position, with their possessions and the call bell within reach. Ask the person to alert you to any changes (sensations, discharge) in the wound following the dressing change. Return to assess pain levels in approximately 30 minutes.

NEGATIVE PRESSURE WOUND THERAPY

Negative Pressure Wound Therapy (NPWT) is a now commonly used therapeutic measure for complex and chronic wounds – that is, those at risk of delayed healing. NPWT is a dressing system that uses a sealed-in foam dressing (within [usually] an infected or non-healing wound, although it is used more frequently now for large clean surgical wounds) and continuous or intermittent sub-atmospheric pressure to reduce the size of the wound, promote blood flow to the wound bed, remove exudate, stimulate granulation tissue and proliferation of cells. NPWT also protects the wound (Holloway & Harding, 2022) and maintains a moist environment (Zaver & Kankanalu, 2023). Using NPWT in clean wounds healing by secondary intention aids in approximating the edges by decreasing lateral tension and oedema to prevent dehiscence; improving tissue perfusion and stimulating granulation. It also isolates the wound from the environment to reduce bacterial contamination (Zukowski & Zukowski, 2022).

The initial NPWT system is applied (usually) in theatre. Under these sterile conditions, the open wound is debrided (if required) and thoroughly irrigated to remove any debris or necrotic material. NPWT systems consist of an open-pore sponge, a protective contact layer, an occlusive adhesive cover, a fluid collection system and vacuum pump (either mechanical or battery operated). The vacuum can be continuous or intermittent.

An expert nurse will care for the person needing NPWT and will be able to show you how the dressing is done and how the system works.

There are many wound vacuum systems, each subtly different. However, the following steps are involved in applying the system. Check the facility's protocol, and seek supervision to undertake this skill.

The equipment for the NPWT is essentially the same as that required for a wound filling (minus the filling and dressing materials). Sterile scissors and a sterile NPWT pack are added. The material you need (adhesive drape material, foam, contact protection layer, seal and connection) will be contained in a sterile pack (except the vacuum pump which is already in situ). This is a sterile procedure – use ANTT throughout along with clinical reasoning and therapeutic interaction (as above).

1. Remove the previous dressing, taking care that all material is removed from the wound (e.g. foam, protective contact layer). Foam may remove granulating tissue (hence the protective contact layer) – be gentle.
2. Assess the wound and determine healing (measure wound, assess edges, assess colour, amount of fluid being removed, odour, peri-wound skin).
3. Cleanse the wound (usually via irrigation).
4. Prepare the peri-wound skin. Cleanse it, dry it and apply a protective skin barrier 5 cm around the entire wound. This improves adherence of the drape and protects the skin from shearing and irritation.
5. Apply extra protection if necessary (e.g. skin fragile, macerated, irritated or abraded skin). To do this, cut a sheet of the transparent drape into 5 cm strips and apply them around the edges of the wound to completely cover the peri-wound skin so the foam does not contact the skin. You may need to shape these strips (i.e. cut to the shape of the edge being covered) if the wound edges are irregular.
6. Cover the wound with (ideally a single piece of) the porous foam dressing, cut exactly to the dimensions of the wound (may be available in a pre-cut formulation). Some fragile wounds will require a protective contact layer to cover the entire wound surface so the foam does not contact the wound directly.
7. Cut the basic shape of the wound out of the foam sheet, then trim to fit. Take care not to get any 'trimmings' in the wound. The foam should fit lightly (not packed) into the wound and sit higher than the skin level. Deep wounds may need extra layers of the foam.
8. Seal the wound with the transparent adhesive drape. Do not compress the foam with the drape. Carefully enclose the foam and adhere it around the edge for about 5 cm. This may need to be done with strips of overlapping drape if the wound is large.
9. Lift the centre of the drape over the foam and cut a 1 cm hole in it.
10. Apply the vacuum seal with the lumen over the hole. Seal it (usually self-adhesive to the underlying drape).
11. Attach the tube to the vacuum pump (usually a Luer Lock connection). Set the pump to the prescribed pressure and start the pump.
12. Listen for leaks (press down on any areas of leaking to secure, may need to apply more strips of drape).

> ?
> If the wound bed is too large for a single piece of foam, multiple pieces are used to adequately cover it. You must document the number of pieces used, so when the dressing is changed no pieces of foam are left inside the wound bed (Zaver & Kankanalu, 2023).

Peri-wound skin breakdown and excoriation can follow removal of the protective adhesive dressing used during NPWT. Greenstein and Moore (2021) demonstrated less skin damage and reduced pain using an acrylic and silicone wound drape.

Post-procedure

As for filling (above), plus returning to assess the seal and vacuum levels. Advise the person not to alter the vacuum levels, which are set to remove maximum exudate and stimulate granulation.

CLEAN, REPLACE AND DISPOSE OF EQUIPMENT

Wear clean gloves to protect yourself from contamination. Seal contaminated material in the disposal bag and then wrap it in the disposable wrapper that has formed the critical aseptic field.

Place it in the contaminated waste bin in the dirty utility room. Wipe down the trolley with the recommended solution. If gross contamination has occurred, use soap and water. Return the trolley to the clean service area of the unit. Wash non-disposable equipment and send to the central sterile services department for resterilisation. Label solutions to be reused with the date and time opened and shelve them in front of unopened solutions so that they are used quickly, avoiding waste. Remove your gloves and perform hand hygiene.

DOCUMENTATION

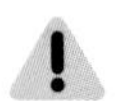

Safety

Relevant information to be documented includes date and time, appearance and measurements of the wound using a diagram indicating areas of granulation, slough, necrosis and undermining (Phillips, 2015). Note the colour of the wound, any drainage, the type and quantity of filling used, number and type of dressings applied and the person's response to the procedure. For any cavity, undermining, sinus tract, or tunnel with a depth greater than 1 cm, count and document the number of filling pieces removed, and the number of filling pieces inserted into the wound (Doyle & McCutcheon, 2015). This validates the care given, gives direction to colleagues and provides a progress report of the person's condition.

Be sure to document and report any of the following to the senior nurse:

- an increase in the amount of exudate
- an increase in the amount of pain in the wound or surrounding area
- increased erythema in or around the wound
- wound tissue that changes colour from pink to white, yellow or black in colour
- odour from the wound
- increase in the size or depth of the wound
- systemic indicators of infection (e.g. fever above 38 °C or shaking chills) (Ayello & Sibbald, 2022; RCHM, 2023).

CLINICAL SKILLS ASSESSMENT

Complex wounds: filling a wound; Negative Pressure Wound Therapy

Demonstrates the ability to effectively and safely fill a wound, or provide Negative Pressure Wound Therapy. Incorporates the *National Safety and Quality Health Service Standards*: 2 Partnering with consumers, 3 Preventing and controlling healthcare-associated infections, 5 Comprehensive care, 6 Communicating for safety, and 8 Recognising and responding to acute deterioration (Australian Commission on Safety and Quality in Health Care [ACSQHC], 2021).

Performance criteria	1	2	3	4	5
(Numbers indicate NMBA *Registered Nurse Standards for Practice*)	(Dependent)	(Marginal)	(Assisted)	(Supervised)	(Independent)
1. Identifies indication (1.1, 3.3, 3.4)	☐	☐	☐	☐	☐
2. Evidence of therapeutic interaction, e.g. gives the person a clear explanation of the procedure (1.4, 1.5, 2.1, 2.2, 3.2)	☐	☐	☐	☐	☐
3. Demonstrates clinical reasoning abilities, e.g. administers analgesia, provides privacy, positions the person appropriately (1.1, 1.2, 1.3, 1.5, 4.1, 4.2, 4.3, 5.1, 6.1)	☐	☐	☐	☐	☐
4. Gathers equipment (1.1, 5.5, 6.1): ■ dressing trolley irrigation tray ■ waterproof bag ■ clean and sterile gloves, personal protective equipment (PPE) ■ sterile scissors, probe and forceps ■ packing material: hydrogel, hydrocolloid alginate or gauze ribbon ■ dressings: sterile moisture-retentive and occlusive ■ tape or tubular mesh	☐	☐	☐	☐	☐
5. Uses appropriate personal protective equipment (1.1, 3.4, 4.3, 6.1)	☐	☐	☐	☐	☐
6. Performs hand hygiene (1.1, 3.4, 6.1)	☐	☐	☐	☐	☐
7. Removes the soiled dressing (1.1, 6.1)	☐	☐	☐	☐	☐
8. Establishes the critical aseptic field and cleanses the wound (1.1, 3.4, 4.3, 6.1)	☐	☐	☐	☐	☐
9. Assesses the wound and wound margins (1.1, 3.4, 4.1, 4.2, 4.3, 6.1)	☐	☐	☐	☐	☐
10. Packs the wound (1.1, 3.4, 4.3, 6.1)	☐	☐	☐	☐	☐
11. Applies a dry dressing and secures it (1.1, 6.1)	☐	☐	☐	☐	☐
12. Cleans, replaces and disposes of equipment appropriately (3.4, 3.6, 6.1)	☐	☐	☐	☐	☐
13. Documents relevant information (1.1, 1.4, 1.6, 2.2, 2.7, 3.5, 3.7, 6.1, 6.2, 6.5, 7.3)	☐	☐	☐	☐	☐
14. Demonstrates the ability to link theory to practice (1.1, 3.3, 3.4, 3.5)	☐	☐	☐	☐	☐

Student:

Clinical facilitator: Date:

REFERENCES

Aljghami, M., Sundas S. & Amini-Nik, S. (2019). Emerging innovative wound dressings. *Annals of Biomedical Engineering, 47*(3), 659–75. https://doi.org/10.1007/s10439-018-02186-w

Alnachoukati, O., Emerson, R. & Muraguri, M. (2019). Non-invasive, zip type skin closure device vs. conventional staples in total knee arthroplasty: Which method holds greater potential for bundled payments? *Cureus, 11*(3), e4281. https://doi.org/10.7759/cureus.4281

Annesley, S. (2019). Current thinking on caring for patients with a wound: A practical approach. *British Journal of Nursing, 28*(5), 290–4. http://nrl.northumbria.ac.uk/38837

Australian Commission on Safety and Quality in Health Care (ACSQHC) (2021). *National safety and quality health service standards* (3rd ed.). Sydney, NSW: ACSQHC.

Ayello, E. & Sibbald, R. G. (2022). Beyond the wound edge: Periwound and regional skin integrity. *Advances in Skin & Wound Care, 35*(10), 527. https://journals.lww.com/aswcjournal/fulltext/2022/10000/beyond_the_wound_edgeperiwound_and_regional_skin.1.aspx

Bahamondez-Canas, T., Heersema, L. & Smyth, H. (2019). Current status of in vitro models and assays for susceptibility testing for wound biofilm infections. *Biomedicines, 7*(2), 34. https://doi.org/10.3390/biomedicines7020034

Boga, S. (2019). Nursing practices in the prevention of post-operative wound infection in accordance with evidence-based approach. *International Journal of Caring Sciences, 12*(2), 1229–36. https://search.proquest.com/docview/2303668811?pq-origsite=gscholar&fromopenview=true

Bonham, J. (2016). Assessment and management of patients with minor traumatic wounds. *Nursing Standard, 31*(8), 60. https://doi.org/10.7748/ns.2016.e10573

Boyce, J. (2023). Best products for skin antisepsis. *American Journal of Infection Control, 51*(11), Supplement A58–A63. https://doi.org/10.1016/j.ajic.2023.02.002

Cochetti, G., Abraha, I., Randolph, J., Montedori, A., Boni, A., Arezzo, A., Mazza, E., Rossi De Vermandois, J. A., Cirocchi, R. & Mearini, E. (2020). Surgical wound closure by staples or sutures? Systematic review. *Medicine (Baltimore), 99*(25), e20573. https://doi.org/10.1097/MD.0000000000020573

Cutting, K., White, R. & Legerstee, R. (2017). Evidence and practical wound care: An all-inclusive approach. *Wound Medicine, 16*, 40–5. https://www.researchgate.net/profile/Keith_Cutting/publication/313885312_Evidence_and_practical_wound_care_-_An_all-inclusive_approach

Daley, B. (2017). Wound care management and treatment. *Medscape, April.* http://emedicine.medscape.com/article/194018-treatment

Denton, A. & Hallam, C. (2020a). Principles of asepsis 1: The rationale for using aseptic technique. *Nursing Times, 116*(5), 38–40. https://www.nursingtimes.net/clinical-archive/infection-control/principles-of-asepsis-1-the-rationale-for-using-aseptic-technique-14-04-2020

Denton, A. & Hallam, C. (2020b) Principles of asepsis 2: Technique for a simple wound dressing. *Nursing Times, 116*(6), 29–31. https://www.nursingtimes.net/clinical-archive/infection-control/principles-of-asepsis-2-technique-for-a-simple-wound-dressing-16-04-2020

Dias, T. A., Fernandes, D. R., dos Santos, B., dos Reis, P., Margatho, A. & Silveira, R. (2023). Dressing to prevent surgical site infection in adult patients with cancer: A systematic review with meta-analysis. *Support Care Cancer, 31*(11). https://doi.org/10.1007/s00520-022-07467-8

Dieter, S. (2023). Dead space in acute and chronic wounds: Causes and treatment approaches. *Sanara MedTech: Clinical Corner.* https://sanaramedtech.com/blog/dead-space-acute-chronic-wounds-causes-treatment

Do, H. T. T., Edwards, H. & Finlayson, K. (2021). Postoperative wound assessment documentation and acute care nurses' perception of factors impacting wound documentation: A mixed methods study. *International Journal of Clinical Practice, 75*, e13668. https://doi.org/10.1111/ijcp.13668

Doyle, G. & McCutcheon, J. (2015) *Clinical procedures for safer patient care.* Open Educational Resource. Vancouver, Canada: University of British Columbia. https://opentextbc.ca/clinicalskills

Earlam, A. & Woods, L. (2020). Obesity: Skin issues and skinfold management. *American Nurse.* https://www.myamericannurse.com/obesity-skin-issues-and-skinfold-management

Falcone, M., De Angelis, B., Pea, F., Scalise, A., Stefani, S., Tasinato, R., Zanetti, O. & Dalla Paola, L. (2021). Challenges in the management of chronic wound infections. *Journal of Global Antimicrobial Resistance, 26*, 140–7. https://doi.org/10.1016/j.jgar.2021.05.010

Fry, D. E. (2019). Operating room hand preparation: to scrub or to rub? *Surgical Infections, 20*(2), 129–34. https://www.liebertpub.com/doi/abs/10.1089/sur.2018.302

Fumarola, S., Allaway, R., Callaghan, R., Collier, M., Downie, S., Geraghty, G., Kiernan, S., Spratt, F., Bianchi, S., Bethell, B., Downe, A., Griffin, A., Hughes, M., King, B., LeBlanc, K., Savine, L., Stubbs, N. & Voegeli, D. (2020). Overlooked and underestimated: Medical adhesive-related skin injuries. *Journal of Wound Care, 29*(Sup3c), S1–S24. https://doi.org/10.12968/jowc.2020.29.Sup3c.S1

Gabriel, A. (2021). Wound irrigation. In *Medscape: Drugs and Diseases > Clinical procedures.* https://emedicine.medscape.com/article/1895071-overview

Gabriel, A., Camardo, M., O'Rorke, E., Gold, R. & Kim, P. (2021). Effects of Negative-Pressure Wound Therapy with instillation versus standard of care in multiple wound types: Systematic literature review and meta-analysis. *Plastic and Reconstructive Surgery, 147*(1S-1), 68S–76S. https://doi.org/10.1097/PRS.0000000000007614

Gajula, B., Munnamgi, S. & Basu, S. (2020). How bacterial biofilms affect chronic wound healing: A narrative review. *International Journal of Surgery: Global Health, 3*(2), e16. https://doi.org/10.1097/GH9.0000000000000016

Gibson, S. & Lillie, A. (2019). Effective drain care and management in community settings. *Nursing Standard.* https://doi.org/10.7748/ns.2019.e11389

Grabowski, G., Pacana, M. & Chen, E. (2020). Keloid and hypertrophic scar formation, prevention, and management: Standard review of abnormal scarring in orthopaedic surgery. *Journal of the American Academy of Orthopaedic Surgeons, 28*(10), e408–e414. https://doi.org/10.5435/JAAOS-D-19-00690

Greenstein, E. & Moore, N. (2021). Use of a novel silicone-acrylic drape with negative pressure wound therapy in four patients with peri-wound skin breakdown. *Wounds, 33*(11), 304–7.

Gupta, A., Kowalczuk, M., Heaselgrave, W., Britland, S., Martin, C. & Radecka, I. (2019). The production and application of hydrogels for wound management: A review. *European Polymer Journal, 111*(Feb.), 134–51. https://doi.org/10.1016/j.eurpolymj.2018.12.019

Haalboom, M., Blokhuis-Arkes, M., Beuk, R., Meerwaldt, R., Klont, R., Schijffelen, M., Bowler, P., Burnet, M., Sigl, E. & van der Palen, J. (2019). Culture results from wound biopsy versus wound swab: Does it matter for the assessment of wound infection? *Clinical Microbiology and Infection, 25*(5), 629.e7–629.e12. https://doi.org/10.1016/j.cmi.2018.08.012

Holloway, S. & Harding, K. (2022). Wound dressings. *Surgery (Oxford), 4*(1), 25–32. https://doi.org/10.1016/j.mpsur.2021.11.002

Holman, M. (2023). Using tap water compared with normal saline for cleansing wounds in adults: A literature review of the evidence. *Journal of Wound Care, 32*(8), 507–12. https://www.magonlinelibrary.com/doi/abs/10.12968/jowc.2023.32.8.507

International Wound Infection Institute (IWII) (2016). Wound infection in clinical practice: Principles of best practice. *Wounds International.* http://www.woundinfection-institute.com/wp-content/uploads/2017/03/IWII-Wound-infection-in-clinical-practice.pdf

Jain, R. & Wairkar, S. (2019). Recent developments and clinical applications of surgical glues: An overview. *International Journal of Biological Macromolecules, 137*, 95–106. https://doi.org/10.1016/j.ijbiomac.2019.06.208

James, R. (2018). *Guidelines on microbial wound swabbing.* National Center for Microbial Stewardship. https://www.vicniss.org.au/media/1926/1500-rod-james-skin-and-soft-tissue-swabs-2.pdf

Kushner, B., Smith, E., Han, B., Otegbeye, E., Holden, S. & Blatnik, J. (2021). Early drain removal does not increase the rate of surgical site infections following an open transversus abdominis release. *Hernia, 25*, 411–18. https://doi.org/10.1007/s10029-020-02362-9

Lalonde, D., Joukhadar, N. & Janis, J. (2019). Simple effective ways to care for skin wounds and incisions. *Plastic and Reconstructive Surgery. Global Open, 7*(10), e2471. https://doi.org/10.1097/GOX.0000000000002471

Le May, S., Tsimicalis, A., Noel, M., Rainville, P., Khadra,C., Ballard, A., Guingo, E., Cotes-Turpin, C., Addab, S., Chougui, K., Francoeur, M., Hung, N., Bernstein, M., Bouchard, S., Parent, S. & Debeurme, M. (2021). Immersive virtual reality vs. non-immersive distraction for pain management of children during bone pins and sutures removal: A randomized clinical trial protocol. *Journal of Advanced Nursing, 77*, 439–47. https://doi.org/10.1111/jan.14607

Lewis, K. & Pay, J. L. (2023). *Wound irrigation.* In *StatPearls [Internet].* StatPearls Publishing. https://www.ncbi.nlm.nih.gov/books/NBK538522

Lockwood, W. (2023). *Wound management comprehensive.* http://www.caceus.com/courses/coursematerial-204.pdf

McCaughan, D., Sheard, L., Cullum, N., Dumville, J. & Chetter, I. (2020). Nurses' and surgeons' views and experiences of surgical wounds healing by secondary intention: A qualitative study. *Journal of Clinical Nursing, 29*, 2557–71. https://doi.org/10.1111/jocn.15279

Morgan-Jones, R., Bishay, M., Hernandez-Hermosa, J., Lantis, J., Murray, J., Pajamaki, J., Pelligrini, A., Tarabichi, S. & Willy, C. (2019). Incision care and dressing selection in surgical wounds: Findings from an international meeting of surgeons. *Wounds International.* https://www.molnlycke.fi/SysSiteAssets/risk-assessment-and-consensus-reports/consensus-reports/incision-care-and-dressing-selection-surgical-wounds-findings-international-meeting-surgeons-1.pdf

Nagle, S. M., Waheed, A. & Wilbraham, S. C. (2020). Wound assessment [Updated 28 April 2020]. *StatPearls [Internet].* Treasure Island (FL): StatPearls Publishing. https://www.ncbi.nlm.nih.gov/books/NBK482198

Ojeh, N., Bharatha, A., Gaur, U. & Forde, A. L. (2020). Keloids: Current and emerging therapies. *Scars, Burns & Healing, 6.* https://journals.sagepub.com/doi/full/10.1177/2059513120940499

Orlov, A. & Gefen, A. (2023). Effective negative pressure wound therapy for open wounds: The importance of consistent pressure delivery. *International Wound Journal, 20*(2), 328–44. https://doi.org/10.1111/iwj.13879

Öztaş, B., Dursun, S. & Öztaş, M. (2020). Determination of nursing practices related to drain care. *Turkish Journal of Colorectal Disease, 30*(2), 128–33. https://doi.org/10.4274/tjcd.galenos.2020.2019-11-3

Parker, C. (2019). Evidence based management of wounds. In *Wound Workshop*, 20 May 2019 (Unpublished). https://eprints.qut.edu.au/132436

Phillips, C. (2015). Skin integrity and wound care. In A. Berman, S. Snyder, T. Levett-Jones, T. Dwyer, M. Hales, N. Harvey, Y. Luxford, L. Moxham, T. Park, B. Parker, K. Reid-Searl & D. Stanley (eds), *Kozier & Erb's fundamentals of nursing* (2nd Australian ed.), vol. 2, pp. 976–1012. Frenchs Forest, NSW: Pearson.

Poeran, J., Ippolito, K., Brochin, R., Zubizarreta, N., Mazumdar, M., Galatz, L. & Moucha, C. (2019). Utilization of drains and association with outcomes: A population-based study using national data on knee arthroplasties. *Journal of the American Academy of Orthopaedic Surgeons, 27*(20), e913–e919. https://doi.org/10.5435/JAAOS-D-18-00408

Rajhathy, E., Vander Meer, J., Valenzano, T., Laing, L., Woo, K., Beeckman, D. & Falk-Brynhildsen, K. (2023). Wound irrigation versus swabbing technique for cleansing noninfected chronic wounds: A systematic review of differences in bleeding, pain, infection, exudate, and necrotic tissue. *Journal of Tissue Viability, 32*(1), 136–43. https://doi.org/10.1016/j.jtv.2022.11.002

Ramesh, B. (2020). *Suction drains.* StatPearls. https://www.ncbi.nlm.nih.gov/books/NBK557687

Royal Children's Hospital Melbourne (RCHM) (2023). *Clinical guidelines: Wound assessment and management.* https://www.rch.org.au/rchcpg/hospital_clinical_guideline_index/Wound_Assessment_and_Management

Rushing, J. (2024). Clinical do's and don'ts: Obtaining a wound culture specimen. *Nursing, 24*, 11, 18. https://doi.org/10.1097/01.NURSE.0000298181.53662.e6

Sadik, K., Flener, J., Gargiulo, J., Post, Z., Wurzelbacher, S., Hogan, A., Hollmann, S. & Ferko, N. (2018). A US hospital budget impact analysis of a skin closure system compared with standard of care in hip and knee arthroplasty. *ClinicoEconomics and Outcomes Research, 11*, 1–11. https://doi.org/10.2147/CEOR.S181630

Sahnan, K., Adegbola, S., Tozer, P., Watfah, J. & Phillips, R. (2017). Perianal abscess. *British Medical Journal (Online), 356.* https://doi.org/10.1136/bmj.j475

Schellack, G. (2020). Wound care in a nutshell. *Professional Nursing Today, 24*(1), 12–15. http://www.pntonline.co.za/index.php/PNT/article/view/1063

Schluer, A. (2021). Wound care in the adult. In S. Probst (ed.), *Wound care nursing: A person-centred approach* (3rd ed.). Elsevier.

Sen, C. (2019). Human wounds and its burden: An updated compendium of estimates. *Advances in Wound Care, 8*(2), 39–48. https://doi.org/10.1089/wound.2019.0946

Shyna, S., Krishna, S., Prabha, A., Nair, D. & Thomas, L. (2020). A nonadherent chitosan-polyvinyl alcohol absorbent wound dressing prepared via controlled freeze-dry technology. *International Journal of Biological Macromolecules, 159*, 129–40. https://doi.org/10.1016/j.ijbiomac.2020.01.292

Sinha, S., Free, B. & Ladlow, O. (2022). The art and science of selecting appropriate dressings for acute open wounds in general practice. *Australian Journal of General Practice, 51*(11). https://doi.org/10.31128/AJGP-06-22-6462

Smith, M. (2020). Moving forward in wound care: Impact of accepting and implementing change. *Journal of Community Nursing, 34*(2), 38–44. https://web.a.ebscohost.com/abstract

Sussman, G. (2023). An update on wound management. *Australian Prescriber, 46*, 29–35. https://doi.org/10.18773/austprescr.2023.006

Tan, G. (2020). Wound care and repair. In P. Cameron, M. Little, B. Mitra & C. Deasy (eds), *Textbook of adult emergency medicine e-book* (5th ed.). Edinburgh, UK: Elsevier.

Tobiano, G., Walker, R., Chaboyer, W., Carlini, J., Webber, L., Latimer, S., Kang, E., Eskes, A., O'Connor, T., Perger, D. & Gillespie, B. (2023). Patient experiences of, and preferences for, surgical wound care education. *International Wound Journal, 20*(5), 1687–99. https://doi.org/10.1111/iwj.14030

Vranešić Bender, D. & Krznarić, Ž. (2020). Nutritional issues and considerations in the elderly: An update. *Croatian Medical Journal, 61*(2), 180–3. https://doi.org/10.3325/cmj.2020.61.180

Williams, E. (2020). Wound dressing techniques. In R. Dehn & D. Asprey (eds), *Essential clinical procedures e-book* (4th ed.). Philadelphia, PA: Elsevier Health Sciences.

Wound Care Centers (2020). *Chronic wounds.* https://www.woundcarecenters.org/article/wound-types/chronic-wounds

Wounds Australia (2016). *Standards for wound prevention and management* (3rd ed.). http://www.woundsaustralia.com.au/2016/standards-for-wound-prevention-and-management-2016.pdf

Zaver, V. & Kankanalu, P. (2023). Negative pressure wound therapy. [Updated 2023 Sep 4]. In *StatPearls [Internet].* Treasure Island (FL): StatPearls Publishing. https://www.ncbi.nlm.nih.gov/books/NBK576388

Zukowski, A. & Zukowski, M. (2022). Surgical site infection in cardiac surgery. *Journal of Clinical Medicine, 11*(23), 6991. https://www.mdpi.com/2077-0383/11/23/6991

APPENDIX A: NMBA *REGISTERED NURSE STANDARDS FOR PRACTICE* 2016

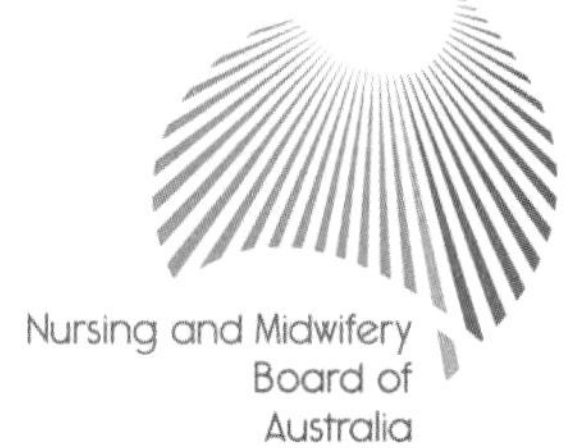

Registered nurse standards for practice

Effective date 1 June 2016

Introduction

Registered nurse (RN) practice is person-centred and evidence-based with preventative, curative, formative, supportive, restorative and palliative elements. RNs work in therapeutic and professional relationships with individuals, as well as with families, groups and communities. These people may be healthy and with a range of abilities, or have health issues related to physical or mental illness and/or health challenges. These challenges may be posed by physical, psychiatric, developmental and/or intellectual disabilities.

The Australian community has a rich mixture of cultural and linguistic diversity, and the *Registered nurse standards for practice* are to be read in this context. RNs recognise the importance of history and culture to health and wellbeing. This practice reflects particular understanding of the impact of colonisation on the cultural, social and spiritual lives of Aboriginal and Torres Strait Islander peoples, which has contributed to significant health inequity in Australia.

As regulated health professionals, RNs are responsible and accountable to the Nursing and Midwifery Board of Australia (NMBA). These are the national *Registered nurse standards for practice* for all RNs. Together with NMBA standards, codes and guidelines, these *Registered nurse standards for practice* should be evident in current practice, and inform the development of the scopes of practice and aspirations of RNs.

RN practice, as a professional endeavour, requires continuous thinking and analysis in the context of thoughtful development and maintenance of constructive relationships. To engage in this work, RNs need to continue to develop professionally and maintain their capability for professional practice. RNs determine, coordinate and provide safe, quality nursing. This practice includes comprehensive assessment, development of a plan, implementation and evaluation of outcomes. As part of practice, RNs are responsible and accountable for supervision and the delegation of nursing activity to enrolled nurses (ENs) and others.

Practice is not restricted to the provision of direct clinical care. Nursing practice extends to any paid or unpaid role where the nurse uses their nursing skills and knowledge. This practice includes working in a direct non-clinical relationship with clients, working in management, administration, education, research, advisory, regulatory, policy development roles or other roles that impact on safe, effective delivery of services in the profession and/or use of the nurse's professional skills. RNs are responsible for autonomous practice within dynamic systems, and in relationships with other health care professionals.

How to use these standards

The *Registered nurse standards for practice* consist of the following seven standards:

1. Thinks critically and analyses nursing practice.
2. Engages in therapeutic and professional relationships.
3. Maintains the capability for practice.
4. Comprehensively conducts assessments.
5. Develops a plan for nursing practice.

6. Provides safe, appropriate and responsive quality nursing practice.
7. Evaluates outcomes to inform nursing practice.

The above standards are all interconnected (see Figure 1). Standards one, two and three relate to each other, as well as to each dimension of practice in standards four, five, six and seven.

Figure 1: Registered nurse standards

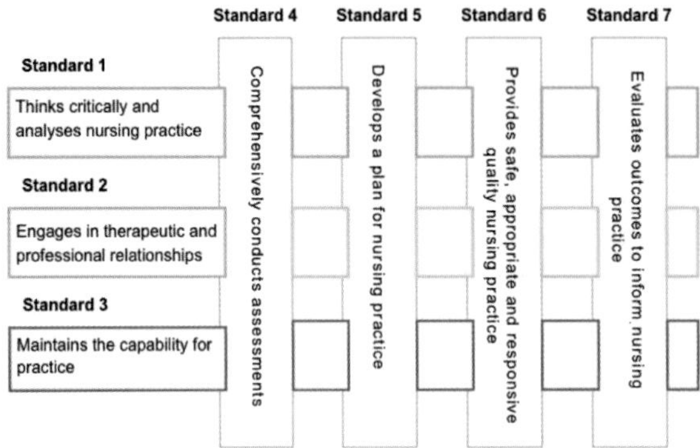

Each standard has criteria that specify how that standard is demonstrated. The criteria are to be interpreted in the context of each RN's practice. For example, all RNs will, at various times, work in partnerships and delegate responsibilities, however not every RN will delegate clinical practice to enrolled nurses. The criteria are not exhaustive and enable rather than limit the development of individual registered nurse scopes of practice.

The *Registered nurse standards for practice* are for all RNs across all areas of practice. They are to be read in conjunction with the applicable NMBA companion documents such as the standards, codes and guidelines, including the *Code of professional conduct for nurses*, *Code of ethics for nurses*, *National framework for the development of decision-making tools for nursing and midwifery practice, Supervision guidelines for nursing and midwifery*, and *Guidelines for mandatory notifications*. The glossary is also important for understanding how key terms are used in these standards.

Registered nurse standards for practice

Standard 1: Thinks critically and analyses nursing practice

RNs use a variety of thinking strategies and the best available evidence in making decisions and providing safe, quality nursing practice within person-centred and evidence-based frameworks.

The registered nurse:

1.1 accesses, analyses, and uses the best available evidence, that includes research findings, for safe, quality practice

1.2 develops practice through reflection on experiences, knowledge, actions, feelings and beliefs to identify how these shape practice

1.3 respects all cultures and experiences, which includes responding to the role of family and community that underpin the health of Aboriginal and Torres Strait Islander peoples and people of other cultures

1.4 complies with legislation, regulations, policies, guidelines and other standards or requirements relevant to the context of practice when making decisions

1.5 uses ethical frameworks when making decisions

1.6 maintains accurate, comprehensive and timely documentation of assessments, planning, decision-making, actions and evaluations, and

1.7 contributes to quality improvement and relevant research.

Standard 2: Engages in therapeutic and professional relationships

RN practice is based on purposefully engaging in effective therapeutic and professional relationships. This includes collegial generosity in the context of mutual trust and respect in professional relationships.

The registered nurse:

2.1 establishes, sustains and concludes relationships in a way that differentiates the boundaries between professional and personal relationships

2.2 communicates effectively, and is respectful of a person's dignity, culture, values, beliefs and rights

2.3 recognises that people are the experts in the experience of their life

2.4 provides support and directs people to resources to optimise health-related decisions

2.5 advocates on behalf of people in a manner that respects the person's autonomy and legal capacity

2.6 uses delegation, supervision, coordination, consultation and referrals in professional relationships to achieve improved health outcomes

2.7 actively fosters a culture of safety and learning that includes engaging with health professionals and others, to share knowledge and practice that supports person-centred care

2.8 participates in and/or leads collaborative practice, and

2.9 reports notifiable conduct of health professionals, health workers and others.

Standard 3: Maintains the capability for practice

RNs, as regulated health professionals, are responsible and accountable for ensuring they are safe, and have the capability for practice. This includes ongoing self-management and responding when there is concern about other health professionals' capability for practice. RNs are responsible for their professional development and contribute to the development of others. They are also responsible for providing information and education to enable people to make decisions and take action in relation to their health.

The registered nurse:

3.1 considers and responds in a timely manner to the health and wellbeing of self and others in relation to the capability for practice

3.2 provides the information and education required to enhance people's control over health

3.3 uses a lifelong learning approach for continuing professional development of self and others

3.4 accepts accountability for decisions, actions, behaviours and responsibilities inherent in their role, and for the actions of others to whom they have delegated responsibilities

3.5 seeks and responds to practice review and feedback

3.6 actively engages with the profession, and

3.7 identifies and promotes the integral role of nursing practice and the profession in influencing better health outcomes for people.

Standard 4: Comprehensively conducts assessments

RNs accurately conduct comprehensive and systematic assessments. They analyse information and data and communicate outcomes as the basis for practice.

The registered nurse:

4.1 conducts assessments that are holistic as well as culturally appropriate

4.2 uses a range of assessment techniques to systematically collect relevant and accurate information and data to inform practice

4.3 works in partnership to determine factors that affect, or potentially affect, the health and wellbeing of people and populations to determine priorities for action and/ or for referral, and

4.4 assesses the resources available to inform planning.

Standard 5: Develops a plan for nursing practice

RNs are responsible for the planning and communication of nursing practice. Agreed plans are developed in partnership. They are based on the RNs appraisal of comprehensive, relevant information, and evidence that is documented and communicated.

The registered nurse:

5.1 uses assessment data and best available evidence to develop a plan

5.2 collaboratively constructs nursing practice plans until contingencies, options priorities, goals, actions, outcomes and timeframes are agreed with the relevant persons

5.3 documents, evaluates and modifies plans accordingly to facilitate the agreed outcomes

5.4 plans and negotiates how practice will be evaluated and the time frame of engagement, and

5.5 coordinates resources effectively and efficiently for planned actions.

Standard 6: Provides safe, appropriate and responsive quality nursing practice

RNs provide and may delegate, quality and ethical goal-directed actions. These are based on comprehensive and systematic assessment, and the best available evidence to achieve planned and agreed outcomes.

The registered nurse:

6.1 provides comprehensive safe, quality practice to achieve agreed goals and outcomes that are responsive to the nursing needs of people

6.2 practises within their scope of practice

6.3 appropriately delegates aspects of practice to enrolled nurses and others, according to enrolled nurse's scope of practice or others' clinical or non-clinical roles

6.4 provides effective timely direction and supervision to ensure that delegated practice is safe and correct

6.5 practises in accordance with relevant policies, guidelines, standards, regulations and legislation, and

6.6 uses the appropriate processes to identify and report potential and actual risk related system issues and where practice may be below the expected standards.

Standard 7: Evaluates outcomes to inform nursing practice

RNs take responsibility for the evaluation of practice based on agreed priorities, goals, plans and outcomes and revises practice accordingly.

The registered nurse:

7.1 evaluates and monitors progress towards the expected goals and outcomes

7.2 revises the plan based on the evaluation, and

7.3 determines, documents and communicates further priorities, goals and outcomes with the relevant persons.

Glossary

These definitions relate to the use of terms in the *Registered nurse standards for practice*.

Accountability means that nurses answer to the people in their care, the nursing regulatory authority, their employers and the public. Nurses are accountable for their decisions, actions, behaviours and the responsibilities that are inherent in their nursing roles including documentation. Accountability cannot be delegated. The registered nurse who delegates activities to be undertaken by another person remains accountable for the decision to delegate, for monitoring the level of performance by the other person, and for evaluating the outcomes of what has been delegated (Nursing and Midwifery Board of Australia 2013). See below for the related definition of 'Delegation'.

Criteria in this document means the actions and behaviours of the RN that demonstrate these standards for practice.

Delegation is the relationship that exists when a RN delegates aspects of their nursing practice to another person such as an enrolled nurse, a student nurse or a person who is not a nurse. Delegations are made to meet peoples' needs and to enable access to health care services, that is, the right person is available at the right time to provide the right service. The RN who is delegating retains accountability for the decision to delegate. They are also accountable for monitoring of the communication of the delegation to the relevant persons and for the practice outcomes. Both parties share the responsibility of making the delegation decision, which includes assessment of the risks and capabilities. In some instances delegation may be preceded by teaching and competence assessment. For further details see the NMBA's National framework for the development of decision-making tools for nursing and midwifery practice (2013).

Enrolled nurse is a person who provides nursing care under the direct or indirect supervision of a registered nurse. They have completed the prescribed education preparation, and demonstrate competence to practise under the Health Practitioner Regulation National Law as an enrolled nurse in Australia. Enrolled nurses are accountable for their own practice and remain responsible to a registered nurse for the delegated care.

Evidence-based practice is accessing and making judgements to translate the best available evidence, which includes the most current, valid, and available research findings into practice.

Person or people is used in these standards to refer to those individuals who have entered into a therapeutic and/or professional relationship with a registered nurse. These individuals will sometimes be health care consumers, at other times they may be colleagues or students, this will vary depending on who is the focus of practice at the time. Therefore, the words person or people include all the patients, clients, consumers, families, carers, groups and/or communities that are within the registered nurse scope and context of practice. The registered nurse has professional relationships in health care related teams.

Person-centred practice is collaborative and respectful partnership built on mutual trust and understanding through good communication. Each person is treated as an individual with the aim of respecting people's ownership of their health information, rights and preferences while protecting their dignity and empowering choice. Person-centred practice recognises the role of family and community with respect to cultural and religious diversity.

Registered nurse is a person who has completed the prescribed education preparation, demonstrates competence to practise and is registered under the Health Practitioner Regulation National Law as a registered nurse in Australia.

Scope of practice is that in which nurses are educated, competent to perform and permitted by law. The actual scope of practice is influenced by the context in which the nurse practises, the health needs of people, the level of competence and confidence of the nurse and the policy requirements of the service provider.

Standards for practice in this document are the expectations of registered nurse practice. They inform the education standards for registered nurses, the regulation of nurses and determination of the nurse's capability for practice, and guide consumers, employers and other stakeholders on what to reasonably expect from a registered nurse regardless of the area of nursing practice or years of nursing experience. They replace the previous *National competency standards for the registered nurse* (2010).

Supervision includes managerial supervision, professional supervision and clinically focused supervision. For further details see the NMBA's, Supervision guidelines for nursing and midwifery (2015).

Therapeutic relationships are different to personal relationships. In a therapeutic relationship the nurse is sensitive to a person's situation and purposefully engages with them using knowledge and skills in respect, compassion and kindness. In the relationship the person's rights and dignity are recognised and respected. The professional nature of the relationship involves recognition of professional boundaries and issues of unequal power. For further details see the NMBA's A nurse's guide to professional boundaries (2010).

References

Nursing and Midwifery Board of Australia (2010) 'A nurse's guide to professional boundaries'. Retrieved 05 January 2015, www.nursingmidwiferyboard.gov.au/Codes-Guidelines-Statements/Professional-standards.aspx

Nursing and Midwifery Board of Australia. (2007) 'National framework for the development of decision-making tools for nursing and midwifery practice'. Retrieved 05 January 2015, www.nursingmidwiferyboard.gov.au/Codes-Guidelines-Statements/Frameworks.aspx

Nursing and Midwifery Board of Australia. (2015) 'Supervision guidelines for nursing and midwifery. Retrieved 25 September 2015', www.nursingmidwiferyboard.gov.au/Registration-and-Endorsement/reentry-to-practice.aspx

APPENDIX B: NMBA DECISION-MAKING FRAMEWORK SUMMARY

Decision-making framework summary: Nursing

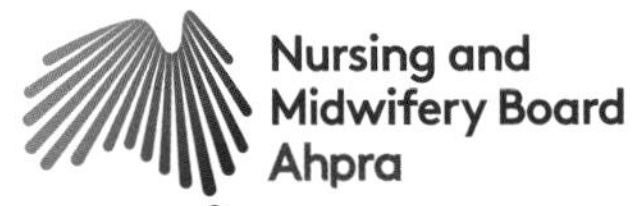

To be read in conjunction with the NMBA *Decision-making framework for nursing and midwifery (2020)*
Note: the order in which these issues are considered may vary according to context

Identify need/benefit

- Has there been a comprehensive assessment by a registered nurse to establish the person's health and cultural needs?
- Has there been appropriate consultation with, and consent by, the person receiving care?
- Is the activity in the best interests of the person receiving care?

Reflect on scope of practice and nursing practice standards

- Is this activity within the current, contemporary scope of nursing practice?
- Have Commonwealth or state/territory legislative requirements (e.g. specific qualification needed) been met?
- If authorisation by a regulatory authority is needed to perform the activity, does the registered nurse, enrolled nurse or health worker have it or can it be obtained before the activity is performed?
- Will performance comply with nursing standards for practice, codes and guidelines, as well as best available evidence?
- If other health professionals should assist, supervise or perform the activity, are they available?

Consider context of practice, governance and identification of risk

- Is this activity/practice/delegation supported by the organisation and/or by the educational institution (for students)?
- Have strategies to avoid or minimise any risk been identified and implemented?
- If organisational authorisation is needed, does the registered nurse, enrolled nurse or health worker have it or can it be obtained before performing the activity?
- Is the skill mix, model of care and staffing levels in the organisation adequate for the level of support/supervision needed to safely perform the activity/delegation?
- If this is a new practice:
  - Is there a system for ongoing education and maintenance of competence in place?
  - Have relevant parties and stakeholders been involved in planning for implementation?

Select appropriate, competent person to perform activities

(Delegation of care is made by a registered nurse)

- Have the roles and responsibilities of registered nurses, enrolled nurses and health workers been considered?
- Does the registered nurse, enrolled nurse or health worker have the necessary educational preparation, experience, capacity, competence and confidence to safely perform the activity either autonomously or with education, support and supervision?
- Are they competent and confident in performing the activity and accepting the delegation?
- Do they understand their accountability and reporting responsibilities?
- Is the required level of education, clinical supervision/support available?

Yes to all

Action

- Perform the activity, **or** delegate to a competent person who then reconfirms consent from the person receiving care, **and**
- document the decision and the actions, **and**
- regular review of the delegation providing guidance, support and clinically focused supervision, **and**
- evaluate outcome.

No to any

Action

- Reconsider decision about whether to implement practice/activity/delegation, **and**
- consult/seek advice/collaborate, **and/or**
- refer if needed to complete the action, **and**
- if appropriate, plan to enable integration/practice changes (including developing/implementing policies, gaining qualifications as needed), **and**
- document the decisions and the actions, **and**
- evaluate outcome.

INDEX

ABCs. *See* airway, breathing and circulation (ABCs)
abdominal assessment, 121
  clean, replace and dispose of equipment, 124
  clinical reasoning, 122–4
  documentation, 124
  evidence of therapeutic interaction, 121
  gastrointestinal history, 121
  post-procedure, 124
ABHR. *See* alcohol-based hand rubs (ABHR)
abstraction, 88
accommodation, 114
accountability, 2
ACORN. *See* Australian College of Operating Room Nurses (ACORN)
acronyms, 153
ACSQHC. *See* Australian Commission on Safety and Quality in Health Care (ACSQHC)
acting, 7
active assisted ROM exercises, 133
active ROM exercises, 133
acute oxygen therapy, 403
ADC. *See* automated dispensing cabinet (ADC)
ADDS. *See* Adult Deterioration Detection System (ADDS)
Adult Deterioration Detection System (ADDS), 49, 60, 64, 82, 107
affect, 87
affective change, 160
airway, breathing and circulation (ABCs), 78
alcohol-based hand rubs (ABHR), 18, 20, 38, 238, 251, 432
  solution procedure, 39–40
alert, voice, pain, unresponsive scale (AVPU scale), 112
analgesia, 360–1
Angle of Louis, 92
ANMAC. *See* Australian Nursing and Midwifery Accreditation Competencies (ANMAC)
ANSAT. *See* Australian Nursing Standards Assessment Tool (ANSAT)
anterior thorax, 106–7
anticipated complications, 350
antimicrobials, 247
antiseptics, 247
ANTT®. *See* Aseptic Non Touch Technique (ANTT®)
appearance, 86–7
artificial airway suctioning, 417
  clean, replace and dispose of equipment, 423
  clinical reasoning, 418–20
  documentation, 423
  evidence of therapeutic interaction, 417–18
  performing, 421–3
  preoxygenate person, 420–1
  suctioning apparatus, 420
aseptic fields, 31–2
aseptic/clinical hand hygiene, 37
  alcohol-based hand rub solution procedure, 39–40
  clinical reasoning, 37
  first five-minute scrub, 38–9
  performing, 37–40
  scrubs of day, 39
  surgical hand wash, 38
Aseptic Non Touch Technique (ANTT®), 19, 31, 42, 179, 217, 224, 296, 309, 328, 335, 421, 431, 436, 449, 479
  background to, 31–32
  clean, replace and dispose of equipment, 35
  clinical reasoning, 33
  documentation, 35
  evidence of therapeutic interaction, 33
  performing, 33–34
assisting with meals, 166
  clean, replace and dispose of equipment, 169
  clinical reasoning, 167–8
  documentation, 169
  evidence of therapeutic interaction, 166–7
  person with meals, 168–9
Australian College of Operating Room Nurses (ACORN), 37
Australian Commission on Safety and Quality in Health Care (ACSQHC), 24, 37, 42, 54, 60, 185, 233
Australian Nursing and Midwifery Accreditation Competencies (ANMAC), 2
Australian Nursing Standards Assessment Tool (ANSAT), 3, 13
Australian Red Cross Blood Service, 443
automated dispensing cabinet (ADC), 234, 276
AVPU scale. *See* alert, voice, pain, unresponsive scale (AVPU scale)
axillary temperature, 52

bed bath, 369
  clean, replace and dispose of equipment, 373
  clinical reasoning, 369–71
  documentation, 373
  evidence of therapeutic interaction, 369
  performing, 371–3
best verbal response, 112–13
BGL. *See* blood glucose level (BGL); blood glucose meter (BGL)
biofilm, 471
blood glucose level (BGL), 72–3, 75
blood glucose measurement, 72
  clean, replace and dispose of equipment, 76
  clinical reasoning, 72–4
  documentation, 76
  evidence of therapeutic interaction, 72
  obtaining, 74–75
blood glucose meter (BGL), 75
blood pressure (BP), 56, 64, 90, 113, 154
  clean, replace and dispose of equipment, 60
  clinical reasoning, 56–8
  documentation, 60
  evidence of therapeutic interaction, 56
  measurement, 59–60
blood products, 443
blood transfusion, 442
  administering, 444–7
  clean, replace and dispose of equipment, 447
  clinical reasoning, 443
  documentation, 447
  evidence of therapeutic interaction, 442–3
BMI. *See* body mass index (BMI)
body mass index (BMI), 126, 286
bolus, 306
  clean, replace and dispose of equipment, 311
  clinical reasoning, 307–8
  documentation, 311
  evidence of therapeutic interaction, 306
  intravenous medication, 308–11
BP. *See* blood pressure (BP)
bronchial sounds, 105
bronchovesicular sounds, 105
buccal administration, 232

C&S. *See* culture and sensitivity (C&S)
cardiovascular health history, 90
  cardiovascular history, 92
  clean, replace and dispose of equipment, 94
  clinical reasoning, 90–91
  conducting, 92–94
  documentation, 94
  evidence of therapeutic interaction, 90
  hand hygiene, 92
  heart assessment, 92–3
  privacy and comfort, 91
  supine position, 91
  vascular system, 93–4
CARE protocol. *See* Connect, Ask, Respond, Empathise protocol (CARE protocol)
carotid arteries, 94
cellulitis, 193
central nervous system (CNS), 109
central sterile services department (CSSD), 35, 468, 475
central stimulation, 112
central venous catheters (CVC), 32
chaperone, 96
character, onset, location, duration, severity, palliation, associated factors (COLDSPA), 82
chemical name, 234
chest drainage system, 435
  assessment, 437
  clean, replace and dispose of equipment, 437
  clinical reasoning, 436–7
  documentation, 437
  evidence of therapeutic interaction, 435
chest drains, 435
clinical decision making, 6
clinical educator, 4–5
clinical handover, 147
  documentation, 150
  environment, 148
  medical terminology, 150
  receiving handover, 150
  safety considerations, 147–8
  teamwork, 148
  template, 148–150
  timeliness, 150
clinical judgement, 6
Clinical Psychomotor Skills, 2

clinical reasoning, 6–7, 349
12-lead electrocardiogram, 96–97
abdominal assessment, 122–4
ANTT, 33
artificial airway suctioning, 418–20
aseptic/clinical hand hygiene, 37
assisting with meals, 167–8
bed bath, 369–71
blood glucose measurement, 72–4
blood pressure, 56–8
blood transfusion, 443
bolus, 307–8
cardiovascular health history, 90–91
chest drainage system, 436–7
drain care, 465
elimination needs, 202–4
enemas, 209–11
enteral medication, 241–3
enteral nutrition, 178–80
filling wound, 477–9
healthcare teaching, 158–9
heat and cold therapy, 321
height, weight and waist circumference measurements, 127
inhaled medication, 279–81
IVT, 185–7, 192–4
mental status assessment, 85
mobilisation, 387–9
musculoskeletal assessment, 132–4
neurological health history, 110
neurovascular observations, 116–117
oral care, hair care, nail care and shaving, 375–6
oral medications, 232–6
oropharyngeal and nasopharyngeal suctioning, 411–13
otic medications, 260–2
oxygen therapy, 405
pain assessment, 67
parenteral medication, 286
patient-controlled analgesia, 326–7
physical assessment, 79
postoperative care, 357–8
preoperative care, 342
pressure injury, 393
pulse oximetry, 62–4
rectal medication, 272–4
reposition, 381–3
respiratory health history, 101
subcutaneous infusion, 334–5
topical medication, 248–51
TPR measurement, 49
urinary catheterisation, 221–3
vaginal medication, 266–7
venipuncture, 449–51
wound irrigation, 471–3
clinical thinking, 6–9
clip removal, 464–5, 467–8
closed gloving method, 43
closed-suctioning technique, 420, 422
closed tracheal suction system, 417
CNS. *See* central nervous system (CNS)
coarse crackles, 105
Codes of Conduct for Nurses and Midwives, 10
cold humidifiers, 406
cold therapy, 320
administering, 321–2
clean, replace and dispose of equipment, 322
clinical reasoning, 321
documentation, 322
evidence of therapeutic interaction, 321
COLDSPA. *See* character, onset, location, duration, severity, palliation, associated factors (COLDSPA)
collaboration, 3
collecting, 6
communication, 13, 427
compartment syndrome, 116
competency, 2, 4
Connect, Ask, Respond, Empathise protocol (CARE protocol), 148
content, 88
continuous glucose monitors (CGMs) test, 73
continuous subcutaneous infusion (CSCI), 333
critical aseptic fields, 32
critical micro aseptic fields, 32
critical thinking, 6
crushing, 243
cryoprecipitate, 443
CSCI. *See* continuous subcutaneous infusion (CSCI)
CSSD. *See* central sterile services department (CSSD)
cultural diversity, 233
cultural safety, 10
culture and sensitivity (C&S), 471
specimen for, 475
CVC. *See* central venous catheters (CVC)

DAR. *See* Data, Action, Response (DAR)
Data, Action, Response (DAR), 154
decerebrate posturing, 110
deciding, 7
decorticate posturing, 110
deep suction, 417
deep vein thrombosis (DVT), 150
deltoid, 290
demonstration coaching, 160–1
diabetes mellitus (DM), 72
diabetes technologies, 73
digital thermometers, 50
disease-related malnutrition, 166
dispersal method, 243
DM. *See* diabetes mellitus (DM)
documentation, 152
by exception, 154
content, 152–3
electronic documentation, 154–5
legal requirements for, 154
narrative, 153
problem-focused, 153–4
structure, 153
written, 153–4
drain care, 464, 466–7
clean, replace and dispose of equipment, 468
clinical reasoning, 465
documentation, 469
evidence of therapeutic interaction, 465
drain removal, 464
dry chest drainage system, 436
dry dressing technique, 458
clean, replace and dispose of equipment, 462
clinical reasoning, 458–9
documentation, 462
evidence of therapeutic interaction, 458
performing, 459–62
dry powder inhaler, 278
DVT. *See* deep vein thrombosis (DVT)
dysphagia, 166

early warning scoring/system (EWS) system, 49, 82
EHR. *See* electronic health record (EHR)
electronic documentation, 154–5
electronic health record (EHR), 154
electronic medication administration record (eMAR), 154, 189, 235, 244, 258, 263, 276, 283, 290, 299, 345–6
electronic medication management (EMM) systems, 235
electronic thermometers, 50
elimination needs, 202
assist with, 204–5
clean, replace and dispose of equipment, 206–7
clinical reasoning, 202–4
documentation, 207
evidence of therapeutic interaction, 202
routine urinalysis, 205–6
stool assessment, 206
eMAR. *See* electronic medication administration record (eMAR)
enemas, 209
administration, 212–13
clean, replace and dispose of equipment, 213
clinical reasoning, 209–11
documentation, 213
evidence of therapeutic interaction, 209
engineered securement devices (ESDs), 189
enteral medication, 241
administering, 243–4
clean, replace and dispose of equipment, 244
clinical reasoning, 241–3
documentation, 244–5
evidence of therapeutic interaction, 241
six rights of administering medication, 243
enteral nutrition, 177
clean, replace and dispose of equipment, 182–3
clinical reasoning, 178–80
documentation, 183
enteral tube feeding, 180–2
evidence of therapeutic interaction, 178
EOMs. *See* extraocular movements (EOMs)
EPUAP. *See* European Pressure Ulcer Advisory Panel (EPUAP)
ESDs. *See* engineered securement devices (ESDs)
European Pressure Ulcer Advisory Panel (EPUAP), 396
evacuant enema, 209
evaluating, 7
evidence-based assessment, 3
extraocular movements (EOMs), 114

face masks, 406
facilitator, 4–5
factual information, 160
falls risk-assessment tool (FRAT), 389
filling wound, 477
clean, replace and dispose of equipment, 481–2
clinical reasoning, 477–9
documentation, 482
evidence of therapeutic interaction, 477
fine crackles on inspiration, 105
flutter valve, 436
formal teaching, 157
FRAT. *See* falls risk-assessment tool (FRAT)
frequency of monitoring, 72

gastrointestinal (GI) problems, 121
gastrostomy tubes, 177
GCS. *See* Glasgow Coma Scale (GCS)
general aseptic field, 32
generic name, 234
Glasgow Coma Scale (GCS), 109, 111
gowning, 43

HAI. *See* hospital-acquired infection (HAI)
hair care, 375
  clean, replace and dispose of equipment, 379
  clinical reasoning, 375–6
  documentation, 379
  evidence of therapeutic interaction, 375
  performing, 377–9
hand health, maintaining, 20–2
hand hygiene, 18, 27, 32
  alcohol-based hand rub, 20
  hand preparation, 19
  hand washing, 20
  maintaining hand health, 20–2
hand preparation, 19
hand washing, 20
HCAIs. *See* healthcare-associated infections (HCAIs)
healthcare-associated infections (HCAIs), 18, 24, 31, 37, 321
healthcare professionals, 10
healthcare teaching, 157
  clinical reasoning, 158–9
  demonstration coaching, 160–1
  documentation, 161
  evidence of therapeutic interaction, 157–8
  teach-back method, 160
  teaching strategies, 159–60
healthcare workers, 11
health literacy, 157
heat and moisture exchanger (HME), 429
heat therapy, 320
  administering, 321–2
  clean, replace and dispose of equipment, 322
  clinical reasoning, 321
  documentation, 322
  evidence of therapeutic interaction, 321
heated humidifiers, 406
height, weight and waist circumference measurements, 126
  clean, replace and dispose of equipment, 130
  clinical reasoning, 127
  conducting, 129–130
  documentation, 130
  evidence of therapeutic interaction, 126
HME. *See* heat and moisture exchanger (HME)
hospital-acquired infection (HAI), 192
humidification, 406–7
hypodermoclysis, 333

ICSs. *See* intercostal spaces (ICSs)
ICU. *See* intensive care unit (ICU)
IDC. *See* indwelling catheter (IDC)
identification of the person, situation and status, background and history, assessment and actions, responsibility, recommendation, risk management and read back (ISBAR), 149–50
independence, 4
indwelling catheter (IDC), 226–7, 362
infiltration, 193
inhaled medication, 278
  administering, 282
  clean, replace and dispose of equipment, 283
  clinical reasoning, 279–81
  documentation, 283
  evidence of therapeutic interaction, 278
  six rights of administering medication, 281–2
initialisms, 153
'in-line' catheter, 417
INR. *See* international normalised ratio (INR)
Institute for Safe Medication Practices (ISMP), 233
intensive care unit (ICU), 345, 357
intercostal spaces (ICSs), 92, 98, 105
intermittent bladder irrigation, 215–16
intermittent infusion, 295
intermittent SC injection, 333
international normalised ratio (INR), 236
interpersonal skills, 12
intradermal (ID) parenteral medication, 285
intramuscular (IM)
  injection, 333
  parenteral medication, 285
intrapleural drains, 435
intravenous (IV)
  infusion, 56, 192
  injection, 333
  therapy, 32
intravenous container, 301
  administering, 303
  clean, replace and dispose of equipment, 303–4
  clinical reasoning, 301–2
  documentation, 304
  evidence of therapeutic interaction, 301
  six rights of administering medication, 302–3
intravenous therapy (IVT), 185, 192
  assist to establish, 188–9
  clean, replace and dispose of equipment, 189, 196
  clinical reasoning, 185–7, 192–4
  documentation, 189–90, 196
  evidence of therapeutic interaction, 185, 192
  general concepts of medication administration and six rights, 188
  local assessment, 193
  management, 194–6
  position person, 188
  systemic assessment, 193–4
ISBAR. *See* identification of the person, situation and status, background and history, assessment and actions, responsibility, recommendation, risk management and read back (ISBAR)
ISMP. *See* Institute for Safe Medication Practices (ISMP)
IVT. *See* intravenous therapy (IVT)

jejunostomy tubes, 177
judgement, 88
jugular veins, 94

key-part and key-site identification and protection, 32
knowledge, 87

language, 88
lateral chest, 106
12-lead electrocardiogram (ECG), 96
  calibrate electrocardiogram machine, 97
  clean, replace and dispose of equipment, 99
  clinical reasoning, 96–97
  documentation, 99
  electrocardiogram reading, 98–9
  evidence of therapeutic interaction, 96
  hand hygiene, 98
  post-procedure, 99
left lower quadrant (LLQ), 123
left sternal border (LSB), 93
left upper quadrant (LUQ), 123
legal requirements for documentation, 154
lesbian, gay, bisexual, transgender, intersex and queer (LGBTIQ+), 11
level of consciousness (LOC), 87, 109, 111–12
LGBTIQ+. *See* lesbian, gay, bisexual, transgender, intersex and queer (LGBTIQ+)
liquid medication, 243–4
LLQ. *See* left lower quadrant (LLQ)
LOC. *See* level of consciousness (LOC)
long-term TT, 426
looking, 6
LSB. *See* left sternal border (LSB)
LUQ. *See* left upper quadrant (LUQ)

malignant hyperthermia (MH), 352
MCL. *See* midclavicular line (MCL)
MDI. *See* measured dose inhaler (MDI)
measured dose inhaler (MDI), 278
  with spacer, 278
medication, 232
  mechanisms of medication administration, 234–6
  six rights of administering, 237–8
Melzack's pain tool, 69
memory, 88
mental status assessment (MSA), 85
  clinical reasoning, 85
  conducting, 86–8
  documentation, 88
  evidence of therapeutic interaction, 85
metered dose inhaler, 282
MH. *See* malignant hyperthermia (MH)
MI. *See* myocardial infarction (MI)
midclavicular line (MCL), 92
mini-tracheostomies, 426
miscommunication, 147
mobilisation, 387
  assist with, 390
  clinical reasoning, 387–9
  documentation, 390
  evidence of therapeutic interaction, 387
monitors, 78–9
mood, 87
motor response, 113
MSA. *See* mental status assessment (MSA)
muscle strength and tone, 114
musculoskeletal assessment, 132, 134–5
  clinical reasoning, 132–4
  documentation, 136
  evidence of therapeutic interaction, 132
  passive range of motion exercises, 135–6
myocardial infarction (MI), 82, 96

nail care, 375
  clean, replace and dispose of equipment, 379
  clinical reasoning, 375–6
  documentation, 379
  evidence of therapeutic interaction, 375
  performing, 377–9
narrative documentation, 153
nasal cannula, 407–8
nasogastric feeding, 177
nasogastric tubes (NGTs), 171, 178, 241, 362
  clean, replace and dispose of equipment, 175
  clinical reasoning, 171–2
  documentation, 175
  evidence of therapeutic interaction, 171
  insertion, 172–5
nasopharyngeal suctioning, 411
  clean, replace and dispose of equipment, 415
  clinical reasoning, 411–13
  documentation, 415
  evidence of therapeutic interaction, 411
  performing, 414–15
National Health and Medical Research Council (NHMRC), 18, 24, 37, 42, 421
National Pressure Ulcer Advisory Panel (NPUAP), 396
NBM. *See* nil by mouth (NBM)
nebulisation, 282

nebulised inhalant, 278
Negative Pressure Wound Therapy (NPWT), 471, 479–81
neurological assessment, 109
neurological health history, 109, 111
clean, replace and dispose of equipment, 114
clinical reasoning, 110
documentation, 114
evidence of therapeutic interaction, 109
GCS, 111–13
hand hygiene, 111
LOC, 111
muscle strength and tone, 114
neurological assessment, 111–14
pupillary activity, 113–14
VS, 113
neurovascular observations, 116
assess person, 117–119
clinical reasoning, 116–117
conducting, 117–19
documentation, 119
evidence of therapeutic interaction, 116
hand hygiene, 117
responsibilities, 119
New Zealand Blood Service (NZBS), 443
NGTs. *See* nasogastric tubes (NGTs)
NHMRC. *See* National Health and Medical Research Council (NHMRC)
nil by mouth (NBM), 152
NMBA. *See* Nursing and Midwifery Board of Australia (NMBA)
non-rebreather mask, 408
non-sterile gloves, 32
non-steroidal anti-inflammatory drugs (NSAIDs), 330
Non Touch Technique (NTT), 31–2
non-viscous effusions, 435
normal saline (NS), 420, 429
NPUAP. *See* National Pressure Ulcer Advisory Panel (NPUAP)
NPWT. *See* Negative Pressure Wound Therapy (NPWT)
NS. *See* normal saline (NS)
NSAIDs. *See* non-steroidal anti-inflammatory drugs (NSAIDs)
NTT. *See* Non Touch Technique (NTT)
Nursing and Midwifery Board of Australia (NMBA), 2, 10, 13, 78, 153
nursing standards, 2
NZBS. *See* New Zealand Blood Service (NZBS)

obesity, 127
obstructive sleep apnoea (OSA), 102
oculocephalic reflex, 114
onset, position and palliating factors, quality and quantity, radiation, setting and associated symptoms, and the timing and treatment (OPQRST), 69, 82
open gloving method, 43–4
open-suction method, 421–2
open tracheal suctioning, 417
operating theatre (OT), 347, 357
OPQRST. *See* onset, position and palliating factors, quality and quantity, radiation, setting and associated symptoms, and the timing and treatment (OPQRST)
optic medication, 254
administering, 256–7
clean, replace and dispose of equipment, 257
clinical reasoning, 254–6
documentation, 258
evidence of therapeutic interaction, 254
six rights of administering medication, 256
oral care, 375
clean, replace and dispose of equipment, 379
clinical reasoning, 375–6
documentation, 379
evidence of therapeutic interaction, 375
performing, 377–9
oral medications, 232, 241
administering, 238–9
clean, replace and dispose of equipment, 239
clinical reasoning, 232–6
documentation, 239
evidence of therapeutic interaction, 232
six rights of administering medication, 237–8
oral temperature, 52
orientation, 87
orogastric tube feeding, 177
oropharyngeal suctioning, 411
clean, replace and dispose of equipment, 415
clinical reasoning, 411–13
documentation, 415
evidence of therapeutic interaction, 411
performing, 414–15
OSA. *See* obstructive sleep apnoea (OSA)
OT. *See* operating theatre (OT)
OTC. *See* over-the-counter (OTC)
other rights, 237–8
otic medications, 260
administering, 262–3
clean, replace and dispose of equipment, 263
clinical reasoning, 260–2
documentation, 263
evidence of therapeutic interaction, 260
six rights of administering medication, 262
over-the-counter (OTC), 247
oxygen delivery system, 405–7
oxygen therapy, 403
clean, replace and dispose of equipment, 409
clinical reasoning, 405
documentation, 409
evidence of therapeutic interaction, 405
safety precautions for oxygen use, 407
via nasal cannula or masks, 407–8

packed red cells, 443
PACU. *See* Post-anaesthetic Care Unit (PACU)
pain assessment, 67
clean, replace and dispose of equipment, 70
clinical reasoning, 67
conducting, 68–70
documentation, 70
evidence of therapeutic interaction, 67
pain, pallor, polar, pulses, paraesthesia, paralysis (6 Ps), 118
pain parameters, 69–70
Pan Pacific Pressure Injury Alliance (PPPIA), 396
parenteral medication, 285
administering, 288–92
clean, replace and dispose of equipment, 292
clinical reasoning, 286
documentation, 293
evidence of therapeutic interaction, 285
six rights of administering medication, 286–8
partial rebreather mask, 408
participation, 3
passive ROM exercises, 133
patient-centred care, 10–11
patient-controlled analgesia (PCA), 324, 342
administering, 328–30
clean, replace and dispose of equipment, 331
clinical reasoning, 326–7
documentation, 331
evidence of therapeutic interaction, 326
general concepts and six rights of administering medication, 328
patient-controlled epidural analgesia (PCEA), 324
administering, 328–30
clinical reasoning, 326
PCA. *See* patient-controlled analgesia (PCA)
PCEA. *See* patient-controlled epidural analgesia (PCEA)
PEEP. *See* positive-end expiratory pressure (PEEP)
PEG. *See* percutaneous endoscopic gastrostomy (PEG); percutaneous epigastric tube (PEG)
PEGJ. *See* percutaneous endoscopic gastrostomy–jejunum (PEGJ)
perception, 9, 349
percutaneous endoscopic gastrostomy (PEG), 177
percutaneous endoscopic gastrostomy–jejunum (PEGJ), 177
percutaneous epigastric tube (PEG), 241
performance-based assessment, 2–3
performance criteria, 4
peripheral intravenous cannulation (PIVC), 185, 192
peripheral pulses, 94
peripheral stimulation, 112
peripherally inserted central cannula (PICC), 32
peripherally inserted venous cannula (PIVC), 309
PERRLA. *See* Pupils are Equal, Round, Reactive to Light and Accommodation (PERRLA)
personal bias, 11
personal protective equipment (PPE), 24, 175, 372
clean, replace and dispose of equipment, 29
evidence of therapeutic interaction, 24–7
hand hygiene, 27
putting on, 27–9
removing, 29
person-centred care, 11
person-centred practice, 10
benefits, 11–12
components, 10
phlebitis, 192–3
physical assessment, 78, 90
cardiovascular history, 92
clean, replace and dispose of equipment, 83, 94
clinical reasoning, 79, 90–1
conducting, 80–2, 92–4
documentation, 83, 94
evidence of therapeutic interaction, 79, 90
hand hygiene, 92
heart assessment, 92–3
post-procedure, 82
primary survey, 79
privacy and comfort, 91
scan, 78
supine position, 91
vascular system, 93–4
PI. *See* pressure injury (PI)
PICC. *See* peripherally inserted central cannula (PICC)
piggyback medication, administering, 298–9
piggyback sets, 295
PIVC. *See* peripheral intravenous cannulation (PIVC); peripherally inserted venous cannula (PIVC)
planning, 7
plasma, 443
platelets, 443
pleural friction rub, 106
POD. *See* postoperative delirium (POD)
PONV. *See* postoperative nausea and vomiting (PONV)
positive-end expiratory pressure (PEEP), 417

post-anaesthesia care, 349
  clean, replace and dispose of equipment, 354
  clinical reasoning, 349–51
  documentation, 355
  evidence of therapeutic interaction, 349
  handover and care, 351–4
  handover to ward staff, 354–5
Post-anaesthetic Care Unit (PACU), 357
posterior thorax, 104
  auscultate for breath sounds, 105–6
  auscultate posterior lung fields, 106
  inspecting, 104
  palpate for tactile and vocal fremitus, 104
  palpate thorax, 104
  percussion, 105
postoperative care, 357
  clean, replace and dispose of equipment, 363
  clinical reasoning, 357–8
  documentation, 363
  evidence of therapeutic interaction, 357
  performing, 359–63
postoperative delirium (POD), 358
postoperative nausea and vomiting (PONV), 362
post-procedure, 82
posturing, 110
potassium chloride (KCl), 192
PPE. *See* personal protective equipment (PPE)
PPPIA. *See* Pan Pacific Pressure Injury Alliance (PPPIA)
preoperative assessment, 342
preoperative care, 341, 344
  blood glucose control, 345
  checklist, 345–6
  clean, replace and dispose of equipment, 347
  clinical reasoning, 342
  documentation, 347
  evidence of therapeutic interaction, 341–2
  person onto the trolley, 347
  person to theatre, 347
  preoperative medication, 346–7
  preoperative routine, 344
  preoperative warming, 345
  surgical site, 344–5
  teaching techniques for preventing complications, 343–4
preoxygenation, 420–1
pressure area care, 394–6
pressure injury (PI), 392
  clean, replace or dispose of equipment, 396–7
  clinical reasoning, 393
  documentation, 397
  evidence of therapeutic interaction, 393
  performing pressure area care, 394–6
primary survey, 79
pro re nata (PRN) administration, 360
problem-focused documentation, 153–4
procedural information, 160
processes, 88
processing, 6–7
professional communication, 13–14
professional standards, 4
psychomotor skills, 2
  assessment, 2–3
  assessment tool, 3–4
  clinical educator or facilitator, 4–5
  nursing standards, 2
  performance criteria, 4
pulse measurement, 52–3
pulse oximetry, 62
  assess and evaluate oxygenation using, 64–5
  clean, replace and dispose of equipment, 65
  clinical reasoning, 62–4
  documentation, 65
  evidence of therapeutic interaction, 62
pulse rate, 113
pupillary activity, 113–14
pupil reactivity, 114
pupil shape, 114
pupil size, 113
Pupils are Equal, Round, Reactive to Light and Accommodation (PERRLA), 114

range of motion (ROM), 132
  exercises, 133
RBCs. *See* red blood cells (RBCs)
rectal medication, 271
  administering, 274–6
  clean, replace and dispose of equipment, 276
  clinical reasoning, 272–4
  documentation, 276
  evidence of therapeutic interaction, 271–2
  six rights of administering medication, 274
rectal temperature, 52
rectal thermometers, 50
rectus femoris site, 290
red blood cells (RBCs), 358, 442
reflecting, 7
Registered Nurse Standards for Practice (2016), 2, 10
registered nurses (RNs), 2, 6, 9–10, 119, 233, 286, 307, 324, 403, 427
relationship-centred care, 11
reliability, 3
reposition, 381
  assist person to, 383–5
  clean, replace and dispose of equipment, 385
  clinical reasoning, 381–3
  documentation, 385
  evidence of therapeutic interaction, 381
resident microorganisms, 18
respiration measurement, 53–4
respiratory health history, 101–3
  and assessment, 102–7
  anterior thorax, 106–7
  clean, replace and dispose of equipment, 107
  clinical reasoning, 101
  documentation, 107
  evidence of therapeutic interaction, 101
  hand hygiene, 102
  lateral chest, 106
  position person for assessing thorax, 103
  post-procedure, 107
  posterior thorax, 104–6
  respiratory system, 103–4
respiratory pattern, 113
retention enema, 209
right documentation, 237
right dose, 237
right lower quadrant (RLQ), 123
right medication, 237
right midclavicular line (MCL), 124
right person, 237
right route, 237
right sternal border (RSB), 93
right time, 237
right upper quadrant (RUQ), 123
RLQ. *See* right lower quadrant (RLQ)
RNs. *See* registered nurses (RNs)
ROM. *See* range of motion (ROM)
RSB. *See* right sternal border (RSB)
RUQ. *See* right upper quadrant (RUQ)

safety, 133
SCRT. *See* subcutaneous rehydration therapy (SCRT)
semi-closed suctioning, 417
sensory and motor skills, 88
sensory information, 159
serum albumin, 443
SG. *See* specific gravity (SG)
shallow suction, 417
shared decision making, 11
shaving, 375
  clean, replace and dispose of equipment, 379
  clinical reasoning, 375–6
  documentation, 379
  evidence of therapeutic interaction, 375
  performing, 377–9
short-term TT, 426
sibilant and sonorous wheezes, 106
simple face mask, 407
situational awareness, 9, 349
SOAP. *See* Subjective, Objective, Assessment, Planning (SOAP)
SOAPIE. *See* Subjective, Objective, Assessment, Planning, Implementation, Evaluation (SOAPIE)
specific gravity (SG), 206
speech, 88
spiritual care, 10
spontaneous pneumothoraxes, 435
SSIs. *See* surgical site infections (SSIs)
SSQCPE. *See* Standards for Safe and Quality Care in the Perioperative Environment (SSQCPE)
standard ANTT procedures, 32
Standards for Safe and Quality Care in the Perioperative Environment (SSQCPE), 37
staple, 464–5, 467–8
sterile gloves, 32
sterile gown's waist ties, 44
stool assessment, 206
stridor, 106
subcutaneous fluid replacement, administering, 336–7
subcutaneous (SC) infusion, 333
  administering, 335–6
  clean, replace and dispose of equipment, 337
  clinical reasoning, 334–5
  documentation, 337
  evidence of therapeutic interaction, 334
  general concepts and six rights of administering medication, 335
subcutaneous (SC) parenteral medication, 285
subcutaneous rehydration therapy (SCRT), 333
Subjective, Objective, Assessment, Planning (SOAP), 150
Subjective, Objective, Assessment, Planning, Implementation, Evaluation (SOAPIE), 150, 154
sublingual administration, 232
suctioning, 417
suctioning apparatus, 420
suprapubic catheters, 215
  clean, replace and dispose of equipment, 219
  documentation, 219
  evidence of therapeutic interaction, 216
  intermittent bladder irrigation, 215–16
  urinary catheter, 217–19
surgical ANTT procedures, 32
surgical gowning and gloving, 42–4
surgically aseptic areas, 44
surgical scrub, 43
surgical site infections (SSIs), 42
suture, 464–5, 467–8

teach-back method, 160
teaching, 157
  strategies, 159–60
  techniques for preventing complications, 343–4

teamwork, 148
temperature, pulse, respiration measurement (TPR measurement), 48, 50, 207
  clean, replace and dispose of equipment, 54
  clinical reasoning, 49
  documentation, 54
  evidence of therapeutic interaction, 49
  hand hygiene, 50
temperature alterations, 113
template, 148–50
temporal artery temperature, 52
therapeutic substances, 233–4
thromboembolism deterrent (TED) stockings, 127, 358
timeliness, 150
tissue perfusion, 116
tissue perfusion, 94
topical medication, 247
  administering, 251–2
  clean, replace and dispose of equipment, 252
  clinical reasoning, 248–51
  documentation, 252
  evidence of therapeutic interaction, 248
  six rights of administering medication, 251
TPR measurement. *See* temperature, pulse, respiration measurement (TPR measurement)
tracheostomy, 426
  care, 430–3
  care for person with, 427
  clean, replace and dispose of equipment, 433
  clinical reasoning, 427–30
  documentation, 433
  emergencies, 427
  evidence of therapeutic interaction, 427
  preventative measures, 428–30
tracheostomy tubes (TTs), 426
trade name, 234
transdermal administration, 247
transient microorganisms, 18
trauma-informed care, 12
TTs. *See* tracheostomy tubes (TTs)
tubes, 78–9
tympanic temperature, 51–2
tympanic thermometer, 50

underwater seal drain (UWSD), 436
urinary catheter, 217–19
urinary catheterisation, 221–6
  clean, replace and dispose of equipment, 227
  clinical reasoning, 221–3
  documentation, 227
  evidence of therapeutic interaction, 221
  indwelling catheter, 226–7
urinary catheters, 221
UWSD. *See* underwater seal drain (UWSD)

vagina, 265
vaginal medication, 265
  administering, 268–9
  clean, replace and dispose of equipment, 269
  clinical reasoning, 266–7
  documentation, 269
  evidence of therapeutic interaction, 265
  six rights of administering medication, 268
validity, 3
vastus lateralis site, 290
venipuncture, 449
  clean, replace and dispose of equipment, 453
  clinical reasoning, 449–51
  documentation, 453
  evidence of therapeutic interaction, 449
  performing, 452–3
ventrogluteal site, 290
Venturi mask, 408
vesicular sounds, 105
vigilance, 9, 349
vital signs (VS), 113
vocabulary, 87
voice sounds, 104
volume-controlled infusion set, 295
  administering, 297–8
  clean, replace and dispose of equipment, 299
  clinical reasoning, 296
  documentation, 299
  evidence of therapeutic interaction, 295
  six rights of administering medication, 297
VS. *See* vital signs (VS)

WHO. *See* World Health Organization (WHO)
World Health Organization (WHO), 64
wound drainage systems, 464
wound irrigation, 471
  clean, replace and dispose of equipment, 475
  clinical reasoning, 471–3
  documentation, 475
  evidence of therapeutic interaction, 471
  performing, 473–4
  specimen for culture and sensitivity, 475
written documentation, 153–4